This edition of Professional Nursing Practice: Concepts and Perspectives *is dedicated in loving memory to Glenora Erb. She, along with her colleague and friend Barbara Kozier, gave birth to this book in its first edition. They placed their faith and trust in us to continue their work into this, the fifth edition. We will always be grateful to them for what they have given us, and through us, have given to our many students and readers.*

Kathleen Koernig Blais
Janice S. Hayes

Brief Contents

Contents

Preface

A dynamic health care system requires growth and change in professional nursing. Skills in communication and interpersonal relations are needed for nurses to be effective members of a collaborative health care team. Critical thinking and creativity are necessary as nurses implement care with clients of diverse cultural and spiritual backgrounds in a variety of settings. Nurses must be prepared to provide care not only in hospital settings but in community residential settings such as occupational sites, faith-based communities, homeless shelters, and prisons. The nurse's unique role demands a blend of nurturance, compassion, sensitivity, caring, empathy, commitment, courage, competence, and skill that comes from a broad knowledge base of the arts, humanities, biological and social sciences, and the discipline of nursing. Nurses need skills in teaching, collaborating, leading, managing, advocacy, political involvement, and applying theory and research to practice. An understanding of holistic healing modalities and complementary therapies is becoming more essential. This book addresses content by which nurses build their repertoire or nursing knowledge. This content includes, but is not limited to, wellness, health promotion, and disease prevention; holistic care; multiculturalism; nursing history; technology and informatics; nursing theories and conceptual frameworks; nursing research; and professional empowerment and politics.

Professional Nursing Practice: Concepts and Perspectives, 5th edition, is intended as a text for registered nurses who are in transition or bridge programs to pursue a baccalaureate degree in nursing. It may also be used in generic nursing programs or in transition or bridge programs for vocational nurses (LPNs or LVNs) to complete the professional nursing baccalaureate degree. This text reflects the areas of knowledge that professional nurses require to be effective in the changing health care system. The organization in the text emphasizes the foundational knowledge related to professional nursing, including nursing history, nursing theory, ethics, and legal aspects; the roles of professional nurses including health promoter and care provider, learner and teacher, leader and manager, research consumer, political advocate, and colleague and collaborator; the processes guiding nursing, including communication, group, change, and technology and informatics; nursing in a changing health care delivery system, including health care economics, cultural and spiritual dimensions of nursing, and nursing in a culture of violence; graduate education and advanced nursing practice; and nursing in the future.

NEW TO THIS EDITION

All chapters have been revised to reflect current professional nursing knowledge based on foundational knowledge. A new chapter, Nursing in a Spiritually Diverse World, provides greater emphasis on the spiritual and religious dimension of the client as it relates to nursing care. New content on bioterrorism has been added to the chapter, Nursing in a Culture of Violence. New content on the international dimensions of the nursing profession have been added throughout the text as appropriate to reflect the global understandings of nursing.

New features include:

- Critical thinking exercises that compel the reader to apply concepts from chapters to situations.
- Reflect on. . . sections in each chapter ask the reader to contemplate the nurse's own practice and beliefs about professional nursing in relation to the chapter content.
- A new and improved Web site that takes readers through the world of cyberspace to connect with nursing, health care, and other sites that provide current information and can serve as ongoing resources for professional nursing practice and health care.

HALLMARK FEATURES

The fifth edition of *Professional Nursing Practice: Concepts and Perspectives* retains several of the features that have been well received by faculty and students who have used previous editions:

- Research boxes from the previous edition have been retitled as Evidence for Practice boxes and describe studies relevant to chapter content and relate them to clinical or professional practice.
- Bookshelf boxes provide additional readings from popular and professional literature that enhance understanding of chapter content. The readings were chosen to pique student interest in exploring additional literary sources outside the classroom. For example, the Bookshelf in Chapter 3, Historical Foundations of

Nursing, includes biographies of nurses who have been instrumental in developing the profession, and in Chapter 21, Nursing in a Culturally Diverse World, the accounts of the personal experiences of people of diverse cultural backgrounds are provided.

■ Practicing nurse interviews occur in two chapters, Chapter 19, Providing Care in the Home and Community, and Chapter 23, Advanced Nursing Education and Practice. The profiles include information about why these practitioners chose their specific practice areas, what qualities they think are necessary to be a nurse in this setting, what their job entails, and what encouragement they would offer a nurse considering practice in this setting. The profiles provide useful first-person perspectives for readers.

ORGANIZATION

This edition is organized into five units, with an introductory chapter preceding the first unit. Units and chapters can be used independently or in any sequence. Some nursing programs use this text for first-semester nursing students in a Professional Socialization course. Other nursing programs use the text at the end of their nursing program in a Professional Transition course. And yet other programs use the text as a primary text in one course and a secondary text in other professional role courses.

■ Chapter 1, Beginning the Transition: Journey to Professionalism, was created to assist registered nurses as they return to school. It provides information regarding factors influencing nurses' return to school for baccalaureate and higher degrees and overcoming barriers that may interfere with student success.

■ Unit I, Foundations of Professional Nursing Practice, focuses on professionalism including socialization, and historical, legal, ethical, and theoretical foundations of nursing.

■ Unit II, Professional Nursing Roles, includes information on the professional roles of health promoter and care provider, learner and teacher, leader and manager, research consumer, advocate, and colleague and collaborator.

■ Unit III, Processes Guiding Professional Practice, focuses on communication process, change process, group process, and the use of technology and informatics.

■ Unit IV, Professional Nursing in a Changing Health Care Delivery System, includes chapters devoted to changes in nursing health care economics, providing care in the home and community, nursing in a culture of violence, nursing in a culturally diverse world, and nursing in a spiritually diverse world.

■ Unit V, Into the Future, looks at the future of nurse and nursing. It includes chapters on advanced nursing education and practice, and concludes with visions for the future of nursing.

We hope this book helps learners from diverse backgrounds appreciate the proud heritage of professional nursing, understand what is meant by professional, view nursing as a profession, and develop knowledge and abilities that will contribute to the advancement of the profession. In addition, we hope the knowledge gained will help nurses provide quality care in a constantly changing health care system.

ACKNOWLEDGMENTS

We extend our sincere thanks to the many talented and committed people who assisted in the birthing of this text:

■ The reviewers, who provided many discerning comments and suggestions that expanded our thinking and writing. Please see page xxv for a list of the reviewers.

■ Maura Conner, Editor-in-Chief, whose commitment to the manuscript, understanding of writing demands, and technical and personal support throughout the project contributed positively to this revision.

■ Pamela Fuller, Acquisitions Editor, who came into the project late in the process and helped bring it to completion.

■ Malgorzata Jaros-White and Eileen Monaghan, editorial assistants, without whose help the book could never have been accomplished. Their organization and capable assistance was invaluable. Their availability to answer questions or find the right person to answer questions was essential to the quality of the text.

■ Robin Reed and Heather Willison, project coordinators, for their contributions to writing style and syntax. They helped make our words and ideas more meaningful.

■ Patricia Jenkins who created the Web site to accompany this text. Her work provides a contemporary dimension to readers' use of the fifth edition.

■ Most importantly, our many students who have challenged and taught us, and in doing so have helped to guide the direction of this book.

Contributors

Barbara A. Happ, PhD, RN
Associate Professor
University of Maryland
Adelphi, Maryland
and
Kellog Distinguished Professor
Hampton University
Hampton, Virginia

Janice Sandiford, EdD, RN
Associate Professor
College of Education
Florida International University
Miami, Florida

Sally Weiss, EdD, RN
School of Nursing
Nova Southeastern University
Davie, Florida

Diane Whitehead, EdD, RN
School of Nursing
Nova Southeastern University
Davie, Florida

Reviewers

Betty Nash Blevins, RN, MSN, CCRN
Associate Professor of Nursing
Bluefield State College
Bluefield, West Virginia

Alice Bernicky, RN, MS
Assistant Clinical Professor
Texas Women's University
College of Nursing
Dallas, Texas

Michelle Buchman, RNC, BSN
Academic Program Director
Springfield College
Springfield, Missouri

Tracy B. Chamblee, RNC, MSN
Associate Professor
St. John Fisher College
Rochester, New York

Pattie Clark, RN, MSN
Associate Professor of Nursing
Nursing Outreach Coordinator
Abraham Baldwin College
Tifton, Georgia

Jennie C. Denker, RN, MSN
Instructor
Spalding University
Louisville, Kentucky

Rebecca Gesler, RN, MSN
Lecturer
Bellarmine University
Louisville, Kentucky

Patricia Leary, MA, Ed
Instructor
Ferris State University
Mecosta-Osceola Career Center
Big Rapids, Michigan

Christine Mihal, RN, MSN, BC, APRN
Assistant Professor
Felician College
Lodi, New Jersey

Jenny Radsma, RN, MN, PhD Candidate
Associate Professor of Nursing
University of Maine
Fort Kent, Maine

Tracy A. Riley, PhD, RN
Assistant Professor
The University of Akron
College of Nursing
Akron, Ohio

Karen J. Saewert, PhD, RN, CPHQ
RN-BSN Program Coordinator
Arizona State University
College of Nursing
Tempe, Arizona

Ann Schmitt, RN, MSN
Instructor
Lewis University
College of Nursing and Health Professions
Romeoville, Illinois

Heidi Taylor, PhD, RN
Associate Professor/Division Head for Nursing
West Texas A&M University
Canyon, Texas

Beginning the Transition:
Journey to Professionalism

Objectives

- Examine changes in society that promote the nurse's return to school and further education.
- Apply models of transition to professional role change.
- Identify strategies that will assist the nurse in returning to an educational setting.
- Identify helpful approaches to academic success.

M E D I A L I N K

Additional online resources for this chapter can be found on the companion Web site at http://www.prenhall.com/blais.

The evolution of nursing has been dramatic in recent history. Most of the changes in nursing are in response to changes in society and in the health care system. There are also changes that are related to the evolution of the profession. The reciprocal relationship between nursing and society requires that nursing must change as society changes.

FACTORS IN SOCIETY THAT PROMOTE THE NURSE'S RETURN TO SCHOOL

Changes in society place new demands on nurses. An aging population results in older patients with more complex health problems. Changing reimbursement practices result in patients being discharged more quickly from hospitals, even though they still need skilled nursing care either in long-term care facilities or in their homes. A more diverse population requires nurses to be more knowledgeable about cultural and social influences on health. New technology and scientific discoveries require nurses to continually update their knowledge and skills. New diseases related to social and environmental problems require nurses to have a greater, integrated knowledge from the biological, psychological, and social sciences to promote health, to prevent illness or injury, and to care for those who are already ill or injured. Many of these societal changes are discussed in more detail in later chapters.

Changing Perceptions of Nursing as a Profession

Changing views of men's and women's roles are at the foundation of some of the profession's internal changes. Historically, nursing was considered a woman's occupation; however, that has gradually changed over the past decades. By 2000, 5.4% of registered nurses were men, up from 2.7% in 1980 (Spratley et al., 2000). As more men entered nursing, the image of the profession changed. Use of traditional identifying symbols of nursing such as caps and white uniforms, declined. There also has been less acceptance of the passive behaviors associated with the historical "handmaiden" role, when the nurse was viewed as the submissive and unquestioning assistant to the physician. Within health care institutions and in interactions with other health care disciplines, nurses are expected to be more accountable and more responsible for their work. This requires a more assertive and proactive role for the contemporary professional nurse as she or he participates in a more collaborative health care system.

Other factors have also accounted for changes in the role of the professional nurse. The average age of working registered nurses has increased. In 2000, the average age of registered nurses was 45.2 years compared to 44.3 years in 1996 (Spratley et al., 2000). Nurses are entering school and pursuing nursing degrees at more mature ages and are working longer, thus bringing more life experiences to the role. Additionally, approximately 14% of registered nurses bring knowledge and skills learned in previous postsecondary academic degrees to their nursing career. In the past, a nurse may have been more likely to

work until having children and then stop working or work only part-time or short term when additional income was needed. Now, about 72% (Spratley et al., 2000) of registered nurses are married and more than half have children living at home. About one third of nurses employed in nursing full-time have children.

The education required for entry into the profession has changed over time. This has been one of the most dramatic changes in the last two decades and has influenced professional identity. Hospital-based diploma training was the mainstay of nursing education until the mid-twentieth century. Between 1980 and 2000 there was a decline in the percentage of nurses who received a diploma in nursing as their entry preparation from 60% to 30% (Spratley et al., 2000). As enrollments in diploma nursing programs declined, enrollment in associate and baccalaureate degree programs increased. Between 1980 and 2000 enrollment in associate degree nursing programs increased from 19% to 40% and the percentage of registered nurses receiving their basic nursing education in baccalaureate degree programs increased from 17% to 29% (Spratley et al., 2000). Educational preparation in institutions of higher learning socialized nurses to formal education and even to the idea of continuing their career development through graduate education.

The practice of nursing has shifted from primarily acute care in the hospital to a more community- and primary-care focus. Between 1980 and 2000 there was a decrease in the percentage of registered nurses working in hospitals from 66% in 1980 to 59% in 2000 (Spratley et al., 2000). This has given nurses more autonomy in institutions with less rigid organizational structure and hierarchy. Many of these positions require a minimum of a baccalaureate degree for employment. See Table 1–1 for a comparison of selected characteristics of nurses between 1980 and 2000.

Specialty certification for nurses created rewards in terms of both recognition by employers and peers and self-fulfillment for the nurse. In recent years, the requirement for taking many specialty certification exams has included having a baccalaureate degree.

The result of all these changes has been a dramatic increase in the number of nurses returning to school. Between 1975 and 1998, the number of registered nurses graduating from BSN programs rose from about 3700 per year to more than 11,000 annually. In 1980, just over half of all registered nurses held hospital diplomas as their highest level of nursing preparation and about 22% held a BSN. According to the American As-

Table 1–1 Comparison of Registered Nurse Characteristics, 1980–2000

Characteristic	1980	2000
Number of RNs	Approximately 1,660,000	2,694,540
Percentage of RNs working in nursing	77%	81.7%
Percentage of RNs working full-time in nursing	52%	59%
Age		
< 40 years of age	52.9%	31.7%
Gender		
Female	1,623,820 (97.3%)	2,547,638 (94.6%)
Male	45,060 (2.7%)	146,902 (5.4%)
Ethnicity		
White nonminority	93%	88%
Minority (including Hispanic; Black, non-Hispanic, Asian/Pacific Islander; American Indian/Alaskan Native; Mixed race)	7%	12%
Educational Preparation		
Diploma	1,050,661 (60%)	800,000 (30%)
Associate Degree	308,616 (19%)	1,087,602 (40%)
Baccalaureate Degree	287,993 (17%)	791,004 (29%)
Master's or Doctoral Degree	86,000 (5%)	275,068 (10%)
Employment Setting		
Hospital	66%	59%
Public and community health, ambulatory care, and other noninstitutional settings	30.3%	38.9%
Education	3.7%	2.1%

Source: The Registered Nurse Population: March 2000: Findings from the National Sample Survey of Registered Nurses, E. Spratley, A. Johnson, J. Sochalski, F. Fritz, and W. Spencer, 2000, Washington, DC: U.S. Department of Health and Human Services.

sociation of Colleges of Nursing (2003) 43% of nurses have a baccalaureate or higher degree. The National Advisory Council on Nurse Education and Practice (NACNEP) (1995) urges that two thirds of the nursing workforce have a baccalaureate or higher degree in nursing by the year 2010.

In 1996, the American Association of Colleges of Nursing issued a position statement recognizing the Bachelor of Science degree in nursing as the minimum educational requirement for professional nursing practice. (See the box on page 4.) It is seen as critical for a career in professional nursing. The BSN nurse is prepared for a broader role; increasingly, the bachelor's degree is required for employment in many health care settings such as community health, case management, and supervisory positions. The

BSN curriculum includes a broad spectrum of scientific, critical thinking, humanistic, communication, and leadership skills (AACN, 2001).

Throughout this book are several features designed to enhance the student's learning experience. A feature integrated into text is titled "Reflect on . . ." Use this feature to reflect on the content of the book as it relates to your own practice. There are no right or wrong answers. The answers may come from professional texts, commercial literature, personal and professional experience, or simply each student's own thoughts, beliefs, or values. "Evidence for Practice" boxes provide a summary of selected current research findings appropriate to the content of the chapter. "Critical Thinking Exercises" provide an activity to encourage the student to use the information in the chapter in a focused way.

American Association of Colleges of Nursing Position Statement: The Baccalaureate Degree in Nursing as Minimal Preparation for Professional Practice

Rapidly expanding clinical knowledge and mounting complexities in health care mandate that professional nurses possess educational preparation commensurate with the diversified responsibilities required of them. As health care shifts from hospital-centered, inpatient care to more primary and preventive care throughout the community, the health system requires registered nurses who can practice across multiple settings—both within and beyond management—providing direct bedside care, supervising unlicensed aides and other support personnel, guiding patients through the maze of health care resources, and educating patients on treatment regimens and adoptions of healthy lifestyles. In particular, preparation of the entry-level professional nurse requires a greater orientation to community-based primary health care and an emphasis on health promotion, maintenance, and cost-effective coordinated care.

Accordingly, the American Association of Colleges of Nursing (AACN) recognizes the Bachelor of Science degree in nursing as the minimum educational requirement for professional nursing practice.

Source: American Association of Colleges of Nursing, approved by the Board of Directors, July 20, 1996. Reprinted with permission.

Reflect on...

■ the changes occurring in your professional life that require a return to school.
■ the changes occurring in your community that require new knowledge about nursing and health care.

FACTORS IN THE PROFESSION THAT PROMOTE THE NURSE'S RETURN TO SCHOOL

Credentialing Requirements

As knowledge and technology increase and nurses are more likely to specialize in specific practice areas, there is an increasing demand to obtain national certification either to obtain jobs in a specialty or to advance in the specialty. At the present time, more than 150,000 registered nurses hold specialty certification through the American Nurses Credentialing Center (2003). Most national certifications now require the baccalaureate degree in nursing (BSN) to sit for the certification examination; for example, the American Nurses Credentialing Center (ANCC) requires the baccalaureate degree as a minimum requirement for specialty certification. Those organizations that do not require the baccalaureate degree at the present time may have future plans to require the BSN for certification.

PROFESSIONAL ROLE TRANSITIONS

As changes in the health care system affect society's expectations of their nursing care and nurses respond to these expectations, nurses are returning to school to acquire new knowledge and skills to be more effective in their changing roles. Changes in nursing roles represent a shift in the view of nursing from an occupation to a profession with a commitment to the role. As nurses transition from novice nurses to expert nurses, they experience challenges related to the change process (Benner, 1984). (See Chapter 6 ⬤ for more discussion of Benner's Model of Nursing Career Transition.) Bridges (2000) and Spencer and Adams (1990) describe models of transition that consider the personal and professional challenges, the internal struggles, and the external influences that occur when people experience change.

Bridges' Model of Transition

Bridges (2000) describes a model of transition that consists of three phases: the ending, the neutral zone, and new beginnings. He believes that individuals move through all three phases as they experience change.

The *ending phase* is the initial stage of transition. In this phase, the individual must "let go" of the past. This occurs with a change in the employment setting or a change in roles within the same employment setting. It occurs whether the nurse makes the choice for change or the change is imposed externally, such as by the employer or by new professional mandates by accrediting agencies (Joint Commission on the Accreditation of Healthcare Organizations [JCAHO]) or professional regulatory agencies (e.g., Boards of Nursing). Even when change is viewed in a positive way, there is an ending of old ways of thinking and behaving with the expectation of new ways of thinking and behaving.

Within the ending phase, Bridges describes four components of "ending": disengagement, disidentification, disenchantment, and disorientation. *Disengagement* occurs when the nurse is separated from previous familiar settings or roles. Previous relationships may also change during this phase; for example, a nurse who was in a peer relationship with colleagues may now assume a managerial role with a responsibility for evaluating those same colleagues. If the change is related to a change in employment settings, supportive relationships in the previous employment setting may be lost and the need to develop new relationships occurs. *Disidentification* is the loss of self-definition. People have a sense of who they are. When one experiences role change, there is a challenge to this sense of self and the need to identify the new self within the context of the new role. This can be difficult if the individual feels uncomfortable in the new role. *Disenchantment* is the understanding that the individual's world has changed. The cause of the change may be minor as defined by the individual (e.g., the retirement of a co-worker, the implementation of a new policy) or major, also defined by the individual. The nurse may initially feel honored at being offered a promotion to a leadership position but may find that after accepting the position there are differences in role requirements that had not been understood. For some nurses, changes in their personal lives may be the impetus for change. The nurse may believe that the birth of a new baby will have minimal effect on her career, but realizes that when the baby arrives, the demands of caring for the new baby require not only organizational changes at home but also at work. The last component of the ending phase is disorientation. *Disorientation* is the sense of confusion that occurs with change, the period of emptiness as one moves from the "old" to the "new." The nurse may question why he or she accepted the new role or his or her ability to handle the new role.

The *neutral zone* is the second phase of transition. The neutral zone is, in itself, a transition between the ending phase and the phase of new beginnings. In this stage the individual has moved from the old to the new, at least superficially. The nurse has outwardly accepted the change, the new role, but the responsibilities and behaviors associated with the new role have not yet been internalized. Old ways of thinking and viewing the world must give way to new values, new ways of thinking, and new ways of viewing the world. This is the inner acceptance of the role change. For example, if the nurse has been promoted from staff nurse to nurse manager, the nurse must not only accept the title but also the responsibilities and behaviors associated with the role change. The superficial transition is the new title. The inner transition requires new perspectives (worldview) on the role (behaviors) of the manager in the effective (values) functioning of the nursing unit. The inner transition also requires an acceptance of the changed relationships with colleagues from a peer to a supervisor.

The final phase of Bridges' model is called *new beginnings*. In this phase there is an acceptance of new knowledge, values, attitudes, and behaviors associated with the role change. The first phase of ending or "letting go" is complete, and the individual is ready to move forward. The challenge in this phase is to keep moving forward and avoid the temptation of going back to old ways of thinking and behaving simply because they are more comfortable. For the nurse returning to school, the challenge of managing work and family and school obligations, and finding the time to accomplish everything, creates the temptation to give up and move back to the former more familiar and, therefore, more comfortable situation. Finding support for the transition in colleagues, family, and faculty can help the nurse overcome these challenges.

Spencer and Adams' Model of Transition

Spencer and Adams (1990) developed a model of transition that includes seven stages: losing focus, minimizing the impact, the pit, letting go of the past, testing the limits, searching for meaning, and integration. The first four stages compare to Bridges' ending phase. In stage 1, *losing focus*, the individual has difficulty keeping things in perspective and experiences feelings of being overwhelmed. Some individuals may feel panic in this stage, whereas others may feel excitement.

In stage 2, *minimizing the impact*, the individual feels the need to go back to what was normal or comfortable. In this stage, the individual tries to avoid the full effect of the change and may question what was wrong with the old ways of doing things. They may resist the change or ignore the need for change. This compares to Bridges' components of disenchantment and disorientation.

In stage 3, *the pit*, the individual experiences self-doubt. She or he may have feelings of depression and grief over losses (the old ways of thinking and behaving, former relationships), anger, or powerlessness. In this stage, the individual must move from powerlessness to strength, from anger and grief to optimism about the new.

In stage 4, *letting go of the past*, there is a move toward optimism. The past has been let go, and there is a focus on the change and the benefits to be obtained by the change. It is a stage of forward vision.

In stage 5, *testing the limits*, the new identity is established. New behaviors and new skills are tried. Success in the new behaviors or roles brings about a sense of self-confidence. New relationships develop with colleagues, family, and friends—all those involved in the change. There is a greater sense of comfort about the change. This stage compares to Bridges' neutral zone phase.

In stage 6, *searching for meaning*, there is a period of self-reflection and finding meaning in the experience. New roles, new relationships, new skills are being established. There may be a reconnection with old friends and colleagues. There may also be a desire to help others who are experiencing a similar situation. For nurses returning to school it may be helpful to share the story of their experience with nurses who are contemplating returning to school, to share the feelings associated with the transition. The final stage, *integration*, is the completion of the transition. The individual experiences satisfaction and self-confidence. They have accepted the change and are willing to consider new risks. The values and behaviors associated with the change are internalized so that new role behaviors occur more automatically. See Table 1–2 for a comparison of behaviors and feelings associated with the various phases and stages of Bridges' and Spencer and Adams' Models of Transition.

Nursing students who are starting their professional nursing education and registered nurses who are returning to school to obtain the baccalaureate degree experience many of the challenges described by Bridges and Spencer and Adams. Students who are starting their professional nursing studies may have difficulty in juggling the dual roles of college student and nursing student. In the college student role, the nursing student attends lectures and simulated laboratory experiences, reads textbooks and other assigned and supplemental readings, and studies new knowledge and skills. As the nursing student, the student also assumes professional role behaviors as she or he provides care to real patients and clients in clinical settings. During this transition, the student nurse also juggles additional roles related to work and family obligations. Often, student nurses must reorganize their schedules to accommodate their many demands in order to be successful in their nursing studies. Sometimes, these many demands result in nursing students questioning their decision to become a nurse.

Table 1–2 Comparison of Bridges' and Spencer and Adams' Models of Transition

Bridges (2000)	Spencer & Adams (1990)	Behaviors and Feelings
Three Phases:	**Seven Stages:**	

1. Ending
  a. Disengagement
  b. Disidentification
	I. Losing focus	Behaviors can be mixed and include inability to think clearly, resistance to change

c. Disenchantment d. Disorientation	II. Minimizing the impact III. The pit IV. Letting go of the past	Feelings can be mixed and include confusion, feeling overwhelmed, loss of sense of self, excitement or disappointment, emptiness, grief, anger, powerlessness, numbness
2. Neutral zone	V. Testing the limits	Behaviors include the establishment of new skills and behaviors associated with the change Feelings include optimism, self-confidence, and a sense of comfort with the change
3. New beginnings	VI. Searching for meaning VII. Integration	Behaviors include self-reflection; greater reinforcement of new roles, skills, and relationships; internalization of new role behaviors Feelings include self-confidence, satisfaction

For registered nurses returning to school, there are similar challenges in managing family and work obligations while attending school. In addition, they may experience additional challenges from other nurses who question their choice to return to school with comments such as "Why are you doing that? You won't get any more money." or "How do you find the time to do that with everything else you are doing?" Nurses may question their own decision, considering that their basic preparation was sufficient to practice as a good nurse or to achieve their current position. Nurses may have to "let go" of beliefs such as "there is no difference between nurses prepared at the diploma, associate degree, or baccalaureate degree level," or "what can I learn that I don't already know," and move to thoughts such as "with more education, I can be a better nurse." Nurses often experience anger about going back to school. At the same time, they may feel excitement with the hope and expectation that something new is happening. As they expand their thinking about the roles of nurses in a changing health care system, they may realize new ways of thinking more holistically about the care of clients. The adage "knowledge is power" may be realized as nurses feel greater power and control over their own roles and the roles of nursing within the changing health care system. Factors that can help the nurse make a successful transition from old ways of thinking and behaving to new ways of thinking and behaving include the following:

- *Choosing a mentor.* Identifying a mentor who has successfully transitioned from one nursing role to another can provide support for the nurse in transition. A mentor can serve as a sounding board for new ideas, a support when negative feelings occur, and a cheerleader when positive successes occur. A mentor can be a senior colleague or a faculty member, one who has the best interests of the nurse in mind.
- *Support from family and friends.* Family and friends can provide emotional support when the nurse experiences self-doubt. Family and friends may also provide physical and financial supports.
- *Celebrating the successes.*

Reflect on...

- the reasons that you have decided to return to school.
- the reactions of colleagues, family, and friends to your decision for change.
- the personal values associated with your desire for change.
- the supports you have to ensure your success in role transition.

WHAT WILL IT TAKE TO GET THERE: OVERCOMING BARRIERS

Returning to school provides the professional advancement that nurses seek. It represents a commitment to goals of both professional and personal growth. Meeting those goals requires lifestyle and role changes. Many students beginning their professional nursing studies may be returning to school to pursue a second career in nursing; they may have been away from the academic setting for many years. Registered nurses returning to school may also have been away from a formal education setting for some time and are anxious about becoming a student again. Fitting into academe represents a substantial transition from work and practice roles. Because many students continue to work, the nurse must become comfortable about fitting into both worlds. Concerns about academic skills, such as library searches, scholarly writing, and test taking, are often a source of stress. Blending the student role with the work role and the family-member role represents great challenges. Learning to deal effectively with the stressors that create barriers to success is important. Some of those barriers include managing time effectively to meet the commitments of family, work, and school; finding the financial resources to pay for tuition, books, and educational supplies; finding and maintaining effective social support systems, including family, work colleagues, and student colleagues; learning to work with faculty who require academic excellence in spite of the many demands on the nurse/student's time; and developing effective study skills.

Time Management

Time-management skills are a necessary tool for survival and success. Organizing, planning, and setting of priorities are keys. Students must learn to balance school, family, work, meals, sleep, exercise, spirituality, and personal time. Keeping balance among physiological needs, professional and personal roles, and expectations is essential and requires clear priorities. Procrastination creates a domino effect when there are multiple tasks related to multiple roles. The ability to handle interruptions goes hand in hand with time-management techniques. Setting limits allows one to be goal-focused and keep the load realistic. This kind of clear focus allows the streamlining of things to be done. Nurses/students who are assuming multiple roles with high expectations of their performance in each of these roles often forget to maintain one of

Critical Thinking Exercise–*Time Management*

Create a schedule that accounts for 24 hours a day, 7 days a week that includes required time for each of the following activities:

- *Work*—How many hours a week do you work? How many days a week do you work? Do you work 8-hour, 10-hour, or 12-hour shifts? Working different time shifts changes the way you can plan the other obligations in your life.
- *School/Study*—How many hours a week do you attend class? Remember to plan a minimum of 1-hour study time for each hour in class. Most experts recommend between 1 and 3 hours of study for each hour spent in class.
- *Sleep*—How many hours of sleep do you need to feel well rested? When do you sleep? Do you take naps? It is important to get adequate sleep so that the body and mind are at the optimum for learning.
- *Family*—What family obligations do you have? Do you have young children that need assistance with their homework, with out-of-school activities such as sports or hobbies? What days do you have family obligations that may prevent study? It's important to plan family time so that you can also plan study time.

- *Meals*—How many meals do you usually eat each day? Do you usually have one meal with family members? It's important to maintain adequate nutrition. Many successful students combine mealtime with family time.
- *Spirituality*—What are your spiritual commitments? Do you attend church, temple, prayer meetings, or other formal spiritual activities? How many hours a week are spent in spiritual activities? Maintaining spiritual activities can help relieve stress related to balancing other roles. Spiritual activities are also an opportunity to spend time with family.
- *Exercise*—Do you exercise routinely? How many hours a day or a week do you exercise? Exercise also can relieve stress related to balancing many responsibilities.
- *Personal time*—Are there activities you do just for yourself (e.g., quiet time, taking a relaxation bath, reading)?

Analyze the time you need for each of the above activities. Do you have the time you need for all your obligations? If not, from which activity will you take the time? What do you sacrifice by taking time from another obligation? Keeping a daily planner will help you manage your time.

---

their major resources—their health. Adequate sleep, good nutrition, and diversion are necessary to keeping the energy level and motivation to succeed. See the accompanying critical thinking exercise to plan your own time.

Reflect on...

- the activities you enjoy that can serve as a break. Which of those could be used as a short-term break to refresh a tired body and mind? Which of these activities are long-term fixes requiring greater planning? Devise a schedule that allows you to take advantage of these.

Money

For students returning to school, money to pay tuition and fees and to purchase textbooks and other supplies is often a concern. Many employers provide tuition reimbursement as a benefit of employment. Informa-

tion can be obtained from human resources or personnel departments. Many civic groups and nursing organizations provide scholarships. There are also various state and federal loan opportunities; some may have forgiveness programs if the nurse works in a specific location or specialty for a period of time after graduation. The university or college financial aid office can provide information on scholarships and other forms of tuition assistance. Students may also want to do their own computer search using key words such as "scholarships" or "nursing scholarships" to identify scholarships that may be available based on unique characteristics related to ethnicity, religion, or other trait.

Social Supports

Although students can be successful on their own, the support of others can make things go more smoothly. The people who can contribute to the success of stu-

Evidence for Practice

Spratley, E., Johnson, A., Sockalski, J., Fritz, M., & Spencer, W. (2000). *The registered nurse population, March 2000: Findings from the national sample survey of registered nurses.* Washington, DC: U.S. Department of Health and Human Services.

This study was conducted with the support of the U.S. Department of Health and Human Services to examine the supply, composition, and distribution of nurses nationally and on the state level. The study identified the characteristics of all registered nurses with active licenses to practice in the United States whether or not they were employed in nursing at the time of the study. Data describe the number of registered nurses, their educational background and specialty areas; their employment settings, position levels, and salaries; their geographic distribution; their personal characteristics, including gender, racial/ethnic background, age, family status, and job satisfaction.

Evidence for Practice

Ohlen, J., & Segesten, K. (1998). The professional identity of the nurse: Concept analysis and development. *Journal of Advanced Nursing, 28*(4),720–727.

The purpose of this qualitative study was to describe the concept of registered nurses' professional identity. Eight Australian registered nurses were interviewed using a semistructured format. Results indicated that the professional and personal identities of the nurse are integrated, consisting of feelings and experience of self as a nurse (subjective part) and other people's image of the nurse (objective part). These identities appear on a maturity continuum, with the opposite poles of strong and weak professional identity. The development takes place in a sociohistorical context through intersubjective processes of growth, maturity, and socialization, where interpersonal relations are important and attained maturity of the nurse influences further growth.

dents include their families and friends, their classmates, and their faculty.

Family and friends might be considered the first level of support and may provide assistance in a variety of ways. This assistance may include financial help, babysitting, cooking meals, typing papers, proofreading papers, being a sounding board for ideas, and helping to study for exams. Some nurses are concerned about whether they can continue to meet the needs of their family, especially young children, when they return to school. The change will require some adjustment on each family member's part, but often the result is positive in ways that were unexpected. For instance, children may learn about the importance of study habits and continuing one's education in the future.

An advantage of returning to school is meeting colleagues from other areas of practice and other health care organizations. This can provide opportunities to broaden perspectives on health care and nursing, as well as to establish important networks. The new colleagues may challenge thinking during discussions of ideas, and they may be the "experts" to consult. This new network can become an informal network for obtaining new jobs based on experience and new knowledge.

Working with Faculty

The faculty is an important resource in increasing knowledge, expanding ways of thinking, and enhancing professional capabilities. According to Twiname and Boyd (2002, p. 43), faculty "are not the enemy. . . . They are there to help you graduate." It's important to use faculty to the fullest while remembering that they are also people. Their suggestions for working with faculty are shown in the box on page 10.

Additionally, do not expect faculty to be mind readers. When having difficulties either personally or related to your coursework, discuss them with the faculty. They may be able to suggest solutions, recommend resources in the college/university, or assist with learning. Sometimes personal circumstances occur that necessitate dropping out of a class before the end of the semester or term. There are usually procedures that must be followed so that there is no negative impact on the student's progression or grade.

Suggestions for Dealing with Faculty

1. *Show your faculty respect.* When you show faculty respect, they will respect you in turn. Respect and courtesy go hand in hand. Find out your faculty's office hours. When you make an appointment, keep it; if you can't, then call to cancel. Don't be afraid to speak up and let your teacher know what you need to meet your goals.

2. *Remember, as human beings, your instructors will have good days and bad days.* Faculty members experience the same life problems as students. Although most of the time faculty will be fully there for students, there may be times when other things, either work-related or personal, may take precedence. Before dropping in for a visit, confirm that it is a convenient time for both you and the faculty member. This will ensure that the faculty member is fully there for you.

3. *Respect your instructor's privacy.* Don't call your instructor at home unless she or he has given you permission to do so. Visit faculty during posted office hours. Faculty have many responsibilities related to teaching, including course preparation, committee work, and grading student assignments. Recognize that faculty members often schedule office time to complete work-related activities, during which they wish not to be disturbed.

4. *Instructors have many different personalities.* Some will be very tough and demanding, whereas others will be very casual. Students will need to learn from a variety of teachers with different teaching styles. Being exposed to a diversity of instructors prepares students for interacting with the various people they will meet in their professional life.

Sources: Adapted from *Student Nurse Handbook: Difficult Concepts Made Easy* (2nd ed.), by B. G. Twiname and S. M. Boyd, 2002. Upper Saddle River, NJ: Prentice Hall; and *How to Study,* by R. Fry, 1994, New York: Career Press.

Study Skills

Study skills may need to be reviewed and enhanced. Unlike many noncredit continuing education activities, there are graded assignments, exams, and grades in college courses. Students need to plan well to balance the many obligations they have. Some suggestions to enhance study skills are found in the accompanying box.

Suggestions for Study-Skills Enhancement

1. *Decide where you will study.* Most people prefer to study in quiet, whereas others find that background noise is helpful. Determine where you will study. Be sure that there is adequate lighting, comfortable seating, and the supplies you need so that you can study without interruption.

2. *Avoid marathon study sessions.* Plan ahead and keep up with readings and other assignments so that you need only to review for exams.

3. *Be prepared for classes.* Read the reading assignments before class and make notes or outline the material. Use class time to clarify information, to ask questions, and to participate in discussion. Don't expect faculty to read the textbook to you. They may assign readings as a foundation and then lecture from other resources to enhance the assigned readings.

4. *Review notes as soon after class as possible.* Make sure you understand your notes. Check your notes against the textbook to determine if there are any discrepancies. Don't wait until the exam to clarify inconsistencies.

5. *Learn how to use the library and how to use computers.* The library is not just a building; it is a collection that is available by computer as well as hard copy. At any time of the day or night, there is access to hundreds of databases where students can locate information related to the area of study. Information from governmental and private organizations is available 24 hours a day by simply going online and using a search engine.

Sources: Adapted from *Student Nurse Handbook: Difficult Concepts Made Easy* (2nd ed.), by B. G. Twiname and S. M. Boyd, 2002. Upper Saddle River, NJ: Prentice Hall; and *How to Study,* by R. Fry, 1994, New York: Career Press.

The challenges of starting professional nursing studies or returning to school to achieve a higher degree in nursing, represented by changes in lifestyle and new demands on time and intellect, can be stimulating and satisfying. Many opportunities will be available for personal and professional growth. New career possibilities will be available, and new perspectives on old views will be considered. The journey is an important one to each student and to nursing as a profession.

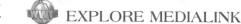 EXPLORE MEDIALINK

Questions, critical thinking exercises, essay activities, and other interactive resources for this chapter can be found on the Web site at http://www.prenhall.com/blais. Click on Chapter 1 to select activites for this chapter.

Bookshelf

Benner, P. (1984). *From novice to expert: Excellence and power in clinical nursing practice.* **Menlo Park, CA: Addison-Wesley Nursing.**

This classic work describes the transition to expert nurse by the new graduate or the experienced nurse who changes to a new practice setting. It describes the roles of nurses in their various stages of development and the challenges they face.

Hudacek, S. (2000). *Making a difference: Stories from the point of care.* **Indianapolis, IN: Sigma Theta Tau International.**

The author discusses the nursing values of caring, courage, comfort, competence, critical thinking, and creativity using nurses' stories to illustrate these values in practice.

Miller, T. W. (2003). *Building and managing a career in nursing: Strategies for advancing your career.* **Indianapolis, IN: Sigma Theta Tau International.**

The author and contributors provide a comprehensive discussion of career management for nurses, including chapters on reclaiming one's career, mentoring, and developing support networks to enhance career growth.

The book also provides information on creating inquiry letters, resumes, and CVs with examples of each.

Smeltzer, C. H., & Vlasses, F. R. (2003). *Ordinary people, extraordinary lives: The story of nurses.* **Indianapolis, IN: Sigma Theta Tau International.**

The authors relate the stories of "ordinary" nurses told by patients, friends, families, and the nurses themselves. The stories portray the qualities of nursing: selflessness, service, hope, courage, authentic presence, and the need to make a difference. When nurses read these stories they may see reflections of their own professional lives and are encouraged to write their own stories.

Twiname, B. G., & Boyd, S. M. (2002). *Student nurse handbook: Difficult concepts made easy* **(2nd ed.). Upper Saddle River, NJ: Prentice Hall.**

This text is written for both basic nursing students and nurses returning to school. It provides suggestions and strategies to help students with study skills, time management, writing papers, getting along with faculty, and managing stress.

REFERENCES

American Association of Colleges of Nursing (AACN). (2001). *Your nursing career: A look at the facts.* http://www.aacn.nche.edu.

American Association of Colleges of Nursing (AACN). (2003). *Fact sheet: The impact of education on nursing practice.* http://www.aacn.nche.edu.

American Nurses Association (ANA). (2004). *Nursing facts.* Retrieved January 3, 2004, http://www.nursingworld.org/readroom/fsdemogrpt .htm.

American Nurses Credentialing Center (ANCC). (2003). *Certification and recertification.* Retrieved December 6, 2003, http://www.nursingworld.org.

Benner, P. (1984). *From novice to expert: Excellence and power in clinical nursing practice.* Menlo Park, CA: Addison-Wesley Nursing.

Bridges, W. (2000). *The way of transition.* Cambridge, MA: Perseus.

McCullough, C. 2003. How to transition: Moving from where you were to where you want to be. In *Building and managing a career in nursing: Strategies for advancing your career,* by T. W. Miller. Indianapolis, IN: Sigma Theta Tau International.

Miller, T. W. (2003). *Building and managing a career in nursing: Strategies for advancing your career.* Indianapolis, IN: Sigma Theta Tau International.

National Advisory Council on Nurse Education and Practice (NACNEP). (1995). *Basic registered nurse workforce.* Washington, DC: U.S. Department of Health and Human Services.

Ohlen, J., & Segesten, K. (1998). The professional identity of the nurse: Concept analysis and development. *Journal of Advanced Nursing, 28*(4), 720–727.

Spencer, S. A., & Adams, J. D. (1990). *Life changes: Growing through personal transitions.* San Francisco: John Adams.

Spratley, E., Johnson, A., Sockalski, J., Fritz, M., & Spencer, W. (2000). *The registered nurse population, March 2000: Findings from the national sample survey of registered nurses.* Washington, DC: U.S. Department of Health and Human Services.

Twiname, B. G., & Boyd, S. M. (2002). *Student nurse handbook: Difficult concepts made easy* (2nd ed.). Upper Saddle River, NJ: Prentice Hall.

C H A P T E R 2
Socialization to Professional Nursing Roles

Objectives

- Discuss professionalism and nursing.
- Describe socialization to professional nursing.
- Analyze elements and boundaries of nursing roles.
- Compare socialization models.
- Discuss ways to manage role stress and strain while enhancing professional identity.

M E D I A L I N K

Additional online resources for this chapter can be found on the companion Web site at http://www.prenhall.com/blais.

Professional socialization is associated with the specialized knowledge, skills, attitudes, values, and norms needed to perform the professional role. There is debate as to whether this socialization is a process or an outcome. When described as a process, it is characterized as "a complex and variable form of learning, highly collaborative in nature" (Weedman, 1998, p. 1). It transmits values, norms, and ways of seeing that are unique to the profession and provides a common ground that shapes the ways in which work is conducted and allows members of the profession to communicate effectively. As an outcome, it is the formation of an individual's professional identity, the self-view as a member of a profession with the requisite knowledge and responsibilities. Socialization as a process or an outcome is interactive, because the knowledge, skills, and values of a profession are passed along to new members.

A profession is generally distinguished from other kinds of occupations by (1) its requirement of prolonged, specialized training to acquire a body of knowledge pertinent to the role to be performed and (2) an orientation of the individual toward service, either to a community or to an organization. The standards of education and practice for the profession are determined by the members of the profession rather than by outsiders. The education of the professional involves a complete socialization process, more far-reaching in its social and attitudinal aspects and its technical features than usually required in other kinds of occupations.

There is debate about whether nursing is a profession or has yet to reach that status. Traditionally, only medicine, law, and theology were considered professions, but nursing has been called a profession for many years.

CHALLENGES AND OPPORTUNITIES

Level of entry. Professional role socialization has been impeded by nursing's multiple levels of entry into the field and the lack of agreement about role differences at these different levels. Nursing is the only major discipline that does not require its members to hold at least a baccalaureate degree to be licensed. Associate degree programs continue to maintain high enrollment and graduate large numbers of individuals (Joel, 2002). Role socialization depends on the way the role is conceptualized, and nurses prepared at multiple levels may not have common language, values, and so on. Thus, nurses may not be in accord with regard to professional practice and may have different perspectives relative to professional practice.

Gaps between education and practice. Adding to the quandary is the lack of agreement between educators and employers of nurses regarding expectations of graduates entering the field. Educators in the professional curriculum provide initial socialization, and they make decisions based on their conception of a beginning-level professional. Employers are looking for graduates who can function independently, require little retraining or orientation, and can supervise a variety of less educated and unlicensed employees. Role incongruity is often experienced in the practice setting.

Professional identity: Job versus career. There is little commitment to a *job* other than going to work, doing what is expected, and collecting a paycheck. A career, on the other hand, is viewed as a person's life work, and it develops over time. There is planning for the future and direction with a career that requires commitment. The practice of nursing is not viewed as a career by all nurses.

Reflect on...

■ What planning brought you to this phase of your career development?

■ Do you think of nursing as an occupation or as a profession? What motivates your commitment?

PROFESSIONALISM

Nursing as a Discipline and Profession

Unlike other professions, nursing has three educational routes leading to eligibility for the licensing exam and becoming a registered nurse. This has created controversy within the profession and confusion for the public. The earliest type of nursing education in the United States took place within hospital-based training schools and awarded a diploma in nursing at the conclusion. Baccalaureate nursing education started at the University of Minnesota in 1909 and exists in 4-year institutions of higher education. Associate degree nursing (ADN) programs began in 1952 in response to a nursing shortage and developed within community colleges. As nursing education began moving into institutions of higher education, the diploma programs began affiliating with nearby colleges and universities.

Associate degree programs focused on preparing bedside nurses and drew large numbers of students. They helped to solve subsequent nursing shortages in the 1960s and 1980s. Baccalaureate degree programs provide a broader background of knowledge from the sciences and liberal arts than the other two programs and prepare the graduates for a greater variety of roles. These roles include community nursing and leadership.

In the 20-year period between 1980 and 2000, the type of program for nursing preparation has shown some shifts in patterns. The percentage of nurses prepared in diploma programs decreased from 60% to 30% while preparation at the associate degree level increased from 19% to 40%. The percentage of nurses prepared at the baccalaureate level increased from

17% to 29%. Between 1996 and 2000 there was a reversal in the trend of preparation at the associate degree and baccalaureate degree levels, with the number of BSN graduates (basic preparation) increasing at a faster rate. In 2000, 34.4% of nurses reported the associate degree as their highest level of education and 32.7% of nurses reported the baccalaureate degree as their highest level (HRSA, 2001).

In 1965, the American Nurses Association published a position paper on educational preparation of nurses that differentiated nurses with baccalaureate degrees and nurses with associate degrees as professional and technical nurses. This issue has been a source of great controversy between those who see all nurses as professional and those who believe professionals should have a minimum of a bachelor's degree. Many changes have occurred since the inception of these programs, allowing for articulation of the programs and making it easier for the ADN graduate to continue for a BSN. RN-BSN transition programs are common today, and many students enter associate degree programs with the intent of continuing for a BSN degree. Some nurse leaders now propose a master's degree as the minimum education for entry into professional practice. As it stands now, nurses have the lowest educational requirement among professional health care providers (Nelson, 2002).

At the core of the controversy over level of entry into professional nursing is the definition of profession. Six different conceptualizations of the criteria, qualities, and behaviors for a profession are shown in the box on page 16. Educational preparation at the baccalaureate level provides a broader education to better address the body of knowledge. Although nursing meets each of the criteria to some extent, some are more adequately addressed than others. The autonomous practice of nursing has been a source of political activism on behalf of nurses. Whether nursing has a sufficiently developed, unique body of knowledge is also in dispute. It may be concluded that nursing has not yet achieved full professional status but is emerging as a profession.

Nursing as a discipline is less controversial. A discipline is "characterized by a unique perspective, a distinct way of viewing all phenomena, which ultimately defines the limits and nature of its inquiry" (Donaldson & Crowley, 1978). Disciplines reflect distinctions among bodies of knowledge; in other words, human knowledge is divided into disciplines. Nursing as a discipline is defined by the essence of nursing.

Disciplines are divided into academic disciplines and professional disciplines. Academic disciplines, such as physics and mathematics, use descriptive theories and do basic and applied research. Professional disciplines are directed toward practical aims using both descriptive and prescriptive theories and add clinical research along with basic and applied research. The practice of academic disciplines is research and education, whereas the practice of professional disciplines adds a component of clinical practice. Thus, nursing has a better fit as a professional discipline.

Standards of Clinical Nursing Practice

Establishing and implementing standards of practice are major functions of a professional organization. The purpose of standards of clinical nursing practice is to describe the responsibilities for which nurses are accountable. The standards (1) reflect the values and priorities of the nursing profession, (2) provide direction for professional nursing practice, (3) provide a framework for the evaluation of nursing practice, and (4) define the profession's accountability to the public and the client outcomes for which nurses are responsible (ANA, 1998, p. 1). In 1991, the ANA developed standards of clinical nursing practice that are generic in nature and provide for the practice of nursing regardless of area of specialization. They were revised in 1998. The ANA and various specialty nursing organizations have further developed specific standards of nursing practice related to the practice of nursing in a specialty area.

Nursing standards clearly reflect the specific functions and activities that nurses provide, as opposed to the functions of other health workers. The ANA's standards of clinical nursing practice consist of both standards of care and standards of professional performance. Standards of professional performance describe the competence level of professional role behaviors. These standards are shown in the box on page 17.

When standards of professional practice are implemented, they serve as yardsticks for the measurements used in licensure, certification, accreditation, quality assurance, peer review, and public policy.

Reflect on...

■ Are the ANA Standards of Professional Practice reflected in your work setting?

Criteria of a Profession

FLEXNER (1915)

Professional activity is basically intellectual.

Activities are practical, not theoretical.

Work can be learned because it is based on a body of knowledge.

Techniques can be taught.

A strong organization is in place.

Work is motivated by altruism.

BIXLER & BIXLER (1945)

Body of knowledge is specialized.

Body of knowledge is increasing.

New knowledge is developed to improve education and practice.

Practice is autonomous.

Education takes place in higher institutions.

Service is considered to be more important than personal gain.

Compensation comes through freedom to act, continuing professional growth, and economic security.

BARBER (1965)

A vast amount of systematic general knowledge.

Oriented primarily to community interest rather than self-interest.

Strong behavioral self-control supported by codes of ethics and internalized through work socialization and through organizing and conducting voluntary associations operated by work specialists.

A system of rewards: monetary and honorary.

PAVALKO (1971)

Work is based on a systematic body of theory and abstract knowledge.

Work has social value.

Work is a service to the public.

Education is required for specialization.

Autonomy.

Commitment to the profession.

Group identity and subculture.

A code of ethics.

MILLER (1993) PROFESSIONAL BEHAVIORS

Educational background.

Adherence to the code of ethics.

Participation in the professional organization.

Continuing education and competency.

Communication and publication.

Autonomy and self-regulation.

Community service.

Theory use, development, and evaluation.

Research development.

JOEL & KELLY (2002) QUALITIES OF A PROFESSION

1. A profession utilizes in its practice a well-defined and well-organized body of knowledge that is intellectual in nature and describes its phenomena of concern.

2. A profession constantly enlarges the body of knowledge it uses and subsequently imposes on its members the life-long obligation to remain current in order to "do no harm."

3. A profession entrusts the education of its practitioners to institutions of higher education.

4. A profession applies its body of knowledge in practical services that are vital to human welfare, and especially suited to the tradition of seasoned practitioners shaping the skills of newcomers to the role.

5. A profession functions autonomously (with authority) in the formulation of professional policy and in the monitoring of its practice and practitioners.

6. A profession is guided by a code of ethics which regulates the relationship between professional and client.

7. A profession is distinguished by the presence of a specific culture, norms, and values that are common among its members.

8. A profession has a clear standard of educational preparation for entry into practice.

Criteria of a Profession (cont.)

9. A profession attracts individuals of intellectual and personal qualities who exalt service above personal gain and who recognize their chosen occupation as a life's work.

10. A profession strives to compensate its practitioners by providing freedom of action, opportunity for continuous professional growth, and economic security.

Sources: Sociology of Occupations & Professions, by R. M. Pavalko, 1971, Itasca, IL: F. E. Peacock; Some Problems in the Sociology of Its Professions, by B. Barber, 1965. In *The Professions in America,* by K. S. Lynu. Boston: Houghton Mifflin; "The Professional Status of Nursing," by G. K. Bixler, and R. W. Bixler, 1945, *American Journal of Nursing 45,* 730; *Is Social Work a Profession? Proceedings of the National Conference of Clarities and Correction,* by A. Flexner, 1915, New York: New York School of Philanthropy; "A Behavioral Inventory for Professionalism in Nursing," by B. K. Miller, D. Adams, and L. Beck, 1993, *Journal of Professional Nursing, 9*(5), 290–295; and *The Nursing Experience: Trends, Challenges, and Transition* (4th ed.), by L. Joel and L. Y. Kelly, 2002, New York: McGraw-Hill.

PROFESSIONAL SOCIALIZATION

Socialization is the process by which people learn social rules and become members of groups. It involves learning to behave in a way that is consistent with other persons occupying the same role. The goal of professional socialization is to internalize a professional identity that includes the norms, values, attitudes, and behaviors of the profession.

An intrinsic aspect of the socialization process is social control—the capacity of a social group to regulate itself through conformity and adherence to group norms to maintain the group's social order and organization. Sanctions are used to enforce norms. Positive sanctions

ANA Standards of Professional Performance

I. Quality of Care
The nurse systematically evaluates the quality and effectiveness of nursing practice.

II. Performance Appraisal
The nurse evaluates his or her own nursing practice in relation to professional practice standards and relevant statutes and regulations.

III. Education
The nurse acquires and maintains current knowledge and competency in nursing practice.

IV. Collegiality
The nurse interacts with, and contributes to the professional development of, peers and other health care providers as colleagues.

V. Ethics
The nurse's decisions and actions on behalf of patients are determined in an ethical manner.

VI. Collaboration
The nurse collaborates with the patient, family, and other health care providers in providing patient care.

VII. Research
The nurse uses research findings in practice.

VIII. Resource Utilization
The nurse considers factors related to safety, effectiveness, and cost in planning and delivering patient care.

Source: From *Standards of Clinical Nursing Practice* (2nd ed.), American Nurses Association, 1998. Washington, DC: ANA. Used by permission.

reward conformity to norms; negative sanctions punish nonconformity. Sanctions may be either externally employed by a source outside the individual (e.g., disciplinary action by a committee) or internally employed from within the individual (e.g., self-congratulations for a job well done). Socialization implies that the individual is induced to conform willingly to the ways of the group. Norms therefore become internalized standards. Professions require both a relatively long period of formal schooling and an informal, internalized system of ethics that guides practice of the professional role. Professional socialization involves exposure to multiple agents of socialization. Agents of socialization are the people who initiate the socialization process; for children, the primary agents of socialization are families, teachers, peers, and the mass media. For adults, the influence of these agents continues but other agents arise, such as superiors and subordinates in the workplace, peers, and people in various other kinds of social groups. Socialization agents that nursing students encounter include clients, faculty, professional colleagues, other health care professionals, family (e.g., a nurse relative), and friends who occupy roles within or outside the formal institutional structure. Professional socialization in nursing occurs formally through the educational experience in the nursing curriculum and later through preceptors, mentors, and staff development on the job. The degree of congruence between the expectations of these multiple agents may either facilitate or hinder socialization. Factors that facilitate the socialization process are listed in the accompanying box.

Reflect on...

■ the agents of professional socialization in your own experience. How have others influenced your development as a nurse?

Critical Values of Professional Nursing

It is within the nursing educational program that the nurse develops, clarifies, and internalizes professional values. Specific professional nursing values are stated in the ANA code of ethics (see Chapter 4 ∞, Ethical Foundations of Professional Nursing), in standards of nursing practice, and in the legal system itself (see Chapter 5 ∞, Legal Foundations of Professional Nursing). Professional values are preferred standards that guide behavior and are used for evaluating behavior.

Weis and Schank (2000) developed an instrument to measure professional nursing values derived from the 1985 ANA Code of Ethics with Interpretive Statements. This tool identified eight value factors; they are caregiving, activism, accountability, integrity, trust, freedom, safety, and knowledge. Caregiving and the nurse's responsibility to the client are related to the first six statements in the Code of Ethics, and the last five statements indicate the social nature of the profession and public responsibility related to activism and accountability.

A study by Tuck, Harris, and Baliko (2000) examined the values expressed in the written philosophies of nursing service in health care organizations. They

Factors That Facilitate the Socialization Process

- Clarity and consensus with which the occupants and aspirants (learners) perceive the roles and positions.

- Degree of compatibility of expectations within role sets—that is, all others who are involved with the learner, such as staff nurses, nurse managers, physicians, clients, and their families or significant others.

- Learning that has occurred before an entry to a position.

- Capability of socialization agents to manage the socialization process.

- Role models who demonstrate the desired characteristics and can enhance internalization of admired qualities.

- A well-developed and extended orientation or internship program that may include preceptors (people who act as teachers).

- Group support from others new to the position to share concerns.

Sources: Adapted from *Role Transition to Patient Care Management* (pp. 64–66) by M. K. Strader and P. J. Decker, 1995, Norwalk, CT: Appleton and Lange; *Role Theory: Perspectives for Health Professionals* (2nd ed.), by M. E. Hardy and M. E. Conway, 1988, Norwalk, CT: Appleton and Lange.

extracted themes and categories using content analysis. The values identified in the philosophy statements were grouped into seven categories: caring, professionalism, individualism, need-fulfillment, culture, well-being or health, and adaptation. Caring, professionalism, and individualism were highly rated values, and the researchers concluded that caring is the core of nursing.

Reflect on...

■ How is caring manifested in your practice?
■ What actions or behaviors demonstrate caring?

The Initial Process of Professional Socialization

Professional socialization is the means of developing a professional identity incorporating values, skills, behaviors, and norms for nursing practice. It is a lifelong process beginning with the curriculum and faculty of the nursing program. Registered nurses who return to school for baccalaureate nursing education experience professional resocialization. Their personal characteristics are diverse and affect resocialization in complex ways. Often they need to overcome prejudices about and resistance to an educational program that may require them to shed habitual ways of thinking. Although professional organizations adhere to the belief that baccalaureate education is the minimum education for professional nursing, there is an absence of agreement within the ranks of practicing nurses. Furthermore, there are others who promote the idea that the graduate level should be the professional level of entry.

Initial socialization prepares the student for the work setting. Several models have been developed to explain the initial process of socialization into professional roles. The models described here include those of Simpson, Henshaw, and Davis. Each model outlines a sequential set of phases or "chain of events" beginning at the role of a layperson and ending at the role of a professional. Table 2–1 summarizes each model.

Simpson Model

Ida Harper Simpson (1967, 1979) outlines three distinct phases of professional socialization. In the first phase, the person concentrates on becoming proficient in specific work tasks. In the second phase, the person becomes attached to significant others in the work or reference group. In the third and final phase, the person internalizes the values of the professional group and adopts the prescribed behaviors.

Table 2–1 Models of Initial Socialization into Professional Roles

Simpson (1967) Model	Hinshaw (1986) Model	Davis (1966) Doctrinal Conversion Model	
Stage 1 Proficiency in specific work tasks	*Phase I* Transition of anticipated role expectations to the role expectations of societal group	*Stage 1* Initial innocence	
		Stage 2 Labeled recognition of incongruity	
Stage 2 Attachment to significant others in the work environment	*Phase II* Attachment to significant others/labeling incongruencies	*Stage 3* "Psyching out" and role simulation	
		Stage 4 Increasing role simulation	
		Stage 5 Provisional internalization	
Stage 3 Internalization of the values of the professional group and adoption of the behaviors it prescribes	*Phase III* Internalization of role values/behaviors	*Stage 6* Stable internalization	

Sources: Adapted from "Patterns of Socialization into Professions: The Case of Student Nurses," by I. H. Simpson, Winter 1967, *Sociological Inquiry,* 37, pp. 47–54, "Socialization and Resocialization of Nurses for Professional Nursing Practice" by A. S. Hinshaw, 1986. In E. C. Hein and M. J. Nicholson (Eds.), *Contemporary Leadership Behavior: Selected Readings* (2nd ed.), Boston: Little, Brown; and "Professional Socialization as Subjective Experiences: The Process of Doctrinal Conversion among Student Nurses," by F. Davis, September 1966, Evian, France: Sixth World Congress of Sociology.

Hinshaw Model

Ada Sue Hinshaw (1986) provides a three-phase general model of socialization that is an adaptation of Simpson's model. During the first phase, individuals change their images of the role from anticipated concepts to the expectations of the persons who are setting the standards for them. Hinshaw states that (1) adults entering a profession have already learned a number of roles and values that help them to evaluate new roles and (2) these individuals are actively involved in the socialization process, having chosen to learn the new role expectations and enter the socialization process.

The second phase has two components: (1) learners attach themselves to significant others in the system, and at the same time (2) they label situations that are incongruent between their anticipated roles and those presented by the significant others. In the initial professional socialization, significant others are usually a group of faculty; in the work setting, they are selected colleagues or immediate supervisors. Hinshaw emphasizes the importance of appropriate role models in both educational programs and work settings. At this stage, individuals are able to verbalize that the expected role behaviors are not what they anticipated. It is a stage that often involves strong emotional reactions to conflicting sets of expectations. Successful resolution of conflicts depends on the existence of role models who demonstrate appropriate behaviors and who show how conflicting systems of standards and values can be integrated.

In the third phase, the student internalizes the values and standards of the new role. The degrees to which values and standards are internalized and the extent of incongruence in role expectations vary.

Kelman (1961, 57) defines three levels of value orientation. Individuals may demonstrate one or a blend of three levels:

■ *Compliance.* The person demonstrates the expected behavior to get positive reactions from others but has not internalized the values. Compliance behavior can be dismissed when it no longer elicits positive responses.
■ *Identification.* The person selectively adopts specific role behaviors that are acceptable to that person. The person may accept only expected behaviors rather than values. Identification behavior usually changes as role models change.
■ *Internalization.* The person believes in and accepts the standards of the new role. The standards are a part of the person's own value system.

Davis Model

Fred Davis (1966) describes a six-stage doctrinal conversion process among nursing students.

STAGE 1: INITIAL INNOCENCE   As students enter a professional program, they have an image of what they expect to become and how they should act or behave. Nursing students usually enter a nursing program with a service orientation and expect to look after sick people. However, educational experiences often differ from what the students expect. During this phase, students may express disappointment and frustration at the experiences they undergo and may question their value.

STAGE 2: LABELED RECOGNITION OF INCONGRUITY   In this phase students begin to identify, articulate, and share their concerns. They learn that they are not alone in their values incongruity; their peers share the same concerns.

STAGES 3 AND 4: "PSYCHING OUT" AND ROLE SIMULATION   At this point, the basic cognitive framework for the internalization of professional nursing values begins to take shape. Students begin to identify the behaviors they are expected to demonstrate and through role modeling begin to practice the behaviors. In Davis's terms, this process becomes a matter of "psyching out" the faculty. The more effectively the role simulation is done, the more authentic the person believes the behavior to be, and it becomes part of the person. However, students may feel they are "playing a game" and are being "untrue to oneself," resulting in feelings of guilt and estrangement.

STAGE 5: PROVISIONAL INTERNALIZATION   In stage 5, students vacillate between commitment to their former image of nursing and performance of new behaviors attached to the professional image. Factors that enhance the students' new image are an increasing ability to use professional language and an increasing identification with professional role models, such as nursing faculty.

STAGE 6: STABLE INTERNALIZATION   During stage 6, the student's behavior reflects the educationally and professionally approved model. However, preparation of the student for the work setting is only the initial process in socialization. New values and behaviors continue to be formed in the work setting.

Kramer's Postgraduate Resocialization Model

STAGE I: SKILL AND ROUTINE MASTERY
The nurse focuses on developing technical expertise and mastering specific skills to overcome feelings of frustration and inadequacy, but may not focus on other important aspects of nursing care.

STAGE II: SOCIAL INTEGRATION
The nurse's major concern is having peers recognize the nurse's competence and accept the nurse into the group.

STAGE III: MORAL OUTRAGE
The nurse recognizes incongruities between conceptions

of the bureaucratic role, which is associated with the rules and regulations and loyalty to agency administration; the professional role, which is committed to continued learning and loyalty to the profession; and the service role, which is concerned with compassion and loyalty to the client as a person.

STAGE IV: CONFLICT RESOLUTION
The nurse resolves conflicts of stage III by surrendering behaviors and/or values or by learning to use both the values and behaviors of the professional and bureaucratic system in a politically astute manner.

Source: Reality Shock: Why Nurses Leave Nursing, by M. Kramer, 1974, St. Louis: Mosby.

Various factors facilitate the socialization process. Absence of these factors interferes with it.

Ongoing Professional Socialization and Resocialization

The process of socialization does not terminate with graduation from a program of study. It continues as the graduate begins a professional career and, in fact, continues throughout life. In school, the nursing student assimilates a central core of values emphasized by the faculty and the profession. In the work setting, the nurse faces the need to put the values of the profession into operation. The transition of the graduate to a full-fledged professional is facilitated if there is congruence between the norms, values, and expectations of the educational program and the realities of the work setting. However, practice settings are often bureaucratic and may not be supportive of professional career development. Three models of career stages or development—those of Benner (1984); Dalton, Thompson, and Price (1977); and Kramer (1974)—follow.

Kramer's Postgraduate Resocialization Model

Kramer (1974) introduced the concept of reality shock to explain discrepancies that arise between the behavioral expectations and values of the educational setting and those of the work setting. Reality shock results when the new graduate is unprepared (ineffec-

tively socialized) to function effectively in the workplace. Kramer describes a four-stage postgraduate resocialization model for the transition of graduates from educational setting to work setting. See the accompanying box.

Dalton's Career Stages Model

Dalton, Thompson, and Price describe a four-stage model that emphasizes the development of competence derived from experience. As the individual's career progresses throughout each stage, activities, relationships, and psychological issues change in focus. For example, the individual's major activities progress from helping, learning, and following directions (stage 1) to shaping direction of the organization (stage 4). The primary relationships progress from that of an apprentice (stage 1) to that of sponsor (stage 4). The major psychological issues progress from a feeling of dependence (stage 1) to a feeling of comfort in exercising power (stage 4). These four stages are summarized in Table 2–2. Only a small percentage of nurses achieve the fourth stage because there are few stage-4 positions available.

Benner's Stages from Novice to Expert

Benner (2001) describes five levels of proficiency in nursing based on the Dreyfus model of skill acquisition derived from a study of chess players and airline

Table 2–2 Dalton, Thompson, and Price Career Stages

Stages	Central Activity	Primary Relationship	Major Psychologic Issue
Stage I	Helping and learning: performs fairly routine duties under the direction of a mentor	Apprentice, subordinate	Dependence
Stage II	Works independently as a competent peer	Colleague	Independence
Stage III	Influences, guides, directs, and helps others to develop	Informal mentor, role model	Assuming responsibility for others
Stage IV	Influences the direction of the organization or a segment of it; has one of three roles: manager, internal entrepreneur, or idea innovator	Sponsor	Exercising power

Source: Adapted from "The Four Stages of Professional Careers—A New Look at Performance by Professionals," by G. W. Dalton, P. H. Thompson, and R. L. Price, Summer 1977, *Organizational Dynamics,* 19–42.

pilots. The five stages, which have implications for teaching and learning, are novice, advanced beginner, competent, proficient, and expert. Benner believes that experience is essential for the development of professional expertise. See the accompanying box.

Benner's Stages of Nursing Expertise

STAGE I: NOVICE
No experience (e.g., nursing student). Performance is limited, inflexible, and governed by context-free rules and regulations rather than experience.

STAGE II: ADVANCED BEGINNER
Demonstrates marginally accepted performance. Recognizes the meaningful "aspects" of a real situation. Has experienced enough real situations to make judgments about them.

STAGE III: COMPETENT PRACTITIONER
Has 2 or 3 years of experience. Demonstrates organizational and planning abilities. Differentiates important factors from less important aspects of care. Coordinates multiple complex care demands.

STAGE IV: PROFICIENT PRACTITIONER
Has 3 to 5 years of experience. Perceives situations as wholes rather than in terms of parts, as in stage II. Uses maxims as guides for what to consider in a situation. Has holistic understanding of the client, which improves decision making. Focuses on long-term goals.

STAGE V: EXPERT PRACTITIONER
Performance is fluid, flexible, and highly proficient; no longer requires rules, guidelines, or maxims to connect an understanding of the situation to appropriate action. Demonstrates highly skilled intuitive and analytic ability in new situations. Is inclined to take a certain action because "it felt right."

Source: From Novice to Expert (Commemorative ed.) (pp. 20–34) by P. Benner, 2001, Upper Saddle River, NJ: Prentice Hall. Reprinted with permission.

Evidence for Practice

Source: McNeese, D. K. "Job stages of entry, mastery, and disengagement among nurses." 2000. *Journal of Nursing Administration, 30*(3), 140–147.

The job stages of entry, mastery, and disengagement are, in theory, related to time on the job, skill development, and attitudes. They reflect levels of identification with the job environment. A descriptive survey queried 412 registered nurses to determine their job stage and job satisfaction. The entry stage is a process of skill development and increasing the congruity of the individual's self-concept and the expected role. It is the time one becomes an "insider." The mastery stage comes with having advanced beginner skills and developing expertise along with growing esteem. At this stage one can become a role model for others. The disengagement stage begins if congruency of the relationship between self-identity and job-identity decline. This may begin in the entry stage or the mastery stage and results in a sense of indifference toward the job. Nurses in the entry stage were primarily new on the job (6 months or less). The number of years as a nurse and years in the institution had a positive influence on mastery but not years in the current job. Longevity in the same job showed an inverse relationship to mastery and a positive relationship to disengagement. Job satisfaction, productivity, and organizational commitment had a positive relationship to mastery, with organizational commitment being the strongest predictor. Disengagement began almost immediately on beginning the job for some nurses. A plan to increase the percentage of nurses in the mastery stage and decrease the move to disengagement will need to include collaboration between nurses and management to facilitate the match between nurses' values and the organizational mission. Plans and support for career mobility are needed for those in their current jobs for extended time to prevent disengagement. Mutual planning to provide nurses a sense of accomplishment, challenge, and purpose hold promise for increasing the number of nurses in the mastery stage.

Reflect on...

- Benner's stages from novice to expert. Where are you on Benner's continuum in relation to your current area of practice? During your nursing career, what have you experienced as you have moved along Benner's continuum? How might you assist a novice nurse to progress successfully to higher levels of practice?

ROLE THEORY

Professional socialization has been based upon role theory, which emerged from the field of sociology. It involves preparation for particular job expectations or roles. A role is a set of expectations associated with a position in society. To understand socialization to a professional role, it is necessary to have an understanding of role theory. What is it that defines a role and how does one make a transition into that role?

Elements of Roles

Any role has three elements: the ideal role, the perceived role, and the performed role.

The ideal role refers to the socially prescribed or agreed-upon rights and responsibilities associated with the role. Persons who assume a certain role are provided with sets of expectations and obligations or norms that can be identified and used as criteria to judge the adequacy of performance in the role. The ideal role concept provides a relatively stable view of roles and role requirements, because the society at large is assumed to have the same or similar expectations about the pattern of behaviors that a person in a particular role should carry out. Although changes may occur in the prescribed rights and responsibilities associated with the ideal role, this ideal role tends to support a static view of role behaviors.

Role expectations are the norms specific to a position that identify the attitudes, cognitions, and behaviors required and anticipated of a person in a particular role. Ideal role expectations may also be determined by culture and education.

The perceived role refers to how a role incumbent (a person who assumes the role) believes she or he should behave in the role. A role incumbent's perceptions of the expected patterns of behavior may differ from the conventional ideal role expectations: Not every person may accept all the norms about a role or perceive them in the same way.

The performed role refers to what the role incumbent actually does. Role performance is defined as the behaviors of or actions taken by a person in relation to the expected behaviors of a particular position. Role mastery is the term used to indicate that a person demonstrates behaviors that meet the societal or cultural expectations associated with the specific role.

The person's perceptions and beliefs about what ought to be done is not the only factor influencing role performance. Other factors include health status, personal and professional values, needs of the client and support persons, and politics of the employing agency. A healthy nurse, for example, may provide care associated with prescribed and perceived roles more effectively than an unhealthy nurse. A nurse who values the client's right to participate in care planning will elicit

the client's thoughts and feelings before planning care. A nurse who must work in a situation in which several of the staff are absent may be required to defer basic aspects of care (e.g., bath, changing bed linen) for some clients in order to meet more critical needs of other clients (Hardy & Conway, 1988).

Role transition is a process by which a person assumes or develops a new role. There are two components associated with role behaviors: norms and values. Norms are the general expectations that support the behaviors, and values justify the behaviors and help the nurse conform to the norms (Strader & Decker 1995). In the new role, the person moves to a new set of responsibilities and, often, to new values as well. Role transition is influenced by many factors, such as individual, interpersonal factors, and organizational factors. A model of role transition is shown in Figure 2–1■.

Figure 2–1

Role Transition

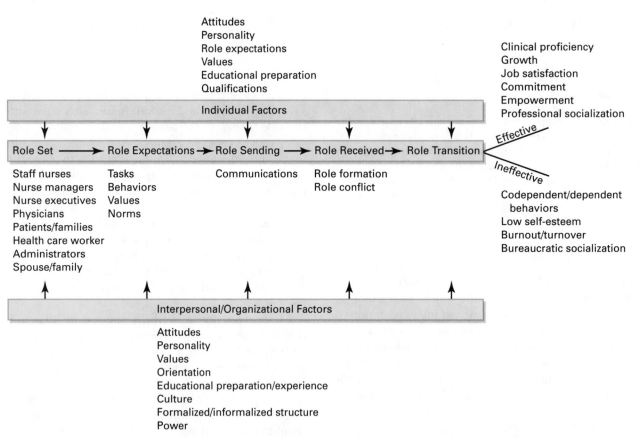

Source: From *Role Transition to Patient Care Management,* (p. 60), by M. K. Strader and P. J. Decker, 1995, Upper Saddle River, NJ: Prentice Hall. Used by permission.

According to this model, the process begins by determining the role set, composed of individuals involved who hold beliefs and attitudes about what should or should not be done in that role, or role expectations. Role sending involves the members of the role set communicating role expectations, and it is at this step that problems may develop. After the role is sent, the next phase is role received, but what is sent may not be received without misunderstanding or distortion. Role formation is affected by such factors as personality, attitudes, qualifications, educational preparation, and clarity of communication. Role conflict may develop when role expectations of the various people involved are incompatible. The actual role transition occurs as the nurse learns role behaviors based on the role received, resulting in two possible outcomes: effective or ineffective. Effective role transitions have associated behaviors within the norms; these can lead to clinical proficiency, personal growth, job satisfaction, organizational commitment, empowerment, and professional socialization. When there is a great deal of role conflict, ineffective role transition is likely to be the outcome, resulting in low self-esteem, a low level of confidence, and burnout.

Transition shock or reality shock may happen when the perceived role comes into conflict with the performed role. Many new graduates experience this as cognitive dissonance; that is, they know what they should do and how they should do it, but circumstances do not allow them to perform the role in that way. The result of this is increased anxiety, which, if not resolved, can result in burnout. Preceptorships, internships, and externships are approaches often found to be helpful in a successful role transition.

Reflect on...

■ the multiple roles you assume and the satisfactions you experience in relation to each. How does your role as a nurse relate to your other roles? In what ways does your choice of nursing as a career enhance or interfere with your other life roles?

Boundaries for Nursing Roles

The following five determinants currently form the boundaries for nursing roles:

1. Theoretical and conceptual frameworks identify the concepts of nursing and specify the relationships among them. Conceptual frameworks provide the nurse with an understanding of the recipient of nursing care, what constitutes health and environment, and how these influence nursing goals and actions. (See Chapter 6 ⟲, Theoretical Foundations of Professional Nursing.)

2. The nursing process, or standard scientific problem-solving method that nurses use in the clinical setting. The nursing process determines nursing actions appropriate for each client. The nursing process consists of five components: assessing, diagnosing, planning, implementing, and evaluating.

3. Standards of nursing practice established by the nursing profession. Standards of practice outline nursing functions and the level of excellence required of the nurse. These standards also define the nurse's ethical and legal obligations to clients and their support persons, to employers, and to society.

4. Nurse practice acts or nursing licensure laws of the specific jurisdiction that legally define the scope of nursing practice. Although nurse practice acts differ in various jurisdictions, they all have a common purpose: to protect the public. (See Chapter 5 ⟲, Legal Foundations of Professional Nursing.)

5. National and international codes of ethics for nurses are fundamental to the practice of nursing. Codes of ethics describe the nurse's relationships to clients, support persons, colleagues, employers, and society. (See Chapter 4 ⟲, Ethical Foundation of Professional Nursing.)

ROLE STRESS AND ROLE STRAIN

People often assume multiple roles, and as the number of roles increases so does role stress, resulting in role strain. This is particularly true for nurses. Role stress occurs when role obligations are unrealistic, vague, conflicting, or irritating. It is generated by the social structure or system; the source is primarily external to the person. Role stress may create role strain, an emotional reaction accompanied by psychological responses, such as anxiety, tension, irritation, resentment, and depression; and social responses, such as withdrawal from interaction, job dissatisfaction, and reduced involvement with colleagues and organizations (Hardy & Hardy 1988; Creasia & Parker 2001). Common role stress problems and descriptions are shown in the box on page 26.

Role ambiguity is often experienced by nurses because of the diversity of their roles and multiple subroles of the nursing role. (In contrast, a technician's role expectations are explicit, and work can often be routinized.) Ambiguity can significantly affect a person's role performance, satisfaction, and commitment.

Role Stress Problems

ROLE AMBIGUITY
Unclear role expectations.

ROLE CONFLICT
Incompatible, competing role expectations within a single role or multiple roles.

ROLE INCONGRUITY
Values are incompatible with role expectations.

ROLE OVERLOAD OR UNDERLOAD
Too much is expected in the time available, or the role is too complex (overload); minimal role expectations that do not use the abilities of the role incumbent (underload).

ROLE OVERQUALIFICATION OR UNDERQUALIFICATION
Nurse's abilities and motivation exceed those required (overqualification); nurse lacks necessary resources (underqualification).

Role conflict is a widely discussed concept in current literature. The primary consequence of role conflict is role stress. If unreconciled, role stress and role strain lead to burnout, a syndrome of mental and physical exhaustion involving negative self-concept, negative job attitude, and loss of concern for clients.

Shead (1991, 737) discusses four major causes of role conflict for nurses. A widely discussed causative factor is professional–bureaucratic work conflict. Nurses who are prepared to provide independent practice and use professional judgment experience conflict in bureaucracies that are more concerned about getting routine tasks completed. The organization's reward systems may contribute to conflict between nurses, who identify with their profession, and supervisors, who identify with the organization. Disproportionate power also creates stress. Increased professionalism often means increased conflict and stress, unless the bureaucratic structure is flexible enough to deal with the professional modality.

A second cause of role conflict arises from different views concerning what nursing is and should be. Role value orientations vary considerably among practitioners; some nurses have a more traditional view of the nurse's role than new managers or new professionals have. The role of the professional nurse continues to change; nurses are becoming increasingly involved in planning and organizing health care activities and are becoming more responsible for delivering total client care services. The nurse's role is becoming one of managing client care activities in general. In this new role, nurses have greater responsibility and accountability and may experience increased stress as a result.

A third cause of conflict is a discrepancy between the nursing and medical view of what the nurse's role should be. Physicians may view the caring ideology of nurses as secondary in importance to their own, idealized curing aspects of care, and view the nurse as a handmaiden. Nurses use behavioral science and communication skills to develop their professional relationship with clients; physicians have traditionally employed a clinical, biological approach. This variance can create role strain if (1) the physician expects the nurse to handle the client as the physician does, or (2) the physician does not listen to the nurse's concerns and suggestions about the client.

A fourth source of conflict arises from the public image of nursing. Personal expectations and self-image may conflict with perceived public expectations. The public may regard the ideal nurse as a dedicated angel of mercy, whereas the media often malign the image by portraying the nurse as a sex symbol or other negative stereotype.

Role stress and strain may be alleviated with appropriate strategies. Priority setting often makes role overload more manageable. When there is role ambiguity, rewriting the job description can provide more clarity about expectations. Integrating multiple roles into a larger whole may be possible in order to reduce role conflict, but when this is not possible, it may be necessary to reduce the number of roles and subroles by eliminating some. A full-time student who is a mother and has a part-time job may need to give up her role as PTA chairman. It is sometimes possible to avoid situations that produce role conflict by changing the setting or the context. A nurse who believes in providing holistic care may look for an employer whose philosophy is more closely aligned with her or his own. Often employment is accepted without evaluating the employer's philosophy and employment policies.

Stress Reduction Strategies

Nurses who seek to maintain or improve both their personal and professional selves are more effective in caring for their clients. They are also more effective in communicating with other health professionals and in promoting a positive image of nursing in the community. Strasen (1992, pg. 2) defines professional self-concept as the set of beliefs and images held to be true as a result of specific professional socialization. The development of professional self-concept is based on one's personal self-concept. An individual's personal self-concept and professional self-concept affect one another. The characteristics of a person who has a positive self-concept include the following (Strader & Decker, 1995, p. 88):

■ Future orientation; ability to minimize past failures
■ Ability to cope with life's problems and disappointments
■ Ability to help and accept help from others
■ Ability to see and value the uniqueness of all individuals
■ Ability to feel all aspects of emotion but not allow the feelings to affect behavior negatively or affect interactions with people who are not responsible for the situation

Because a person's subconscious mind acts positively or negatively on the information it receives, nurses can change their self-concept by controlling what goes into the subconscious mind. Nurses who perceive themselves as successful will use their energy and creativity to explore ways to become even more successful. Positive thoughts help them to succeed.

To develop a positive self-concept, Strader and Decker (1995, pp. 88–89) suggest the following steps:

■ Accept your present self but have a better self in mind.
■ Set goals that are high but attainable.
■ Develop expertise in some area to increase your value to yourself and to your employing agency. This may involve continuing education or obtaining certification in a specialized area of practice.

Managing Role Stress and Role Strain

Prevention of burnout in professional nursing can be approached by stress reduction. A number of approaches can be applied, but common threads among them are personal goal setting, problem identification, and problem-solving strategies. Personal goals should include both long-term and short-term goals. Being goal-directed reduces the erratic activity that frequently keeps the person busy and working hard without accomplishing much and leading to frustration. These goals can be applied to personal life choices, as well as professional career development. An important step in implementing a plan to pursue goals is identification of the problems that produce stress. Correctly identifying a problem allows the development of a plan to appropriately and positively create a solution. Problem solving is applied to the development of solutions that will result in stress reduction.

Time-management skills can be a valuable tool in stress reduction and may result in improvement in the nurse's personal life, as well as in the practice setting. Assuming multiple roles creates heavy demands on time, and multitasking tends to fragment attention and concentration. Delegation is one tool the nurse can use in time management. Overcoming procrastination is another time-management strategy. Simply starting a task is one of the best ways to overcome procrastination. Once begun, a task is usually completed. Prioritization may be needed when the number or scope of tasks seems insurmountable.

Taking care of one's self is important in stress management. Nurses must care for themselves before they can care for others effectively. Decompression is an important component, and the nurse can reduce tension by taking time for those things that meet personal needs and are pleasurable and restorative. Nursing support groups are also helpful. Using these techniques prevents stress and keeps problems from becoming overwhelming.

A summary of stress reduction activities for the working nurse is shown in Table 2–3. It is divided into personal stress reduction strategies and strategies to employ in the work setting.

Reflect on...

■ your own strategies for dealing with role stress. Which strategies have been effective? Which have not?
■ how your practice setting supports nurses dealing with role stress. What resources are needed for the institution to provide a work environment that minimizes role stress and strain?

Table 2–3   Strategies for Stress Reduction and Time Management

Personal	Professional
Care for yourself	**Select employment thoughtfully**
Exercise regularly	Compare your values to the agency's mission
Have a healthy diet	Know your competencies and make a match
Get adequate sleep and rest	**Participate in policy development opportunities**
Examine your lifestyle	Join committees that contribute to governance
Build time for relaxation activities such as meditation and yoga	Participate in organizational structure to target problematic job and role design
Reflect on what has been helpful in the past	Use negotiation skills
Budget time according to priorities	Seek win-win resolutions to conflict
Develop new coping skills	**Manage your role positively**
Let go of perfectionism	Network with colleagues
Let go of the need to do it all	Communicate clearly
Attend time-management workshop	Support excellence in practice
Attend assertiveness program	Be a self-advocate; use positive self-talk
Continue education to develop expertise in areas that give you satisfaction	Develop good delegation skills
	Participate in support groups

Evidence for Practice

Santos, S. R. Carol, C. A., Cox, K. S., Teasley, S. L., Simon, S., Bainbridge, L., Cunningham, M. and Ott, L. "Baby boomer nurses bearing the burden of care: A four-site study of stress, strain, and coping for inpatient registered nurses." 2003. *Journal of Nursing Administration* 33(4), 243–250.

Today's nursing workforce faces a myriad of stress and strain requiring coping skills. Six hundred ninety-four inpatient registered nurses participated in a study to identify the stressors and the influence of age of the nurse upon experiencing the stressors. Age cohorts were grouped as Mature (born 1919–1945), Baby Boomers (born 1946–1964), and Generation X (born 1965–1979). The physical demands and responsibility were the most problematic for all groups. The Baby Boomers were more stressed than the other two groups by role overload (in-creased work load), role insufficiency (poor fit between skills and the job), role ambiguity (unclear expectations), and role boundary (conflicting demands and factions). Focus groups with these nurses identified that the stressors were amplified for the Baby Boomers who were caught between many competing demands as part of the sandwich generation caring for both the younger and older generation at home. Coping was poorer for this group, who indicated a lack of social support available to them while they were the source of social support for others. The Mature group showed better coping in self-care and recreation. Institutions may need to begin to incorporate benefits targeted to these different age groups. Eldercare may be as necessary to the workforce as childcare. New staffing models may be necessary to accommodate a wider age range of nurses.

EXPLORE MEDIALINK

Questions, critical thinking exercises, essay activities, and other interactive resources for this chapter can be found on the Web site at http://www. prenhall .com/blais. Click on Chapter 2 to select activites for this chapter.

Critical Thinking Exercise

Marcia is an RN who recently finished the RN-BSN transition program at Sierra University. In the cafeteria, she runs into a former classmate, Brenda, from her ADN program, and Marcia tells Brenda about completing her BSN. Brenda then says to her, "I've thought about doing that, but it just doesn't seem worth it. We all do the same things anyway, and I have so many other things to do in the evenings. What difference does it make?"

Using the information in this chapter on criteria of a profession, socialization, and role theory, develop a response to Brenda that Marcia could use in responding to her friend's question.

Bookshelf

Canfield, J., Thieman, L., & Mitchell-Autio, N. (2001). *Chicken soup for the nurse's soul: 101 stories to celebrate, honor, and inspire the nursing profession.* **Deerfield Beach, FL: Health Communications, Inc.** This book celebrates and honors nursing as a profession with a collection of touching and humorous anecdotes.

Nicolson, P. (1996). *Gender, power, and organization: A psychological perspective.* **Westport, CT: Routledge.** This book looks at the professional socialization of women to the business world.

Goodman-Draper, J. (1995). *Health care's forgotten majority: Nurses and their frayed white collars.* **New York: Greenwood Publishing.** This book is a class analysis of nurses within the white-collar workforce.

SUMMARY

Nurses must understand the roles they and others play and societal expectations associated with those roles. Any role consists of three elements: the ideal role, the perceived role, and the performed role. Role performance is influenced by such factors as health status, values, and situational pressures. Five determinants form boundaries for nursing roles: conceptual frameworks, the nursing process, standards of practice, nurse practice acts, and a code of ethics.

Socialization is a lifelong process by which people become functioning participants of a society or a group. It is a reciprocal learning process that is brought about by interaction with other people and establishes boundaries of behavior. Socialization to professional nursing practice is the process whereby the values and norms of the nursing profession are internalized into the nurse's own behavior and self-concept. The nurse acquires the knowledge, skills, and attitudes characteristic of the profession.

Socialization for professional nursing requires the development of critical values, including a strong com-

mitment to the service that nursing provides to the public, a belief in the dignity and worth of each person, a commitment to education, and autonomy.

Socialization into professional nursing has been challenging because of the different educational routes available. Controversy exists as to the appropriate level of entry into professional nursing, although professional organizations have stated that it is at the baccalaureate level.

Various models of the socialization process have been developed. Such models may serve as guidelines to establish the phase and extent of an individual's socialization.

Nurses are prone to role stress and strain for a variety of reasons unique to their role in the health care and social systems. Common problems are role conflict, role ambiguity, role overload, and role incongruity. Strategies to handle role stress differ from strategies to manage role strain. Nurses can positively influence their self-concepts and role images to improve work satisfaction and provide quality care.

REFERENCES

American Nurses Association (ANA). (1998). *Standards of clinical nursing practice*. Washington, DC: ANA.

Benner, P. (1984). *From novice to expert: Excellence and power in clinical nursing practice*. Menlo Park, CA: Addison-Wesley Nursing.

Benner, P. (2001). *From novice to expert: Excellence and power in clinical nursing practice* (Commerative ed.). Upper Saddle River, NJ: Prentice Hall.

Creasia, J. L., & Parker, B. (2001). *Conceptual foundations: The bridge to professional nursing practice* (3rd ed.). St. Louis: Mosby.

Dalton, G. W., Thompson, P. H., & Price, R. L. (1977, Summer). The four stages of professional careers—A new look at performance by professionals. *Organizational Dynamics*, 19–42.

Davis, F. (1966, September). *Professional socialization as subjective experiences: The process of doctrinal conversion among student nurses*. Paper. Evian, France: Sixth World Congress of Sociology.

Donaldson, S. K., & Crowley, D. M. (1978). The discipline of nursing. *Nursing Outlook*, 113–120.

Hardy, M. E., & Conway, M. E. (1988). *Role theory: Perspectives for healthy professionals* (2nd ed.). Norwalk, CT: Appleton and Lange.

Hardy, M. E., & Hardy, W. L. (1988). Role stress and strain. In M. E. Hardy & M. E. Conway (Eds.), *Role theory: Perspectives for health professionals* (2nd ed., pp. 159–239). Norwalk, CT: Appleton and Lange.

Health Resources and Services Administration. (2001). *The registered nurse population: March 2000 Findings from the National Sample Survey of Registered Nurses*. Rockville, MD: U.S. Department of Health and Human Services.

Hinshaw, A. S. (1986). Socialization and resocialization of nurses for professional nursing practice. In E. C. Hein & M. J. Nicholson (Eds.), *Contemporary leadership behavior: Selected readings* (2nd ed.). Boston: Little, Brown.

Joel, L. (2002). Education for entry into nursing practice: Revisited for the 21st century. *Online Journal of Issues in Nursing, 7*(2), manuscript 4. Retrieved from http://www.nursingworld.org/ojin/topic181/tpc18_4.htm.

Kelman, H. (1961). Process of opinion changes. *Public Opinion Quarterly, 25*(1), 57.

Kramer, M. (1974). *Reality shock: Why nurses leave nursing*. St. Louis: Mosby.

Nelson, M. A. (2002). Education for professional nursing practice: Looking backward into the future. *Online Journal of Issues in Nursing, 71*(3), manuscript 3. Retrieved from http://www.nursingworld.org/ojin/topic18/tpc18_3.htm.

Shead, H. (1991, June). Role conflict in student nurses: Towards a positive approach for the 1990s. *Journal of Advanced Nursing, 16*, 736–740.

Simpson, I. H. (1967), Winter. Patterns of socialization into professions: The case of student nurses. *Sociological Inquiry, 37*, 47–54.

Simpson, I. H. (1979). *From student to nurse: A longitudinal study of socialization*. New York: Cambridge University Press.

Strader, M. K., & Decker, P. J. (1995). *Role transition to patient care management*. Norwalk, CT: Appleton and Lange.

Strasen, L. L. (1992). *The image of professional nursing: Strategies for action*. Philadelphia: Lippincott.

Tuck, I., Harris, L. H., & Baliko, B. (2000). Values expressed in philosophies of nursing services. *Journal of Nursing Administration, 30*(4), 180–184.

Weedman, J. (1998, May). *Burglar's tools: The use of collaborative technology in professional socialization*. Paper presented at meeting of American Society for Information Science, Orlando, FL.

Weis, D., and Schank, M. J. (2000). An instrument to measure professional nursing values. *Journal of Nursing Scholarship, 32*(2), 201–204.

CHAPTER 3

Historical Foundations of Professional Nursing

Outline

Objectives

- Discuss the historical development of nursing from ancient times to the present.

- Discuss the role of religion in the development of nursing.

- Discuss the influence of war on the development of nursing.

- Describe the contributions of selected nurses to nursing and society.

- Analyze the contributions of selected nurses and the nursing profession to society from a historical perspective.

- Discuss the development of professional nursing organizations and their role in advocating for nurses and health care.

- Compare and contrast the history of nursing and the history of caring.

M E D I A L I N K

Additional online resources for this chapter can be found on the companion Web site at http://www.prenhall.com/blais.

One of the irrefutable laws of nature is dynamism, or change. Individual and group elements of society respond and adapt to historical events that may alter the behaviors, values, laws, beliefs, and even the daily living habits of society. Influencing events may be related to natural disasters, such as floods, earthquakes, famine, or epidemic disease, or they may be invented by people, such as the discovery of fire, the wheel, the printing press, the microscope, and penicillin. War, political upheaval, religious intolerance, and economic instability are systemic events that can alter individuals' lives and group progress.

As a subgroup of society, nursing must also respond and adapt to the influences of society. Nursing has been a continuous thread linking the past with the present—from the tribal groups of early societies to modern societies linked by jet-powered transportation and instant telecommunications. Just as human history has shown tremendous progress over the centuries, so has nursing evolved from the art of comforting, caring for, and nurturing the sick to a synthesis of this art with the science and technology of contemporary thinking.

CHALLENGES AND OPPORTUNITIES

Studying the history of nursing can lead to an appreciation of the development of the discipline and profession that challenges nurses to honor the leaders and carry forward the best of the values and traditions. The perspective provided by knowing the roots of nursing can contribute to professional identity. Although nursing is facing a time of change and challenge, the depth and breadth of nursing's historical foundations provide a broad base of experience to draw on as the profession evolves. One challenge is to continue the leadership within the profession in furthering the traditional values by understanding where nursing has been and how it got there as well as where it needs to go in the future. It is important to convey to new nurses a knowledge and value of the past. In a profession that can be intensely involved in immediate decision making, knowing the past may seem to be of low priority.

Knowing the past and understanding the roles of early nursing leaders provides an opportunity to use the experience and lessons learned to create the future. The mistakes and successes of the past provide examples and can help guide decisions of today. Appreciation of what has been contributed by the pioneers of nursing and the social influences of the past provides the opportunity to celebrate the accomplishments, take pride in what has been done, and carry the best of the past into the future.

NURSING IN PRIMITIVE SOCIETIES

It is impossible to describe nursing practice or the role of the nurse before recorded history. It is also difficult to differentiate between the role of the physician and that of the nurse or even to determine if there were two distinctly different roles. It is likely that any differentiation that existed was based on male-female role proscriptions, such as medicine man or herb woman. It may be postulated that individuals provided care or cure based on experience and oral transmission of available knowledge about health and illness. Traditional female roles of wife, mother, daughter, and sister always included the care and nurturing of other family members. The term *nurse* derives from the care mothers gave to their helpless infant children. Donahue (1996, p. 2) suggests that the very survival of the human race is evidence of the existence of nursing throughout history and is "inextricably intertwined with the development of nursing."

NURSING IN ANCIENT CIVILIZATIONS

In the early recordings of ancient civilizations, there is little information about those who cared for the sick. It is known that midwives provided care for the mother and infant during birthing and wet nurses often suckled and cared for infant children of wealthy families. Often, these roles were filled by female slaves. This fact contributes to the lack of recorded information about nursing, because slaves had no status and thus their work was not thought worthy of documentation. The slave-nurse depended on the master, healer, or priest for instruction or direction in the care of her charge. Often the care provided for the sick was related to physical maintenance and comfort.

During this time, beliefs about the cause of disease were imbedded in superstition and magic, so treatment often required magical cures. The priest or witch doctor enjoyed great status in ancient societies. But as these societies evolved, practical theories of medical care emerged as nonmagical causes of disease were observed. The earliest recording of healing practices is a 4000-year-old clay tablet attributed to the Sumerian civilization. It contains healing prescriptions but, unfortunately, neglects to describe the illnesses for which they were prescribed.

The earliest documentation of law governing the practice of medicine is the Code of Hammurabi, attributed to the Babylonians and dating to 1900 B.C. The code recorded regulations related to sanitation and public health, the practice of surgery, the differentiation between the practice of human and veterinary medicine, a table of fees for operations, and penalties for violators of the code. There is no specific record of nursing in the Babylonian civilization; however, there are references to tasks and practices traditionally provided by nurses. Medical illustrations from that period often include a nurse-like figure providing patient support or comfort.

Important historic findings related to the Egyptian culture include the Ebers papyrus and the practice of mummification. The Ebers papyrus, which dates to approximately 1550 B.C., is believed to be the oldest medical text in the world. It describes many diseases known today and identifies specific symptomatology. It also lists more than 700 substances that were used as drugs and describes their preparation and medicinal use.

Mummification, or embalming, derived from the belief in life after death. The development of effective solutions to preserve the body from decay and the subsequent ability for modern-day anthropologists to examine the mummified body indicate a high level of knowledge of human anatomy, physiology, and pathophysiology.

The ancient Hebrew culture contributed the Mosaic Health Code to the history of health care. This code is considered the first sanitary legislation and contains the first record of public health requirements. The code, which covered every aspect of individual, family, and community health, differentiated between clean and unclean. Principles of personal health related to rest, sleep, and cleanliness were also provided. There were rules for women related to menstruation and childbearing. Dietary laws were a significant part of the Mosaic Code and provided for the "kosher" slaughter of animals, as well as preparation and preservation of animal and plant foods.

The use of quarantine as a prevention against the transmission of communicable diseases, such as leprosy and diphtheria, is recorded in the Bible. Nurses are mentioned occasionally in the Old Testament as women who provided care for infants, children, the sick, and the dying and as midwives who assisted during pregnancy and at delivery.

In ancient African cultures, the nurturing functions of the nurse included roles as midwives, herbal-ists, wet nurses, and caregivers for children and the elderly (Dolan, Fitzpatrick, and Herrmann, 1983, p. 19). In ancient India, early hospitals were staffed by male nurses who were required to meet four qualifications: (1) "knowledge of the manner in which drugs should be prepared for administration, (2) cleverness, (3) devotedness to the patient, and (4) purity of mind and body" (Donahue, 1996, p. 47). Indian women served as midwives and nursed ill family members. There is no mention of the nurse role in ancient China; however, the contribution of ancient China to health care knowledge includes the effects of some 365 herbal remedies in the Pen Tsao (ca. 2700 B.C.), the use of acupuncture as a treatment method, and the publication of the Nei Ching (Canon of Medicine), which detailed the four steps of examination: look, listen, ask, and feel.

In the histories of ancient Greece and Rome, care of the sick and injured was advanced in mythology and reality. The Greek mythic God Asklepios was the chief healer; his wife, Epigone, was the soother. Hygeia, the daughter of Asklepios, was the goddess of health and was revered by some as the embodiment of the nurse. Temples built to honor Asklepios became centers of healing, and the priests of Asklepios provided healing through natural and supernatural remedies (Donahue, 1996, p. 54). The ancient Greek physician Hippocrates is honored today as the father of medicine. He believed that disease had a natural cause, in contrast to the magical and mystical causes pronounced by the priest healers of the temples.

After they conquered Greece in 200 B.C., the Romans borrowed gods from the Greeks, including Aesculapius (Asklepios) and Hygeia. Greek physician-slaves brought medical practices to the Roman empire. The Romans' contribution to health care was in public sanitation, the draining of marshes, and the building of aqueducts, public and private baths, drainage systems, and central heating.

THE ROLE OF RELIGION IN THE DEVELOPMENT OF NURSING

Many of the world's religions encourage benevolence, but it was the Christian value of "love thy neighbor as thyself" that significantly influenced the development of Western nursing. The principle of caring was established with Christ's parable of the Good Samaritan providing care for a tired and injured stranger. Converts to Christianity who were considered embodiments of early nursing during the third and fourth

Dedicated Women of the Roman Empire

- Marcella converted her palace into a monastery and encouraged other Roman matrons to join her in caring for the sick poor. She is considered by some to be the first nurse educator, because she taught her followers how to care for the sick. She was also literate in Latin, Greek, and Hebrew and encouraged the education of women.

- Fabiola, a follower of Marcella, also contributed her great wealth to the care of the poor and sick. She is credited with establishing the first public hospital in Rome in 390 A.D. She is said to have personally nursed patients whose wounds and sores were ugly and repugnant. She was considered the patron saint of nursing.

- Paula was a wealthy and learned friend of Fabiola. Upon the death of her husband, she converted to Christianity. She, too, studied with Marcella. In 385 A.D. she moved with her daughter to Palestine, where she built hospitals for the sick and hospices for the pilgrims who followed the road to Bethlehem. She also provided direct care to the sick.

centuries included several wealthy women of the Roman Empire. See the accompanying box.

Women were not the sole providers of nursing services; in the third century in Rome there was an organization of men called the Parabolani brotherhood. This group of men provided care to the sick and dying during the great plague in Alexandria. During the Crusades, knighthood orders, such as the Knights Hospitallers of St. John of Jerusalem, the Teutonic Knights, and the Knights of Lazarus, often comprised brothers in arms who provided nursing care to their sick and injured comrades. These orders were responsible for building great hospitals, the organization and management of which set a standard for the administration of hospitals throughout Europe at that time.

As the Christian church grew, more hospitals were built, as were specialized institutions providing care for orphans, widows, the elderly, the poor, and the sick. It is unfortunate that the religious beliefs of the church were in conflict with scientific thought and education during this period. The church encouraged care and comfort of the sick and poor but did not allow for the advancement of knowledge in preventing illness or curing disease. This attitude pervaded the period known as the Dark Ages, which endured for approximately 500 years.

During the Middle Ages (A.D. 500–1500), male and female religious, military, and secular orders with the primary purpose of caring for the sick were formed. Conspicuous among them were the Knights Hospitallers of St. John, the Alexian Brotherhood (organized in 1431), and the Augustinian sisters, which was the first purely nursing order.

A brief discussion of nursing in the Islamic world can be found in Bryant's text, *Women in Nursing in Islamic Societies* (2003). Muslim women prepared food, established tent hospitals, and attended the sick and wounded during the time of the Prophet Mohammad in battles during the sixth century. Rufida, the daughter of Saad al-Aslamy, a prominent healer in Arabia, is identified as the first nurse in Islam. She is believed to have started the first nursing school in Islam when she taught women and girls the art of nursing the sick and wounded. She is described to have set down the first code of Nursing Rules and Ethics in the world and is still considered a symbol of noble deeds and self-denial in the modern Islamic world. The need for women care providers in the Islamic world is dictated by the custom of purdah, which makes it difficult for women to receive care from men and for men to receive care from women other than their family members.

In 1633, the Sisters of Charity was founded by St. Vincent de Paul in France. It was the first of many such orders organized under various Roman Catholic Church auspices and largely devoted to caring for the sick.

The deaconess groups, which had their origins in the Roman Empire of the third and fourth centuries under Marcella, Fabiola, and Paula, were suppressed during the Middle Ages by the Western churches. However, these groups of nursing providers reoccurred occasionally throughout the centuries, most notably in 1836 when Theodor Fliedner reinstituted the Order of Deaconesses and opened a small hospital and training school in Kaiserswerth, Germany. Florence Nightingale received her "training" in nursing at the Kaiserswerth School.

THE DEVELOPMENT OF MODERN NURSING

In the eighteenth and nineteenth centuries, the world underwent a renaissance. The discoveries of Copernicus, Galileo, Newton, Kepler, Briggs, and Descartes precipitated an intellectual revolution. Vesalius, Harvey, Hooke, and van Leeuwenhoek contributed to the scientific revolution in medicine. With the discovery and exploration of new continents, an economic revolution evolved, after which nations became more interdependent through trade and mercantilism. The Industrial Revolution displaced workers from cottage craftspeople to factory laborers. With these changes came stressors to health. New illnesses, transmitted in the holds of ships by sailors and stowaway rodents, jumped national boundaries and continents. The closeness of factory work, the long hours, and the unhealthy working conditions led to the rapid transmission of communicable diseases such as cholera and plague. Lack of prenatal care, inadequate nutrition, and poor delivery techniques resulted in a high rate of maternal and infant mortality. Orphaned children died in workhouses of neglect or cruelty. These conditions have been effectively portrayed in the writings of Dickens, including Oliver Twist and David Copperfield.

During the early nineteenth century women's roles were dictated by their gender and included daughter, wife, and mother. Howell (2001, p. 80) states that "as men gave in to "selfish passions" [work] outside the home, women came to be seen as those most responsible for the common good—for caring." A "proper" woman's role in life was to maintain a gracious and elegant home for her family. A common woman worked as a servant in a private home or was dependent on her husband's wages. The provision of care for the sick in hospitals or private homes fell to the uncommon women, often prisoners or prostitutes who had little or no training in nursing and even less enthusiasm for the job. Because of this, nursing had little acceptance and no prestige. The only acceptable nursing role was within a religious order, wherein services were provided to the hospital for little or no cost.

The development of the Deaconess Institute at Kaiserswerth, Germany, changed all this. Associated with a religious organization, the Order of Deaconesses ignited recognition of the need for the services of women in the care of the sick, the poor, children, and female prisoners. The training school for nurses at Kaiserswerth included care of the sick in hospitals, instruction in visiting nursing, instruction in religious doctrine and ethics, and pharmacy. The deaconess movement eventually spread to four continents, including North America, North Africa, Asia, and Australia.

Florence Nightingale, the most famous Kaiserswerth pupil, was born to a wealthy and intellectual family. Her education included the mastery of several ancient and modern languages, literature, philosophy, history, science, mathematics, religion, art, and music. It was expected that she would follow the usual path of a wealthy and intelligent woman of the day: marry, bear children, and maintain an elegant home. She was determined, however, to become a nurse in order to diminish the suffering of the helpless. As a well-traveled young woman of the day, in 1847 she arranged to visit Kaiserswerth, where she received 3 months' training in nursing. In 1853 she studied in Paris with the Sisters of Charity, after which she returned to England to assume the position of superintendent of a charity hospital for ill governesses.

During the Crimean War, there was public outcry about the inadequacy of care for the soldiers. The death rate, estimated at 43%, was attributed to wounds, infection, cholera, inadequate nutrition, lack of drugs, and lack of care. Florence Nightingale was asked by Sir Sidney Herbert of the War Department to recruit a contingent of female nurses to provide care to the sick and injured in the Crimea. In spite of opposition from the Army medical officers, she and her nurses transformed the environment by setting up diet kitchens, a laundry, recreation centers, and reading rooms and organizing classes. She trained the orderlies to scrub the wards and empty wastes. In the course of 6 months, the mortality rate decreased to 2% (Donahue, 1996, p. 204).

When she returned to England, Nightingale was given an honorarium of £4500 by a grateful English public. She later used this money to develop the Nightingale Training School for Nurses, which opened in 1860. The school served as a model for other training schools. Its graduates traveled to other countries to manage hospitals and institute nurse-training programs. The efforts of Florence Nightingale and her nurses changed the status of nursing to a respectable occupation for women.

THE DEVELOPMENT OF NURSING IN THE AMERICAS

Between the American Revolution and the Civil War nursing in America probably paralleled nursing in Europe. Early public hospitals developed in the colonies included The Philadelphia Almshouse (1731) and Bellevue Hospital in New York (1658). These early "hospitals" provided care for the sick, indigent, insane, infirm, prisoners, and orphans. Caregivers or attendants were described as paupers or prisoners, who were often drunk.

In 1639 the Augustinian Sisters migrated to Canada and eventually established the first hospital, the Hotel Dieu, in Quebec City. In 1809 in the United States, Mother Elizabeth Seton established the first American order of the Sisters of Charity of St. Joseph's in Maryland. Eventually, other orders or branches of orders in the Roman Catholic Church evolved under the name of Sisters of Charity throughout the eastern United States and Canada. These religious orders developed programs of nursing education and provided nursing service. Following the westward expansion of the United States, Roman Catholic religious orders established hospitals in New Orleans, Chicago, and San Francisco. Religious sisterhoods of Protestant churches, including the Episcopal Sisterhood of the Holy Communion and the English Lutheran Church, also established hospitals and provided nursing care.

Much of nursing's development is related to the need to provide care to sick and injured soldiers during times of war. This fact is true in the development of nursing in the United States. During the Civil War, Dorothea Dix was appointed superintendent of the first nurse corps of the United States Army. She recruited only women who were over 30 and plain-looking. She was able to recruit 2000 women to care for the armed forces. These nurses dressed wounds, gave medicines, and attended to diets. In addition to war wounds, the soldiers suffered from dysentery and smallpox, and many nurses died as a result of disease contracted in the line of duty.

As with Nightingale in the Crimea, the nurses in the Civil War met with much opposition from the male physicians. Hospital ships were used to transport the wounded to hospitals, and nurses provided care along with medical orderlies. Many assertive women, known not only for their ability to nurse but also for their influence in other arenas, provided nursing service during the Civil War. Some of the most influential were Louisa May Alcott, who eventually became an important literary figure; Harriet Tubman, who as a nurse and abolitionist provided care and comfort to her fellow African Americans on the Underground Railroad; and Sojourner Truth, another African American nurse who provided care for the wounded soldiers of the Union Army and was active in the early roots of the women's movement.

During World War I approximately 23,000 nurses were assigned to military service. After the war, many of these nurses continued to provide care with relief programs in Europe and Asia. The need for trained nurses placed a strain on the supply of nurses, resulting in a fear that the admission and graduation standards of nurse training would be lowered. Rather than sacrifice the quality of nurses, a committee composed of M. Adelaide Nutting, Annie Goodrich, and Lillian Wald met to develop an alternative training program combining university and hospital training. The first such program was the "Vassar Training Camp," under the direction of Isabel Stewart. In 1918, in response to the need for trained nurses, the Secretary of War authorized the Army School of Nursing, with Annie Goodrich as its first dean.

World War II had a tremendous influence on nursing. Nurses served at the war front in field hospitals, on hospital ships, and in air ambulances. Again the need for nurses influenced nursing education, resulting in the development of the United States Cadet Nurse Corps, a training program for nurses funded by federal funds under the Bolton Act of 1943. This was a forerunner of federal funding programs aiding nursing education. Provisions of this act forbade discrimination on the basis of race and marital status, required minimum educational standards, and forced nursing schools to review and revise their curricula (Kelly & Joel, 1999, p. 59).

As nursing developed its practice and training schools proliferated, nurse leaders considered the need to establish minimum standards for educational programs and for safe practice. In 1903, North Carolina, New Jersey, New York, and Virginia enacted voluntary licensure laws. These laws did not require licensure but regulated the use of the title Registered Nurse (RN). In 1915, the American Nurses Association drafted a model nurse practice act. By 1923, all 48 states had passed laws to regulate nursing licensure or registration. Licensure was still voluntary or permissive. It was not until 1935 that the first mandatory licensure act was passed in New York, but it did not go

Evidence for Practice

Fairman, J., & Kagan, S. (1999). Creating critical care: The case of the hospital of the University of Pennsylvania 1950–1965. *Advances in Nursing Science, 22*(1), 63–77. This study uses social history to study the development of critical-care nursing using oral history interviews, archival material, and secondary sources. This critical-care unit was the third of its kind in 1955, preceded by North Carolina Memorial Hospital in 1953 and Chestnut Hill Hospital in Philadelphia in 1954.

Architectural changes were implemented at hospitals to create semiprivate and private rooms in response to social trends that placed high value on privacy. Because of their reliance financially on income from patients, hospitals depended on the loyalty of the local community to support the facilities. Patients also wanted to be sure they received adequate care, and so they wanted private-duty nurses when they were ill. These three factors were major influences in the development of critical-care units.

An acute nursing shortage greatly reduced the availability of private-duty nurses. As more severely ill people required more complicated care, the demand for nurses further increased. By the 1950s, the hospital was having difficulty caring for the growing complexity of its patient population in semiprivate rooms. Having a special room for desperately ill patients that was well-staffed with nurses was proposed as a solution. Critical care was a response to the dangers posed by traditional staffing and was thought to be an economical strategy.

The study concludes that social factors, such as workforce and economic issues, architectural changes, and a more complex hospital population, rather than new technology led to the development of critical care. Many of the workforce issues parallel contemporary nurse workforce issues.

into effect until 1949. Now, licensure is mandatory throughout the United States and Canada. In 1971 Idaho became the first state to recognize advanced nursing practice in its Nurse Practice Act, and in 1986 North Dakota became the first state to require the baccalaureate degree for licensure as a registered nurse (Ellis & Hartley, 2001).

Social change has continued to influence change within the profession. At the same time nurses change society through their education and practice. In 1992, Eddie Bernice Johnson was the first nurse elected to the United States House of Representatives. Today many nurses have been elected to local, state, and national office. These nurses effect change in the social systems in which nurses work and live. Nurses are involved in professional and civic organizations to effect change in society.

HISTORICAL LEADERS IN NURSING

Throughout the history of nursing, individuals have come forward to influence the profession and society. Many of the names are familiar. The people discussed are not the only leaders in nursing but are presented to provide a perspective of nurses as women and men, founders, risk takers, and social reformers.

The Founders

It is usually difficult to identify who was the first nurse in a specific country. Often the first person to provide nursing care was an unnamed slave, convict, pilgrim, rebel, mother, daughter, wife, or other unknown. Nurses as founders have established schools of nursing, hospitals, and organizations to promote the good health of the public. The box on page 38 describes some of nursing's founders.

The Men

Although nursing is often thought of as a woman's profession, men have been influential in nursing's history. Often male caregivers were not called nurses; however, their activities of caring for and nurturing the sick and injured reflect the values and activities of nursing. For example, knighthood orders of the Middle Ages combined religion, chivalry, militarism, and charity. Their original purpose was to

Nurses as Founders

- *Rufida* (sixth century), considered the "First Nurse in Islam," started the first nursing school in Islam to teach women and girls the art of nursing the sick and wounded.
- *Jeanne Mance* (1606–1673), founder of the Hotel Dieu hospital in Montreal, Quebec, Canada, is credited with being the first lay nurse not only in Canada, but also in North America.
- *Florence Nightingale* (1830–1910) is considered the founder of modern nursing. Her achievements in improving standards for the care of war casualties in the Crimea earned her the title "Lady of the Lamp." She was the first nurse to exert political pressure on government to improve health conditions. Through her contributions to nursing education, she is also recognized as nursing's first scientist/theorist for her work *Notes on Nursing: What It Is, and What It Is Not.*
- *Mary Seacole* (1805–1881) learned about nursing from her mother in Jamaica, British West Indies. When she learned about the war in the Crimea, she offered to go to the Crimea to tend the soldiers. Her request was denied, so she traveled at her own expense to the Crimea, where she opened a lodging house in which she cared for wounded and sick officers.
- *Clara Barton* (1821–1912) nursed in federal hospitals during the Civil War. Following the war she went to Europe, where she learned about the International Red Cross. She served with the Red Cross during the Franco-Prussian War. She returned to the United States, where she was instrumental in founding the American Red Cross in 1882.
- *Lucy Osborne* (1835–1891) was a Nightingale-trained nurse who arrived in Australia in 1868 as superin-

tendent of nurses, along with five head nurses, to provide nursing care to patients at the Sydney Hospital. She is credited with founding the Sydney training school, the first training school for nurses in Australia using the Nightingale model (Burchill, 1992).
- *Linda (Melinda) Richards* (1841–1930) is considered the first trained nurse in the United States. She received her nursing certificate October 1, 1873, from the New England Hospital for Women and Children. She went to England in 1877 to study nursing with Florence Nightingale. She then went to Japan, where she organized the first nurse-training school.
- *Mary Mahoney* (1845–1926) is considered America's first African American professional nurse, receiving her nursing certificate from the New England Hospital for Women and Children in 1879.
- *Cecilia Makiwane* (1880–unknown) became South Africa's first Black African professional nurse in 1908. She was a pioneer for nurses in Africa (Carnegie, 1995).
- *Lillian Wald* (1858–1940) is considered the founder of public health nursing. She and Mary Brewster were the first to offer trained nursing services to the poor in the New York slums. Their home among the poor on the upper floor of a tenement, called the Henry Street Settlement and the Visiting Nurse Service, provided nursing services, social services, and organized educational and cultural activities.
- *Mary Breckinridge* (1881–1965) established the Frontier Nursing Service in 1925 to provide health care to the people of rural America. Within this organization, Breckinridge started one of the first midwifery training schools in the United States.

carry the wounded from the battlefield to the hospitals and to provide care. During the period of the Crusades, the organization and management of their battlefield hospitals became the standard for the development of hospitals throughout Europe. The American Assembly for Men in Nursing was established in 1974. Some specific men who have been identified with their nursing roles are described in the box on page 39.

The Risk Takers

Many nurses have taken personal risks to uphold the values of nursing. Caring for those who are ill exposes nurses to the obvious risks of contagious illnesses or work-related injuries. Some nurses have risked loss of status, danger to family and friends, and even death. Some of these risk takers are described in the box on page 40.

Evidence for Practice

Mackintosh, C. 1997. A historical study of men in nursing. *Journal of Advanced Nursing* **26(2): 232–236.**

This study uses primary archival sources, oral history, and secondary sources to outline a brief history of men as nurses in the United Kingdom. Men have had a place in nursing for as long as records have been available. Their place is detailed in records of the monastic movement in 1095, when St. Antonines was founded to nurse sufferers of erysipelas and the mentally ill. The Knight Hospitallers of St. John of Jerusalem was founded in 1200 and records male nurses, as does the Knights of Lazarus, founded in 1490 to care for lepers. However, once the monasteries went through dissolution in the 1600s, records of organized nursing disappear.

Workhouses with attached infirmaries appeared in the mid-nineteenth century using inmates to nurse each other. Men worked in a strictly sex-segregated setting; however, they were referred to as attendants or keepers rather than nurses.

Nursing at this point in history was a low-status occupation, and nurses had dubious reputations. Reformers were influenced by the religious sisterhoods, so the occupation was placed in a female sphere that was furthered by Nightingale. The assumption was that this new nursing was more natural for females. Male nurses continued to fill roles outside the reformed sphere in private sectors. In the early 1900s the Royal Army Medical Corp was another avenue for employment.

In the mid-1920s, a chronic shortage of nurses allowed male nurses into the workforce. The Society of Registered Male Nurses was established in 1937; in 1949 formal legislative discrimination was ended, and 108 schools of nursing opened their doors to male students. The expansion of males in nursing has been dramatic since that time.

Stereotypes and assumptions regarding male nurses, their characteristics, employment, and role must be viewed within the historical perspective. Male nurses are a product of many years of biased and discriminatory employment practices. This is a by-product of moral squeamishness of earlier times. The contributions men have made to nursing history should be more positively recognized.

The Social Reformers

Nurses have assumed roles in social reform throughout recorded history. Many of their efforts have been to improve the plight of the poor, the sick, the abandoned, or the hopeless. Often the focus has been on the particular difficulties experienced by women and children who did not have the support of male family members. It must be remembered that it has only been during the twentieth century that women and minorities achieved the right to vote or to own property in many of the Western nations. The box on page 40 describes the work of some these social reformers.

Men in Nursing

- *John Ciudad* (1495–1550) founded the order of the Brothers of St. John of God, or the Brothers of Mercy in 1538. He opened a hospital in Granada and asked a group of friends to assist in providing nursing care to the mentally ill, homeless vagrants, crippled, derelicts, and abandoned children. Men of this order also visited the sick in their homes.

- *St. Camillus de Lellis* (1550–1614) founded the Nursing Order of Ministers of the Sick. Men of this order cared for the dying, people stricken with the plague, and alcoholics. St. Camillus opened a hospital for alcoholics in Germany.

- *James Derham* (1762–unknown) was an African American man who worked as a nurse in New Orleans in 1783. He was able to save enough money to buy his freedom from slavery. He went on to become the first African American physician in the United States (Carnegie, 1995).

- *Walt Whitman* (1819–1892), poet and writer, served as a volunteer hospital nurse in Washington, DC, during the Civil War. He recorded his experiences in a collection of poems called *Drumtaps* and in his diary, *Specimen Days and Collect*.

Nurses as Risk Takers

- *Clara Maass* (1876–1901) volunteered to go to Havana, Cuba, where experiments on yellow fever were being conducted. She provided nursing care for victims of yellow fever through the spring of 1901. She allowed herself to be bitten by a mosquito to prove a theory that yellow fever was caused by mosquitoes. She experienced a mild attack of the fever in June but offered to be bitten again. She died following the second bite in August 1901, demonstrating that mosquitoes were indeed the cause of yellow fever.

- *Edith Cavell* (1865–1915) was an English nurse during World War I who had founded a training school for nurses in Belgium. During the war, her hospital cared for both Allied and German soldiers. She also assisted Allied soldiers who were prisoners of the Germans in escaping. She was charged by the Germans with harboring British and French soldiers and aiding them in escape. She was shot on October 12, 1915.

- *Sharon Lane* (1943–1969), an Army nurse during the Vietnam conflict, was the only nurse to die as a result of enemy fire. She died on June 8, 1969, of wounds received while on duty.

- *Barbara Fassbinder* (1951–1994) was an advocate for mandatory HIV testing of health care workers. She was infected with HIV in 1986 while caring for a patient with AIDS. She is recognized as the first health care provider to acquire AIDS on the job. She died in 1994 of AIDS.

Nurses as Social Reformers

- *Sojourner Truth* (1767–1881) was an early feminist and abolitionist who identified the similarity between the problems of African Americans and women. She was significant in helping African American women overcome the oppression caused by their race and sex.

- *Dorothea Lynde Dix* (1802–1887) was an early crusader for humane care for the mentally ill in the United States. She also advocated for humane care for criminals in prison after finding that many of them suffered from mental illness. Before her efforts, it was not uncommon to find mentally ill people imprisoned in jails along with criminals. Through her efforts, standards of care for the mentally ill were improved, and more than 30 psychiatric hospitals were established in the United States.

- *Harriet Tubman* (1820–1913) was called the "Moses of her people." She made numerous trips between the South and the North to assist slaves in their quest for freedom. She was an abolitionist who became active with the Underground Railroad. She provided nursing care to the sick and suffering slaves and former slaves.

- *Lavinia Dock* (1858–1956) was a feminist, prolific writer, political activist, and suffragette. She actively participated in protest movements for women's rights that resulted in the passage of the Nineteenth Amendment to the U.S. Constitution in 1920, which granted women the right to vote. She also campaigned for legislation to allow nurses rather than physicians to control the nursing profession. In 1893, she founded, with the assistance of Mary Adelaide Nutting and Isabel Hampton Robb, the American Society of Superintendents of Training Schools for Nurses of the United States and Canada, a forerunner of the National League for Nursing.

- *Margaret Sanger* (1879–1966) worked as a public health nurse in New York City. In 1912, she was called to care for a woman who had attempted to abort herself and who later died. It was illegal at the time to provide information about contraception and family planning. However, Sanger learned everything she could about contraception and family planning and published information about it in a journal. She was arrested, convicted, and sentenced to 30 days in a workhouse. She continued to provide information on family planning and lobbied to change the laws. She founded the National Committee on Federal Legislation for Birth Control, the forerunner of the Planned Parenthood Federation.

Reflect on...

- how the history of nursing has affected your own nursing practice.
- who the nursing leaders in your community or your area of practice are. What have they done to enhance the profession or the society in which we live?
- issues in health care today that ask nurses to become risk takers to uphold the values of nursing. What risks are you willing to take to uphold the values of nursing?

NURSING: A HISTORY OF CARING

Most students, when studying nursing history, focus on the most recent history, starting with Nightingale because of her influences on nursing care and nursing education today. However, the notion of caring has spanned not only centuries but millennia going back to prerecorded history. Nursing has created a history starting in ancient times before the word *nurse* had the meaning it has today. Rather, the basis for this "modern" history is the idea of caring: caring for and caring about. What did it mean to care for family or those who were not family? What were the issues that these individuals cared about: care for the poor, care for wounded soldiers, care for the sick, care for the aged, care for society in times of increased urbanization that led to disease?

More contemporary thinking about the history of nursing suggests that rather than looking at history in the context of specific individuals and their influences on nursing at a specific time, one should look at the reasons why individuals did what they did in the past

and why people do what they do in the present. In analyzing the reasons for actions, one can better understand the symbiotic relationship between the history of nursing, the history of caring, and the history of women. For example, every student nurse in the western world knows who Florence Nightingale was and her influence on nursing. But if one looks at the actions of Nightingale in the context of what was expected of a young wealthy woman of the mid-eighteenth century, one sees the influence of Nightingale on society as a whole, as an early feminist, as a nurse, and as a hospital administrator. She wanted to do something meaningful. She connected meaning to the needs of poor women and children, to suffering soldiers in the Crimean and "cared" in such a way as to improve their plight. Much of Nightingale's work is not only the foundation for nursing, but also the foundation for hospital administration, social services, and public health, all "caring" professions. When we look at other "nursing" leaders, we see that the connection between them is not that they were nurses, but that they cared deeply about the society in which they lived and wanted to make change. Most of these individuals have other descriptors attached to their names besides nurse, descriptors such as suffragette (Lillian Wald), abolitionist (Sojourner Truth), mental health advocate (Dorothea Dix), and so on. Maggs (1996) suggests that analysis of nurses' "memoirs" provides information about nurses choices to do what they do, and the decisions they make about practice and caring. Memoirs also give context to the time in which the decisions were made.

Evidence for Practice

Neal, L. J. (2002). Elder RNs: Learning from their experiences. *Geriatric Nursing, 23*(5), 244–249.
This study used grounded theory to explore the perceptions of elderly registered nurses about the nursing profession. The 17 participants ranged in age from 65 to 90 years of age, with the average age of 69 years. They came from a variety of educational (diploma through doctoral education) and nursing backgrounds. Participants shared their personal stories about the reasons they chose nursing school, ways they felt that they made a difference in the lives of others based on their nursing practice, and their views of nursing today as elderly patients. The older participants described gender barriers related

to the roles of women from the 1920s to the 1960s, financial barriers, and the image of nursing by some people. Participants described experiences of caring for particular patients "who touched them and influenced them as nurses." All participants had recently been either patients themselves or the close friend or relative of a patient. They described a greater focus of nurses today on technology with a decreased focus on the "basics of comfort, care, and listening." Knowledge gained from this study can be used by nurses to examine their own reasons for choosing nursing as a career, their own patient experiences, and their own views of caring in a technology focused health system.

Critical Thinking Exercise

Interview nurses who have varying career lengths: 5, 10, 15, 20, 25 years in the profession. What are the reasons they chose nursing for their career? What nursing situations or experiences have provided the most gratification for them? How do they relate their personal life experiences to their professional life experiences?

Interview nurses from various nursing specialties: critical care, community health, home health, pediatrics, oncology (end-of-life) care, anesthesia, midwife, education. What are the reasons they chose their specialties? What nursing situations or experiences have provided the most gratification for them? How do they relate their personal life experiences to their professional life experiences?

Reflect on...

■ your own thoughts abut the meaning of caring. Within the context of nursing, what does it mean to care?

■ your own nursing history. What were the reasons that you chose nursing as a career? What are the factors that influence you as a nurse? How do your beliefs about caring and nursing influence your practice? How do you see your own influence as a nurse?

■ the stories of your nurse colleagues or other nurses that you know. What were their reasons for choosing nursing as a career? How do their beliefs about caring and nursing influence their practice?

THE DEVELOPMENT OF PROFESSIONAL NURSING ORGANIZATIONS

As nursing has developed, an increasing number of nursing organizations have formed. These organizations function at the local, regional, national, and international levels. When nurses participate in the activities of nursing organizations, they enhance their own professional growth and help all nurses collectively as they influence policies affecting nursing, nursing practice, and the health of the community. Nursing organizations can be divided into three types: organizations that represent all nurses (e.g., the American Nurses Association and the National League for Nursing), organizations that meet the needs of nurses within specific nursing specialties (e.g., the American Association for Critical Care Nurses, the Emergency Nurses Association, the Association of Operating Room Nurses), and organizations that represent special interests, such as the National Black Nurses Association or the National Hispanic Nurses Association. Some of these organizations are discussed on the following pages.

American Nurses Association

The American Nurses Association (ANA), with its headquarters in Washington DC, is the national professional organization representing all registered nurses in the United States. It was founded in 1896 as the Nurses Associated Alumnae of the United States and Canada. In 1911, the name was changed to the American Nurses Association. It was a charter member of the International Council of Nurses in 1899, along with nursing organizations in Great Britain and Germany.

In 1982, the ANA became a federation of state nurses' associations. Nurses participate in the ANA by joining their state nurses' associations. The official journal of the ANA is the *American Journal of Nursing*, and *American Nurse* is the official newspaper.

The purposes of the ANA are to foster high standards of nursing practice, to promote the economic and general welfare of nurses in the workplace, to project a positive and realistic view of nursing, and to lobby Congress and regulatory agencies on health care issues affecting nurses and the public (ANA, 2004). Affiliate groups of the ANA are the American Nurses Credentialing Center (ANCC), which conducts the certification process at the nurse generalist and the advanced practice levels in many nursing specialties; the United American Nurses (UAN), which acts as the agent for those nurses who are organized for collective bargaining; the American Nurses Foundation (ANF), which supports nursing research and scholarship; and the American Academy of Nursing (AAN), which recognizes nursing leaders.

National Student Nurses Association

The National Student Nurses Association (NSNA) was established in 1952. The mission of NSNA is to "organize, represent and mentor students preparing for initial licensure as registered nurses, as well as those enrolled in baccalaureate completion programs; convey the standards and ethics of the nursing profession; promote development of the skills that students will need as responsible and accountable members of the nursing profession; advocate for high-quality health care; and advocate for and contribute to advances in nursing education." The organization "promotes self-governance, advocates for students' rights and the rights of patients, and advocates for collective, responsible action on vital social and political issues" (NSNA, 2004). The official journal of the NSNA is *Imprint*.

National League for Nursing

The National League for Nursing (NLN) is an organization whose mission is "to advance quality nursing education that prepares the nursing workforce to meet the needs of diverse populations in an ever-changing health care environment" (NLN, 2004). The National League for Nursing began in 1893 as part of the American Society of Superintendents of Training Schools for Nurses. In 1912, the society was renamed the National League for Nursing Education (NLNE). In 1952, the NLNE, the National Organization for Public Health Nursing, and the Association for Collegiate Schools of Nursing combined to form the National League for Nursing (NLN, 2004).

The NLN also provides professional development for nursing faculty; provides support for research related to nursing education; and provides information, services, and products to support nursing education. The official publication of the NLN is *Nursing and Health Care Perspectives*. The National League for Nursing Accrediting Commission (NLNAC), an affiliate of the NLN, serves as a national accreditation body for schools of nursing at the vocational, associate degree, baccalaureate, and graduate levels. The official publication of the National League for Nursing is *Nursing Education Perspectives*.

American Association of Colleges of Nursing

The American Association of Colleges of Nursing (AACN) is the national voice for baccalaureate- and higher-degree nursing education programs in the United States. The purpose of the AACN is to "establish standards for bachelor's and graduate degree nursing programs, to assist deans and directors to implement those standards, to influence the nursing profession to improve health care, and to promote public support of baccalaureate and graduate education, research, and practice in nursing" (AACN, 2004). To fulfill its purpose, AACN serves as an accrediting organization for baccalaureate- and higher-degree nursing programs. The official publication of AACN is the *Journal of Professional Nursing*.

International Council of Nurses

The International Council of Nurses (ICN) was formed in 1899 as the world's first and widest international organization for health professionals. The goals of the ICN are to "bring nursing together worldwide, advance nurses and nursing worldwide, and to influence health policy. The five core values of ICN are visionary leadership, inclusiveness, flexibility, partnership, and achievement." (ICN, 2004). The ICN Code for Nurses is the "foundation for ethical nursing practice throughout the world. ICN standards, guidelines and policies for nursing practice, education, management, research and socioeconomic welfare are used globally as the basis for nursing policy." In 2004, ICN represented nurses in more than 120 countries. The official journal of the ICN is *International Nursing Review*.

Sigma Theta Tau International

Sigma Theta Tau is the international honor society for nursing. It was founded in 1922 at the University of Indiana in Indianapolis. The Greek letters stand for the Greek words *storga*, *tharos*, and *tima*, meaning "love," "courage," and "honor." The society is a member of the Association of College Honor Societies. The mission of the society is to "provide leadership and scholarship in practice, education and research to enhance the health of all people." The society supports the learning and professional development of members who strive to improve nursing care worldwide (STTI, 2004). The official publication of Sigma Theta Tau is the *Journal of Nursing Scholarship*.

Specialty Nursing Organizations

There are many organizations that represent the special interests of nurses from a practice perspective. Examples of such organizations include the Association for peri-Operative Registered Nurses (AORN), the

American Association of Critical Care Nurses (AACCN), the Emergency Nurses Association (ENA), Academy of Medical-Surgical Nurses, Association of Women's Health, Obstetric and Neonatal Nurses (AWHONN), Society of Pediatric Nurses, Association of Rehabilitation Nurses (ARN), and Association for Nurses in AIDS Care (ANAC). Most of these organizations have Internet websites that can be accessed using any computer search engine. Specialty nursing organizations usually provide educational opportunities for their members specific to the specialty, including national or international conferences that provide information related to current research findings in the specialty, information about new equipment used in the specialty, and general information about professional issues and issues in health care policy related to the specialty or to the nursing profession as a whole.

Special Interest Organizations

There are also several organizations that represent nurses of specific ethnic groups or other special interests. Some of these organizations address the special needs of nurses from minority groups such as the Aboriginal Nurses Association of Canada, the National Alaska Native American Indian Nurses Association (NANAINA), the National Black Nurses Association (NBNA), the National Hispanic Nurses Association, the Philippine Nurses Association (PNA), and the Jamaican Nurses Association. Another special interest group is the American Assembly of Men in Nursing. These organizations represent the issues and concerns of these nurses and the populations they serve. These organizations often conduct activities to provide service to their own ethnic groups; for example, the National Black Nurses Association provides education and conducts research to understand the health problems that adversely affect African Americans.

Reflect on...

■ your involvement in professional nursing organizations. Which organizations are you a member of? If you do not belong to any professional organizations, why not? How might being a member of a professional organization help you become more connected with the profession?

■ why many nurses choose not to be involved in nursing organizations.

■ how involvement in professional nursing organizations can assist nurses in managing the stresses of the changing and challenging health care system.

■ the nursing organizations you are involved in. What benefits do you obtain from membership in these organizations?

EXPLORE MEDIALINK

Questions, critical thinking exercises, essay activities, and other interactive resources for this chapter can be found on the Web site at http://www.prenhall.com/blais. Click on Chapter 3 to select activites for this chapter.

Bookshelf

Dossey, B. M. (2000). *Florence Nightingale: Mystic, visionary, healer.* **Springhouse, PA: Springhouse.**
This biography of Florence Nightingale describes her life as a social activist and visionary whose ideas about public health, holistic health, and women's place in society were decades ahead of their time.

Gollaher, D. (1995). *Voice for the mad: The life of Dorothea Dix.* **New York: The Free Press.**
This biography of Dorothea Dix describes her life as a social activist for people with mental health problems and for the homeless.

Oates, S. B. (1994). *A woman of valor: Clara Barton and the Civil War.* **New York: The Free Press.**
Clara Barton's role in advocating care for soldiers during the American Civil War is described in this biography of her life. The outcome of her experience was the founding of the American Red Cross.

Schorr, T. M., & Zimmerman, A. (1988). *Making choices, taking chances: Nurse leaders tell their stories.* **St. Louis: Mosby.**
This book includes autobiographies of more than 40 nursing leaders of the twentieth century. These very personal stories, written by the leaders themselves, are rich in knowledge, history, and inspiration.

Ulrich, L. T. (1991). *A midwife's tale: The life of Martha Ballard, based on her diary, 1785–1812.* **New York: Vintage Books.**
Ms Ulrich describes the life and society of a midwife and healer named Martha Ballard who provided care in colonial Maine between 1785 and 1812. The book provides information about medical practices, religious issues, and sexual mores of the time.

SUMMARY

Nursing has existed throughout the history of humankind. From primitive to contemporary societies, care of the sick has been influenced by many factors, such as superstition and magic, Greek and Roman mythology, religion, male-female role proscriptions, legislation, wars, and other societal events. Male-female role proscriptions traditionally attributed the care and nurturing functions to women. In the third century in Rome, however, the Parabolani Brotherhood provided care to the sick and dying during the great plague in Alexandria, and early hospitals in India were staffed largely by male nurses.

The first sanitary legislation, the Mosaic Health Code, was contributed by the ancient Hebrew culture. This code differentiated between clean and unclean.

The Christian value of "love thy neighbor as thyself" and the parable of the Good Samaritan influenced the development of Western nursing. During the Dark Ages, religious beliefs of the church encouraged comfort of the sick and poor, but little was done to prevent illness or cure disease. During the Middle Ages, male and female religious, military, and secular orders, with the primary purpose of caring for the sick, were established. Examples are the Knights Hospitallers of St. John, the Alexian Brotherhood, the Augustinian Sisters, and the Sisters of Charity, founded by St. Vincent de Paul in France. Nursing developed in a parallel world of Islam in the Middle East or Arabian countries from the time of the Prophet Mohammad.

In 1835, the Order of Deaconesses operated a small hospital and training school in Kaiserswerth, Germany, where Florence Nightingale trained. Nightingale went to the Crimea with several nurses to provide care to the ill and wounded soldiers. As a result of a grateful English public, Nightingale opened her training school for nurses in London.

The development of nursing in the Americas started with the Augustinian Sisters in Canada. Jeanne Mance founded the Hotel Dieu in Montreal in 1644, and Mother Elizabeth Seton established the first American order of the Sisters of Charity of St. Joseph in Maryland.

Nursing education, knowledge, and practice have developed as a result of societal events, including wars, civil strife, changes in women's roles, and so on. Nurses have demonstrated leadership as founders, risk takers, and social reformers.

The history of nursing is connected with the history of caring and the history of feminism. The basic roles of caring and nursing were often associated with women's roles of daughter, wife, and mother.

Nursing organizations have developed to meet the professional needs of nurses and the health care needs of the public. There are several types of nursing organizations: organizations that represent and influence all of nursing, organizations that represent the needs of nurses practicing in specialty areas, organizations that represent the needs of nurses of specific ethnic groups, and organizations that represent nurses' special interests.

REFERENCES

American Association of Colleges of Nursing (AACN). (2004). Retrieved from http://www.aacn.nche.edu.

American Nurses Association (ANA). (2004). Retrieved from http://www.nursingworld.org.

Baer, E. D., D'Antonio, P., Rinker, S., & Lynaugh, J. E. (2002). *Enduring issues in American nursing.* New York: Springer Publishing Company.

Baly, M. E. (1986). *Florence Nightingale and the nursing legacy.* London: Croom Helm.

Bryant, N. H. (2003). *Women in nursing in Islamic societies.* Oxford, England: Oxford University Press.

Burchill, E. (1992). *Australian nurses since Nightingale: 1860–1990.* Richmond, Victoria, Australia: Spectrum Publications.

Carnegie, M. E. (1995). *The path we tread: Blacks in nursing worldwide, 1854–1994* (3rd ed.). New York: NLN Press.

Cluff, L. E., & Binstock, R. H. (2001) (Eds.). *The lost art of caring: A challenge to health professionals, families, communities, and society.* Baltimore: Johns Hopkins University Press.

Dolan, J. A., Fitzpatrick, M. L., & Herrmann, E. K. (1983). *Nursing in society: A historical perspective* (15th ed.). Philadelphia: W. B. Saunders.

Donahue, M. P. (1996). *Nursing: The finest art* (2nd ed.). St. Louis: Mosby.

Donahue, M. P. (2004). Turning points in nursing history. In L. C. Haynes, H. K. Butcher, & T. A. Boese

(Eds.), *Nursing in contemporary society: Issues, trends, and transition to practice.* Upper Saddle River, NJ: Prentice Hall.

Dossey, B. M. (2000). *Florence Nightingale: Mystic, visionary, healer.* Springhouse, PA: Springhouse.

Ellis, J. R., & Hartley, C. L. (2001). *Nursing in today's world: Challenges, issues, and trends* (7th ed.). Philadelphia: Lippincott.

Fairman, J., & Kagan, S. (1999). Creating critical care: The case of the hospital of the University of Pennsylvania 1950–1965. *Advances in Nursing Science, 22*(1), 63–77.

Howell, J. D. (2001). A history of caring in medicine. In L. E. Cluff & R. H. Binstock (Eds.), *The lost art of caring: A challenge to health professionals, families, communities, and society.* Baltimore: Johns Hopkins University Press.

International Council of Nurses (ICN). (2004). http://www.icn.org.

Kalisch, P. A., and Kalisch, B. J. (1995). *The advance of American nursing* (3rd ed.). Philadelphia: Lippincott.

Kelly, L. Y., and Joel, L. A. 1999. *Dimensions of professional nursing* (8th ed.). New York: McGraw-Hill.

Kozier, B., Erb, G., and Blais, K. (1992). *Concepts and issues in nursing practice* (2nd ed.). Redwood City, CA: Addison-Wesley.

Locsin, R. C. (Ed.). (2001). *Advancing technology, caring, and nursing.* Westport, CT: Auburn House.

Mackintosh, C. (1997). A historical study of men in nursing. *Journal of Advanced Nursing, 26*(2), 232–236.

Maggs, C. (1996). A history of nursing: A history of caring? *Journal of Advanced Nursing, 23,* 630–635.

National League for Nursing (NLN). (2004). Retrieved from http://www.nln.org.

National Student Nurses' Association (NSNA). (2004). http://www.nsna.org.

Neal, L. J. (2002). Elder RNs: Learning from their experiences. *Geriatric Nursing, 23*(5), 244–249.

Sigma Theta Tau International (STTI). (2004). Retrieved from http://www.stti.iupui.edu.

Schorr, T. M. (1999). *100 years of American nursing: Celebrating a century of caring.* Philadelphia: Lippincott.

Small, H. (1998). *Florence Nightingale: Avenging angel.* New York: St. Martin's Press.

Ethical Foundation of Professional Nursing

Objectives

- Explain how nurses can help clients clarify their values to facilitate ethical decision making.
- Explain the uses and limitations of professional codes of ethics.
- Discuss how cognitive development, values, moral frameworks, and codes of ethics affect moral decisions.
- Discuss common bioethical issues currently facing health care professionals.
- Analyze ways in which nurses can enhance their ethical decision-making abilities.
- Identify the moral principles involved in ethical decision making.
- Describe the advocacy role of the nurse.

M E D I A L I N K

Additional online resources for this chapter can be found on the companion Web site at http://www.prenhall.com/blais.

Professional nurses must attend to the ethical responsibilities and conflicts they may experience as a result of their unique relationships in professional practice. Advances in medical and reproductive technology, clients' rights, social and legal changes, and the allocation of scarce resources are among the things that have contributed to an increase in ethical concerns. Standards of conduct for nurses are set forth in codes of ethics developed by international, national, and state or provincial nursing associations. Nurses need to be able to apply ethical principles in decision making and consider their own values and beliefs and the values and beliefs of clients, of the profession, and of all other concerned parties. Nurses have a responsibility to protect the rights of clients by acting as client advocates. Advocacy derives from the ethical principles of beneficence (the duty to do good) and nonmaleficence (the duty to do no harm).

CHALLENGES AND OPPORTUNITIES

VALUES CONFLICTS   Nursing has long advocated a nonjudgmental approach to care. However, nurses come into the profession with established values and beliefs, which may conflict with the values and beliefs of clients. Nurses sometimes feel compromised when they must provide care in such a situation. Beliefs may be so strong that it is difficult not to judge the other person and act or react in a way that might compromise care. The nursing profession must be able to identify ways and means of assisting members of the profession so that values are not compromised by either party.

ETHICAL-LEGAL CONFLICTS   Ethical and legal are not synonymous. There are times in professional practice when the legal requirement does not appear compatible with the ethical approach. Nurses may place themselves in legal jeopardy when they opt for what they see as the ethical, or "right" thing to do, in spite of what is inherent in the laws that apply. A similar conflict may occur with institutional policy that may place the nurse in a similar position of risk at the work place. Advocacy for the profession is needed when such a conflict arises so that laws and/or policies may better serve the public.

VALUES

Values are freely chosen, enduring beliefs or attitudes about the worth of a person, object, idea, or action. Freedom, courage, family, and dignity are examples of values. Values frequently derive from a person's cultural, ethnic, and religious background; from societal traditions; and from the values held by peer group and family.

Values form a basis for behavior. Once a person becomes aware of his or her values, those values become an internal control for behavior; thus, a person's real values are manifested in consistent patterns of behavior.

Values exist within a person and affect the person's relationship to others. A value system is the organization of a person's values along a continuum, that is, from most important to least important. Values form the basis of purposive behavior, which refers to actions that a person performs "on purpose," with the intention of reaching some goal or bringing about a certain result. Thus, purposive behavior is based on a person's decisions or choices, and these decisions or choices are based on the person's underlying values.

Values Transmission

Values are learned and are greatly influenced by a person's sociocultural environment. They are learned through observation and experience. Early influences come from the family and gradually widen to include extended groups in the community. Cultural influences can be particularly influential. For example, if a parent consistently demonstrates honesty in dealing with others, the child will probably begin to value honesty. Acquiring values is a gradual process, usually occurring at an unconscious level. For example, some cultures value the treatment of a folk healer over that of a physician. For additional information about cultural values relative to health and illness, see Chapter 21 ⊙, Nursing in a Culturally Diverse World.

Although people derive some values from the society or subgroup of society in which they live, a person may internalize some or all of these values and perceive them as personal values. People need societal values to feel accepted, and they need personal values to produce a sense of individuality. See the box on page 49 for examples of personal and societal values.

Professional values often reflect and expand on personal values. Nurses acquire professional values during socialization into nursing from nursing experiences, teachers, and peers. As members of a caring profession, nurses hold values that relate to both competence and compassion.

Nurses often need to behave in a value-neutral way, which means being nonjudgmental. This outlook permits nurses to establish effective relationships with clients who have diverse values. Although nurses cannot and should not ignore or deny their own and the profession's values, they need to be able to accept a client's values and beliefs rather than assume their own are the "right ones." This acceptance and nonjudgmental approach requires nurses to be aware of their own values and how they influence behavior.

Examples of Societal and Personal Values

SOCIETAL VALUES	PERSONAL VALUES
• Human life	• Family unity
• Individual rights	• Worth of others
• Individual autonomy	• Independence
• Liberty	• Religion
• Democracy	• Honesty
• Equal opportunity	• Fairness
• Power	• Love
• Health	• Sense of humor
• Wealth	• Safety
• Youth	• Peace
• Vigor	• Beauty
• Intelligence	• Harmony
• Imagination	• Financial security
• Education	• Material things
• Technology	• Property of others
• Conformity	• Leisure time
• Friendship	• Work
• Courage	• Travel
• Compassion	• Physical activity
• Family	• Intellectual activity

Reflect on...

■ what values you hold about life, health, illness, and death. How do your values influence the nursing care you provide?

■ whether a nurse who smokes can effectively help a client stop smoking or whether a nurse who is overweight can effectively help a client who needs to lose weight.

■ whether a nurse whose religious beliefs oppose the use of contraceptives can effectively teach a client about family planning.

■ how your values influence the career choices you make (e.g., your initial choice to become a nurse, your choice of practice setting, your choice of specialty).

Values Clarification

Values clarification is a process by which people identify, examine, and develop their own individual values. A principle of values clarification is that no one set of values is right for everyone. When people are able to identify their values, they can retain or change them and thus act on the basis of freely chosen rather than unconscious values. Values clarification promotes personal growth by fostering awareness, empathy, and insight.

A widely used theory of values clarification was developed in 1966 by Raths, Harmin, and Simon. This "valuing process" includes cognitive, affective, and behavioral components, referred to as choosing, prizing, and acting. See the accompanying box.

Identifying Personal Values

Nurses need to know specifically what values they hold about life, health, illness, and death. Beginning as students, nurses should explore their own values and beliefs regarding such situations as the following:

■ An individual's right to make decisions for self when conflicting with medical advice
■ Abortion
■ End-of-life care
■ Domestic violence, child discipline
■ Cloning and genetic engineering
■ Having a child to provide a bone marrow transplant

Values Clarification

PROCESSES	DOMAINS	ACTIONS
Choosing	Cognitive	Reflection and consideration of alternatives result in freely choosing beliefs.
Prizing	Affective	Chosen beliefs are cherished.
Acting	Behavioral	Chosen beliefs are incorporated into behaviors that are affirmed to others and repeated consistently.

Behaviors That May Indicate Unclear Values

BEHAVIOR	EXAMPLE
Ignoring a health professional's advice	A client with heart disease who values hard work ignores advice to exercise regularly.
Inconsistent communication or behavior	A pregnant woman says she wants a healthy baby but continues to drink alcohol and smoke tobacco.
Numerous admissions to a health agency for the same problem	A middle-aged, obese woman repeatedly seeks help for back pain but does not lose weight.
Confusion or uncertainty about which course of action to take	A woman wants to obtain a job to meet financial obligations, but also wants to stay at home to care for an ailing husband.

Identification of personal values helps nurses understand why certain situations bother them and decide whether they can accept the difference in values when providing care.

Because nurses are called upon to provide care to individuals who may have made decisions that conflict with the nurse's values, self-awareness is important. Nurses must be aware of their own values and attitudes in order to recognize when a situation might affect the care they are able to provide. Often, the awareness of the conflict of values allows nurses to hold their personal values in check and provide effective care. In those instances when nurses feel they cannot be effective because of their conflicting values, they need to be able to discuss the situation with colleagues who may be able to assist with providing care.

Helping Clients Identify Values

Nurses need to help clients identify values as they influence and relate to a particular health problem. Examples of behaviors that may indicate the need for values clarification are listed in the accompanying box.

The following steps may help clients clarify their values.

1. *List alternatives.* Make sure that the client is aware of all alternative actions and has thought about the consequences of each. Ask, Are you considering other courses of action?

2. *Examine possible consequences of choices.* Ask, What do you think you will gain by doing that? What benefits do you foresee from doing that? What might you lose by doing that? What are the risks of doing that?

3. *Choose freely.* To determine whether the client chose freely, ask, Did you have any say in that decision? Did you have a choice?

4. *Feel good about the choice.* To determine how the client feels, ask, How do you feel about that decision (or action)? Because some clients may not feel satisfied with their decision, a more sensitive question may be, Some people feel good after a decision is made; others feel bad. How do you feel?

5. *Affirms the choice.* Ask, What will you say to others (family, friends) about this?

6. *Act on the choice.* To determine whether the client is prepared to act on the decision, ask, for example, Will it be difficult to tell your wife about this?

7. *Act with a pattern.* To determine whether the client consistently behaves in a pattern, ask, How many times have you done that before? or Would you act that way again?

When implementing these seven steps, the nurse assists the client to think each question through, never imposing personal values. When clarifying values, the nurse never offers an opinion (e.g., "It would be better to do it this way") or offers a judgment (e.g., "That's not the right thing to do"). The nurse offers an opinion only when the client asks the nurse for it, and then only with careful consideration. The nurse may provide information in a nonjudgmental way that would assist a client to make an informed decision.

MORALS

Morality (morals) is similar to ethics, and many people use the two words interchangeably. Morality usually refers to an individual's personal standards of what is right and wrong in conduct, character, and attitude. Ethics usually refers to the moral standards of a particular group, such as nurses. (See Table 4–1 for a comparison of morals and ethics.)

Sometimes the first clue to the moral nature of a situation is an aroused conscience, or an awareness of feelings such as guilt, hope, or shame. The tendency to respond to the situation with words such as *ought, should, right, wrong, good,* and *bad* is another indicator. Finally, moral issues are concerned with important social values and norms; they are not about trivial things.

Moral Development

Moral development is a complex process that is not fully understood. It is more than the imprinting of parents' rules and virtues or values upon children; rather, moral development is the process of learning what ought to be done and what ought not to be done. The terms *morality, moral behavior,* and *moral development* need to be distinguished. **Morality** refers to the requirements necessary for people to live together in society; **moral behavior** is the way a person perceives those requirements and responds to them; **moral development** is the pattern of change in moral behavior with age. Lawrence Kohlberg and Carol Gilligan are two researchers who have studied and developed theories about moral development.

Table 4–1 Comparison of Morals and Ethics

Morals	Principles and rules of right conduct
	Private, personal
	Commitment to principles and values is usually defended in daily life
Ethics	Formal responding process used to determine right conduct
	Professionally and publicly stated
	Inquiry or study of principles and values
	Process of questioning, and perhaps changing, one's morals

Kohlberg

The research of Lawrence Kohlberg has provided one of the most well-known approaches to moral development. He was directly affected by Jean Piaget's theory of cognitive development. Kohlberg's theory focuses on the structure of thought about moral issues rather than the specific content of moral values. It applies ways of thinking about issues that depend upon the specific issue and whether the person is very familiar with the topic. According to Kohlberg, moral development progresses through three levels and six stages, and they are not always linked to a specific age or growth and development phase. Some people progress to a higher level of moral development than others. The levels and stages range from egocentric actions to behaviors that show concern for society and rightness.

At Kohlberg's first level, called the *premoral* or *preconventional level,* children are responsive to cultural rules and labels of good and bad, right and wrong. However, children interpret these in terms of the physical consequences of their actions, that is, punishment or reward. At the second level, the *conventional level,* the individual is concerned about maintaining the expectations of the family, group, or nation and sees this as right. The emphasis at this level is conformity and loyalty to one's own expectations as well as society's. The third level is called the *postconventional, autonomous,* or *principled level.* At this level, people make an effort to define valid values and principles without regard to outside authority or to the expectations of others. For additional information about Kohlberg's levels, see Table 4–2.

With reference to Kohlberg's six stages, Munhall (1982, p. 14) writes that stage four, the "law-and-order" orientation, is the dominant stage of most adults. It is recognized that there is a difference in action between nurses who act at the conventional level (level II) and those who act at the postconventional or principled level (level III). Refer to examples in Table 4–2.

Progression through the stages is determined by one's exposure to social complexity and the opportunity to question and discuss ethical decisions. Theoretically, formal operations (Piaget) are associated with stage 4; the ability to think abstractly is necessary to consider such things as social order. It is rare for an adult to reach stage 6. In his later writings, Kohlberg questioned the validity of including it as a stage.

There are questions about whether Kohlberg's stages, particularly 5 and 6, are universal across cultures. There is research supporting the sequence and

Table 4–2 Kohlberg's Stages of Moral Development

Level and Stage	Definition	Example
Level I Preconventional		
Stage 1: Punishment and obedience orientation	The activity is wrong if one is punished, and the activity is right if one is not punished.	A nurse follows a physician's order so as not to be fired.
Stage 2: Instrumental-relativist orientation	Action is taken to satisfy one's needs.	A client in hospital agrees to stay in bed if the nurse will buy the client a newspaper.
Level II Conventional		
Stage 3: Interpersonal concordance (good boy, nice girl)	Action is taken to please another and gain approval.	A nurse gives older clients in hospital sedatives at bedtime because the night nurse wants all clients to sleep at night.
Stage 4: Law and order orientation	Right behavior is obeying the law and following the rules.	A nurse does not permit a worried client to phone home because hospital rules stipulate no phone calls after 9:00 P.M.
Level III Postconventional		
Stage 5: Social contract, legalistic orientation	Standard of behavior is based on adhering to laws that protect the welfare and rights of others. Personal values and opinions are recognized, and violating the rights of others is avoided.	A nurse arranges for an East Indian client to have privacy for prayer each evening.
Stage 6: Universal-ethical principles	Universal moral principles are internalized. Person respects other humans and believes that relationships are based on mutual trust.	A nurse becomes an advocate for a hospitalized client by reporting to the nursing supervisor a conversation in which a physician threatened to withhold assistance unless the client agreed to surgery.

Source: Adapted from *Moral Development: A Guide to Piaget and Kohlberg,* by Ronald Duska and Mariaellen Whelan. Copyright © 1975 by The Missionary Society of St. Paul the Apostle in the State of New York. Used by permission of Paulist Press. http://www.paulistpress.com.

achievement of these stages among various groups, such as South African blacks and whites, Chinese, Buddhists, British, and Hong Kong Chinese (Lei, 1994; Tudin, Straker, & Mendolsohn, 1994). Others question whether the universal ethical principle at stage 6 reflects Western ways of thinking (Heubner & Garrod, 1993; Miller, 1994).

Kohlberg developed this theory by conducting interviews using hypothetical dilemmas. Each dilemma described a character who finds himself or herself in a difficult situation and has to choose from conflicting values. The participant is asked how the character should resolve the problem in the right way. Analysis of the responses resulted in the formulation of Kohlberg's levels and stages (Colby & Kohlberg, 1987).

Unfortunately, all the subjects in the study were male, which has led to serious criticism of the theory.

Gilligan

Carol Gilligan (1982) has been one of the major critics of Kohlberg's theory, particularly in its application to females. She contends that Kohlberg's stage sequence places the qualities most often stressed in the socialization of females in stage 3; these qualities are compassion, responsibility, and obligation. Men, who are taught to organize social relationships in a hierarchical order and subscribe to a morality of right, will be included in Kohlberg's higher stages of moral judgment.

After more than 10 years of research with women subjects, she found that women often considered the

Comparison of Moral Justice and Care Orientations

JUSTICE ORIENTATION

Focuses on the moral vision of "not to treat others unfairly."

Requires understanding of what "fairness" means.

Draws attention to problems of inequality and oppression.

Holds up an ideal of reciprocal rights and equal respect for individuals.

CARE ORIENTATION

Focuses on the moral vision of "not to turn away from someone in need."

Requires understanding of what constitutes "care."

Draws attention to problems of detachment or abandonment.

Holds up an ideal of attention and response to need.

situations that Kohlberg used in his research to be irrelevant. Women scored consistently lower on his scale of moral development, in spite of the fact that they approached moral situations with considerable sophistication. Gilligan maintains that most frameworks do not include the concepts of caring and responsibility.

In contrast to Kohlberg's theory of moral development, which emphasizes fairness, rights, and autonomy in a *justice framework*, Gilligan focuses on a *care perspective*, which is organized around the notions of responsibility, compassion (care), and relationships. Gilligan contends that for women, moral maturity is less a matter of abstract, impersonal justice and more an ethic of caring relationships.

The ethic of *justice*, or fairness, is based on the idea of equality: that everyone should receive the same treatment. This is the development path usually followed by men. By contrast, the ethic of *care* is based on a premise of nonviolence: that no one should be harmed or abandoned. This is the path typically followed by women. Distinctions between a justice orientation and a care orientation are shown in the accompanying box.

Gilligan feels that a blend of justice and care perspectives is necessary for a person to reach maturity. The blending of these two perspectives could give rise to a new view of human development and a better understanding of human relations. To Gilligan, two intersecting dimensions characterize human relationships: equality and attachment. All relationships can be described as unequal or equal and as attached or detached. Most people have been vulnerable both to oppression and to abandonment. Thus, two moral visions—one of justice and one of care—recur in human experience.

Gilligan describes three stages in the process of developing an "ethic of care" (1982, pg. 74). Each stage ends with a transitional period. A *transitional period* is a time when the individual recognizes a conflict or discomfort with some present behavior and considers new approaches.

- *Stage 1. Caring for oneself.* In this first stage of development, the person is concerned only with caring for the self. The individual feels isolated, alone, and unconnected to others. There is no concern or conflict with the needs of others because the self is the most important. The focus of this stage is survival. The end of this stage occurs when the individual begins to view this approach as selfish. At this time, the person also begins to see a need for relationships and connections with other people.
- *Stage 2. Caring for others.* During this stage, the individual recognizes the selfishness of earlier behavior and begins to understand the need for caring relationships with others. Caring relationships bring with them responsibility. The definition of responsibility includes self-sacrifice, in which "good" is considered to be "caring for others." The individual now approaches relationships with a focus of not hurting others. This approach causes the individual to be more responsive and submissive to others' needs, excluding any thoughts of meeting one's own. A transition occurs when the individual recognizes that this approach can cause difficulties with relationships because of the lack of balance between caring for oneself and caring for others.
- *Stage 3. Caring for oneself and others.* During this last stage, a person sees that there is a need for a balance between caring for others and caring for the self. One's concept of responsibility is now defined as including responsibility for both the self and other

Critical Thinking Exercise

Situations may arise in health care in which the cultural practices of a family conflict with the values of the dominant culture. For instance, child discipline practices that are accepted as appropriate by some may be interpreted as severe or abusive by others. How might the nurse respond to the dilemma of mandatory reporting to a child protection agency at each stage or level of Kohlberg's and Gilligan's theories?

people. In this final stage, care still remains the focus on which decisions are made. However, the person now recognizes the interconnections between the self and others and thus realizes that it is important to take care of one's own needs, because if those needs are not met, other people may also suffer.

Moral Frameworks

General moral theories or frameworks include teleology and utilitarianism, deontology and natural law including intuitionism, pragmatism and virtue-based, and the ethic of caring. **Teleology** looks to the consequences of an action in judging whether that action is right or wrong. **Utilitarianism**, one specific teleologic theory, is summarized in the ideas "the greatest good for the greatest number" and "the end justifies the means."

Deontology emphasizes duty, rationality, and obedience to rules and proposes that the morality of a decision is not determined by its consequences. For instance, a nurse might believe it is necessary to tell the truth no matter who is hurt. There are many deontologic theories; each justifies the rules of acceptable behavior differently. For example, some state that the rules are known by divine revelation; others refer to a natural law or social contract; still others propose both of these as sources.

The difference between teleology and deontology can be seen when each approach is applied to the issue of abortion. A person taking a teleologic approach might consider that saving the mother's life (the end, or consequence) justifies the abortion (the means, or act). A person taking a deontologic approach might consider any termination of life as a violation of the rule "Do not kill" and, therefore, would not abort the fetus, regardless of the consequences to the mother. It is important to note that the approach, or framework, guides making the moral decision; it does not determine the outcome (e.g., the person taking a teleologic approach might

have considered that saving the life of the fetus justified the death of the mother).

A third framework, **pragmatism** and **virtue-based**, proposes that trial and error serves to determine what is right and wrong, good and bad. Intent is the distinguishing factor. If the intent is good, the act is moral regardless of the outcome.

Benner and Wrubel (1989) proposed **caring** as the central goal of nursing as well as a basis for nursing ethics. Unlike the preceding theories, which are based on the concept of fairness (justice), an ethic of caring is based on relationships. Caring theories stress courage, generosity, commitment, and responsibility. Caring is a force for protecting and enhancing client dignity. Caring is of central importance in the client-nurse relationship. For example, guided by this ethic, nurses use touch and truth-telling to affirm clients as persons rather than objects and to assist them to make choices and find meaning in their illness experiences.

Moral Principles

Moral principles are statements about broad, general philosophic concepts such as autonomy and justice. They provide the foundation for **moral rules**, which are specific prescriptions for actions. For example, "People should not lie" (rule) is based on the moral principle of respect for people's autonomy. Principles are useful in ethical discussions because even people who do not agree on which action to take may be able to agree on the principles that apply. That agreement can serve as the basis for an acceptable solution. For example, most people would agree that nurses are obligated to respect their clients (a principle), even if they disagree about whether a nurse should deceive a client about the client's prognosis (action).

Several moral concepts have special relevance to nursing practice. They include autonomy, nonmaleficence, beneficence, justice, fidelity, and veracity. These concepts form the basis of ethical principles for bioethics and nursing (Schroeter, Derse, Junkerman, & Schiedermayer, 2002).

Autonomy refers to the self-determination and the right to make one's own decisions. Respect for person is incorporated and means that nurses recognize the individual's uniqueness, the right to be who the person is, and the right to choose personal goals. Nurses who follow the principle of autonomy respect a client's right to make decisions even when those choices seem not to be in the client's best interest.

Respect for people also means treating others with consideration. In a health care setting, this principle is violated when a nurse disregards clients' subjective accounts of their symptoms (e.g., pain). The application of this principle requires that clients give informed consent before tests and procedures are carried out.

Nonmaleficence means the duty to do no harm. This principle is the basis of most codes of nursing ethics. Although this would seem to be a simple principle to follow in nursing practice, in reality it is complex. Harm can mean deliberate harm, risk of harm, and unintentional harm. In nursing, intentional harm is always unacceptable. However, the risk of harm is not always clear. A client may be at risk of harm during a nursing intervention that is intended to be helpful. For example, a client may react adversely to a medication. Sometimes, the degree to which a risk is morally permissible can be in dispute.

Beneficence refers to doing good. Nurses are obligated to act in the best interest of the clients and their support persons. However, in an increasingly technologic health care system, doing good can also pose a risk of doing harm. For example, a nurse may advise a client about an intensive exercise program to improve general health, but should not do so if the client is at risk of cardiovascular compromise.

Justice is often referred to as fairness and treating people equally. Nurses frequently face decisions in which a sense of justice should prevail. For example, a nurse is alone on a hospital unit, and one client arrives to be admitted at the same time another client requires a medication for pain. Instead of running from one client to the other, the nurse weighs the situation and then acts based on the principle of justice. It also means that the nurse provides the same level of care regardless of a person's socioeconomic background.

Fidelity means to be faithful to agreements and responsibilities one has undertaken. If a nurse tells a client she will return in an hour to check on the effectiveness of the pain medication, she should be faithful to that promise. Nurses have responsibilities

---

Critical Thinking Exercise

You are caring for a client who is contemplating an abortion but has moral distress about doing so. She tells you her boyfriend is strongly opposed to an abortion. She, however, feels she is too young to be a mother but feels guilty about having an abortion. Applying the moral principles of beneficence, nonmaleficence, veracity, autonomy, justice, and fidelity, decide how you would care for her and give your rationale.

---

to clients, employers, government, society, the profession, and to themselves. It also refers to maintaining confidentiality.

Veracity refers to telling the truth. Most children are taught always to tell the truth, but for adults, the choice is often less clear. Does a nurse tell the truth when it is known that doing so will cause harm? Does a nurse tell a lie when it is known that the lie will relieve anxiety and fear? Bok (1992) concludes that lying to sick and dying people is rarely justified. The loss of trust in the nurse and the anxiety caused by not knowing the truth, for example, usually outweigh any benefits derived from lying.

ETHICS

The term **ethics** derives from the Greek *ethos*, meaning custom or character. It has several meanings in common usage. First, it refers to a method of inquiry that assists people to understand the morality of human behavior; that is, ethics is the study of morality. When used in this sense, ethics is an activity; it is a way of looking at or investigating certain issues about human behavior. Second, ethics refers to the practices, beliefs, and standards of behavior of a certain group (e.g., physicians' ethics, nursing ethics). These standards are described in the group's code of professional conduct. **Bioethics** is ethics as applied to life (i.e., to life and death decision making). Because of technologic advances, bioethics is receiving increased attention in literature and discussions. Nursing ethics refers to ethical issues involved in nursing practice.

Nurses are accountable for their ethical conduct. In 2004, the American Nurses Association (ANA) published the revised *Scope and Standards of Practice*. Standard 12 relates to ethics; see the box on page 56.

ANA Standard of Nursing Practice 12: Ethics

The registered nurse integrates ethical provisions in all areas of practice.

MEASUREMENT CRITERIA

The registered nurse:

Uses the *Code of Ethics for Nurses with Interpretive Statements* (ANA, 2001) to guide practice.

Delivers care in a manner that preserves and protects patient autonomy, dignity, and rights.

Maintains patient confidentiality within legal and regulatory parameters.

Serves as a patient advocate assisting patients in developing skills for self-advocacy.

Maintains a therapeutic and professional patient-nurse relationship with appropriate professional role boundaries.

Demonstrates a commitment to practicing self-care, managing stress, and connecting with self and others.

Contributes to resolving ethical issues of patients, colleagues, or systems as evidenced in such activities as participating on ethics committees.

Reports illegal, incompetent, or impaired practice.

Additional Measurement Criteria for the Advanced Practice Registered Nurse:

The advanced practice registered nurse:

Informs the patient of the risks, benefits, and outcomes of health care regimens.

Participates in interdisciplinary teams that address ethical risks, benefits, and outcomes.

Additional Measurement Criteria for the Nursing Role Specialty:

The registered nurse in a nursing role specialty:

Participates on multidisciplinary and interdisciplinary teams that address ethical risks, benefits, and outcomes.

Informs administrators or others of the risks, benefits, and outcomes of programs and decisions that affect health care delivery.

Source: Nursing: Scope and Standards of Practice, American Nurses Association, 2004, Washington, DC: ANA.

Nurses need to understand their own values related to moral matters and to use ethical reasoning to determine and explain their moral positions. Sometimes it is not enough for nurses to be aware of an ethical issue; they also need moral principles and reasoning skills to explain their position. Otherwise they may give emotional responses, which often are not helpful.

Nursing Codes of Ethics

A **code of ethics** is a formal statement of a group's ideals and values. It is a set of ethical principles that is shared by members of the group, reflects their moral judgments over time, and serves as a standard for their professional actions. Codes of ethics are usually higher than legal standards, and they can never be less than the legal standards of the profession.

International, national, state, and provincial nursing associations have established codes of ethics. The International Council of Nurses (ICN) developed and adopted their first code of ethics in 1953. The ICN Code was revised in 1965 and again in 1973. The ANA

first adopted a code of ethics in 1950; it was revised in 1968, 1976, 1985, and 2001 and is simply referred to as the *Code for Nurses*. It is published in booklet form called *Code of Ethics for Nurses with Interpretive Statements* (2001). The code has nine provisions, and they are shown in the box on page 57. The code serves the following purposes (ANA, 2001, p. 5):

- It is a succinct statement of the ethical obligations and duties of every individual who enters the nursing profession.
- It is the profession's nonnegotiable ethical standard.
- It is an expression of nursing's own understanding of its commitment to society.

The first three provisions describe the most fundamental values and commitments, the next three address boundaries of duties and loyalty, and the remaining three address duty beyond individual nurse-patient encounters. The code provides a basis for ethical analysis and decision making and establishes the ethical standard for the profession in the United States.

American Nurses Association *Code of Ethics for Nurses*

1. The nurse, in all professional relationships, practices with compassion and respect for the inherent dignity, worth, and uniqueness of every individual, unrestricted by considerations of social or economic status, personal attributes, or the nature of health problems.

2. The nurse's primary commitment is to the patient, whether an individual, family, group, or community.

3. The nurse promotes, advocates for, and strives to protect the health, safety, and rights of the patient.

4. The nurse is responsible and accountable for individual nursing practice and determines the appropriate delegation of tasks consistent with the nurse's obligation to provide optimum patient care.

5. The nurse owes the same duties to self as to others, including the responsibility to preserve integrity and safety, to maintain competence, and to continue personal and professional growth.

6. The nurse participates in establishing, maintaining, and improving health care environments and conditions of employment conducive to the provision of quality health care and consistent with the values of the profession through individual and collective action.

7. The nurse participates in the advancement of the profession through contributions to practice, education, administration, and knowledge development.

8. The nurse collaborates with other health professionals and the public in promoting community, national, and international efforts to meet health needs.

9. The profession of nursing, as represented by associations and their members, is responsible for articulating nursing values, for maintaining integrity of the profession and its practice, and for shaping social policy.

Source: Used by permission of the American Nurses Association from the *Code of Ethics for Nurses with Interpretive Statements,* American Nurses Association, 2001, Washington, DC: ANA.

In 1980, the Canadian Nurses Association (CNA) adopted a code of ethics; it was revised in 1991, 1996, and 2002. It is based on eight primary values central to ethical nursing practice. The *Code of Ethics for Nurses in Australia* was first published in 1993 and revised in 2002. It is based on six broad values statements to guide reflection on practice. The values from these codes are compared in Table 4–3. Increasingly, professional nursing associations are taking an active part in improving and enforcing standards. Nurses are responsible for being familiar with the code that governs their practice.

Nursing codes of ethics have the following purposes:

1. To inform the public about the minimum standards of the profession and to help them understand professional nursing conduct

2. To provide a sign of the profession's commitment to the public it serves

3. To outline the major ethical considerations of the profession

4. To provide general guidelines for professional behavior

5. To guide the profession in self-regulation

6. To remind nurses of the special responsibility they assume when caring for clients

Because the wording in a code of ethics is intentionally vague, such codes can serve as general guides. They do not give direction for actions to take in specific cases. For example, the first item in the ANA *Code for Nurses* refers to respect for human dignity and states that in caring for clients, nurses should be "unrestricted by considerations of the nature of health problems." Does that mean that it is wrong for a pregnant nurse to refuse to care for a client with active herpes? Or that it is wrong to refuse to care for a client who uses rude language? When making ethical decisions, nurses should consider their code of ethics together with a more unified ethical theory, ethical principles, and the relevant data about each situation.

Reflect on...

■ a situation in which your personal code of ethics might conflict with the client's. What would guide your practice?

Table 4–3 Comparison of Values from the Canadian Nurses Association *Code of Ethics* and the Values Statements from the *Code of Ethics for Nurses in Australia*

Canada	Australia
Nurses value the ability to provide safe, competent, and ethical care.	Nurses respect the individual's needs, values, culture, and vulnerability in the provision of nursing care.
Nurses value health promotion and well-being and assisting persons to achieve their optimum level of health.	Nurses accept the rights of individual's informed choices in relation to their care.
Nurses respect and promote the autonomy of persons and help them to express their health needs and values, and also to obtain desired information and services so they can make informed decisions.	Nurses promote and uphold the provision of quality nursing care for all people.
Nurses recognize and respect the inherent worth of each person and advocate for respectful treatment of all persons.	Nurses hold in confidence any information obtained in a professional capacity, use professional judgment where there is a need to share information for the therapeutic benefit and safety of a person, and ensure that privacy is safeguarded.
Nurses safeguard information learned in the context of a professional relationship and ensure it is shared outside the health care team only with the person's informed consent, or as may be legally required, or where the failure to disclose would cause significant harm.	Nurses fulfill the accountability and responsibility inherent in their roles.
Nurses uphold principles of equity and fairness to assist persons in receiving a share of health services and resources proportionate to their needs and in promoting social justice.	Nurses value environmental ethics and a social, economic, and ecologically sustainable environment that promotes health and well-being.
Nurses are answerable for their practice, and they act in a manner consistent with their professional responsibilities and standards of practice.	
Nurses value and advocate for practice environments that have the organizational structures and resources necessary to ensure safety, support, and respect for all persons in the work setting.	

Sources: Code of Ethics for Registered Nurses, Ottawa, Canadian Nurses Association, 2002; and *Code of Ethics for Nurses in Australia,* Australian Nursing Council, 2002, http://www.anci.org.au.

Types of Ethical Problems

Nurses encounter two broad types of problems: decision-focused problems and action-focused problems. Each requires a different approach (Wilkinson, 1993, p. 4).

In decision-focused problems, the difficulty lies in deciding what to do. The question is, What should I do? For example:

Because Leon is committed to the sanctity of life, he wishes his client to have artificial nutrition and hydration. As a nurse, Leon also believes in relieving suffering, so when he sees that the tube-feedings are prolonging the client's pain and even contributing to her discomfort, he wishes to have the feedings discontinued. He is not comfortable with either choice.

In this case, two principles clearly apply, so no matter what the nurse does, an important value must be sacrificed. This is the typical **ethical dilemma** that people commonly refer to as "being between a rock and a hard place." The nature of a dilemma dictates that there are no easy solutions. However, because the difficulty is personal and internal, nurses can address decision-focused problems by engaging in activities developed to enhance decision-making skills, for example, by reviewing their own personal value systems, taking advantage of continuing education offerings, and attending ethics rounds.

In **action-focused problems**, the difficulty lies not in making the decision, but in implementing it. In these situations, nurses usually feel secure in their judgment about what is right but act on their judgment only at personal risk. The central question is, What can I do? or What risks am I willing to take to do what is right? **Moral distress**, one type of action-focused problem, occurs when the nurse knows the right course of action but cannot carry it out because of institutional policies or other constraints (Jameton, 1984, p. 6). This results in feelings of anger, guilt, and loss of integrity on the part of the nurse and can affect client care. For example:

> A resident physician has told the nurses to order complete blood count (CBC) and urinalysis on all clients and to get the results before calling him to the emergency room to examine the clients. The nurses believe this is unethical because it is wasteful and poses unnecessary discomfort and possible risks for clients. However, they do not have the authority or the access to decision-making channels needed to change the situation. So they order the tests, but they feel guilty and upset because they believe what they are doing is wrong.

Unlike decision-focused problems, action-focused problems cannot be resolved by improving one's decision-making skills. Even after a nurse decides what is right to do, the issue becomes what the nurse actually can do given the conditions of practice. Nurses' actions are influenced by such constraints as lack of support from both peers and administrators and consequently fear of losing their jobs or their nursing licenses and fear of legal action. Action-focused problems require knowledge, experience, communication, and the ability to make integrity-preserving compromises. To deal successfully with these problems, nurses must shift their attention away from "making the right decision" and focus on the factors that are preventing the "right

action" (Wilkinson, 1993, p. 5). Applying the professional code of ethics provides support for "doing the right thing" in many situations.

Ethical conflicts also arise from nurses' unresolved questions about the nature and scope of their practice. High-technology and specialty roles (intensive care nurses, advanced practice nurses) have expanded the scope of nursing practice, often causing nursing and medical activities to overlap. This creates value conflicts for nurses. For example:

- Although nurses value health promotion and wellness, many still work in hospitals and many are involved in high-tech treatment of illness.
- Although the profession values a humanistic, caring approach and emphasizes nurse-client relationships, many nurses spend much of their time attending to the client's machines.

Because of their unique position in the health care system, nurses experience conflicting loyalties and obligations to clients, families, physicians, employing institutions, and licensing bodies. The client's needs may conflict with institutional policies, physician preferences, needs of the client's family, or even laws of the state. According to the nursing code of ethics, the nurse's first allegiance is to the client. However, it is not always easy to determine which action best serves the client's needs. For instance, a nurse may believe that the client's interests require telling the client a truth that others have been withholding. But this might damage the client-physician relationship, in the long run causing harm to the client rather than the intended good.

Making Ethical Decisions

Responsible ethical reasoning is rational thinking. It is also systematic and based on ethical principles and civil law. It should not be based on emotions, intuition, fixed policies, or precedent. (A *precedent* is an earlier similar occurrence. For example, "We have always done it this way" is a statement reflecting a decision based on precedent.)

Catalano (2000) has developed an ethical decision-making algorithm for the nurse. See Figure 4–1■. It involves five steps, beginning with the identification of a potential ethical delimma and resulting in either a resolution or a decision to take no action. Many components enter into the decision-making process. These include the following:

- Facts of the specific situation
- Ethical theories and principles
- Nursing codes of ethics

Figure 4–1

Ethical Decision-Making Algorithm

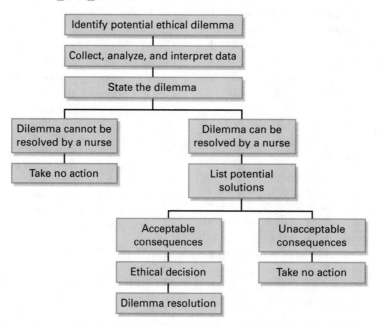

Source: Nursing Now! Today's Issues, Tommorow's Trends, (2nd ed.), by J. T. Catalano, 2000, Philadelphia: F. A. Davis.

■ The client's rights
■ Personal values
■ Factors that contribute to or hinder one's ability to make or enact a choice, such as cultural values, societal expectations, degree of commitment, lack of time, lack of experience, ignorance or fear of the law, and conflicting loyalties

Ethical decision making that entails a person's choices, values, and actions begins in desire: people are inspired by a desire to pursue the good as they each see it. However, to know that what they are pursuing truly is good, people must rely on reason. Ethical choices, values, and actions then become a reasoned desire (Husted & Husted, 2001, pp. 178–183).

Nurses are responsible for deciding on their own actions and for supporting clients who are making ethical decisions or coping with the results of decisions that other people have made. A good decision is one that is in the client's best interest and at the same time preserves the integrity of all involved. Nurses have multiple obligations to balance in moral situations.

Ethical decision making requires that the nurse understand the differences among problems, dilemmas, and quandaries. A problem may be hard to understand and to deal with but it is solvable in principle. A **quandary** is a perplexed state with uncertainty over alternatives. A **dilemma** is a specific situation involving a choice between undesirable alternatives and where

Examples of Nurses' Obligations in Ethical Decisions

• Maximizing the client's well-being

• Balancing the client's need for autonomy with family members' responsibilities for the client's well-being

• Supporting each family member and enhancing the family support system

• Carrying out hospital policies

• Protecting other clients' well-being

• Protecting the nurse's own standards of care

there are no precedents or rules to follow (Thompson, Melia, & Boyd, 2000, p. 7). Moral dilemmas bring into sharper focus the moral values and principles that matter. Ethical decision making applies problem solving and involves reflecting on alternatives and justification of actions chosen.

In some cases, the most important question is who should make the decision. When the decision maker is the client, the nurse functions in a supportive role. Clients need knowledge about the probability and nature of consequences attending various courses of action. Nurses share their special knowledge and expertise with clients to enable them to make informed decisions.

The following questions may help the nurse determine who owns a problem:

- For whom is the decision being made?
- Who should be involved in making the decision, and why?
- What criteria (social, economic, psychological, physiological, or legal) should be used in deciding who makes the decision?
- What degree of consent is needed by the subject?

The box on page 62 shows an example using a bioethical decision-making model.

Because they have ethical obligations to their clients, to the agency that employs them, and to the other members of the health care team, nurses weigh competing factors when making ethical decisions. In many health care settings, nurses are not given the autonomy to act on their moral or ethical choices.

The goal of settling moral conflict is to ensure that the conflicting values of all parties are respected and sometimes concessions are made. When compromises are necessary the most desirable outcome is the preservation of each person's integrity, with no one forced to give up values, principles, or moral integrity. In the process all parties are encouraged to discuss personal values, their assessment of the situation, and the perceived "best decision" for the client. For example, a nurse who is opposed to abortion provides physical care and emotional support for a woman having an elective abortion because there was no one else available to provide adequate care. The outcome of moral compromise strives to preserve each party's integrity by reaching a decision that respects the values held by all the decision makers; the outcome does not necessarily fall in line with what any one person thinks should be done. Each participant needs to recognize reasonable differences of opinion, see things from others' points of view, and reach an agreement that is mutual and peaceful for all concerned.

Evidence for Practice

Ahern, K., McDonald, S. (2002). The beliefs of nurses who were involved in a whistleblowing event. *Journal of Advanced Nursing, 38*(3), 303–309.
A descriptive survey was used to explore the beliefs of nurses in Western Australia about involvment in "whistleblowing" events. Statements from current codes of ethics, traditional views of nursing, and statements of beliefs about the participant's whistleblowing experience were rated on a five-point Likert scale by a sample of 95 nurses. Factor analysis identified four clusters of items; these clusters were named Rational/Advocacy, Advocacy Role, Traditional Role, and Traditional/Conformity. The whistleblowers agreed more strongly with the Advocacy items than did non-whistleblowers. The non-whistleblowers agreed more strongly with the Traditional statements. This has implications for the profession. Nursing codes of ethics require nurses to safeguard patients from incompetent, unethical, or illegal practices, yet those who do not hold patient advocacy beliefs may hesitate to act if it means opposing authority or tradition. Nurse managers and nursing boards need to provide support for nursing advocacy actions and reward the nurse who blows the whistle on misconduct.

According to Winslow and Winslow (1991, pp. 309, 315–320), an **integrity-preserving moral compromise** is one in which the following elements are present:

1. *Some basic moral language must be shared.* Currently, moral and ethical issues are expressed in the language of client care, client rights, autonomy, and client advocacy. One task of institutional ethics committees is to provide a setting in which a mutual moral language can be built.

2. *A context of mutual respect must exist.* All parties must listen with respect to those with whom they differ. Coercive measures are not used. Without mutual respect, compromise becomes capitulation or persuasion. Everyone's views must be considered.

3. *The moral perplexity of the situation must be honestly acknowledged.* Each person should retain a sense of humility, remembering that there are elements of uncertainty and that he or she could be wrong.

Clinical Application Bioethical Decision-Making Model

SITUATION

Mrs. LaVesque, a 67-year-old woman, is hospitalized with multiple fractures and lacerations caused by an automobile crash. Her husband, who was killed in the crash, was taken to the same hospital. Mrs. LaVesque, who had been driving the automobile, constantly questions Kate Murillo, her primary nurse, about her husband. The surgeon, Dr. Mario Gonzales, has told the nurse not to tell Mrs. LaVesque about the death of her husband; however, he does not give the nurse any reason for these instructions. Ms. Murillo expresses concern to the charge nurse, who says the surgeon's orders must be followed. Ms. Murillo is not comfortable with this and wonders what she should do.

NURSING ACTIONS	CONSIDERATIONS
1. Identify the moral aspects.	In this situation, the ethical dilemma is either to tell the truth or to withhold it. There is conflict between the values of honesty and loyalty. The primary nurse wants to be honest with Mrs. LaVesque without being disloyal to the surgeon and the charge nurse. Her choice will probably be affected by her concern for Mrs. LaVesque and perhaps by the surgeon's incomplete communication with her.
2. Gather relevant facts related to the issue.	Data should include information about the client's health problems. Determine who is involved, the nature of their involvement, and their motives for acting. In this case, the people involved are the client (who is concerned about her husband), the husband (who is deceased), the surgeon, the charge nurse, and the primary nurse. Motives are not known. Perhaps the nurse wishes to protect her therapeutic relationship with Mrs. LaVesque; possibly the physician believes he is protecting Mrs. LaVesque from psychologic trauma and consequent physical deterioration.
3. Determine ownership of the decision.	In this case, the decision is being made for Mrs. LaVesque. The surgeon obviously believes that he should be the one to decide, and the charge nurse agrees. It would be helpful if caregivers agreed on criteria for deciding who the decision maker should be.
4. Clarify and apply personal values.	We can infer from this situation that Mrs. LaVesque values her husband's welfare, that the charge nurse values policy and procedure, and that Ms. Murillo seems to value a client's right to have information. Ms. Murillo needs to clarify her own and the surgeon's values, as well as confirm the values of Mrs. LaVesque and the charge nurse.
5. Identify ethical theories and principles.	For example, failing to tell Mrs. LaVesque the truth can negate her autonomy. The nurse would uphold the principle of honesty by telling Mrs. LaVesque. The principles of beneficence and nonmaleficence are also involved because of the possible effects of the alternative actions on Mrs. LaVesque's physical and psychologic well-being.
6. Identify applicable laws or agency policies.	Because Dr. Gonzales simply "gave instructions" rather than an actual order, agency policies might not require Ms. Murillo to do as he says. She should clarify this with the charge nurse. She should also be familiar with the nurse practice act in her state or province.
7. Use competent interdisciplinary resources.	In this case, Ms. Murillo might consult literature to find out whether clients are harmed by receiving bad news when they are injured. She might also consult with the chaplain.

Clinical Application Bioethical Decision-Making Model (cont.)

8. Develop alternative actions and project their outcomes on the client and family. Possibly because of the limited time available for ethical deliberations in the clinical setting, nurses tend to identify two opposing, either-or alternatives (e.g., to tell or not to tell) instead of generating multiple options. This creates a dilemma even when none exists.

   Two alternative actions, with possible outcomes, follow:
   1. Follow the charge nurse's advice and do as the surgeon says. Possible outcomes: (a) Mrs. LaVesque might become increasingly anxious and angry when she finds out that information has been withheld from her; or (b) by waiting until Mrs. LaVesque is stronger to give her the bad news, the health care team avoids harming Mrs. LaVesque's health.
   2. Discuss the situation further with the charge nurse and surgeon, pointing out Mrs. LaVesque's right to autonomy and information. Possible outcomes: (a) The surgeon acknowledges Mrs. LaVesque's right to be informed, or (b) he states that Mrs. LaVesque's health is at risk and insists that she not be informed until a later time.

   Regardless of whether the action is congruent with Ms. Murillo's personal value system, Mrs. LaVesque's best interests take precedence.

9. Apply nursing codes of ethics to help guide actions. Codes of nursing usually support autonomy and nursing advocacy.

   If Ms. Murillo believes strongly that Mrs. LaVesque should hear the truth, then, as a client advocate, she should choose to confer again with the charge nurse and surgeon.

10. For each alternative action, identify the risk and seriousness of consequences for the nurse.

   If Ms. Murillo tells Mrs. LaVesque the truth without the agreement of the charge nurse and surgeon, she risks the surgeon's anger and a reprimand from the charge nurse. If Ms. Murillo follows the charge nurse's advice, she will receive approval from the charge nurse and surgeon; however, she risks being seen as unassertive and she violates her personal value of truthfulness. If Ms. Murillo requests a conference, she may gain respect for her assertiveness and professionalism, but she risks the surgeon's annoyance at having his instructions questioned.

11. Participate actively in resolving the issue.

   The appropriate degree of nursing input varies with the situation. Sometimes nurses participate in choosing what will be done; sometimes they merely support a client who is making the decision. In this situation, if an action cannot be agreed upon, Ms. Murillo must decide whether this issue is important enough to merit the personal risks involved.

12. Implement the action.

13. Evaluate the action taken.

   Ms. Murillo can begin by asking, "Did I do the right thing?" Involve the client, family, and other health members in the evaluation, if possible. Ms. Murillo can ask herself whether she would make the same decisions again if the situation were repeated. If she is not satisfied, she can review other alternatives and work through the process again.

Source: Model adapted from "Preparing Students to be Moral Agents in Clinical Nursing Practice," by J. Cassells and B. Redman, June 1989, *Nursing Clinics of North America, 24*(2), 463–473.

4. *Legitimate limits to compromise must be admitted.* There are times when one cannot compromise. Compromise is more likely when there is factual uncertainty, ambiguity, and an extremely complex situation. The more certain a person is of the facts and the more clearly convinced he or she is about the morality of a course of action, the less room there is for compromise. The limits of compromise are reached when a person is so certain about a particular course of action that to compromise on that point would be to compromise the sense of self as a moral agent.

Specific Ethical Issues

The changing scope of nursing practice has led to an increasing incidence of conflicts between clients' needs and expectations and nurses' professional values. Some of these conflicts involve end-of-life care, elective abortion, organ transplantation, and the allocation of health care resources. With the development of sophisticated technology that affects the course and outcome of illness, nurses and clients face more complex ethical decisions. Because today's public is better informed about medical advances and issues, it is important that nurses become comfortable in dealing with clients, families, and peers facing ethical decisions. Nurses are ethically obligated to maintain a nonjudgmental attitude, be honest, and protect the client's right to privacy and confidentiality.

ELECTIVE ABORTION   Abortion is a highly publicized issue about which many people, including nurses, feel very strongly. Debate continues, pitting the principle of the sanctity of life against the principle of autonomy and the woman's right to control her own body. This is an especially volatile issue because no public consensus has yet been reached.

Most state and provincial laws have provisions known as conscience clauses, which permit individual physicians and nurses, as well as institutions, to refuse to assist with an abortion if doing so violates their religious or moral principles. However, nurses have no right to impose their values on a client, and nursing codes of ethics support clients' rights to information and counseling regarding abortion.

END-OF-LIFE CARE   Advances in health care technology have made it possible to sustain life much longer than previously possible. Some people want everything possible done to maintain life, and others do not. Competent adults have a legal right to refuse or have withdrawn any medical treatment. Often family members of the dying patient cannot make end-of-life decisions or have conflicting desires about the care that should be provided. Advance directives and living wills allow people to indicate their desires about end-of-life care. A durable power of attorney can designate a decision maker in the event that the patient is unable to make the choice. Information about advance directives are mandated for individuals admitted to health care facilities. Nurses are often called upon to present information and provide explanations.

Active and passive euthanasia are also end-of-life issues. Active euthanasia involves the administration of a lethal agent to end life and alleviate suffering; this approach can result in criminal charges of murder. Passive euthanasia involves the withdrawal of extraordinary means of life support, such as removing ventilator support and withholding resuscitation (DNR orders). The concept of death with dignity and the concerns about quality of life have brought about right-to-die legislative actions. These statutes absolve health care personnel from possible liability when they support a client's wishes not to prolong life. However, these statutes are complex and varied. Nurses are advised to familiarize themselves with the statutes in their particular state or province.

Withdrawing or withholding food and fluids and terminating or withholding treatment present difficult decisions. It is generally accepted that providing food and fluids is part of nursing practice and, therefore, a moral duty. A nurse is morally obligated, however, to withhold food and fluids when it is more harmful to administer them than to withhold them.

Clients may specify that they wish to have life-sustaining measures withdrawn, they may have advance directives on this matter, or they may specify a surrogate decision maker. When these decisions are made, the nurse, as the primary caregiver, must ensure that sensitive care and comfort measures are given as the client's illness progresses. A decision to withdraw treatment is not a decision to withdraw care.

ORGAN DONATION   Organs for transplantation may come from living donors or from donors who have just died. Ethical issues related to organ transplantation include the allocation of organs, the selling of body parts, the involvement of children as potential donors and recipients, and cloning for the manufacture of organs. Ethical decision making related to these issues is complex. In some situations, religious beliefs may be a source of conflict; for example, the mutilation of the body even for the benefit of another person may be forbidden.

Many people are choosing to become donors by giving consent under the Uniform Anatomical Gift Act. Making these decisions in advance can be helpful. When there is a death resulting from injury and organs are healthy enough to be harvested, it often falls upon the nurse and other members of the health care team to approach the grieving family about the possibility of organ donation. Many nurses feel uncomfortable about discussing this topic with the family. Some nurses have strong feelings about organ donation that make it difficult to remain neutral when a family faces that decision.

ALLOCATION OF HEALTH RESOURCES

Allocation of health care goods and services, including such things as organ transplants, the services of medical specialists, and care involving expensive technology, has become an especially urgent issue as medical costs continue to rise and more stringent cost-containment measures are implemented. For example, decisions about the number of office visits and the length of hospital stay are increasingly being influenced not by medical considerations but by administrative policies of health care facilities and funding entities, such as insurance companies, HMOs, and Medicare. Third-party coverage of some expensive and/or experimental treatments is being denied.

Critics dispute that health care is a scarce resource in North America; instead, they contend that access to health care is limited for segments of the population. Increasing people's access to health care is costly, however, and makes decisions about providing and financing health care difficult. An ethical argument arises as to whether health care is a right or a privilege.

Reflect on...

- whether there should be a level of "essential" care that is provided for all individuals and a higher level that must be financed privately.
- whether preventive care services should receive the same financing as illness services.
- your views about organ donation from someone under the age of 18 years.

Strategies to Enhance Ethical Decision Making

Rodney and Starzomski (1993, p. 24) and Davis and Aroskar (1991, p. 65) describe several strategies to help nurses overcome possible organizational and social constraints that may hinder the ethical practice of nursing and create moral distress for nurses. These strategies encompass areas of education, administration, practice, and research.

Become aware of one's own values and the ethical aspects of nursing situations. Much of this chapter has been devoted to discussions of nursing values and ethical situations. Most nursing programs include information about these topics at the undergraduate and graduate levels. Continuing education, in the form of in-service programs or other activities, also helps practicing professionals learn more about ethics.

Be familiar with nursing codes of ethics. The content and intent of these codes focus on supporting nursing practice based on ethical principles.

Evidence for Practice

Oberle, K., Hughes, D. (2001). Doctors' and nurses' perceptions of ethical problems in end-of-life decisions. *Journal of Advanced Nursing, 33*(3), 707–715.
This qualitative study was done to identify and compare the perceptions of doctors and nurses regarding ethical problems in end-of-life decisions. Seven doctors and 14 nurses working in acute care adult medical-surgical areas, including intensive care units, were interviewed and asked to describe ethical problems that they frequently encounter in practice. The interview data were analyzed using the constant comparative technique of Grounded Theory and themes were identified as they emerged from the data. All the participants described ethical problems around decision making at the end of life. The core problem was witnessing suffering, which brought out a moral obligation to reduce the suffering. The themes that emerged were uncertainty about the best course of action for the patient and family, competing values when the patients are unable to speak for themselves, allocation of scarce resources, and communication with the patient and family (what to tell them). Differences between doctors' and nurses' ethical concerns were related to their differing perspectives; doctors bore the burden of making decisions, and nurses were burdened by living with the decision made by someone else. The nurses experienced moral distress resulting from the inability to influence decisions. The researchers suggest that doctors and nurses need to engage in discourse regarding the ethical burdens each one experiences, and that administrators should provide opportunities for the discourses.

Understand the values of other health care professionals. An understanding of the values that other health care professionals hold enables nurses to appreciate and respect values, opinions, and responsibilities similar to and different from their own. For example, nurses may find it helpful to know that the American Medical Association considers it morally permissible to refrain from exercising or to discontinue extraordinary efforts to prolong life. In this context, the choice of action is decided on the basis of doing good and avoiding harm.

Some educational institutions now include interdisciplinary ethics education at both undergraduate and graduate levels to enhance the understanding of beliefs, responsibilities, and values among various members of the health care team. For example, nursing students and medical students take classes together on bioethics, professional ethics, and business ethics. The goal of this type of interdisciplinary education is to bring about better team communication in the practice setting.

Participate on ethics committees. Because nurses have more contact with the client and family than other members of the health care team, they know the client better and have access to special kinds of information not available to other health care professionals. Nurses offer unique perspectives that can greatly improve the quality of the ethical decisions made in health care settings. One important way for nurses to provide input is to serve on institutional ethics committees. Standards established by the Joint Commission on Accreditation of Healthcare Organizations (JCAHO) support this involvement.

Ethics committees typically review cases, write guidelines and policies, and provide education and counseling. They ensure that relevant facts are brought out; provide a forum in which diverse views, such as views on resource allocation, can be expressed; reduce stress for caregivers; and can reduce legal risks. These factors tend to produce better decisions than would otherwise be made.

Institutional policies and guidelines about such issues as informed consent, the withdrawal or withholding of life-sustaining treatment, and do-not-resuscitate (DNR) orders provide direction for all health care practitioners to resolve ethical conflicts. To encourage the most effective functioning, ethics committees need to include representatives of all parties involved—consumers, hospital administrators, nurses, physicians, attorneys, hospital chaplains, social workers, and bioethicists.

Participate in or establish a nursing ethics group. A nursing ethics group can address the specific ethical issues of nursing practice and explore ethical choices nurses consider on a daily basis. Nurses are most commonly involved in issues of client refusal of treatment, informed consent, discontinuation of life-saving treatment, withholding of information from clients, confidentiality, client competence, and allocation of resources.

Nursing ethics committees also can provide an opportunity for nurse-to-nurse collaboration, facilitating effective cooperation among nurses and increasing nurses' power or capacity to produce change and to implement the care they believe to be most beneficial

to their clients. For nurses to act freely as moral agents within any institution, collaboration among and support of peers are essential. Discussions with peers during difficult ethical situations help to reduce nurses' moral distress.

Participate in or establish educational ethics rounds. Ethics rounds using hypothetical or real cases can be used to explore ethical principles and discuss ethical dilemmas. Ethics rounds incorporate the traditional teaching approach for clinical rounds, but the focus is on the ethical dimensions of client care rather than the client's clinical diagnosis and treatment. Discussions may be held at the bedside, where health care professionals can speak directly to the client. Consent from the client must first be obtained.

Ethics rounds help all those involved to articulate their own views, encourage discussion of value conflicts, and help individuals apply decision-making skills. There are various formats. The situations to be discussed may be presented by staff nurses, advanced nursing students, clinical nurse specialists, or ethics consultants, among others. Rounds serve as examples for future situations the nurse may confront. Each health care facility establishes the format and procedure of ethics rounds to fit its particular situation.

ADVOCACY

An **advocate** is one who pleads the cause of another, and a **client advocate** is an advocate for clients' rights. The origin of the word *advocate* derives from the Latin *advocatus,* meaning "one summoned to give evidence." The focus of the client advocacy role is to respect client decisions and enhance client autonomy. Values basic to client advocacy are shown in the box on page 67.

The Advocacy Role

The nurse needs self-knowledge as well as professional knowledge about nursing and health care or needs to know where to obtain such knowledge to assist clients in their decision making. Nurses as knowledgeable professionals share their unique knowledge with the community when needed. Today's health care crises of AIDS, homelessness, teenage pregnancy, child and spouse abuse, drug and alcohol abuse, and increasing health care costs all demand the nurse to fulfill the role of advocate in the community.

Professional/Public Advocacy

Gates (1995, p. 32) states that advocacy encompasses a range of approaches including legal, self-, collective

Nursing Values Basic to Client Advocacy

- The client is a holistic, autonomous being who has the right to make choices and decisions.
- Clients have the right to expect a nurse-client relationship that is based on shared respect, trust, collaboration in solving problems related to health and health care needs, and consideration of their thoughts and feelings.
- Clients are responsible for their health.
- Nurses are responsible for helping clients use their strengths to achieve the highest level of health possible.
- It is the nurse's responsibility to ensure the client has access to health care services that meet health needs.
- The nurse and client are equally able and responsible for the outcomes of care.

(class), and citizen advocacy. Citizen advocacy may be likened to client advocacy. See Table 4–4. Political advocacy will be discussed in detail in Chapter 11 ⃝ The Nurse as Advocate.

The defining attributes of patient advocacy include the following (Baldwin, 2003):

- ■ A therapeutic nurse-patient relationship in which to secure patients' freedom and self-determination
- ■ Promoting and protecting patients' rights to be involved in decision making and informed consent
- ■ Acting as an intermediary between patients and their families or significant others, and between them and health care providers

Table 4–4 Types of Advocacy

Type	Description	Example
Legal advocacy	Related to various tribunals and other court case work.	Limited to the work of attorneys or other court-appointed agents.
Self-advocacy	Individual people or groups speaking or acting on behalf of other people on issues that are of mutual interest. Individuals are encouraged to speak for themselves in order to encourage an element of self-empowerment.	Individual clients or family members telling the physician their own requirements related to treatment. Nurses behaving assertively in describing their own needs to administrators.
Collective or class advocacy	Refers to relatively large organizations that pursue the interests of a category of people. Such organizations usually have a national resource that provides full-time officers, as well as volunteers who are able to act as advocates.	American Association for Retired Persons (AARP), National Association for the Advancement of Colored People (NAACP). Professional organizations: American Nurses Association (ANA), Canadian Nurses Association (CNA).
Citizen or client advocacy	Concerned primarily with empowering people through an individual relationship. One person represents, as if they were his or her own, the interests of another person who has needs that are unmet and are likely to remain unmet without special intervention.	Nurse, social worker, court appointed temporary guardian.

These attributes involve valuing patients as unique individuals and informing, advising, and educating them to help in their reasoning and deliberations. The nurse may need to intercede and help them overcome barriers to meeting their needs. This happens in a context of vulnerability, in which the nurse is needed for assistance in facing a conflict or making a decision.

An advocate supports clients in their decisions. Support can involve action or nonaction. An advocate must know how to provide support in an objective manner, being careful not to convey approval or disapproval of the client's choices. Advocacy involves accepting and respecting the client's right to decide, even if the nurse believes the decision is wrong. As advocates, nurses do not make decisions for clients; clients must make their own decisions freely. For example, after being fully informed about the chemotherapy treatment, the alternative treatments, and the possible consequences of the available choices, Mr. Rae decides against further chemotherapy for his cancer. The client advocate supports Mr. Rae in his decision. Underlying client advocacy are the beliefs that individuals have the following rights (Donahue, 1985, p. 1037):

- The right to select values they deem necessary to sustain their lives
- The right to decide which course of action will best achieve the chosen values
- The right to dispose of values in a way they choose without coercion by others

There are many occasions when the nurse may speak up for clients. Examples include issues of resuscitation status, inadequate pain control, lack of information, or the client's desire to refuse a treatment. It is often stated that nurses are in a unique position to be client advocates because they spend more time with clients and their families than any other health care professionals. However, a number of challenges face nurses who wish to act as client advocates. To be a client advocate involves the following:

- Being assertive
- Recognizing that the rights and values of their clients and families must take precedence when they conflict with those of health care providers
- Ensuring that clients and families are adequately informed to make decisions about their own health and health care
- Being aware that potential conflicts may arise over issues that require consultation, confrontation, or negotiation between the nurses and administrative personnel or between the nurse and physician
- Working with unfamiliar community agencies or lay practitioners

Advocacy may also require political action—communicating a client's health care needs to government and other officials who have the authority to do something about these needs.

Reflect on...

- risks the nurse takes when assuming an advocacy role. What benefits might the nurse realize when acting as an advocate?
- factors that would make the nurse an appropriate or inappropriate advocate for a client. In what situations might you feel personally compromised as the client's advocate?
- what client advocacy needs may be required as a result of changes in technology.
- what societal situations require professional nursing advocacy.

Evidence for Practice

Foley, B. J., Minick, M., & Kee, C. (2002). How nurses learn advocacy. *Journal of Nursing Scholarship,* *34*(2), 181–186.

A phenomenologic study was done to describe how nurses develop the skill of advocating for patients. Interviews were done with U.S. Army nurses who cared for patients associated with the military operation in Bosnia. Sixty-two nurses participated, representing seven Army hospital units; 24 were in active duty and 38 were in the Army reserves. Each interview lasted about 1½ hours beginning with a request for stories that reflected their experiences during the military operation when they assumed a patient advocate role. Following their stories, the nurses were asked how they believed that they had learned patient advocacy skills. The interviews were transcribed and analyzed using interpretive hermeneutics. Three themes arose from the analysis. The first was that advocacy was rooted in who they were rather than resulting from a learning process. The second was that by watching other nurses interact with patients and talking with them about what they did, they also learned advocating practices. The third theme was that confidence was acquired from working with mentors and gaining experience in a supportive environment. The researchers suggest that the use of clinical preceptors may help new nurses practice advocacy.

EXPLORE MEDIALINK

Questions, critical thinking exercises, essay activities, and other interactive resources for this chapter can be found on the Web site at http://www.prenhall.com/blais. Click on Chapter 4 to select activities for this chapter.

SUMMARY

Values give direction and meaning to life and guide a person's behavior. They are freely chosen, prized and cherished, affirmed to others, and consistently incorporated into one's behavior. Most people derive some values from the society or subgroup of society in which they live. A person may internalize some or all of these values and perceive them as *personal values. Professional values* often reflect and expand on personal values. They are acquired during socialization into nursing—from codes of ethics, nursing experiences, teachers, and peers.

Values clarification is a process in which people identify, examine, and develop their own values. Nurses need to help clients clarify their values as they influence and relate to a particular health problem or to end-of-life issues.

Morality refers to what is right and wrong in conduct, character, or attitude—that is, the requirements necessary for people to live together in society. *Moral behavior* is the way a person perceives those requirements and responds to them. *Moral development* is the pattern of change in moral behavior that occurs with age. According to Kohlberg, moral development progresses through three levels: the premoral or preconventional level; the conventional level; and the postconventional, autonomous, or principled level. Each level has two stages. Gilligan describes three stages in the process of developing an "ethic of care": caring for oneself, caring for others, and caring for self and others.

There are general moral frameworks: teleology, deontology, pragmatism, and caring. Moral principles, such as autonomy, beneficence, nonmaleficence, justice, fidelity, and veracity, are broad, general philosophical concepts. Moral rules, by contrast, are specific prescriptions for actions. Moral issues are those that arouse conscience, are concerned with important values and norms, and evoke words such as *good, bad, right, wrong, should,* and *ought.*

Nursing codes of ethics are formal statements of the profession's ideals and values that serve as a standard for professional actions and inform the public of its commitment.

Ethical problems are created as a result of changes in society, advances in technology, conflicts within the nursing role itself, and nurses' conflicting loyalties and obligations to clients, families, employees, physicians, and other nurses. Decision-focused problems are those in which it is difficult to arrive at a decision; they can be relieved by improving one's decision-making skills. Action-focused problems arise when nurses believe they know the right action but cannot act on their judgment without great personal risk; improved decision-making skills will not relieve the effects of these problems. Nurses's ethical decisions are influenced by their role perceptions, moral theories and principles, nursing codes of ethics, level of cognitive development, and personal and professional values. The goal of ethical reasoning, in the context of nursing, is to reach a mutual, peaceful agreement that is in the best interests of the client; reaching the agreement may require compromise. Integrity-preserving moral compromise requires shared moral language, a context of mutual respect, and acknowledgment of a situation's moral complexity.

In all situations, nurses are ethically obligated to maintain a nonjudgmental attitude, be honest, and protect the client's right of privacy and confidentiality. To enhance their ethical decision making, nurses can gain a better understanding of their own values and those of other health care professionals; participate on ethics committees, nursing ethics groups, and educational rounds; and help establish an ethical research base. Ethics committees are multidisciplinary bodies that review cases, write guidelines and policies, and provide education and counseling.

The focus of client advocacy is to respect client decisions and enhance client autonomy. Its goal is to protect the rights of clients. Various levels and types of client advocacy include advocacy for self, advocacy for the client, and advocacy for the community of which the nurse is a part. Advocacy is also needed for the profession, which benefits not only nursing but also the public. Its goal is to achieve better health care. A number of challenges face nurses who assume the role of client advocacy.

Bookshelf

Bohjalian, C. (1997). *Midwives.* **New York: Harmony Books.**
This book is a novel about a lay midwife accused of killing a patient during a difficult delivery. The story centers around her ethical dilemmas.

Caplan, A. L. (1997). *Am I my brother's keeper? The ethical frontiers of biomedicine.* **Bloomington, IN: Indiana University Press.**
This book discusses the need for compassion in relation to the needs of others. It suggests that an excessive reliance on defense of rights and adversarial roles means that a moral framework is overlooked.

Ikeda, D., Bourgeault, G., & Simard, R. (2003). *On being human: Where ethics, medicine and spirituality converge.* **Chicago, IL: Middleway Press.**
It explores what it means to be healthy in a holistic way from the perspectives of Western humanism, Japanese Buddhism, and modern science. A number of ethical issues are examined.

Irving, J. (1999). *The Cider House Rules.* **New York, NY: Ballantine Books.**
This is a fictional story of Dr. Wilbur Larch, an obstretician and founder of an orphanage in rural Maine. Dr. Larch, who is also an ether addict and abortionist, raises an orphan, Homer Wells.

Kidder, R. M. (1996). *How good people make tough choices: Resolving the dilemmas of ethical living.* **New York: Simon and Schuster.**
A good book for beginners in ethical analysis, it uses a practical approach.

Reed, D., & Moore, K. (1988). *Deadly medicine.* **New York: St. Martins Press.**
This book describes why heart patients died in a disastrous clinical trial of a drug.

REFERENCES

American Nurses Association (ANA). (2001). *Code of ethics for nurses with interpretive statements.* Washington, DC: ANA.

American Nurses Association. (2004). *Nursing: Scope and standards of practice.* Washington, DC: ANA.

Australian Nursing Council, Inc. (2004). *Code of Ethics for Nurses in Australia* http://www.anci.org.au.

Baldwin, M. (2003). Patient advocacy: A concept analysis. *Nursing Standard, 17*(21), 33–39.

Benner, P., and Wrubel, J. (1989). *The primacy of caring.* Redwood City, CA: Addison-Wesley Nursing.

Bok, S. (1992). *Moral choice in public and private life.* New York: Pantheon Books. As cited in J. R. Ellis & C. L. Hartley, 1992, *Nursing in today's world* (4th ed.). Philadelphia: Lippincott.

Canadian Nurses' Association (CNA). (1996). *Code of ethics for nursing.* CRNA. Ottawa: CNA.

Cassells, J., & Redman, B. (1989, June). Preparing students to be moral agents in clinical nursing practice. *Nursing Clinics of North America, 24,* 463–473.

Catalano, J. (2000). *Nursing now: Today's issues, tomorrow's trends* (2nd ed.). Philadelphia: F. A. Davis.

Colby, A., & Kohlberg, L. (1987). *The measurement of moral judgment: Theoretical foundations and research validation* (Vol. 1). New York: Cambridge University Press.

Davis, A., & Aroskar, M. (1991). *Ethical dilemmas and nursing practice* (3rd ed.). Norwalk, CT: Appleton and Lange.

Donahue, M. P. (1985). The viewpoints. Euthanasia: An ethical uncertainty. In J. C. McClosky & H. K. Grace, *Current issues in nursing* (2nd ed.). Boston: Blackwell Scientific Publications.

Duska, R., & Whelan, M. (1975). *Moral development: A guide to Piaget and Kohlberg.* New York: Paulist Press.

Foley, B. J., Minick, M., & Kee, C. (2002). How nurses learn advocacy. *Journal of Nursing Scholarship, 34*(2), 181–186.

Fry, S., & Veatch, T. (2000). *Case studies in nursing ethics* (2nd ed.). Boston: Jones and Bartlett.

Gates, B. (1995). Advocacy: Whose best interest? *Nursing Times, 91*(4), 31–32.

Gilligan, C. (1982). *In a different voice*. Cambridge, MA: Harvard University Press.

Gilligan, C., & Attanucci, J. (1988, July). Two moral orientations: Gender differences and similarities. *Merrill-Palmer Quarterly, 34*(3), 223–237.

Hamric, A. B. (1999). Ethics: The nurse as moral agent in modern health care. *Nursing Outlook, 47*(3), 106.

Heubner, A. M., & Garrod, A. C. (1993). Moral reasoning among Tibetian monks: A study of Buddhist adolescents and young adults in Nepal. *Journal of Cross Cultural Psychology, 24*(2), 167–185.

Husted, G. L., & Husted, J. H. (2001). *Ethical decision-making in nursing and healthcare* (3rd ed.). New York: Springer Publishing Co.

International Council of Nurses. (1973). *ICN code for nurses: Ethical concepts applied to nursing*. Geneva: Imprimeries Populaires.

Jameton, A. (1984). *Nursing practice: The ethical issues*. Upper Saddle River, NJ: Prentice Hall.

Lei, T. (1994). Being and becoming moral in a Chinese culture: Unique or universal? *Cross-Cultural Research: The Journal of Comparative Social Science, 28*(1), 59–91.

Miller, J. (1994). Cultural diversity in the morality of caring: Individually oriented versus duty-based interpersonal moral codes. *Cross-Cultural Research: The Journal of Comparative Social Science, 28*(1), 3–39.

Munhall, P. L. (1982, June). Moral development: A prerequisite. *Journal of Nursing Education, 21*, 11–15.

Raths, L., Harmin, M., & Simon, S. (1978). *Values and teaching* (2nd ed.). Columbus, OH: Merrill.

Raths, L., Harmin, M., & Simon, S. (1966). Values clarification. In M. D. M. Fowler & J. Levine-Ariff, 1987, *Ethics at the bedside*. Philadelphia: Lippincott.

Rodney, P., and Starzomski, R. (1993, October). Constraints on the moral agency of nurses. *Canadian Nurse, 89*, 23–26.

Schroeter, K., Derse, A., Junkerman, C., & Schiedermayer, D. (2002). *Practical ethics for nurses and nursing students*. Hagerstown, MD: University Publishing Group.

Steele, S. M., & Harmon, V. M. (1983). *Values clarification in nursing* (2nd ed.). Norwalk, CT: Appleton-Century-Crofts.

Thompson, I., Melia, K., & Boyd, K. (2000). *Nursing ethics*. (4th ed.). New York: Churchill Livingstone.

Tudin, P., Straker, G., & Mendolsohn, M. (1994). Social and political complexity and moral development. *South African Journal of Psychology, 24*(3), 163–168.

Watson, J. (1985). *Nursing: Human science and human care*. Norwalk, CT: Appleton-Century-Crofts.

Wilkinson, J. (1993, January). All ethics problems are not created equal. *The Kansas Nurse, 68*(1), 4–6.

Winslow, B. J., and Winslow, G. R. (1991, June). Integrity and compromise in nursing ethics. *The Journal of Medicine and Philosophy, 16*, 307–323.

Legal Foundations of Professional Nursing

Objectives

- Identify primary sources of law and types of legal actions.
- Describe how nurse practice acts direct nursing.
- Discuss essential legal aspects of malpractice, informed consent, adverse event reports, DNR orders, euthanasia, and death-related issues.
- Examine the nurse's role in identifying and assisting the chemically impaired nurse.
- Examine the problem of sexual harassment in nursing.
- Consider how the collective bargaining process is used to improve nursing practice.

M E D I A L I N K

Additional online resources for this chapter can be found on the companion Web site at http://www.prenhall.com/blais.

Knowledge of legal rights and responsibilities related to nursing practice is essential for the nurse. In the past, nurses were not considered responsible for their actions. In fact, the hospital, physician, or clinic assumed responsibility for a nurse's actions. In the nineteenth century, life was fairly simple, and questions were uncomplicated. Medical advances were few. The roles of physicians and nurses were to support patients through times of illness, helping them toward recovery or keeping them comfortable until death. The nurse acted as a caregiver and physician-helper. However, as nursing practice became more autonomous, nurses have held increasing responsibility for their actions as well as the actions of those they supervise. Understanding one's own rights and responsibilities as a registered nurse, as well as those of others, is essential for competent and safe nursing practice. Standards of practice, codes of ethics, and established laws act as guides for nursing practice.

In 1938, New York State passed the first nurse practice act, which was implemented in 1949. By 1952, all states had nurse practice acts. Nurse practice acts control the practice of nursing through licensing. They legally define the practice of nursing within the specific state, thereby describing the scope of nursing and protecting the public. They also set the requirements for licensure, including educational requirements, and they describe the legal titles and abbreviations that a nurse may use.

CHALLENGES AND OPPORTUNITIES

The latter part of the twentieth century introduced life-saving technology. The creation of critical care units, new surgical techniques for organ transplants and the development of medications to prevent rejection, and the ability to keep individuals alive on life support presented challenges for nurses. These advances led to the development of advance directives, such as living wills, and the creation of health care surrogates. In many situations, nurses needed to act as client advocates.

Scientific development and new technological advances in the 21st century will create situations and questions that may be resolved only in courts of law. Genetic engineering and the identification of disease-carrying genes present problems regarding confidentiality and possible discrimination. As client advocates, nurses find themselves on the front line in many of these situations. Analysis, discussion, and debate among nurses, other health care providers, ethicists, and attorneys will take place to develop an under-

standing and agreement on public policy and laws regarding these scientific advances.

Changes in the health care system have provided new opportunities for nursing. The roles of the advanced practice nurse (APN) and clinical specialist have taken on new dimensions. APNs act as primary care providers in areas such as emergency care, critical care, and community health. Many work as first surgical assistants. Additionally, APNs work as nurse midwives and nurse anesthetists. With these expanded roles come added responsibilities and legal issues.

Nurses will need to understand the legalities involved with these new technologies to practice safely and effectively. Dock (1907, p. 896) emphasized, "it is essential that nurses as trained workers exercise social awareness." Scientific achievements have opened up new ground for nursing exploration. Nurses can find career opportunities as forensic nurses, legal nurse consultants, and nurse-attorneys.

THE JUDICIAL SYSTEM

The judicial systems in both the United States and Canada have their origins in the English common law system. Three primary sources of law are constitutions, statutes, and decisions of court (common law).

Constitutions

The constitution of a country constitutes the supreme laws of the country. The Constitution of the United States, which was ratified in 1787, establishes the general organization of the federal government into the executive, legislative, and judicial branches; grants certain powers to each branch; and places limits on what federal and state governments may do. Constitutions create legal rights and responsibilities and are the foundation for a system of justice. The individual states also have constitutions, but state statutes and regulations must be consistent with the principles contained in the Constitution of the United States (Monarch, 2002).

Legislation (Statutes)

Laws enacted by any legislative body are called statutory laws. When federal and state laws (or, in Canada, provincial laws) conflict, federal law supersedes. Likewise, state or provincial laws supersede local laws.

The regulation of nursing is a function of state or provincial law. State or provincial legislatures pass statutes that define and regulate nursing; these statutes are known as nurse practice acts. These acts, however, must be consistent with constitutional and federal provisions. The Patient Self-Determination Act of 1991 enables clients to participate in decisions about their care, including the right to refuse treatment, even if such treatment is necessary to preserve life. This act requires that hospitals and other health care organizations receiving payment through Medicare and Medicaid do the following:

- Tell clients that they have the right to declare their personal wishes regarding treatment decisions, including the right to refuse medical treatment.
- Inform the client regarding the hospital's policy on how advance directives are honored.
- Provide a written statement on the client's chart indicating whether the client has an advance directive. A copy of the advance directive should be included on the client's chart.
- Provide staff and community education on advance directives.

Nurse practice acts, Good Samaritan laws, and laws regarding spouse or child abuse are other examples of statutes that affect nurses.

Common Law

The body of principles that evolves from court decisions is referred to as common law, or *decisional law*. Common law is continually being adapted and expanded. To arrive at a ruling in a particular case, a court applies the same rules and principles applied in previous, similar cases; this practice is known as following precedent. Courts may depart from precedent when slight differences are noted between cases or when it is thought that a particular common law rule no longer applies to the needs of society. See Table 5–1 for types of laws that affect nurses.

Types of Legal Actions

There are two kinds of legal actions: civil (private) actions and criminal actions. Civil actions deal with conflicts between individuals; for example, a man may file a suit against a person he believes cheated him. Criminal actions deal with disputes between an individual and the society as a whole: for example, if a man shoots a person, society, through the actions of the court, brings him to trial.

SAFEGUARDING THE PUBLIC

The first laws applicable to nursing in the United States were passed in the 1890s. These were "permissive" laws because they placed no restrictions on nurs-

Table 5–1 Types of Laws Affecting Nurses

Category	Examples
Constitutional	Due process Equal protection
Statutory (legislative)	Nurse practice acts Good Samaritan acts Child and adult abuse laws Living wills Sexual harassment laws Americans with Disabilities Act
Criminal (public)	Homicide, manslaughter Theft Arson Active euthanasia Sexual assault Illegal possession of controlled drugs
Contracts (private/civil)	Nurse and client Nurse and employer Nurse and insurance Client and agency
Torts (private/civil)	Negligence Libel and slander Invasion of privacy Assault and battery False imprisonment Abandonment

ing practice, stating that the registered nurse (RN) title could be used by individuals who were registered and paid the required fee. By 1923 all states had nurse registration laws.

In 1981 the ANA published a document, *The Nursing Practice Act: Suggested State Legislation*, to serve as a guide for states in developing their nurse practice acts. This document described nursing practice as including but not limited to "administration, teaching, counseling, supervision, delegation, and evaluation of practice and execution of the medical regimen, including the administration of medications and treatments prescribed by any person authorized by state law to prescribe" (ANA, 1981, p. 6).

The state authority that has responsibility for the regulation of nursing practice within a state is the state board of nursing. The boards of nursing are authorized to develop administrative rules, regulations and responsibilities related to the nurse practice act and to enforce the rules to obtain and maintain licensure. The boards are appointed by the governor and usually consist of RNs, licensed practical nurses (LPNs), and consumers of nursing. State boards may be independent agencies of the state government or part of a bureau or department, such as the department of licensure and regulation. The National Council of State Boards of Nursing (NCSBN) comprises all the state boards of nursing. The Nursing Practice and Education Committee of the NCSBN is working to develop uniform core licensure requirements and to develop collaborative licensure agreements between states (NCSBN, 2004). In 1990, the American Nurses Association published *A Guideline for Suggested State Legislation* to help state nurses' associations revise their nurse practice acts. In 2002, the NCSBN updated the Model Nursing Practice Act to recognize that nursing is an evolving profession that has overlapping functions with other health care providers. This document also identifies that nurses practice based on established standards and evidence-based practice guidelines developed by recognized authorities. State boards of nursing and state nurses associations usually collaborate in the development or revision of the state nurse practice act. The nurse practice act usually:

■ Defines the authority of the board of nursing, its composition, and its powers
■ Defines nursing and the boundaries of the scope of nursing practice
■ Identifies types of licenses and titles
■ States the requirements for licensure
■ Protects titles
■ Identifies grounds for disciplinary action.

Because registered nurses not only provide care to patients and clients directly but also supervise the care given by others, state nurse practice acts permit professional nurses to delegate, but they do not permit delegating by licensed vocational/practical nurses. An important aspect of the delegation process is the ethical responsibility of delegatees to refuse any responsibilities for activities that they do not have the expertise to carry out safely and competently. This applies even if hospital policies, physicians, and other nurses request these activities be carried out.

CREDENTIALING

Credentialing is the process of determining and maintaining competence in nursing practice. The credentialing process is one way in which the nursing profession maintains standards of practice and accountability for the educational preparation of its members. Credentialing includes licensure, registration, certification, and accreditation.

Licensure

Licensure is defined by the National Council of State Boards of Nursing as the "process by which an agency of state government grants permission to an individual to engage in a given profession upon finding that the applicant has attained the essential degree of competency necessary to perform a unique scope of practice" (NCSBN, 2004). Licenses are legal permits a government agency grants to individuals to engage in the practice of a profession and to use a particular title. A particular jurisdiction or area is covered by the license.

There are two types of licensure: mandatory and permissive. Under *mandatory licensure*, anyone who practices nursing must be licensed. Under *permissive licensure*, the title RN is reserved for licensed or, in Canada, registered practitioners, but the practice of nursing is not prohibited to others who are not licensed or registered. In the United States, nursing licensure is mandatory in all states.

In each state there is a mechanism by which licenses (or registration in Canada) can be revoked for just cause, for example, incompetent nursing practice, professional misconduct, or conviction for a crime, such as using illegal drugs or selling drugs illegally. In each situation, all the facts are generally reviewed by a committee at a hearing. Nurses are entitled to be represented by legal counsel at such a hearing. If the nurse's license is revoked as a result of the hearing, either the nurse can appeal the decision to a court of law, or, in some states, an agency is designated to review the decision before any court action is initiated.

In recent years, changes in the delivery of nursing and health care and increasing use of communication technology, for example, telehealth, have led to questions about one state licensure. Nurses who are licensed in one state may be providing direct care or patient education to clients in another state. Additionally, emergency situations such as earthquakes, hurricanes, or man-made disasters have resulted in states having unexpected and abrupt needs for increased numbers of professional staff from outside the state to assist victims. In response to these changes, the National Council of State Boards of Nursing is developing two mechanisms to assist states meet these situations: Mutual Recognition Model and Interstate Compact. In the Mutual Recognition Model, nurses would be able to practice electronically or in person across state lines with one license. An Interstate Compact is an agreement between two or more states to create mutual recognition among the states. Nurses can obtain information about these licensure innovations from the NCSBN Web site.

For advanced nursing practice, many states require a different license or have an additional clause that pertains to actions that may be performed only by nurses with advanced education. For example, an additional license may be required to practice as a nurse midwife, nurse anesthetist, or nurse practitioner. The advanced practice nurse also requires a license to be able to prescribe medication or order treatment from physical therapists or other health professionals. There is some controversy about the requirement for additional licensure for advanced practice. The ANA's position is that it is the function of the professional association, not the law, to establish the scope of practice for advanced nursing practice and that the state boards of nursing can regulate advanced nursing practice within each state (ANA, 1993b).

Reflect on...

- the nurse practice act in your state or province. What are the actions of the nurse that are permitted under your nurse practice act? What actions are prohibited? What actions of nurse colleagues are you responsible for reporting? What are the requirements for initial licensure? Renewal of licensure? How do you feel about the regulation of nursing practice in your state? What changes would you suggest? Why?
- the nurse practice act in your state as it regulates advanced practice. Is there separate licensure or certification required for advanced practice? What are the criteria to practice in an advanced practice role in your state? How do you feel about the regulation of advanced practice in your state? What changes would your suggest? Why?

Registration

Registration is the listing of an individual's name and other information on the official roster of a governmental or nongovernmental agency. Nurses who are registered are permitted to use the title "Registered Nurse."

In the United States, all registered nurses are licensed by the board of nursing of the state; in Canada, they are licensed or registered by the provincial nursing association or college of nursing. The requirements for licensure vary by state and province. In the United States, all nursing candidates write the National Council Licensure Examinations (NCLEX) for registered nursing or practical nursing.

In Canada, applicants take the Canadian Registered Nurse Examination (CRNE) to obtain registration/licensure. Nurses from other countries are granted registration by endorsement after successfully completing this examination. Both licensure and registration must be renewed on an annual basis (in some states, every two years) to remain valid.

Certification

Certification is the voluntary practice of validating that an individual nurse has met minimum standards of nursing competence in specialty or advanced practice areas, such as maternal-child health, pediatrics, mental health, and gerontology. Certification programs are conducted by the American Nurses Credentialing Center (an affiliate organization of the American Nurses Association) and by specialty nursing organizations. In Canada, the Canadian Nurses Association (CNA) certifies nurses in a number of specialized fields of nursing.

Reflect on...

- specialty certification in your practice setting. What are the requirements for certification in your practice area? Are you certified in a specialty area of practice? What are the personal and professional benefits of certification in your practice setting?

Accreditation

Accreditation is a process by which a voluntary organization, such as the National League for Nursing Accrediting Commission (NLNAC) or the American Association of Colleges of Nursing (AACN), or governmental agency, such as the state board of nursing, appraises and grants accredited status to institutions and/or programs or services that meet predetermined standards and measurement criteria. Minimum standards for basic nursing education programs are established in each state of the United States and in each province in Canada. State accreditation or provincial approval is granted to schools of nursing meeting the minimum criteria.

According to the American Association of Colleges of Nursing, accreditation is intended to "hold nursing education programs accountable to the community of interest—the nursing profession, consumers, employers, higher education, students and their families . . . " and "to foster continuing improvement in nursing education programs"—thereby resulting in improvement in professional practice (AACN, 2004). Achievement of accreditation indicates to the general public and to the educational community that a nursing program has clear and appropriate educational objectives and is providing the conditions under which its objectives can be fulfilled. The NLNAC provides accreditation for schools of nursing from practical or vocational nursing through master's level nursing education. The American Association of Colleges of Nursing accredits nursing programs at the baccalaureate and master's levels.

Standards of Care

Another way the nursing profession attempts to ensure that its practitioners are competent and safe to practice is through the establishment of standards of practice. These standards are often used to evaluate the quality of care nurses provide. In addition to this basic set of standards, which are applicable in any practice setting, the ANA has developed standards of nursing practice for specific areas such as maternal-child, medical-surgical, geriatric, psychiatric, and community health nursing.

Standards have also been developed for Medicare and Medicaid clients. The Joint Commission for Accreditation of Healthcare Organizations (JCAHO) has developed accreditation standards that help ensure specific levels of care in hospitals and other health care organizations. In addition, individual health care agencies have developed standard care plans intended to reflect a standard of care. Specific nursing measures that promote safe nursing practice are shown in the accompanying box.

POTENTIAL LIABILITY AREAS

Malpractice

Malpractice is defined as "professional misconduct, or the failure to meet the requisite standard of care. The alleged misconduct may be intentional or unintentional" (Monarch, 2002, p. 74). The elements of proof for nursing malpractice are (1) a duty of the nurse to the client to provide care and follow an acceptable standard, (2) a breach of the duty on the part of the nurse, (3) an injury to the client, and (4) a causal relationship between the breach of the duty and the client's subsequent injury. A nurse could be liable for malpractice if the nurse injures a client while performing a procedure differently from the way other nurses would have done it.

Malpractice suits may result from untoward patient outcomes or injury related to patient falls, operating room errors, medication errors, or other negligent acts on the part of the health care provider. "According to the Institute of Medicine (IOM), 44,000 to 98,000 deaths occur from medical errors each year" (Kohn, 2000). This report suggested a mandatory medical-error reporting system, including a national patient safety center. The reporting system and safety center would work together to decrease system errors. To create this system, *error* must be defined. The IOM defines error "as the failure of a planned action to be completed as intended or the use of a wrong plan to achieve an aim" (Kohn, 2000). In court, error is not necessarily equated with legal liability. Therefore, an error in judgment may not necessarily have the elements necessary to constitute professional negligence.

Nursing Measures That Protect Nurses and Clients

- Know your job description.
- Follow the policies and procedures of the agency in which you are employed.
- Always identify clients before implementing nursing activities.
- Report all incidents or accidents involving clients.
- Maintain your clinical competence.
- Know your own strengths and weaknesses.
- Question any order a client questions.
- Question any order if a client's condition has changed since it was written.
- Question and record verbal orders to avoid miscommunication.
- Question standing orders if you are inexperienced in the particular area.

Nurses are responsible for their own actions, whether they are independent practitioners or employees of a health agency. The descriptions of malpractice do not mention good intentions; it is not pertinent that the nurse did not intend to be negligent. If a nurse administers an incorrect medication, even in good faith, the fact that the nurse failed to read the label correctly indicates malpractice if all the conditions of negligence are met.

Another significant aspect of malpractice is that it encompasses both omissions and commissions; that is, a nurse can be negligent by forgetting to give a medication as well as by giving the wrong medication.

To avoid charges of malpractice, nurses need to recognize nursing situations in which negligent actions are most likely to occur and to take measures to prevent them. The most common situations are medication errors, burning a client, client falls, and failure to assess and take appropriate action. The Agency for Healthcare Research and Quality (AHRQ, 2004, p. 4) has suggested several strategies to reduce medical errors. Strategies related to nursing care include:

- Those that help to increase staffing levels of licensed and unlicensed nurses in both acute-care hospitals and nursing homes will likely lead to improved patient outcomes.
- The duration of experience of the health professional is associated with better patient outcomes for some types of clinical care.
- Those systems that reduce interruptions and distractions will likely reduce the incidence of medical errors.
- Those systems that improve information exchange, transfer of responsibility, and continuity of care between hospital and nonhospital settings decrease medication errors and, in some settings, hospital readmissions.

Medication errors account for a large number of deaths each year (Kohn, 2000). Many individuals receive either the wrong medication or the right medication but the wrong dosage. Some patients never receive their ordered medication. In addition to medication errors, other causes of medical errors include diagnostic errors resulting in misdiagnosis; equipment failure; infections, such as nosocomial and post-surgical wound infections; blood transfusion–related injuries; and misinterpretation of medical orders such as failing to provide a therapeutic diet as ordered to a client.

Because of the increase in the number of malpractice lawsuits against health professionals, nurses are advised in many areas to carry their own liability insurance. Most hospitals have liability insurance that covers all employees, including all nurses. However, some smaller facilities, such as "walk-in" clinics, may not. Thus the nurse should always check with the employer at the time of hiring to see what coverage the facility provides. A physician or a hospital can be sued because of the negligent conduct of a nurse, and the nurse can also be sued and held liable for negligence or malpractice. Because hospitals have been known to counter-sue nurses when they have been found negligent and the hospital was required to pay, nurses are advised to obtain their own insurance coverage and not rely on hospital-provided insurance.

Liability insurance coverage usually defrays all costs of defending a nurse, including the costs of retaining an attorney. The insurance also covers all costs incurred by the nurse up to the face value of the policy, including a settlement made out of court. In return, the insurance company may have the right to make the decisions about the claim and the settlement.

In the United States, insurance can be obtained through the ANA or private insurance companies; in Canada, it can usually be obtained through provincial nurses' associations. Nursing students in the United States can also obtain insurance through the National Student Nurses Association. In some states, hospitals do not allow nursing students to provide nursing care without liability insurance.

Documentation

The old adage, not documented-not done, holds true in nursing. According to the law, if something is not documented, then the responsible party did not do whatever needed to be done. If the nurse did not carry out or complete an activity or documented it incorrectly, he or she is open to a charge of negligence or malpractice. Nursing documentation needs to be legally credible; that is, it must give an accurate accounting of the care the client received. Tappen, Weiss, and Whitehead (2004) assert that documentation is credible when it is the following:

- *Contemporaneous*—care is documented at the time it is provided.
- *Accurate*—a factual account is given of what the nurse did and how the client responded.
- *Truthful*—documentation includes an honest account of what was actually done or observed.
- *Appropriate*—only what one would be comfortable discussing in a public setting is documented.

The client's medical record is a legal document and can be produced in court as evidence. Often, the record is used to remind a witness of events surrounding a lawsuit, because several months or years usually

Guidelines for Documentation

MEDICATIONS

- Always chart the time, route, dose, and response.
- Always chart prn medications and the client response.
- Always chart when a medication was not given, the reason, and the nursing intervention.
- Chart all medication refusals and report them to the appropriate person.

PHYSICIANS

- Document each time a call to a physician is made, even if he or she is not reached. Include the exact time of the call. If the physician is reached, document the details of the message and the physician's response.
- Read verbal orders back to the physician and clarify the client's name on the chart to confirm the client's identity.
- Chart verbal orders only if you have heard them, not those told to you by another nurse or unit personnel.

FORMAL ISSUES IN CHARTING

- Before writing, check to be sure you have the correct client record.
- Check to make sure each page has the client's name and date stamped in the appropriate area.
- If you forget to make an entry, chart "late entry" and place the date and time at the entry.
- Correct all charting mistakes according to the policy and procedures of your institution.
- Chart in an organized fashion following the nursing process.
- Write legibly and concisely, avoiding subjective statements.
- Write specific and accurate descriptions.
- When charting a symptom or situation, chart the interventions taken and the client response.
- Document your own observations, not those that were told to you.
- Chart frequently to demonstrate ongoing care, and chart routine activities.
- Chart client and family teaching and the response.

Source: Essentials of Nursing Leadership and Management (3rd ed., p. 216), by R. M. Tappan, S. A. Weiss, and D. K. Whitehead, 2004. Philadelphia: F. A. Davis.

elapse before the suit goes to trial. The effectiveness of a witness's testimony can depend on the accuracy of such records. Therefore, nurses need to keep accurate and complete records of nursing care provided to clients. Failure to keep proper records can constitute negligence and be the basis for tort liability. Insufficient or inaccurate assessments and documentation can hinder proper diagnosis and treatment and result in injury to the client. The accompanying box provides guidelines for appropriate documentation.

Delegation

The American Nurses Association *Code of Ethics for Nurses with Interpretive Statements* (2001, p. 17) states, "since the nurse is accountable for the quality of nursing care given to patients, nurses are accountable for the assignment of nursing responsibilities to other nurses and the delegation of nursing care activities to other health care workers." The nurse is accountable for the care given to his or her clients even if that care

has been delegated to a subordinate. In 1990 the National Council of State Boards of Nursing (NCSBN) defined delegation as the "transferring to a competent individual the authority to perform a selected nursing task in a selected situation" (NCSBN, 1997, p. 2). This definition was reaffirmed in 1995. To delegate tasks safely, nurses must delegate appropriately and supervise adequately (Barter & Furmidge, 1994).

In 1997, the NCSBN developed the *Delegation Decision-Making Grid* to help nurses delegate appropriately. The grid provides a scoring instrument for seven categories the nurse should consider when making delegation decisions. The categories for the grid are listed in the box on page 81. The scoring of the components helps the nurse evaluate situations, client needs, and health care personnel available to meet client needs. A low score on the grid states that the activity may be safely delegated to personnel other than the registered nurse, whereas a high score indicates that delegation may not be advisable.

Components of the *Delegation Decision-Making Grid*

- Level of client acuity
- Level of unlicensed assistive personnel (UAP) capability
- Level of licensed nurse capability
- Possibility for injury

- Number of times the skill has been performed by the UAP
- Level of decision making needed for the activity
- Client's ability for self-care

Source: Adapted from the National Council of State Boards of Nursing *Delegation Decision-Making Grid,* by the National Council of State Boards of Nursing, Inc., 1997. Retrieved from http://www.ncsbn.com.

Nurses who delegate tasks to unlicensed assistive personnel should evaluate the activities being considered for delegation (Herrick et al., 1994). The American Association of Critical Care Nurses (AACN) (1990) recommends consideration of five factors affecting the decision to delegate: (1) potential for harm, (2) complexity of task, (3) problem solving and necessary innovation, (4) unpredictability of outcome, and (5) level of interaction with the client required.

It is the responsibility of the nurse to be well acquainted with the state nurse practice acts and regulations issued by the state board of nursing regarding unlicensed assistive personnel. State laws and regulations supersede any publications or opinions set forth by professional organizations.

Reflect on...

- the responsibilities for delegation in your practice setting. What policies exist in your practice setting to ensure responsible delegation of nursing care? What are the qualifications of your colleagues to whom you delegate aspects of nursing care?

Informed Consent

Informed consent is an agreement by a client to accept a course of treatment or a procedure after complete information, including the risks of treatment and facts relating to it, has been provided by the physician. Informed consent, then, is an exchange between a client and a physician. Usually, the client signs a form provided by the agency. The form is a record of the informed consent, not the informed consent itself.

Obtaining informed consent for specific medical and surgical treatments is the responsibility of a physician. Although this responsibility is delegated to nurses in some agencies and there are no laws that prohibit the nurse from being part of the information-giving process, the practice nevertheless is highly undesirable (Aiken & Catalano, 1994, p. 104). Often, the nurse's responsibility is to witness the giving of informed consent. This involves the following:

- Witnessing the exchange between the client and the physician
- Establishing that the client really did understand, that is, was really informed
- Witnessing the client's signature

If a nurse witnesses only the client's signature and not the exchange between the client and the physician, the nurse should write "witnessing signature only" on the form. If the nurse finds that the client really does not understand the physician's explanation, the physician must be notified.

There are three major elements of informed consent:

1. The consent must be given voluntarily.
2. The consent must be given by an individual with the capacity and competence to understand.
3. The client must be given enough information to be the ultimate decision maker.

To give informed consent voluntarily, the client must not feel coerced. Sometimes fear of disapproval by a health professional can be the motivation for giving consent; such consent is not voluntarily given.

To give informed consent, the client must receive sufficient information to make a decision; otherwise, the client's right to decide has been usurped. Information needs to include the purpose and expected outcomes of the treatment, benefits, risks, and alternative procedures. It is also important that the client

Evidence for Practice

Anthony, M. K., Standing, T., & Hertz, J. E. (2000). Factors influencing outcomes after delegation to unlicensed assistive personnel. *Journal of Nursing Administration*, 30(10), 474–481.
The purpose of the study was to examine factors related to the outcomes of delegated nursing activities. There were four research questions: (1) How do characteristics of the practice setting influence outcomes of delegated nursing activities? (2) How do the educational and experiential backgrounds of licensed nurses and unlicensed assistive personnal (UAPs) influence the outcomes of delegated nursing activities? (3) How do factors related to supervision influence outcomes of delegated nursing activities? (4) Is there a pattern among critical factors related to practice, education, supervision, and the outcome of delegated nursing activities?

A cross-sectional sample of 516 licensed nurses (both registered nurses and licensed practical nurses) working in long-term care, home health care, and acute-care settings across the United States were sent questionnaires; 148 were returned. The respondents were asked to write about two events of which they had personal knowledge that involved delegation to and supervision of UAPs. One event resulted in a positive outcome, and the other had a potential or actual negative outcome. Several questions asking for specific information about the events were included. A chi-square analysis showed no significant differences between patient conditions and positive or negative outcomes. There was no significant difference between positive and negative outcomes and the nurse's educational preparation. The manner in which the UAP was supervised was significantly different between positive and negative events; no direct observation was associated with more negative outcomes. Routine observations resulted in more positive outcomes. The greater the length of time the UAP had worked in the area was also associated with greater frequency of positive outcomes. In the delegation process, outcomes were affected by the experience of the UAP and the supervisory behaviors of the nurse.

---

understand. Technical words and language barriers can inhibit understanding. If a client cannot read, the consent form must be read to the client before it is signed. If the client does not speak the same language as the health professional who is providing the information, an interpreter must be acquired. See Chapter 21 ⚭, Nursing in a Culturally Diverse World to see guidelines for using an interpreter.

If given sufficient information, the client can make decisions regarding health. To do so, the client must be competent and an adult. A competent adult is a person over 18 years of age who is conscious and oriented. A person under 18 years who is considered "an emancipated minor" (i.e., self-supporting or married) can also give consent. A client who is confused, disoriented, or sedated is not considered functionally competent at that time.

There are three groups of people who cannot provide consent. The first is *minors*. In most areas, a parent or guardian must give consent before minors can obtain treatment. The same is true for adults who are not mentally competent to make decisions for themselves and have a legal guardian. In some states, however, minors are allowed to give consent for such procedures as blood donations, treatment for drug dependence and sexually transmitted disease, and procedures for obstetric care. The second group is *persons who are unconscious or injured* in such a way that they are unable to give consent. In these situations, consent is usually obtained from the closest adult relative if existing statutes permit. In a life-threatening emergency, if consent cannot be obtained from the client or a relative, then the law generally agrees that consent is assumed. This is referred to as implied consent. The third group is *mentally ill persons* who have been judged to be incompetent. State and provincial mental health acts or similar statutes generally provide definitions of mental illness and specify the rights of the mentally ill under the law as well as the rights of the staff caring for such clients.

Adverse Events and Risk Management

An adverse event report, also called an unusual occurrence or incident report, is an agency record of an adverse event or unusual occurrence that is required by JCAHO. Adverse events include medication errors, patient falls, equipment malfunction, surgical errors, and other incidents that may be preventable. Adverse

Information to Include in an Adverse Event Report

- Identify the client by name, initials, and hospital or identification number.
- Give the date, time, and place of the incident.
- Describe the facts of the incident. Avoid any conclusions or blame. Describe the incident as you saw it even if your impressions differ from those of others.
- Identify all witnesses to the incident.
- Identify any equipment by number and any medication by name and number.
- Document any circumstance surrounding the incident, for example, that another client was experiencing cardiac arrest.

event reports are used to make all the facts about an unusual occurrence available to agency personnel, to contribute to statistical data about adverse events, and to help health care personnel prevent future incidents. All adverse events are usually reported on adverse event report forms and are usually filed with the agency's risk-management department. The accompanying box lists information to be included in an adverse event report. The report should be completed as soon as possible, always within 24 hours of the incident, and filed according to agency policy. Because adverse event reports are not part of the client's medical record, the facts of the incident should also be noted in the medical record. Adverse event reports are used not only to report incidents related to direct client care, but also to report occupational injuries of employees, such as needle-stick or back injuries, and injuries to visitors to the agency, such as falls.

The risk-management department reviews all adverse event reports. The purpose of risk management is to "identify risks, control occurrences, prevent damage, and control legal liability" (Huber, 2000, p. 628). The risk-management department decides whether to investigate the incident further. It is important to conduct investigations of adverse events in a nonpunitive atmosphere so that all facts of an incident can be identified. If health care providers feel that they will be punished because an error occurred, they might not reveal facts that might be self-incriminating. When this occurs, ways in which the event could be prevented

may not be realized and corrective action does not occur. The nurse may be required to answer such questions as what the nurse believes precipitated the incident, how it could have been prevented, and whether any equipment should be adjusted. The process of determining the underlying cause of an adverse event is called "root cause analysis." Nurses who believe they may be dismissed or that a suit may be brought against them should obtain legal advice. Even if the risk-management department clears the nurse of responsibility, the client or the client's family may file suit. The plaintiff, however, bears the burden of proving that the incident occurred because reasonable care was not taken. Even if the accepted standard of care was not met, the plaintiff must prove that the incident was the direct result of failure to meet the acceptable standards of care and that the incident caused physical, emotional, or financial injury.

When an adverse event occurs, the nurse should first assess the client and intervene to prevent injury. If the client is injured, nurses must take steps to protect the client, themselves, and their employer. Most agencies have policies regarding incidents. It is important to follow these policies and not to assume someone is negligent. Although negligence may be involved, incidents can and do happen even when every precaution has been taken to prevent them.

Wills

A **will** is a declaration by a person about how the person's property is to be disposed of after death. For a will to be valid the following conditions must be met:

- The person making the will must be of sound mind, that is, able to understand and retain mentally the general nature and extent of the person's own property, the relationship of the beneficiaries and of relatives to whom portions of the estate will be left, and the disposition being made of the property. A person, therefore, who is seriously ill and unable to carry out usual roles but is mentally competent may still be able to direct preparation of a will.
- The person must not be unduly influenced by anyone else. Sometimes a client may be persuaded by someone who is close at that particular time to make that person a beneficiary. Clients sometimes are persuaded to leave their estates to persons looking after them rather than to their relatives. Frequently, the relatives contest the will in such situations and take the matter to court, claiming undue influence.

Nurses may be requested from time to time to witness a will, although most agencies have policies that nurses not do so. In most states and provinces, a will must be signed in the presence of two witnesses. In some situations, a mark can suffice if the person making the will cannot write a signature. When witnessing a will, the nurse (1) attests that the client signed a document that is stated to be the client's last will and (2) attests that the client appears to be mentally sound and appreciates the significance of their actions (Bernzweig, 1996).

If a nurse witnesses a will, the nurse should note on the client's chart the fact that a will was made and the nurse's perception of the physical and mental condition of the client. This record provides the nurse with accurate information if the nurse is called as a witness later. The record may also be helpful if the will is contested. If a nurse does not wish to act as a witness—for example, if in the nurse's opinion undue influence has been brought on the client, then it is the nurse's right to refuse to act in this capacity.

Do-Not-Resuscitate Orders

Physicians may order "no-code" or **do-not-resuscitate (DNR)** for clients who are in a stage of terminal, irreversible illness or expected death. DNR orders require that no effort be made to resuscitate the client in the event of a respiratory or cardiac arrest. The ANA believes that "the appropriate use of DNR orders can prevent suffering for many clients who choose not to extend their lives after experiencing cardiac arrest" (ANA, 1992a, p. 2). The ANA makes the following recommendations related to DNR orders:

- The competent client's values and choices should always be given highest priority, even when these wishes conflict with those of the family or health care providers.
- When the client is incompetent, an advance directive or the surrogate decision makers acting for the client should make health care treatment decisions.
- A DNR decision should always be the subject of explicit discussion between the client, family, any designated surrogate decision maker acting on the client's behalf, and the health care team.
- DNR orders must be clearly documented, reviewed, and updated periodically to reflect changes in the client's condition. Such documentation is required to meet standards of the Joint Commission on Accreditation of Healthcare Organizations (JCAHO, 1996).
- A DNR order is separate from other aspects of a client's care and does not imply that other types of care should be withdrawn, for example, nursing care to ensure comfort or medical treatment for chronic but non–life-threatening illnesses.
- If it is contrary to a nurse's personal beliefs to carry out a DNR order, the nurse should consult the nurse-manager for a change in assignment.

The ANA also recommends that each health care organization put into place mechanisms to resolve conflicts between clients, their families, and health care professionals, or between different health care professionals. Institutional ethics committees usually deal with such conflicts. It is important that nurses be represented on these institutional ethics committees, so that nursing perspectives can be heard and nurses can be involved in developing DNR policies.

Advance Medical Directives

An **advance medical directive** is a statement the client makes before receiving health care, specifying the client's wishes regarding health care decisions. There are three types of advance medical directives, the **living will**, the **health care proxy** or **surrogate**, and the **durable power of attorney for health care**. The living will states what medical treatment the client chooses to omit or refuse in the event that the client is unable to make those decisions and is terminally ill. For example, the client can indicate a wish not to be kept alive by artificial means such as cardiopulmonary resuscitation (CPR), respiratory ventilation, or intravenous or tube feeding. With a health care proxy, the client appoints a proxy, usually a relative or trusted friend, to make medical decisions on the client's behalf in the event that the client is unable to do so. The health care proxy is not limited to terminal situations but can apply to any illness or injury in which the client is incapacitated. Similar to a health care proxy, durable power of attorney is a notarized statement appointing someone else to manage health care treatment decisions when the client is unable to do so.

The specific requirements of advance medical directives are directed by individual state legislation. In most states, advance directives must be witnessed by two people but do not require review by an attorney. Some states do not permit relatives, heirs, or physicians to witness advance directives.

The ANA (1991) supports the client's right to self-determination and believes that nurses must play a primary role in implementation of the law. The nurse is often the facilitator of discussions between clients and their families about health care and end-of-life decisions. The ANA recommends that the following questions be part of the nursing admission assessment regarding advance directives:

- Does the client have basic information about advance care directives, including living wills and durable power of attorney?
- Does the client wish to initiate an advance care directive?

- If the client has prepared an advance care directive, did the client bring it to the health care agency?
- Has the client discussed end-of-life-choices with the family and/or designated surrogate, physician, or other health care team worker?

Nurses should learn the law regarding client self-determination for the state in which they practice, as well as the policy and procedures for implementation in the institution where they work.

Euthanasia

Euthanasia is the act of painlessly putting to death persons suffering from incurable or distressing disease. It is commonly referred to as "mercy killing." Regardless of compassion and good intentions or moral convictions, euthanasia is *legally wrong* in both Canada and the United States and can lead to criminal charges of homicide or to a civil lawsuit for withholding treatment or providing an unacceptable standard of care. Because advanced technology has enabled the medical profession to sustain life almost indefinitely, people are increasingly considering the meaning of quality of life. For some people, the withholding of artificial life-support measures or even the withdrawal of life support is a desired and acceptable practice for clients who are terminally ill or who are incurably disabled and believed unable to live their lives with some happiness and meaning.

Voluntary euthanasia refers to situations in which the dying individual desires some control over the time and manner of death. All forms of euthanasia are illegal except in states where right-to-die statutes and living wills exist. Currently, the legality of assisted suicide in the United States is being tested in the court of law. Right-to-die statutes legally recognize the client's right to refuse treatment.

In 1994, Oregon approved the first physician-assisted suicide law in the United States. This law permits physicians to prescribe lethal doses of medications. The Oregon Death with Dignity Act was challenged in court and was not finally enacted until November 1997 (Kirk, 1998). Since the enactment of Oregon's law, several other states have proposed similar laws. Right-to-die statutes legally acknowledge a client's right to refuse treatment.

Reflect on...

- your own beliefs about death and dying. How do you feel about terminating ventilator support, intravenous or tube feedings, or other life-maintaining strategies on terminally ill clients? What are the policies in place in your practice setting that cover the termination of life support?

Death and Related Issues

Legal issues surrounding death include issuing the death certificate, labeling of the deceased, autopsy, organ donation, and inquest. By law, a death certificate must be completed when a person dies. It is usually signed by the attending physician and filed with a local health or other government office. The family is usually given a copy to use for legal matters, such as insurance claims.

Nurses have a duty to handle the deceased with dignity and label the body appropriately. Mishandling can cause emotional distress to survivors. Mislabeling can create legal problems if the body is inappropriately identified and prepared incorrectly for burial or a funeral. Usually, the deceased's wrist identification tag is left on, and another tag is tied to the client's ankles, in case one of the tags becomes detached. Tags tied to the ankles are preferred, because any tissue damage they cause will be concealed by bed linen or clothing. A third tag is attached to the shroud. All identification tags should include the client's name, hospital number, and physician's name.

An **autopsy**, or **postmortem examination**, is an examination of the body after death. It is performed only in certain cases. The law describes under what circumstances an autopsy must be performed, for example, when death is sudden or occurs within 48 hours of admission to a hospital. The organs and tissues of the body are examined to establish the exact cause of death, to learn more about a disease, and to assist in the accumulation of statistical data.

It is the responsibility of the physician or, in some instances, of a designated person in the hospital to obtain consent for autopsy. Consent must be given by the decedent (before death) or by the next of kin. Laws in many states and provinces prioritize the family members who can provide consent as follows: surviving spouse, adult children, parents, siblings. After autopsy, hospitals cannot retain any tissues or organs without the permission of the person who consented to the autopsy.

Organ Donation

Under the Uniform Anatomical Gift Act in the United States or the Human Tissue Act in Canada, any person 18 years or older and of sound mind may make a gift of all or any part of the body for the following purposes: for medical or dental education, research, advancement of medical or dental science, therapy, or transplantation. The donation can be made by a provision in a will or by signing a wallet-sized form in the presence of two witnesses. This form is usually carried at all times by the person who signed it. In some states, organ donation permission is recorded on the driver's license. In most states and provinces, organ donation can be revoked either by destroying the form or by oral revocation in the presence of two witnesses. Nurses may serve as witnesses for persons consenting to donate organs. In some states health care workers are required to ask survivors for consent to donate the deceased's organs.

Inquest

An **inquest** is a legal inquiry into the cause or manner of a death. When a death is the result of a motor-vehicle crash, for example, an inquest is held into the circumstances of the crash to determine any blame. The inquest is conducted under the jurisdiction of a coroner or medical examiner. A coroner is a public official, not necessarily a physician, appointed or elected to inquire into the causes of death, when appropriate. A medical examiner is a physician who usually has advanced education in pathology or forensic medicine. Agency policy dictates the individual who is responsible for reporting deaths to the coroner or medical examiner.

THE IMPAIRED NURSE

An impaired nurse is one whose practice has deteriorated because of substance abuse, specifically the use of alcohol and/or drugs. Chemical dependence in health care workers has become a problem because of the high levels of stress involved in many health care settings and the easy access to addictive drugs. In addition to substance abuse, mental illnesses such as depression or secondary post-traumatic stress disorder may also affect the nurse's ability to deliver safe, competent care (Tappen, Weiss, & Whitehead, 2004). The ANA *Code of Ethics for Nurses* states that "nurses must be vigilant to protect the patient, the public, and the profession from potential harm when a colleague's practice, in any setting, appears to be impaired" (ANA, 2001, p. 15).

Impaired nurses adversely affect client care, staff retention, and morale (Damrosch & Scholler-Jacquish, 1993). There are three victims of the nurse who is impaired: the client, whose care may be compromised by the nurse whose judgment and skills are impaired; the nurse's colleagues, who must pick up after the impaired worker; and the impaired nurse, whose illness may go undetected and untreated for years. The primary concern is for the protection of clients, but it is also critically important that the nurse's problem be identified quickly so that appropriate treatment can be instituted. In 1981 the ANA appointed a task force on addiction and psychological disturbance to develop guidelines for identifying, treating, and assisting nurses impaired by alcohol or drug abuse or psychological disturbance. The accompanying box lists behaviors that may be seen in the impaired nurse.

Danis (2004) describes the following actions the nurse should take when he or she suspects a colleague of being chemically impaired:

- Do not permit a visibly impaired coworker to care for patients. The safety of patients and staff must be protected.
- Report behaviors of unsafe practices or impaired behavior immediately to the appropriate supervisor.
- Document accurately and completely any suspicious behaviors or incidents that have occurred.

Behavioral Indicators of Chemical Abuse

- Increasing isolation from colleagues, friends, and family
- Frequent reports or illness, minor accidents, and emergencies
- Complaints about poor work performance
- Inability to meet schedules and deadlines
- Tendency to avoid new and challenging assignments
- Mood swings, irritability, and depression
- Request for night shifts
- Social avoidance of staff
- Illogical and sloppy charting
- Excessive errors
- Increasing carelessness about personal appearance
- Medication "errors" that require many changes in charting
- Arriving on duty early or staying late for no reason
- Volunteering to administer client medications, especially pain medications

- The nurse suspected of substance abuse should be confronted by a supervisor or manager in the presence of at least one other person.
- The nurse's right to confidentiality and privacy must be respected during the investigative process.
- Avoid being judgmental. Be supportive and recognize that substance abuse is an illness that can be treated.

Several programs have been developed to assist impaired nurses to recovery. In many states, impaired nurses who enter an intervention program for treatment do not have their nursing license revoked, but their practice is closely supervised within the limitations placed by the intervention program.

Reflect on...

- the factors in nursing that may lead to nurses being impaired. Have you worked with a nurse you suspected of being impaired? How did you feel about that situation? Under your state nurse practice act and your agency policies, what is your responsibility if you suspect a nursing colleague is impaired? How do you feel about this responsibility?

SEXUAL HARASSMENT

Sexual harassment is a violation of the individual's rights and a form of discrimination. The Equal Employment Opportunity Commission (EEOC) defines sexual harassment as "unwelcome sexual advances, requests for sexual favors, and other verbal or physical conduct of a sexual nature" occurring in the following circumstances (EEOC, 1980, sections 3950.10–3950.11):

- When submission to such conduct is considered, either explicitly or implicitly, a condition of an individual's employment
- When submission to or rejection of such conduct is used as the basis for employment decisions affecting the individual
- When such conduct interferes with an individual's work performance or creates an "intimidating, hostile, or offensive working environment"

In 1993, the Supreme Court determined that a plaintiff is not required to prove any psychological injury to establish a harassment claim. A proven hostile or abusive environment was sufficient for a claim.

In health care, both clients and health care professionals may experience sexual harassment. Because sexual harassment is generally related to a power imbalance, female nurses are more likely to experience sexual harassment from male colleagues.

Nurses may report having been "sexually propositioned," "suggestively touched," or "sexually insulted" by physicians during their career. Such behavior is considered sexual harassment and can negatively affect client care. For example, to avoid uncomfortable situations, the nurse may refuse to care for the clients of a particular offensive physician or work on a unit with an offensive administrator, or the nurse may avoid calling a physician to report changes in client status or to suggest changes to improve client care.

The victim of the harasser may be male or female. The victim does not have to be of the opposite sex. Moreover, the victim does not have to be the person harassed; anyone who is affected by the offensive conduct may be considered a victim (ANA, 1992b, p. 2). Nurses must be familiar with the sexual harassment policy and procedures in their employing agency. Many organizations provide educational programs to provide information about sexual harassment, including what incidents are considered sexual harassment and how to prevent them. They also review sexual harassment policies and procedures, including grievance procedures, determine to whom incidents should be reported, and provide the process for resolution. See the accompanying box for strategies to deter sexual harassment.

Strategies to Deter Sexual Harassment

- Confront the harasser, repeatedly if necessary, and clearly ask that the behavior stop.
- Report the harassment to authorities, using the "chain of command" and whatever formal complaint channels are available.
- Document the harassment, recording in detail the "who," "what," "where," and "when" of the situation and how you responded. Include witnesses if any.
- Seek support from others, such as friends, colleagues, relatives, or an organized support group.

Source: Reprinted with permission from *Sexual Harrassment: It's Against the Law,* © 1993 American Nurses Association, Washington, DC.

NURSES AS WITNESSES

A nurse may be called to testify in a legal action for a variety of reasons. The nurse may be a defendant in a malpractice or negligence action or may have been a health professional that provided care to the plaintiff. It is advisable that any nurse who is asked to testify in such a situation obtain the advice of an attorney before providing testimony. In most cases, the attorney for the institution will provide support and counsel during the legal case. If the nurse is the defendant, however, it is advisable for the nurse to retain an attorney to protect her or his own interests.

A nurse may also be asked to provide testimony as an expert witness. An **expert witness** is one who has special training, experience, or skill in a relevant area and who is allowed by the court to offer an opinion on some issue within the nurse's area of expertise (Bernzweig, 1996). Such a witness is usually called to help a judge or jury understand evidence pertaining to the extent of damage and the standard of care.

When called into court as a witness, the nurse has a duty to assist justice as far as possible. The nurse should always respond directly and truthfully to the questions asked. The nurse is not expected to volunteer additional information, nor is the nurse expected to remember completely all the details of a situation that may have occurred months or even years before the legal action. The nurse may ask to refer to the client record or to personal notes related to the incident. If the nurse does not remember the details of the incident, it is advisable to say so rather than to report an inaccurate recollection. In any case, it is the nurse's professional responsibility to provide accurate testimony, both during the pretrial discovery phase and the trial phase of a legal action.

COLLECTIVE BARGAINING

Collective bargaining is the formalized decision-making process between representatives of management and representatives of labor to negotiate wages and conditions of employment, including work hours, working environment, and fringe benefits of employment (e.g., vacation time, sick leave, and personal leave). Through a written agreement, both employer and employees legally commit themselves to observe the terms and conditions of employment. Collective bargaining is a controversial issue among nurses. Some nurses consider collective bargaining to be unprofessional and contrary to the altruistic nature of nursing. Others argue that collective bargaining is necessary to obtain control of nursing practice and economic security.

The collective bargaining process involves the recognition of a certified bargaining agent for the employees. This agent can be a union, a trade association, or a professional organization. The agent represents the employees in negotiating a contract with management.

In the 1930s, the National Labor Relations Act (NLRA) established the regulation of collective bargaining. In nursing, the NLRA provides guidelines for the resolution of conflicts between nurse employees and their employers. Nurses who are supervisors are not covered by the NLRA. There is still debate regarding whether all nurses who oversee the nursing care provided by other nurses, such as team leaders, are supervisors as defined by the NLRA (Brent, 1997).

In 1999 the ANA established the United American Nurses as the labor union for registered nurses in the United States. As a subsidiary of the ANA, the UAN is

Critical Thinking Exercise

You are called as a witness in a malpractice case. The incident occurred more than three years ago. The case is against the health care institution and a nurse whom you know was overtly negligent. This negligence resulted in harm to the client in question. On several previous occasions you observed the nurse violating standards of care. You reported these incidents to the administration. At the time of the incident in question, you kept personal anecdotal notes because you were concerned about a possible lawsuit in the future. You are still an employee of the health care institution involved. You are asked if you have ever witnessed other incidents of negligence performed by this nurse and, if so, what you did. What is your responsibility to your employer, the nurse being sued, the client in question, and the institution's clients? What do you do? To whom is your obligation?

the largest labor union for registered nurses in the country (UAN, 2004). Examples of resolutions approved at the 2000 National Labor Assembly included "Documenting the Relationship Between Working Conditions Related to Patient Safety and Working Conditions Related to Nurses' Safety," "Emergency Action to Prevent Musculoskeletal Disorders," and "Preventing Violence in the Healthcare Workplace."

When collective bargaining breaks down because an agreement cannot be reached, the employees usually call a strike. A **strike** is an organized work stoppage by a group of employees to express a grievance, enforce a demand for changes in conditions of employment, or solve a dispute with management.

Because nursing practice is a service to people (often ill people), striking presents a moral dilemma to many nurses. Actions taken by nurses can affect the safety of people. When faced with a strike, each nurse must make an individual decision to cross or not to cross a picket line. Nursing students may also be faced with decisions about crossing picket lines in the event of a strike at a clinical agency used for learning experiences. The ANA supports striking as a means of achieving economic and general welfare.

Collective bargaining is more than the negotiating of salary terms and hours of work; it is a continuous process in which day-to-day working problems and relationships can be handled in an orderly and democratic manner. Day-to-day difficulties or grievances are handled through the grievance procedure, a formal plan established in the contract that outlines the channels for handling and settling grievances through progressively higher levels of administration. A grievance is any dispute, difference, controversy, or disagreement arising out of the terms and conditions of employment. Grievances fall into four main categories, outlined in Table 5–2.

Reflect on...

- your own opinions about collective bargaining. Do you believe nurses should be able to strike or have a work stoppage?
- what would happen if your workplace downsized and closed several units. The administration is requesting nurses to take leave days without pay when the census drops. At the same time, administration is asking nurses to work 4 to 6 hours overtime to cover units when staffing is inadequate. Nurses are also being floated to areas where they have no expertise. The nurses want to organize for collective bargaining. What is your position? What can be gained by organizing? Are there disadvantages to organizing in a union?
- health care settings where nurses choose not to organize for collective bargaining. What are the characteristics of these employment settings?
- health care settings where nurses choose to organize for collective bargaining. What are the characteristics of these employment settings?

Table 5–2 Categories and Examples of Grievances

Category	Examples
Contract violations	Shift or weekend work is assigned inequitably.
	A nurse is dismissed without cause.
Violations of federal and state law	A female nurse is paid less than a male nurse for the same work.
	Appropriate payment is not given for overtime work.
	Minority group nurses are not promoted.
Management responsibilities	Appropriate locker room facilities are not provided.
	Safe client care is jeopardized by inadequate staffing.
Violation of agency rules	Performance evaluations are conducted only at termination of employment, but the contract requires annual evaluations.
	A vacation period is assigned without the nurse's agreement, as required in personnel policies.

Source: The Grievance Procedure (pp. 2–4), American Nurses Association, 1985, Washington, DC. Used by permission.

EXPLORE MEDIALINK

Questions, critical thinking exercises, essay activities, and other interactive resources for this chapter can be found on the Web site at http://www.prenhall.com/blasis. Click on Chapter 5 to select activities for this chapter.

Bookshelf

Cook. (1990). *Harmful intent.* **New York: J. P. Putnam.** The ethical principle to do no harm guides medical and nursing practice. In this fictional novel, a mother dies during delivery and the baby is born with brain damage. The anesthesiologist is blamed and charged with malpractice. He believes that he did nothing wrong. The author blends legal and medical issues together in this medical mystery.

Cook. (1995). *Acceptable risk.* **New York: J. P. Putnam.** The use of personality-altering drugs raises complex moral and legal issues, particularly pertaining to research and informed consent. The enormous profits available from marketing these drugs acts as a strong motivator for both the pharmaceutical companies and the researchers. In this novel, the author describes how far an individual and the medical community will go regarding testing and marketing.

Levy, H. (1999). *Chain of custody.* **New York: Random House.** When a highly respected deputy district attorney is found murdered, her physician husband becomes suspect. Forensic evidence connects him to the crime scene. The author pursues the legal issues regarding forensic evidence discovered at crime scenes and how such evidence is used to confirm the guilt or innocence of an individual.

SUMMARY

Accountability is an essential concept of professional nursing practice under the law. Nurses need to understand laws that regulate and affect practice to ensure that their actions are consistent with current legal principles and to protect themselves from liability. Nurse practice acts legally define and describe the scope of nursing practice that legislation seeks to regulate. Competence in nursing practice is determined and maintained by various credentialing methods, including licensure, registration, certification, and accreditation. The purpose of these credentialing methods is to protect the public's welfare and safety. Standards of practice published by national and state or provincial nursing associations and agency policies, procedures, and job descriptions further delineate the scope of a nurse's practice.

Negligence or malpractice of nurses can be established when (1) the nurse (defendant) owed a duty to the client, (2) the nurse failed to carry out that duty, (3) the client (plaintiff) was injured, and (4) the client's injury was caused by the nurse's failure to carry out that duty. When a client is injured or involved in an unusual incident, the nurse's first responsibility is to take steps to protect the client and then to notify appropriate agency personnel.

The nurse is responsible for ensuring that informed consent from clients (or from the closest relative in emergencies or from parents or guardians when the client is a minor) are in the medical record before treatment regimens and procedures begin. Informed consent implies that (1) the consent was given voluntarily; (2) the client was of age and had the capacity and competence to understand; and (3) the client was given enough information on which to make an informed decision.

Nurses must be knowledgeable about their responsibilities in regard to legal issues surrounding death: ensuring completion of the death certificate, labeling of the deceased, autopsy, organ donation, and inquest. Physicians may order no-code or do-not-resuscitate (DNR) for clients who are in a stage of terminal, irreversible illness or expected death. Nurses need to know their responsibility to clients who have a DNR order.

Nurses need to be aware of their responsibility when identifying a colleague who is impaired. Nurses also need to know the legal protections available for them when confronted with sexual harassment. Nurses may be called as witnesses for a variety of reasons. When called as a witness, a nurse has a duty to assist justice. Nurses also must be knowledgeable about collective bargaining as a means of ensuring just compensation, including wages and benefits and a safe and positive work environment.

REFERENCES

Agency for Healthcare Research and Quality (AHRQ). (2004). *Medical errors and patient safety.* Retrieved January 20, 2004, http://www.ahrq.gov.

Aiken, T. D., & Catalano, J. T. (1994). *Legal, ethical, and political issues in nursing.* Philadelphia: F. A. Davis.

American Association of Colleges of Nursing. (2004). *Mission statement and goals: Commission on collegiate nursing education.* Retrieved January 20, 2004, http://www.aacn.nche.edu.

American Association of Critical Care Nurses. (1990). *Delegation of nursing and non-nursing activities in critical care: A framework for decision-making.* Irvine, CA: AACN.

American Nurses Association. (1981). *The Nursing Practice Act: Suggested state legislation.* Kansas City, MO: ANA.

American Nurses Association. (1985). *The grievance procedure.* Washington, DC: ANA.

American Nurses Association. (1990). *A guideline for suggested state legislation.* Kansas City, MO: ANA.

American Nurses Association. (1991). *Position statement on nursing and the Patient Self-Determination* Act. Washington, DC: ANA.

American Nurses Association. (1992a). *Position statement on nursing care and do-not-resuscitate decisions.* Washington, DC: ANA.

American Nurses Association. (1992b). *Report to the Constituent Assembly on Sexual Harassment in the Workplace.* Washington, DC: ANA.

American Nurses Association. (1993a). *Sexual harassment: It's against the law.* Washington, DC: ANA.

American Nurses Association. (1993b). Regulation of advanced nursing practice. In *Summary of proceedings, 1993, House of Delegates.* Washington, DC: ANA.

American Nurses Association. (1995). *Registered professional nurses and unlicensed assistive personnel.* Washington, DC: ANA.

American Nurses Association. (2001). *Code of ethics for nurses with interpretive statements.* Washington, DC: ANA.

Anthony, M. K., Standing, T. & Heitz, J. E. (2000). Factors influencing outcome after delegation to unlicensed assistive personnel. *Journal of Nursing Administration, 30*(10), 474–481.

Barter, M., & Furmidge, M. L. (1994). Unlicensed assistive personnel: Issues relating to delegation and supervision. *Journal of Nursing Administration, 24,* 36–43.

Bernzweig, E. P. (1996). *The nurse's liability for malpractice: A programmed course* (6th ed.). St. Louis: Mosby.

Brent, N. J. (1997). *Nurses and the law.* Philadelphia: W. B. Saunders.

Damsrosch, S., & Scholler-Jaquish, A. (1993). Nurses' experiences with impaired coworkers. *Applied Nursing Research, 6*(4), 154–160.

Danis, S. J. (2004). *The impaired nurse.* Nursing Spectrum-Career Fitness Online, http://nsweb.nursingspectrum.com/ce/ce153.htm. Retrieved December 10, 2004.

Diaz, A. L., & McMillin, F. D. (1991, February). A definition and description of nurse abuse. *Western Journal of Nursing Research, 13,* 97–109.

Dock, L. L. (1900). What we may expect from the law. *American Journal of Nursing, 1*(1): 8–12.

Dock, L. L. (1907). Some urgent social claims. *American Journal of Nursing, 7*(11), 895–911.

Equal Employment Opportunity Commission. (1980). Sex discrimination guideline. In *EEOC Rules and Regulations.* Chicago: Commerce Clearing House.

Hall, J. K. (1990, October). Understanding the fine line between law and ethics. *Nursing, 90*(20), 34–39.

Health Match BC. (2004). *Registered nurse registration.* Retrieved January 20, 2004, http://www.healthmatchbc.org.

Herrick, K., Hansten, R., O'Neill, L., Hayes, P., & Washburn, M. (1994). My license is on the line: The art of delegation. *Nursing Management, 25*(2), 48–50.

Huber, D. (2000). *Leadership and nursing care management,* (2nd ed.). Philadelphia: W. B. Saunders.

International Nurses Society on Addictions (IntNSA). (2004). *Addictive disorders among nurses and nursing students in academic settings.* Retrieved January 22, 2004, http://www.intnsa.org.

Joint Commission on the Accreditation of Healthcare Organizations. (1996). *1997 accreditation manual for hospitals.* Oak Bluffs Terrace, IL: JCAHO.

Joint Commission on the Accreditation of Healthcare Organizations. (2002). *Sentinel event policy and procedure.* Retrieved January 20, 2003, http://www.jcaho.org/sentinel.

Kentucky Peer Assistance Program for Nurses, Inc. (2004). *Signs and symptoms.* Retrieved January 22, 2004, http://www.kpapn.org.

Kirk, K. (1998). How Oregon's Death with Dignity Act affects practice. *American Journal of Nursing, 98*(8), 54–55.

Kohn, L. T. (2000). *To err is human: Building a safer health system.* Washington, DC: National Academy Press.

Lee, N. G. (2000). Proving nursing negligence. *American Journal of Nursing, 7*(11), 55–56.

Monarch, K. (2002). *Nursing & the law: Trends and issues.* Washington, DC: American Nurses Association.

National Council of State Boards of Nursing. (1995). *Delegation concepts and decision making process.* Retrieved January 12, 2004, http://www.ncsbn.org.

National Council of State Boards of Nursing (NCSBN). (1997). *Delegation Decision-Making Grid.* Retrieved January 12, 2004, http://www.ncsbn.org.

National Council of State Boards of Nursing. (2004). *Nursing regulation.* Retrieved January 12, 2004, http://www.ncsbn.org.

Nguyen, B. Q. (2000). If you are replaced by a younger nurse. *American Journal of Nursing, 100*(3), 82.

Sheehy, S. B. (2000). Law and the emergency room nurse: Infections in pregnant women. *Journal of Emergency Nursing, 26,* 155–157.

Tappen, R. M., Weiss, S. A., & Whitehead, D. K. (2004). *Essentials of nursing leadership and management* (3rd ed.). Philadelphia: F. A. Davis.

United American Nurses. (2004). Retrieved January 22, 2004, http://www.ana.org/uan.

CHAPTER 6

Theoretical Foundations of Professional Nursing

Objectives

- Describe the nature of knowledge development.
- Differentiate among the terms *concept, conceptual framework, conceptual model, theory, construct, proposition,* and *hypothesis.*
- Analyze the development of theory in nursing.
- Compare the theoretical approach of selected nurse theorists.
- Identify the relationship between nursing process and nursing theory.

M E D I A L I N K

Additional online resources for this chapter can be found on the companion Web site at http://www.prenhall.com/blais.

Knowledge development in nursing has proliferated since the 1960s. To be meaningful, this knowledge must be organized and information must be linked in a way that can be understood and used to continue to generate new knowledge. Theory and conceptual frameworks allow that organization and linking of data in the building of a body of knowledge for nursing. This chapter presents the development of theoretical foundations for professional nursing practice.

Purposes of Nursing Theories and Conceptual Frameworks

Provide direction and guidance for (1) structuring professional nursing practice, education, and research; and (2) differentiating the focus of nursing from other professions.

IN PRACTICE

- Assist nurses to describe, explain, and predict everyday experiences.
- Serve to guide assessment, intervention, and evaluation of nursing care.
- Provide a rationale for collecting reliable and valid data about the health status of clients, which is essential for effective decision making and implementation.
- Help establish criteria to measure the quality of nursing care.
- Help build a common nursing terminology to use in communicating with other health professionals. Ideas are developed and words defined.

- Enhance autonomy (independence and self-governance) of nursing through defining its own independent functions.

IN EDUCATION

- Provide a general focus for curriculum design.
- Guide curricular decision making.

IN RESEARCH

- Offer a framework for generating knowledge and new ideas.
- Assist in discovering knowledge gaps in the specific field of study.
- Offer a systematic approach to identify questions for study; select variables, interpret findings, and validate nursing interventions.

CHALLENGES AND OPPORTUNITIES

Traditionally there has been a gap between academia and practice. As a result, nursing theories have been developed and articulated by academicians who proposed those theories to guide clinical practice in nursing. The collegial contact and communication between nurse educators and nurses in practice has been limited, and as a result nursing theory has been viewed by the practicing nurse as ethereal and unrelated to the "real world" of nursing. This gap must be bridged to achieve theory-based practice. Nursing theories must be seen as supporting and guiding practice and must be communicated in ways that are compelling to nurses who must apply them in a clinical setting.

The development of nursing theory has resulted in multiple diverse approaches with a language all its own. Theories have been drawn from a number of other disciplines and have been developed at varying levels of abstraction. This has the advantage of allowing nurses to match their own thinking and reasoning styles with the theory that is the "best fit." But is this diverse approach one that best serves the profession? Should nursing continue on its current course of numerous theories from which to choose, or should nursing theorists now begin to converge on one theoretical approach?

WORLD VIEWS AND KNOWLEDGE DEVELOPMENT

Einstein is credited with saying that there is nothing so practical as a good theory. Theory is defined as a system of ideas proposed to explain something. Theory helps provide knowledge to improve practice by describing, explaining, predicting, and controlling phenomena. It guides practice, education, and research and provides professional autonomy as knowledge is systematically developed, producing practices that are more likely to be successful. The study of theory helps nurses develop analytical skills and critical thinking ability. Each nurse uses concepts and theories daily, which may or may not be articulated or perceived as such, to guide nursing action. Each time a decision is made based on ideas that explain the situation or event, theory is used, even though it may not be formalized as such. Nursing theory has not been formally integrated at an everyday level. The gap between nurse theorists and practicing nurses can be attributed, at least in part, to the devel-

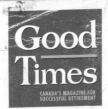

Good Times

CANADA'S MAGAZINE FOR
SUCCESSFUL RETIREMENT

USEFUL INFORMATION

HEALTH CANADA
(613) 957-2991

VICTORIAN ORDER OF NURSES
1-888-866-2273

CANADIAN MEDICAL ASSOCIATION
1-800-267-9703

CANADIAN HUMAN RIGHTS
COMMISSION
1-888-214-1090

CANADIAN BAR ASSOCIATION
1-800-267-8860

CANADA MORTGAGE AND
HOUSING CORPORATION (CMHC)
(416) 221-2642

BETTER BUSINESS BUREAU
(613) 237-4856

CONSUMER'S ASSOCIATION
OF CANADA INC.
(613) 238-2533

SERVICE CANADA
1-800-277-9914

CANADA REVENUE AGENCY
1-800-959-8281

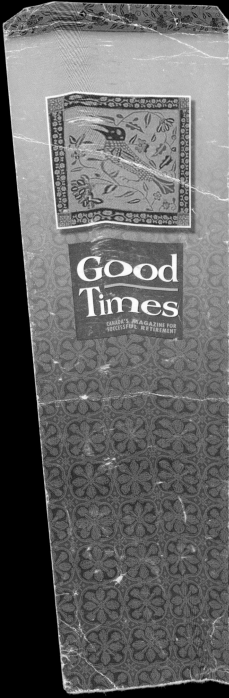

Good
Times

CANADA'S MAGAZINE FOR
SUCCESSFUL RETIREMENT

Table 6–1 Nursing Theorists and Their Theoretical Scope

Philosophies	Grand Theory	Middle-Range Theory
Florence Nightingale	Dorothea Orem	Hildegard Peplau
Ernestine Wiedenbach	Myra Levine	Ida Orlando
Virginia Henderson	Martha Rogers	Joyce Travelbee
Faye Abdellah	Dorothy Johnson	Kathryn Barnard
Lydia Hall	Callista Roy	Madeleine Leininger
Jean Watson	Betty Neuman	Rosemarie Parse
Patricia Benner	Imogene King	Margaret Newman
		Nola Pender

Source: Based upon *Nursing Theorists and Their Work,* by A. M. Tomey and M. R. Alligood, (5th ed.), 2002, St. Louis: Mosby.

opment of nursing theories in the 1960s by nurses who were pursuing graduate degrees in nursing and related fields. Few other nurses knew or cared about such matters; it was not part of nursing education at that time. Until the 1950s nursing practice was based on principles and traditions passed on through an apprenticeship form of education and common sense that came from years of experience. Florence Nightingale, in the mid-1800s, proposed that nursing knowledge was based on knowledge of persons and their environment and was different and distinct from medical knowledge. It was nearly a century later that nursing theory began to emerge and be valued by the profession.

Different theories represent different worldviews, which are different ways of conceiving of knowledge. Theories are not discovered; individuals who think and see the world in different ways create them. These worldviews provide contrasting paradigms (structure for organizing theory) and provide different traditions and approaches to science and knowledge development.

One paradigm is derived from the positivist approach that comes from the nineteenth century Age of Enlightenment and represents what many people regard as hard science. It deals with natural law and assumes that there is a body of facts and principles to be discovered and understood that is independent of the context. This approach is linear and attempts to look at cause and effect using experimental research methods. The theories generated by quantitative methods are normative, and they suggest propositions to explain relationships. They start with a generalization

and bring it to a more specific level. Hypotheses are deduced from the theory to be tested in research.

The second paradigm began as a countermovement to positivism and sees science as necessarily embedded in time because truth is dynamic. That is, reality is not a fixed entity but, instead, is relative. Truth is found in one's experiences, and research uses naturalistic settings and observational methods to describe phenomena. This approach is sometimes referred to as constructivist. These theories are inductively constructed and give insights in social contexts and personal meanings; they start with a specific observation or relationship and make generalizations from it.

Theories differ in their scope and have been categorized as philosophies, grand theories, or middle-range theories. These theories can all be used to explain more specific situations. Table 6–1 lists theorists whose work can fall into these categories.

A *philosophy* looks at the nature of things and aims to provide the meaning of nursing phenomena. Philosophies represent the early works leading to nursing theory. A *grand theory* is broad and complex and tends to be very general; grand theories are abstract but may provide insights useful for practice. They are conceptual and have concepts, definitions, and propositions. *Middle-range theory* has a narrower focus and is derived from earlier works, such as philosophies and grand theories, or from works in other disciplines. Middle-range theories may be refined through a series of studies, each providing increased focus. The accompanying boxes describe two such middle-range theories.

Middle-Range Theory of Caregiver Stress

The middle-range theory of caregiver stress is based on Roy's Adaptation Model and hypothesizes that objective burden in caregiving will be the most important stimulus leading to the caregiver stress. Higher perceived stress and depression will result in ineffective responses: poor physical functioning, lower self-esteem and mastery, lower role enjoyment, and less marital satisfaction. The concepts are derived from the Input-Control Process (Throughput)-Output structure. Input consists of three stimuli: focal, contextual, and residual and are operationalized as follows:

Focal stimuli–Objective burden in caregiving

Contextual stimuli–Stressful life events, social support, and social roles

Residual stimuli–Race, age, gender, relationship with the care recipient

Each of these stimuli begin the pathway to an adaptive mode and are acted upon by the control process (coping mechanism) of regulator and cognator. In this middle-range theory, the coping mechanism comes from the cognator and is operationalized as perceived caregiver stress and depression, and they control the stimuli as the person moves to output in four adaptive modes. The four adaptive modes from Roy's model are operationalized in the following way:

Physiological function–Physical function

Self-concept–Self-esteem/mastery

Role-function–Role enjoyment

Interdependence–Marital satisfaction

This middle-range theory identifies variables that can be used to guide nursing assessment and then assist in identifying interventions that would promote adaptation as well as identifying behaviors that may be used to evaluate outcomes.

Source: "A Middle-Range Theory of Caregiver Stress," by P.-F. Tsai, 2003. *Nursing Science Quarterly, 16*(2), 137–145.

DEFINING TERMS

Before specific theories and conceptual frameworks can be understood, the terms *concept, conceptual framework, conceptual model,* and *theory* must be clarified. **Concepts**, the building blocks of theory, are abstract ideas or mental images of phenomena. Concepts are words that bring forth mental pictures of the properties and meanings of objects, events, or things. Concepts may be (1) readily observable, or *concrete*, ideas such as thermometer, rash, and lesion; (2) indirectly observable, or *inferential*, ideas such as pain and temperature; or (3) nonobservable, or *abstract*, ideas such as equilibrium, adaptation, stress, and powerlessness.

Four concepts have been identified as the *metaparadigm* of nursing—the most global philosophical or conceptual framework of a profession. The term originates from two Greek words: *meta*, meaning "with"; and *paradigm*, meaning "pattern." The four concepts are as follows:

1. *Person or client*, the recipient of nursing care (includes individuals, families, groups, and communities)
2. *Environment*, the internal and external surroundings that affect the client, including people in the physical environment, such as families, friends, and significant others
3. *Health*, the degree of wellness or well-being that the client experiences
4. *Nursing*, the attributes, characteristics, and actions of the nurse providing care on behalf of or in conjunction with the client

Each nurse theorist's definitions of these four concepts vary in accordance with philosophy, scientific orientation, experience, and view of nursing held by the theorist. At the time the metaparadigm was conceived, it assisted nurse scholars and students of nursing to analyze, compare, and contrast theories within a nursing framework. Not all theorists embrace the four concepts as distinct concepts. The theories representing more holistic and phenomenological ap-

The Middle-Range Theory of Experiencing Transitions

Changes in health and illness create transitions, and clients in transition tend to be more vulnerable to risks that may affect their health. Examples of transitions are illness experiences, developmental and lifespan transitions, and social and cultural transitions. This theory was developed by reviewing inductively and deductively studies of the experiences of the following: pregnancy and childbirth, menopause, diagnostic events, migration, and family care giving. A theoretical framework emerged, consisting of types and patterns of transitions, properties of transition experiences, transition conditions (facilitators and inhibitors), process indicators, outcome indicators, and nursing therapeutics.

Transitions are complex and multidimensional. Several properties have been identified: awareness, engagement, change and difference, time span, and critical points and events. Several conditions affect transitions; these are personal, community, and societal. Personal conditions include meanings attributed to the event, cultural beliefs and attitudes, socioeconomic status, and preparation for the transition and knowledge about what to expect.

Patterns of response are feeling connected, interacting, location and being situated, developing confidence, and coping. Outcome indicators are mastery and fluid integrative identities. Understanding the process allows nursing therapeutics congruent with the unique experience of the client to promote a healthy transition.

Source: "Experiencing Transitions: An Emerging Middle-Range Theory," by A. I. Meleis, L. M. Sawyer, E. Im, D. K. Hilfinger-Messias, and K. Schumacher, *Advances in Nursing Science, 23*(1), 12–28.

proaches do not necessarily separate person from environment or health.

THEORY DEVELOPMENT IN NURSING

The terms *theory* and *conceptual framework* are often used interchangeably in nursing literature. Strictly speaking, they differ in their levels of abstraction; conceptual framework is more abstract than theory. A **conceptual framework**, viewed simply, is a group of related concepts. It provides an overall view or orientation to focus thoughts. A conceptual framework can be thought of as an umbrella under which many concepts can exist. A **conceptual model**, a term also used interchangeably with *conceptual framework*, is a graphic illustration or diagram of a conceptual framework. A **theory** is a supposition or system of ideas that is proposed to explain a given phenomenon. For example, Newton proposed his theory of gravity to explain why objects always fall from a tree to the ground. A *theory* goes one step beyond a *conceptual framework*; a theory relates concepts by using definitions that state significant relationships between concepts.

Knowledge development may use a deductive or inductive approach. These two approaches represent the-

ory testing or theory generation. Theory testing compares observed outcomes with the relationship predicted by the hypothesis that was drawn from the theory and linked the concepts. Theory generation comes from descriptive data that result in new concepts that may be related to other concepts. Generally speaking, theory testing uses a deductive approach and applies quantitative research methods. Theory generation uses an inductive approach and is a result of qualitative research.

Not all knowledge comes about as a result of research. Ways of knowing have been identified and described that include but are not limited to empirical methods. Kneller (1971) described the following five kinds of knowledge:

> *Revealed knowledge*—that disclosed by God
>
> *Intuitive knowledge*—that coming from a process of discovery nurtured by experience with the world
>
> *Rational knowledge*—that using principles of formal logic
>
> *Empirical knowledge*—information tested by observation or experiment
>
> *Authoritative knowledge*—that vouched for by authorities in the field

Carper (1978) organized ways of knowing according to the following framework: empirical, esthetic, personal, and ethical. *Empirical knowing* represents the science of nursing that emphasizes generation of theory that is systematic and controllable by factual evidence. *Esthetic knowing* represents the art of nursing and emphasizes expressiveness, creativity, perceptions, subjectivity, and empathy. *Personal knowing* focuses on interpersonal processes and the therapeutic use of self. *Ethical knowing* represents a pattern of knowing related to what ought to be done and focuses on matters of obligation.

Efforts to develop theory in nursing have resulted in discussion and debate about what is unique to nursing. Do nurses need basic scientific knowledge that they apply in practice, or is there a distinct body of knowledge for the discipline? Historically, nursing practice has been linked to the use of medical knowledge and has embraced the scientific bases of social and behavioral sciences as well as education.

Some have suggested that theories in nursing are borrowed and shared theories. Other disciplines have provided the foundation of nursing theory more unique to nursing. Nurse theorists have borrowed from others and applied these theories to nursing. Some theories are shared with other disciplines. For instance, Maslow's hierarchy of needs and Erikson's psychosocial development are applied to nursing without modification to the theories. This has resulted in a diversity of theories. An overview of some selected nursing theories representing a range of scope and worldviews is included in this chapter. For further examination of particular theories, the student is referred to one of the many books available on nursing theory.

OVERVIEW OF SELECTED NURSING THEORIES

Nursing theories have been developed by nurses who were, in most instances, involved in their own graduate education at a time when there were few doctoral programs in nursing. Therefore, they were studying in related fields and, consequently, their developing theories were influenced by and borrowed from disciplines, such as anthropology and sociology, and applied to nursing. This can be seen in the description of the selected theories discussed here.

Nightingale's Environmental Theory

Florence Nightingale, often considered the first nurse theorist, defined nursing more than 100 years ago as utilizing the environment of the patient to assist him in his recovery (Nightingale, 1860). She linked health with five environmental factors: (1) pure or fresh air, (2) pure water, (3) efficient drainage, (4) cleanliness, and (5) light, especially direct sunlight. Deficiencies in these five factors produced lack of health or illness.

These factors are especially significant when one considers that sanitation conditions in hospitals of the mid-1800s were extremely poor and that women working in the hospitals were often unreliable, uneducated, and incompetent to care for the ill.

In addition to the preceding factors, Nightingale also stressed the importance of keeping the client warm, maintaining a noise-free environment, and attending to the client's diet in terms of assessing intake, timeliness of the food, and its effect on the person.

Nightingale set the stage for further work in the development of nursing theories. Her general concepts about ventilation, cleanliness, quiet, warmth, and diet remain integral parts of nursing and health care today.

Peplau's Interpersonal Relations Model

Hildegard Peplau, a psychiatric nurse, introduced her interpersonal concepts in 1952 (Peplau, 1952) and based them on available theories at the time: psychoanalytic theory, principles of social learning, and concepts of human motivation and personality development. *Psychodynamic nursing* is defined as the nurse understanding his or her own behavior in order to help others identify felt difficulties. Principles of human relations are applied to problems arising during the nursing experience.

Peplau views nursing as a maturing force that is realized as the personality develops through educational, therapeutic, and interpersonal processes. Nurses enter into a personal relationship with an individual when a felt need is present. This nurse-client relationship evolves in four phases:

1. *Orientation.* During this phase, the client seeks help, and the nurse assists the client to understand the problem and the extent of the need for help.
2. *Identification.* During this phase, the client assumes a posture of dependence, interdependence, or independence in relation to the nurse (relatedness). The nurse's focus is to ensure the person that the nurse understands the interpersonal meaning of the client's situation.
3. *Exploitation.* In this phase, the client derives full value from what the nurse offers through the relationship. The client uses available services on the

basis of self-interest and needs. Power shifts from the nurse to the client.

4. *Resolution.* In this final phase, old needs and goals are put aside and new ones adopted. Once older needs are resolved, newer and more mature ones emerge.

During the nurse-client relationship, nurses assume many roles: stranger, teacher, resource person, surrogate, leader, and counselor. Today, Peplau's model continues to be used by clinicians when working with individuals in psychiatric and mental health settings.

Henderson's Definition of Nursing

Virginia Henderson is well known for her *Textbook on the Principles and Practices of Nursing*, coauthored with Canadian nurse Bertha Harmer (Harmer & Henderson, 1955); her subsequent publications include *The Nature of Nursing* (1966) and numerous scholarly papers. She was motivated to develop her ideas because she was dissatisfied with the emphasis that nursing education programs placed on technical competence and mastery of nursing procedures; her experiences in psychiatric, pediatric, and community health nursing were other major influences.

In 1955, Henderson formulated a definition of the unique function of nursing. This definition was a major stepping-stone in the emergence of nursing as a discipline separate from medicine. She wrote, "The unique function of the nurse is to assist the individual, sick or well, in the performance of those activities contributing to health or its recovery (or to peaceful death) that he would perform unaided if he had the necessary strength, will, or knowledge, and to do this in such a way as to help him gain independence as rapidly as possible" (Henderson, 1966, p. 3). Like Nightingale, Henderson described nursing in relation to the client and the client's environment. Unlike Nightingale, Henderson saw the nurse as concerned with both well and ill individuals, acknowledged that nurses interact with clients even when recovery may not be feasible, and mentioned the teaching and advocacy roles of the nurse.

Basic to her definition are various assumptions about the individual: namely, that the individual (1) needs to maintain physiological and emotional balance, (2) requires assistance to achieve health and independence or a peaceful death, and (3) needs the necessary strength, will, or knowledge to achieve or maintain health. These needs give direction to the nurse's role.

Henderson conceptualized the nurse's role as assisting sick or well individuals in a supplementary or complementary way. The nurse needs to be a partner with the client, a helper to the client, and, when necessary, a substitute for the client. The nurse's focus is to help individuals and families (which she viewed as a unit) to gain independence in meeting the following 14 fundamental needs (Henderson, 1966):

1. Breathing normally
2. Eating and drinking adequately
3. Eliminating body wastes
4. Moving and maintaining a desirable position
5. Sleeping and resting
6. Selecting suitable clothes
7. Maintaining body temperature within normal range by adjusting clothing and modifying the environment
8. Keeping the body clean and well groomed to protect the integument
9. Avoiding dangers in the environment and avoiding injuring others
10. Communicating with others in expressing emotions, needs, fears, or opinions
11. Worshipping according to one's faith
12. Working in such a way that one feels a sense of accomplishment
13. Playing or participating in various forms of recreation
14. Learning, discovering, or satisfying the curiosity that leads to normal development and health, and using available health facilities

Henderson continues to be cited in current nursing literature. Her emphasis on the importance of nursing's independence from and interdependence with other health care disciplines is well recognized.

Reflect on...

■ the relationship between Henderson's 14 fundamental needs and Maslow's hierarchy of needs. How might one have built upon the other?

Rogers' Science of Unitary Human Beings

Martha Rogers first presented her theory of unitary human beings in 1970. It contains complex conceptualizations related to multiple scientific disciplines. Her theory was influenced by Einstein's theory of relativity, which introduced the four coordinates of space-time; Burr and Northrop's electrodynamics theory of life, which revealed the pattern and organization of the electrodynamics field; Von Bertalanffy's general systems theory; and many other disciplines, such as anthropology, psychology, sociology, astronomy, religion, philosophy, history, biology, and literature. She was a pioneer in her focus on human beings and their environments as equally important, and she traced that influence to Florence Nightingale (Fawcett, 2003).

Rogers views the person as an irreducible whole, the whole being greater than the sum of its parts. *Whole* is differentiated from *holistic*, the latter often being used to mean only the sum of all the parts. She states that humans are dynamic energy fields in continuous exchange with environmental fields, both of which are infinite. Both human and environmental fields are characterized by pattern, a universe of open systems, and pandimensionality. According to Rogers, *unitary human being* exhibits the following:

- Is an irreducible energy field identified by pattern
- Manifests characteristics different from the sum of the parts
- Interacts continuously and creatively with the environment
- Behaves as a totality
- As a sentient being, participates creatively in change

Key concepts Rogers uses to describe the individual and the environment are energy fields, openness, pattern and organization, and pandimensionality. *Energy fields* are the fundamental level of humans and the environment (all that is outside a given human field). Energy fields are dynamic, constantly exchanging energy from one to the other. The concept of *openness* holds that the energy fields of humans and the environment are open systems, that is, infinite, integral with one another, and in continuous process. *Pattern* refers to the unique identifying behaviors, qualities, and characteristics of the energy fields that change continuously and innovatively. *Pandimensionality* expresses the idea of unitary whole; it provides for an infinite domain without limits.

To Rogers, the life process in humans is homeodynamic, involving continuous and creative change. She provides three principles of homeodynamics to offer a way of perceiving how unitary human beings develop: integrality (formerly complementarity), resonancy, and helicy. According to the principle of *integrality*, the human and environmental fields interact mutually and simultaneously. *Resonancy* means the wave pattern in the fields change continuously and from lower- to higher-frequency patterns. *Helicy* is spiral development, that is, continuous and nonrepeating.

When Rogers' theory is applied in practice, nurses (1) focus on the person's wholeness, (2) seek to promote symphonic interaction between the two energy fields (human and environment) to strengthen the coherence and integrity of the person, (3) coordinate the human field with the rhythmicities of the environmental field, and (4) direct and redirect patterns of interaction between the two energy fields to promote maximum health potential. Her theory has been applied in holistic nursing.

Some find Rogers' concepts difficult to understand, but a specific example can help clarify them. Nurses' use of therapeutic touch is based on the concept of human energy fields. The human energy field is identified by pattern. The qualities of the field vary from person to person and are affected by pain and illness. Although the field is infinite, realistically it is most clearly "felt" within several feet of the body. The nurse trained in therapeutic touch can assess and feel the energy field and manipulate it to help a person manage pain and illness.

Orem's General Theory of Nursing

Dorothea Orem's theory, first published in 1971, has been widely accepted by the nursing community and has resulted from the work of the Nursing Development Conference Group. This general theory of nursing is referred to as the *self-care deficit theory of nursing*, and it consists of the articulation of the theories of self-care, self-care deficit, and nursing systems. It provides a way of looking at and investigating what nurses do.

SELF-CARE Self-care theory postulates that self-care and the self-care of dependents are learned behaviors that individuals initiate and perform on their own behalf to maintain life, health, and well-being. Self-care theory is based on four concepts: self-care, self-care agency, self-care requisites, and therapeutic self-care demand. *Self-care* refers to those activities an individual performs independently throughout life to promote and maintain personal well-being. *Self-care agency* is the individual's ability to perform self-care activities. It consists of two agents: a *self-care agent* (an individual who performs self-care independently) and a *dependent-care agent* (a person other than the individual who provides the care). Adults care for themselves, whereas infants, the aged, the ill, and the disabled require assistance with self-care activities.

Self-care requisites are measures or actions taken to regulate functioning and development. They are the goals of self care. There are three categories of self-care requisites:

1. *Universal requisites* are common to all people. They include maintaining intake and elimination of air, water, and food; balancing rest, solitude, and social

interaction; preventing hazards to life and well-being; and promoting normal human functioning.

2. *Developmental requisites* result from maturation and are related to stage of development or are associated with conditions or events, such as adjusting to a change in body image or to the loss of a spouse.

3. *Health deviation requisites* result from illness, injury, or disease or its diagnosis and treatment. They include actions such as seeking health care assistance, carrying out prescribed therapies, and learning to live with the effects of illness or treatment.

Therapeutic self-care demand refers to all self-care activities required to meet the requisites for certain conditions and circumstances, such as an illness.

SELF-CARE Self-care deficit theory asserts that people benefit from nursing because they have health-related limitations in providing self-care. These limitations may result from illness, injury, or the effects of medical tests or treatments. Two variables affect these deficits: self-care agency (ability) and the therapeutic self-care demands (the measures of care required to meet the existing requisites). *Self-care deficit* results when the self-care agency is not adequate to meet the known self-care demand. Orem's self-care deficit theory explains not only when nursing is needed but also how people can be assisted through five methods of helping: acting or doing for, guiding, teaching, supporting, and providing an environment that promotes the individual's abilities to meet current and future demands.

NURSING SYSTEMS Nursing systems theory postulates that nursing systems form when nurses prescribe, design, and provide nursing that regulates the individual's self-care capabilities and meets therapeutic self-care requirements. Orem identifies three types of nursing systems:

1. *Wholly compensatory* systems are required for individuals who are unable to control and monitor their environment and process information.

2. *Partly compensatory* systems are designed for individuals who are unable to perform some (but not all) self-care activities.

3. *Supportive-educative* systems are designed for persons who need to learn to perform self-care measures and need assistance to do so.

Development of the theory continues with contributions from researchers, scholars, nursing faculty, nursing students, and practicing nurses (Orem, 1995).

Evidence for Practice

Wilson, F. L., Mood, D. W., Risk, J., & Kershaw, T. (2003). **Evaluation of education materials using Orem's self-care deficit theory.** *Nursing Science Quarterly, 16* (1), 68–76.

A conceptual framework based on Orem's self-care deficit nursing theory was developed and tested to guide nurses in the selection of appropriate educational materials to use for patient education. The model offers nurses a tool to judge the suitability of materials for the individual client based on assessment guided by self-care concepts. Nurses have a critical role in educating people to care for themselves; this is a particular challenge when working with individuals who have low literacy.

The model consists of two components: assessment of the patient and his or her environment and the evaluation of the written educational materials. Three major concepts of Orem's theory guide the assessment of the patient and environment: self-care agency (the patient's ability to engage in self-care activities), basic conditioning factors (background and health status), and therapeutic self-care demand (the activities needed to meet the requirements for self-care). The assessment data are needed to make a judgment about self-care abilities and guide the selection of materials appropriate to the client. The second part of the model is evaluation of the materials to see that they match with the assessment of the client. It looks for factors congruent with patient assessment, such as age, gender, ability to comprehend, socioeconomic status, and so on.

The model was tested with 238 randomly selected patients receiving radiation therapy. Findings indicated that nearly half of the sample would need supplemental instructions in order to understand the educational materials they were given to read. There were indications that the organization of educational materials should begin with "need to know" information rather than the usual explanation of an illness as an introduction.

This model offers a framework for judging the appropriateness of patient teaching materials. It can guide nurses in determining whether materials are congruent with therapeutic self-care needs and self-care abilities. Working in tandem with literacy experts, nurses can choose and design the most effective patient educational materials.

King's Goal-Attainment Theory

Imogene King's theory of goal attainment is based on systems theory, the behavioral sciences, and deductive and inductive reasoning. She first published *Toward a Theory of Nursing: General Concepts of Human Behavior* in 1971. Initially, King formulated her theory as a conceptual framework for nursing when, as an associate professor of nursing at Loyola University in Chicago, she developed a master's degree program in nursing. King refined her concepts in her 1981 publication *A Theory for Nursing: Systems, Concepts, Process*. Important in King's theory is mutual goal setting based on nursing assessment, nurse's and patient's perceptions, and their information sharing in order to attain the identified mutual goals.

King's theory consists of three dynamic interacting systems: (1) personal systems (individuals), (2) interpersonal systems (groups), and (3) social systems (society). Key concepts are identified for each system as follows:

1. *Personal-system concepts*: coping, spirituality, perception, self, body image, growth and development, space and time
2. *Interpersonal-system concepts*: interaction, communication, transaction, role, stress, and coping
3. *Social-system concepts*: organization, authority, power, status, and decision making

The client and nurse are personal systems or subsystems within interpersonal and social systems. To identify problems and to establish goals, the nurse and client perceive one another, act and react, interact, and transact. *Transactions* are defined as purposeful interactions that lead to goal attainment. Transactions have the following characteristics:

- They are basic to goal attainment and include social exchange, bargaining and negotiating, and sharing a frame of reference toward mutual goal setting.
- They require perceptual accuracy in nurse-client interactions and congruence between role performance and role expectation for nurse and client.
- They lead to goal attainment, satisfaction, effective care, and enhanced growth and development.

King postulates seven hypotheses in goal-attainment theory:

1. Perceptual congruence in nurse-client interactions increases mutual goal setting.
2. Communication increases mutual goal setting between nurses and clients and leads to satisfaction.
3. Satisfaction in nurses and clients increases goal attainment.
4. Goal attainment decreases stress and anxiety in nursing situations.
5. Goal attainment increases client learning and coping ability in nursing situations.
6. Role conflict experienced by clients, nurses, or both decreases transactions in nurse-client interactions.
7. Congruence in role expectations and role performance increases transactions in nurse-client interactions.

King's theory highlights the importance of the participation of all individuals in decision making and deals with the choices, alternatives, and outcomes of nursing care. The theory offers insight into nurses' interactions with individuals and groups within the environment.

Neuman Systems Model

Betty Neuman, a pioneer in mental health nursing, began developing her model while teaching at the University of California at Los Angeles. She did so in response to the expressed needs of her students for content that would present a general picture of nursing before content on specific nursing problems. The model is based on numerous theories, including Gestalt theory, Selye's stress theory, and general systems theory. It adapts the concept of levels of prevention from Caplan's conceptual model and relates these levels to nursing; they are primary, secondary, and tertiary prevention. Neuman's model was first published in 1972 in *Nursing Research* in an article coauthored by R. J. Young, "A Model for Teaching Total Person Approach to Patient Problems." Refinements were published as the Neuman Systems Model in 1974, 1982, 1989, and 1995.

Neuman Systems Model focuses on the wellness of the client system in relation to environmental stressors and reactions to stressors. It guides the nurse to consider five client system variables and four levels of environmental influence on the client system. The five client system variables are physiological, psychological, sociocultural, developmental, and spiritual. The four levels of environmental influence are internal, external interpersonal, external extrapersonal, and created.

Neuman views the client as an open system consisting of a basic structure or central core of energy resources (physiological, psychologic, sociocultural, developmental, and spiritual) surrounded by two lines of resistance. The *lines of resistance* represent internal factors that help the client defend against a stressor; one example is an increase in the body's leukocyte count to combat an infection. Outside the lines of resistance are two lines of defense. The inner line of defense, or *normal line of defense*, depicted as a solid line, represents the person's state of equilibrium or the state of adaptation developed and maintained over time and considered normal for that person. The *flexible line of defense* is dynamic and can be rapidly altered over a short period of time. It is a protective buffer that prevents stressors from penetrating the normal line of defense. Certain variables (e.g., sleep deprivation) can create rapid changes in the flexible line of defense.

Neuman describes a stressor as any environmental force that alters the system's stability. Stressors are categorized as *internal stressors*, those that occur within the individual (e.g., an infection); *interpersonal stressors*, those that occur between individuals (e.g., unrealistic role expectations); *extrapersonal stressors*, those that occur outside the person (e.g., financial concerns); and *created stressors*, those that are unconsciously mobilized toward system integration, stability, and integrity. The individual's reaction to stressors depends on the strength of the lines of defense. When the lines of defense fail, the resulting reaction depends on the strength of the lines of resistance. As part of the reaction, a person's system can adapt to a stressor, an effect known as reconstitution.

Nursing interventions focus on retaining or maintaining system stability. These interventions are carried out on the following three preventive levels.

1. *Primary prevention* identifies risk factors, attempts to eliminate the stressor, and focuses on protecting the normal line of defense and strengthening the flexible line of defense. A reaction has not yet occurred, but the degree of risk is known.
2. *Secondary prevention* relates to interventions or active treatment initiated after symptoms have occurred. The focus is to strengthen internal lines of resistance, reduce the reaction, and increase resistance factors.
3. *Tertiary prevention* refers to intervention following that in the secondary stage. It focuses on readaptation and stability and protects reconstitution or return to wellness following treatment. The nurse emphasizes educating the client in strengthening resistance to stressors and ways to help prevent recurrence of reaction or regression.

Betty Neuman's model of nursing has been widely accepted by the nursing community, nationally and internationally. It is applicable to a variety of nursing practice settings involving individuals, families, groups, and communities.

Roy's Adaptation Model

Callista Roy, a nurse and sociologist, based her theory on Harry Helson's work in psychophysics and on her observations of the great resilience of children and their ability to adapt to major physical and psychological changes. Roy's Adaptation Model, widely used by nurse educators, researchers, and practitioners, was introduced in *Nursing Outlook* as "Adaptation: A Conceptual Framework in Nursing" (Roy, 1970). The model was published in book form in 1976 and 1984 as *Introduction to Nursing: An Adaptation Model* (Roy, 1976, 1984) and in 1991 and 1999 as *The Roy Adaptation Model* (Roy & Andrews, 1991, 1999).

Roy focuses on the individual as a biopsychosocial adaptive system that employs a feedback cycle of input, throughput, and output. Both the individual and the environment are sources of stimuli that require modification to promote adaptation, an ongoing purposive response. Adaptive responses contribute to health, which she defines as the process of being and becoming integrated; ineffective or maladaptive responses do not contribute to health. Each person's adaptation level is unique and constantly changing.

As an open system, an individual receives input or stimuli from both the self and the environment. Roy identifies the following three classes of stimuli:

1. *Focal stimuli:* the internal or external stimuli most immediately confronting the person and contributing to behavior
2. *Contextual stimuli:* all other internal or external stimuli present
3. *Residual stimuli:* beliefs, attitudes, or traits having an indeterminate effect on the person's behavior but whose effects are not validated

Throughput makes use of a person's (1) *processes*, which are control mechanisms that a person uses as an adaptive system, and (2) *effectors*, which refer to the physiological function, self-concept, and role function involved in adaptation. *Output* of the system refers to the individual's behaviors, which can be either adaptive responses promoting the system's integrity or ineffective responses, such as not following a prescribed therapy. These outputs or responses provide feedback for the system.

Roy's adaptive systems consist of two interrelated subsystems. The *primary subsystem* is a functional or

Roy's Adaptation Model: Scientific Assumptions for the 21st Century

- Systems of matter and energy progress to higher levels of complex self-organization.
- Consciousness and meaning are constitutive of person and environment integration.
- Awareness of self and environment is rooted in thinking and feeling.
- Human decisions are accountable for the integration of creative processes.
- Thinking and feeling mediate human action.

- System relationships include acceptance, protection, and fostering interdependence.
- Persons and the earth have common patterns and integral relations.
- Person and environment transformations are created in human consciousness.
- Integration of human and environment meanings results in adaptation.

Source: From "Future of the Roy Model: Challenge to Redefine Adaptation," by C. Roy, 1997. *Nursing Science Quarterly, 10*(1), 42–48.

internal control process that consists of the regulator and the cognator. The *regulator* processes input automatically through neural-chemical-endocrine channels. The *cognator* processes input through cognitive pathways, such as perception, information processing, learning, judgment, and emotion. Roy views the regulator and cognator as methods of coping.

The *secondary subsystem* is an effector system that manifests cognator and regulator activity. It consists of the following four adaptive modes:

1. The *physiological mode* involves the body's basic physiological needs and ways of adapting in regard to fluid and electrolytes, activity and rest, circulation and oxygen, nutrition and elimination, protection, the senses, and neurological and endocrine function.

2. The *self-concept mode* includes two components: the *physical self*, which involves sensation and body image, and the *personal self*, which involves self-ideal, self-consistency, and the moral-ethical self.

3. The *role-function mode* is determined by the need for social integrity and refers to the performance of duties based on given positions within society.

4. The *interdependence mode* involves one's relations with significant others and support systems that provide help, affection, and attention.

These adaptive modes include people as individuals or in groups.

Roy's work has been shaped by the current influences in nursing of holism and spiritualism. She has proposed some changes to guide nursing through the

21st century. Adaptation has been redefined as "the process and outcome whereby the thinking and feeling person uses conscious awareness and choice to create human and environmental integration" (Roy, 1997, p. 42). Two sets of assumptions of the Roy model, scientific and philosophic, have been examined for applicability in the 21st century. These are listed in the accompanying boxes on pages 104 and 105.

Benner's Novice to Expert

Patricia Benner was a medical-surgical nurse who worked as a research assistant with Richard Lazarus and did research on stress, coping, and health. Her thinking in nursing was influenced by Virginia Henderson. Herbert Dreyfus, a philosophy professor at Berkley University, introduced her to phenomenology and to the Dreyfus model of skill acquisition. Both of these were influential in her development of Novice to Expert. Her book *From Novice to Expert: Excellence and Power in Clinical Nursing Practice* was published in 1984. A continuation and expansion of those ideas were subsequently published in *Expertise in Nursing Practice: Caring, Clinical Judgment, and Ethics* (Benner, Tanner, and Chesla, 1996). She has published extensively on the model and on expertise in clinical practice including a later book, *Clinical Wisdom in Critical Care: A Thinking-in-Action Approach* (Benner, Hooper-Kyriakidis, & Stannard, 1999).

Benner studied clinical nursing practice to examine knowledge embedded in nursing practice that accrues over time. She was interested in the difference between practical and theoretical knowledge and believed that knowledge development came about by ex-

Roy's Adaptation Model: Philosophical Assumptions for the 21st Century

- Persons have mutual relationships with the world and with a God figure.
- Human meaning is rooted in an omega point convergence of the universe.
- God is intimately revealed in the diversity of creation and is the common destiny of creation.

- Persons use human creative abilities of awareness, enlightenment, and faith.
- Persons are accountable for the processes of deriving, sustaining, and transforming the universe.

Source: From "Future of the Roy Model: Challenge to Redefine Adaptation," by C. Roy, 1997. *Nursing Science Quarterly, 10*(1), 42–48.

tending practical knowledge, or know-how, through theory-based scientific investigations. She emphasized the charting of practices and clinical observations. She described "knowing how" as skill acquisition that is different from "knowing that."

Benner adapted the Dreyfus and Dreyfus Model of Skill Acquisition and Skill Development to clinical nursing practice. The model is situational and consists of five levels: (1) novice, (2) advanced beginner, (3) competent, (4) proficient, and (5) expert. As one moves through the levels, the following four aspects of performance change:

- Movement from a reliance on abstract principles and rules to use of past concrete experiences
- A shift from reliance on analytical, rule-based thinking to intuition
- Change in perception of the situation from a compilation of equally relevant bits to viewing it as a more complex whole, with some aspects being more or less relevant than other aspects
- Passage from a detached observer to someone fully engaged and involved in the situation

The concept of experience is important to the progression. As the nurse gains experience, clinical knowledge becomes a blend of practical and theoretical knowledge.

The model was based upon qualitative, hermeneutic research involving 1200 nurses. Descriptions from observations and narratives of nursing practice were interpreted and described the following five levels of skill acquisition.

1. *Novice:* No background understanding of the situation is present. This is represented by nursing students as they enter their programs of study.

2. *Advanced beginner:* At this level, there is enough experience to grasp aspects and meaningful components of the situation. An example is the new graduate nurse.

3. *Competent:* The nurse is beginning to be able to determine which aspects of a situation are important and which are not.

4. *Proficient:* The nurse is now able to perceive the situation as a whole and is guided by principles and rules of conduct. There is an intuitive grasp on the situation.

5. *Expert:* Judgment is based on understanding, and the nurse focuses on the salient part of the problem. The nurse is no longer reliant on rules, guidelines, and principles.

The model is situational, and so a nurse who is expert in one set of circumstances may not perform at that level in a different situation. These levels are fluid and do not have set boundaries.

The Caring Theorists

Several nursing theories are based on the concept of caring. This movement grew out of humanism and was given considerable impetus by the work of Mayeroff (1971), a philosopher who provided much of the foundational work on the concept of caring. The nursing caring theories provide a link between generic caring and the uniqueness of caring in nursing. In 1998, the American Association of Colleges of Nursing (AACN, 1998) published *The Essentials of Baccalaureate Education for Professional Nursing Practice*, a document prepared to guide education for practice in the 21st century. It defines caring as a concept central to the practice of professional nursing and identifies it as a core value encompassing altruism, autonomy, human dignity, integrity, and social justice.

Caring as a central concept in nursing has its own substantive area of nursing science and has been a focus of scholarly inquiry. Jean Watson (1979, 1985, 1988) may be the best known and most widely recognized caring theorist. However, Madeleine Leininger (1978, 1980, 1984) was a forerunner in the caring movement, although her work may be better known for its transcultural focus. Roach (1992) and Boykin and Schoenhofer (1993) further developed the concepts of caring. Each of these theorists identifies caring as the essence of nursing and a central and unifying feature. Table 6–2 shows a comparison of four caring theories.

Table 6–2   Comparison of Caring Models and Theories

	Mayeroff	Leininger	Roach	Watson	Boykin & Schoenhofer
Perspective on caring	To care for another person is to help that person grow and actualize.	Care is the essence of nursing.	Caring is the human mode of being.	Individual healing processes can be strengthened through authentic caring relationships.	Caring is an essential feature and expression of being human.
Unique focus	Major ingredients of caring: Knowing, alternating rhythms, patience, honesty, trust, humility, hope, and courage.	Inextricably linked with culture.	Caring is not unique to nursing but is unique in nursing.	Caratis processes based on the carative factors. Transpersonal caring relationship through the processes of caring and healing and being in authentic relation, in the moment.	Nurturing persons living and growing in caring.
Expression in nursing	Assists the nurse in developing a sense of self as caring person.	Provide culturally acceptable care.	Professionalization of caring expressed through the 5 C's of caring: Compassion Competence Confidence Conscience Commitment	Watson's theory stresses the importance of the lived experience not only of the client but of the nurse. Both the nurse and the client come together in a caring moment.	Caring is the intentional and authentic presence of the nurse with another who is recognized as a person living and growing in caring.
Discipline of origin	Philosophy	Anthropology	Philosophy	Humanism and Metaphysics	Philosophy, Human Science, and Nursing

Sources: Based on "Caring: Theoretical Perspectives of Relevance to Nursing," by T. V. McCance, H. P. McKenna, and J. R. P. Boore, 1999, *Journal of Advanced Nursing, 30*(6), 1388–1395; *On Caring,* by Milton Maycroff, 1971, New York: Harper Perennial; *Nursing as Caring: A Model for Transforming Nursing Practice,* by A. Boykin and S. Schoenhofer, 1993, National League for Nursing Press. Boston: Jones and Bartlett: Theory of Human Caring, by J. Watson. In *Nursing Theories and Nursing Practice* (pp. 344–354), by M. Parker, 2001, Philadelphia: F. A. Davis.

Critics of caring theory question whether practitioners can use these theories with a limited understanding of the existential-phenomenological-spiritual philosophies that underpin and contribute to the language used in describing them. Nurses from mainstream nursing curricula often find the theories to be abstract and difficult to understand. However, few nurses will deny that caring is essential to professional practice.

The caring movement has produced an organization dedicated to the dissemination of research and scholarly activity in caring. The International Association for Human Caring was first convened by Madeleine Leininger in 1978, and it continues to meet on an annual basis.

Leininger and Watson's theories are the best known of the caring theories and have had the most exposure in nursing literature and critical review. They are the least abstract and have been the basis of research and clinical applications. Both of these theories will be briefly described.

Reflect on...

■ whether caring is the essence of nursing. If so, should it be studied and have its own body of knowledge? How does this knowledge apply in situations where fast responses and highly technological care are critical to outcomes?

Watson's Human Caring Theory

Jean Watson was educated in psychiatric and mental health nursing and received her doctorate in educational psychology and counseling. Her theory of the science of caring was first published in *Nursing: The Philosophy and Science of Caring* (Watson, 1979). She refined her ideas in *Nursing: Human Science and Human Care* (Watson, 1985, 1988, 1999). Watson believes the practice of caring is central to nursing; it is the unifying focus for practice. Two major assumptions underlie human care values in nursing: (1) care and love constitute the primal and universal psychic energy, and (2) care and love are requisite for our survival and the nourishment of humanity. Watson's major assumptions about caring are shown in the accompanying box.

The major conceptual elements of the theory are carative factors, transpersonal caring relationship, and caring moment/caring occasion. The *carative factors* provide a focus for nursing phenomena; these factors are evolving into *caritas processes*. The word *caritas* comes from the Greek word meaning "to cherish." This newer focus includes a greater spiritual dimension and allows for caring and love to transform the self and others being cared for. The original ten caring factors and the evolution to caratas are shown in Table 6–3. *Transpersonal caring relationships* convey a

Watson's Assumptions of Caring

- Human caring in nursing is not just an emotion, concern, attitude, or benevolent desire. Caring connotes a personal response.

- Caring is an intersubjective human process and is the moral ideal of nursing.

- Caring can be effectively demonstrated only interpersonally.

- Effective caring promotes health and individual or family growth.

- Caring promotes health more than does curing.

- Caring responses accept a person not only as they are now but also for what the person may become.

- A caring environment offers the development of potential while allowing the person to choose the best action for the self at a given point in time.

- Caring occasions involve action and choice by nurse and client. If the caring occasion is transpersonal, the limits of openness expand, as do human capacities.

- The most abstract characteristic of a caring person is that the person is somehow responsive to another person as a unique individual, perceives the other's feelings, and sets one person apart from another.

- Human caring involves values, a will and commitment to care, knowledge, caring actions, and consequences.

- The ideal and value of caring is a starting point, a stance, and an attitude that has to become a will, an intention, a commitment, and a conscious judgment that manifests itself in concrete acts.

Table 6–3   Jean Watson's Ten Caring Factors and Caritas

Caring Factors	Caritas
Formation of a humanistic-altruistic system of values	Practice of loving-kindness and equanimity within context of caring consciousness
Instillation of faith-hope	Being authentically present and enabling and sustaining the deep belief system and subjective life world of self and one-being-cared-for
Cultivation of sensitivity to one's self and to others	Cultivation of one's own spiritual practices and transpersonal self, going beyond ego self
Development of a helping-trusting, human caring relationship	Developing and sustaining a helping-trusting, authentic caring relationship
Promotion and acceptance of the expression of positive and negative feelings	Being present to, and supportive, of the expression of positive and negative feelings as a connection with the deeper spirit of self and the one-being-cared-for
Systematic use of a creative problem-solving caring process	Creative use of self and all ways of knowing as part of the caring process; to engage in artistry of caring-healing practices
Promotion of transpersonal teaching-learning	Engaging in a genuine teaching-learning experience that attends to unity of being and meaning, attempting to stay within the other's frame of reference
Provision for a supportive, protective, and/or corrective mental, physical, sociocultural, and spiritual environment	Creating healing environment at all levels, (physical as well as nonphysical), subtle environment of energy and consciousness whereby wholeness, beauty, comfort, dignity, and peace are potentiated
Assistance with gratification of human needs	Assisting with basic needs, with an intentional caring consciousness, administering "human care essentials," which potentiates alignment of mind-bodyspirit, wholeness, and unity of being in all aspects of care; tending to both embodied spirit and evolving spiritual emergence
Allowance for existential-phenomenological-spiritual force	Opening and attending to spiritual-mysterious existential dimensions of one's own life-death; soul care and the one-being-cared-for

concern for the inner life world and subjective meaning for another, and it reaches to the deeper connections to spirit and with the broader universe; it calls for authenticity of being. *Caring moment/caring occasion* occurs whenever the nurse and another come together in a given moment for human-to-human transaction. It involves action and choice by both nurse and other.

Watson considers her work to be a philosophical and moral/ethical foundation for professional nursing and part of the central focus for nursing at the disciplinary level. It includes a call for both art and science that embraces and intersects with art, science, humanities, spirituality, and new dimensions of mind-bodyspirit medicine and nursing.

Leininger's Culture Care Diversity and Universality Theory

Madeleine Leininger, a well-known nurse anthropologist, has written extensively on transcultural nursing concepts and is a proponent of the science of human caring. She first published her cultural care diversity and universality theory in 1985 in the journal *Nursing and Health Care*, explained it further in 1988 and then in 1991, in her book *Culture Care Diversity and Univer-*

Leininger's Descriptions of Care and Caring

- Caring includes assistive, supportive, and facilitative acts toward or for another individual or group with evident or anticipated needs.

- Caring serves to ameliorate or to improve human conditions or life ways. It emphasizes healthful, enabling activities of individuals and groups that are based on culturally defined, ascribed, or sanctioned helping modes.

- Caring is essential to human development, growth, and survival.

- Caring behaviors include comfort, compassion, concern, coping behavior, empathy, enabling, facilitating, interest, involvement, health consultative acts, health maintenance acts, helping behaviors, love, nurturance, presence, protective behaviors, restorative behaviors, sharing, stimulating behaviors, stress alleviation, succor, surveillance, tenderness, touching, and trust.

sality: A Theory of Nursing (Leininger, 1984, 1988, 1991). In this book she produced the sunrise model to depict her theory. (See also Chapter 21 ⬤, Nursing in a Culturally Diverse World.)

Leininger postulates that caring and culture are inextricably linked. Educated in cultural and social anthropology, Leininger observed a marked number of differences between Western and non-Western cultures in caring and health practices. She defines transcultural nursing as a major area of nursing that focuses on comparative study and analysis of different cultures and subcultures in the world, with respect to their caring behavior, nursing care, health values, beliefs, and patterns. The goal of transcultural nursing is to develop a scientific and humanistic body of knowledge in order to provide culture-specific and culture-universal nursing practices. Central to her theory is the belief that cultures have differences in their ways of perceiving, knowing, and practicing care but that there are also commonalities about care among cultures. Thus, her theory focuses on diversity and universality.

Leininger states that care is the essence of nursing and the dominant, distinctive, and unifying feature of nursing. She says that there can be no cure without caring, but that there may be caring without curing. She emphasizes that human caring, although a universal phenomenon, varies among cultures in its expressions, processes, and patterns; it is largely culturally derived. These differences in caring values and behaviors lead to differences in the expectations of those seeking care. For example, cultures that perceive illness primarily as a personal and internal body experience—caused by physical, genetic, and intrabody stresses—tend to use more medications and physical techniques than cultures that view illness as an extrapersonal experience.

Leininger identifies many caring constructs (see the accompanying box). Leininger believes that the goal of health care personnel should be to work toward an understanding of care and the values, health beliefs, and lifestyles of different cultures, which will form the basis for providing culture-specific care.

Critical Thinking Exercise

How does Leininger's description of caring compare and contrast to Watson's description of caring? In providing care to an infant with diarrhea and dehydration, would nursing practice based on these two theories of caring each lead to differing or similar nursing interventions? Would they lead to different outcomes?

ONE MODEL VERSUS SEVERAL MODELS

Many nurses believe that having a single, universal model for nursing would offer the following advantages:

■ Further the development of nursing as a profession.
■ Give all nurses a common framework, enhancing communication and research.
■ Promote understanding about the nurse's role in nontraditional nursing settings, such as independent nurse practitioner practices, self-help clinics, and health maintenance organizations (HMOs), correcting the common misconception that nurses provide care only for sick persons.

In contrast, advocates of several different conceptual models point out the following:

■ Most disciplines have several conceptual models, which allow members to explore phenomena in different ways and from different viewpoints.
■ Several models increase an understanding of the nature of nursing and its scope.
■ Several models foster development of the full scope and potential of the discipline.

It is possible that in the 21st century more models for nursing will be developed and that existing ones will be refined in accordance with societal needs and with their tested usefulness. More research on existing theory may result in the development of middle-range theories that have the potential to direct practice in more specific situations. This direction would help narrow the gap between theory and practice.

RELATIONSHIP OF THEORIES TO THE NURSING PROCESS AND RESEARCH

Conceptual models for nursing are abstractions that are operationalized, or made real, by the use of the nursing process. Each step is guided by the selected theory.

1. *Assessing.* The specific data collected about a client's health needs relate directly to the theorist's view of the client. These views will identify the focus of the assessment. For example, if the client is seen as having 14 fundamental needs, the nurse collects data about these 14 needs.

2. *Diagnosing.* In this step, the nurse analyzes assessment data to identify actual, potential, and possible nursing diagnoses. The nurse outlines or writes the client's actual or potential health problems as a nursing diagnostic statement in accordance with the terminology and focus of the nursing model used. Some models would look at problems that are fairly specific, whereas others would look more holistically.

3. *Planning.* Planning also relates directly to the conceptual nursing model. The nurse establishes goals for resolution of client problems, nursing interventions aimed at achieving those goals, and outcome criteria by which the nurse can evaluate whether or not the goals are met. These goals, interventions, and criteria are established in accordance with the modes of intervention outlined in the conceptual model. Some models will direct the nurse to plan care in partnership with the client, for instance.

4. *Implementing.* Implementing the planned interventions draws on scientific knowledge from many sources. The nursing model instructs the nurse what to do and directly influences what nursing interventions are planned, but it does not tell the nurse how to do it. Implementation in Orem's theory, for instance, would have the nurse work within a wholly compensatory, partially compensatory, or education-supportive system.

5. *Evaluating.* Evaluating is a continuous nursing function. How is the client adjusting and reacting? What does the client see as needs? How does the client see these needs changing? Has the client achieved the desired consequences? The answers to these questions help the nurse evaluate the effectiveness of the total nursing process and the nursing model. In Roy's model this would be part of the output and throughput.

Table 6–4 outlines how two selected nurse theorists have addressed the nursing process.

The conceptual models for nursing drive nursing research and provide a way to organize findings of research in a meaningful way. Variables selected for study are selected according to the suggested relationships drawn from theories; research then validates theory and confirms the presence of the

Table 6–4 Selected Nursing Theories and the Nursing Process

Theory	Nursing Process	Application
Orem's general theory of nursing	Assessing	Involves collecting data about the client's capacities (knowledge, skills, and motivation) to perform universal, developmental, and health-deviation self-care requisites; determines self-care deficits.
	Diagnosing	Stated in terms of the client's limitations to maintain self-care (a deficit in self-care agency).
	Planning	Involves considering and designing, with the client's participation, an appropriate nursing system (wholly compensatory, partially compensatory, and/or supportive-educative) that will help the client achieve an optimal level of self-care (i.e., enhance the client's self-care agency).
	Implementing	Assisting the client by acting for or doing for, guiding, supporting, providing a developmental environment, and teaching.
	Evaluating	Determining the client's level of achievement in resolving self-care deficits and in performing self-care.
Roy's adaptation model	Assessing	Involves two levels: *First-level assessment* includes collecting data about output behaviors related to the four adaptive modes (physiologic, self-concept, role function, and interdependence modes); *second-level assessment* includes collecting data about internal and external stimuli (focal, contextual, or residual) that are influencing the identified behaviors.
	Diagnosing	Focuses on adaptation problems and uses one of three alternative methods: 1. Stating behaviors within one mode with their most relevant influencing stimuli. 2. Clustering behavioral information and labeling it according to indicators of positive adaptation and a typology of common adaptation problems related to each mode. Roy provides a typology of indicators of positive adaptation and a typology of commonly recurring adaptation problems according to each of the four modes. 3. Labeling a behavioral pattern when more than one mode is being affected by the same stimuli.
	Planning	Setting goals in terms of behaviors the client is to achieve and planning nursing interventions to promote the effectiveness of the client's coping mechanisms and adaptive behaviors.
	Implementing	Altering and manipulating the focal, contextual, and residual stimuli by increasing, decreasing, or maintaining them.
	Evaluating	Determining the client's output behaviors with those identified in the goals.

proposed relationships. Research also can be theory generating by describing concepts and suggesting relationships between and among variables that have not previously been proposed. For more discussion of the relationship between research and theory, see Chapter 10 ⬭, The Nurse as Research Consumer.

 EXPLORE MEDIALINK

Questions, critical thinking exercises, essay activities, and other interactive resources for this chapter can be found on the Web site at http://www.prenhall.com/blais. Click on Chapter 6 to select activities for this chapter.

Bookshelf

Nightingale Songs. http://www.fau.edu/divisions/collegeofnursing.
Esthetic expressions of caring written by students in nursing.
O'Brien, J., & Kollock, P. (1997). *The production of reality: Essays and readings on social interaction.* **Thousand Oaks, CA: Pine Forge Press.**
A collection of essays written by well-known authors. These essays focus on perceptions of reality from a variety of perspectives in an entertaining way.

SUMMARY

Nursing is deeply involved in identifying its own unique knowledge base, the body of knowledge needed for practice. Knowledge development in nursing comes from science generated by varying worldviews. Theories and conceptual frameworks help to unify the knowledge into a science of nursing. They offer ways of conceptualizing a discipline in clear, explicit terms that can be easily communicated. Because opinions about the nature and structure of nursing vary, theories continue to be developed. Some theories are broad in scope and others are limited. They vary in level of abstraction, conceptualization, and ability to describe, explain, or predict. A major distinction between a theory and a conceptual framework or model is the level of abstraction with the conceptual framework being more abstract than the theory. A conceptual model is a system of related concepts or a conceptual diagram. Its major purpose is to give clear and explicit direction to the three areas of nursing: practice, education, and research. A theory generates knowledge in a field. Theories can be categorized as philosophy, grand theory, and middle-range theory based upon the scope and structure.

Theory development in nursing had its origins with Florence Nightingale, but it was about a century later when theory development accelerated. The 1960s produced a flurry of activity as nurses pursued graduate education in nursing and related fields. Much of the early theory was inspired by related science in other fields. A current focus in nursing theory development is caring, which has been identified by the AACN as a core value for the profession. It is identified by some as the essence of nursing, a view that is growing in popularity.

Challenges in the 21st century include making theory-based practice a reality. Direct application of theory to clinical situations will depend upon the ability to develop models that are operationalized with the nursing process. A question for the future is whether there should be one grand theory for nursing or the continued use of multiple theories and models. To be considered professionals, nurses must be able to communicate about the science of nursing. Theory can offer a way of communicating to others what is unique about nursing and direct practice in a meaningful way. Theory can be either generated by or tested by research.

REFERENCES

American Association of Colleges of Nursing. (1998). *The essentials of baccalaureate education for professional nursing practice.* Washington, DC: AACN.

Benner, P. (1984). *From Novice to Expert: Excellence and power in clinical nursing practice.* Menlo Park, CA: Addison-Wesley.

Benner, P., Tanner, C., & Chesla, C. (1996). *Expertise in nursing practice: Caring, clinical judgment, and ethics.* New York: Springer.

Benner, P., Hooper-Kyriakidis, P., & Stannard, D. (1999). *Clinical wisdom in critical care: A thinking-in-action approach.* Philadelphia: W. B. Saunders.

Booth, K., Kenrick, M., & Woods, S. (1997). Nursing knowledge, theory, and method revisited. *Journal of Advanced Nursing, 26*(4): 804–811.

Boykin, A., & Schoenhofer, S. (1993). *Nursing as caring: A model for transforming practice.* New York: National League for Nursing Press, Pub. No. 15–2549.

Carboni, J. T. (1995, Spring). A Rogerian process of inquiry. *Nursing Science Quarterly, 7*(3), 128–133.

Carper, B. (1978). Fundamental patterns of knowing in nursing. *Advances in Nursing Science, 1,* 33–54.

Gaut, D. A. (1995). *Historical review of the IAHC 1978–1995.* Royal Palm Beach, FL: International Association for Human Caring.

Fawcett, J. (2002a). The nurse theorists: 21st century updates—Betty Neuman. *Nursing Science Quarterly, 14*(3), 211–214.

Fawcett. J. (2002b). The nurse theorists: 21st century updates—Madeleine M. Leininger. *Nursing Science Quarterly, 15*(2), 131–136.

Fawcett, J. (2003). The nurse theorists: 21st century updates—Martha E. Rogers. *Nursing Science Quarterly, 16*(1), 44–51.

Frey, M., Sieloff, C., & Norris, D. (2002). King's conceptual system and theory of goal attainment: Past, present, and future. *Nursing Science Quarterly, 15*(2), 107–112.

Harmer, B., & Henderson, V. (1955). *Textbook of the principles and practice of nursing,* (5th ed.). Riverside, NJ: Macmillan.

Henderson, V. (1966). *The nature of nursing: A definition and its implications for practice, research, and education.* Riverside, NJ: Macmillan.

Henderson, V. (1991). *The nature of nursing: Reflections after 25 years.* New York: National League for Nursing Press, Pub. No. 15–2346.

King, I. M. (1971). *Toward a theory for nursing: General concepts of human behavior.* New York: Wiley.

King, I. M. (1981). *A theory for nursing: Systems, concepts, process.* New York: Wiley.

Kneller, G. F. (1971). *Introduction to the Philosophy of Education.* (2nd ed.). New York: Wiley.

Leininger, M. M. (1978). *Transcultural nursing: Concepts, theories, and practices.* New York: Wiley.

Leininger, M. M. (1980, October). Caring: A central focus of nursing and health care services. *Nursing and Health Care, 1*(3): 135–143.

Leininger, M. M. (1984). *Care: The essence of nursing and health,* Thorofare, NJ: Charles B. Slack.

Leininger, M. M. (1985, April). Transcultural care diversity and universality: A theory of nursing. *Nursing and Health Care, 6*(4), 208–212.

Leininger, M. M. (1988, November). Leininger's theory of nursing: Cultural care, diversity and universality. *Nursing Science Quarterly, 1*(4), 152–160.

Leininger, M. M. (Ed.). (1991). *Culture care diversity and universality: A theory of nursing.* New York: National League for Nursing Press, Pub. No. 15–2402.

Madrid, M., & Barrett, E. A. M. (Eds.). (1994). *Rogers' scientific art of nursing practice.* New York: National League for Nursing Press, Pub. No. 15–2610.

McCance, T. V., McKenna, H. P., & Boore, J. R. P. (1999). Caring: Theoretical perspectives of relevance to nursing. *Journal of Advanced Nursing, 30*(6), 1388–1395.

Mayeroff, M. (1971). *On caring.* London: Harper Row.

Meleis, A. I., Sawyer, L. M., Im, E., Hilfinger-Messias, D. K., & Schumacher, K. (2000). Experiencing transitions: An emerging middle-range theory. *Advances in Nursing Science, 23*(1), 12–28.

Neuman, B. (1974). The Betty Neuman health-care systems model: A total person approach to patient problems. In J. P. Riehl & C. Roy (Eds.), *Conceptual models for nursing practice.* New York: Appleton-Century-Crofts.

Neuman, B. (1982). *The Neuman systems model: Applications to nursing education and practice.* New York: Appleton-Century-Crofts.

Neuman, B. (1989). *The Neuman systems model: Applications to nursing education and practice* (2nd ed.). Norwalk, CT: Appleton and Lange.

Neuman, B. 1995. *The Neuman systems model* (3rd ed.). Norwalk, CT: Appleton and Lange.

Neuman, B., & Young, R. J. (1972, June). A model for teaching total person approach to patient problems. *Nursing Research, 21,* 264–269.

Nicoll, L. H. (1997). *Perspectives on nursing theory* (3rd ed.). Philadelphia: Lippincott.

Nightingale, F. (1860). *Notes on nursing.* Philadelphia: Lippincott. (Reprint 1957).

Orem, D. E. (1971). *Nursing: Concepts of practice.* Hightstown, NJ: McGraw-Hill.

Orem, D. E. (1980). *Nursing: Concepts of practice* (2nd ed.). Hightstown, NJ: McGraw-Hill.

Orem, D. E. (1985). *Nursing: Concepts of practice* (3rd ed.). Hightstown, NJ: McGraw-Hill.

Orem, D. E. (1991). *Nursing: Concepts of practice* (4th ed.). Hightstown, NJ: McGraw-Hill.

Orem, D. E. (1995). *Nursing: Concepts of practice* (5th ed.). Hightstown, NJ: McGraw-Hill.

Orem, D. E., & Vardiman, E. M. (1995, Winter). Orem's theory and positive mental health: Practical considerations. *Nursing Science Quarterly, 8*(4), 165–173.

Peplau, H. E. (1952). *Interpersonal relations in nursing.* New York: Putnam.

Peplau, H. E. (1963, October/November). Interpersonal relations and the process of adaptations. *Nursing Science, 1*(4), 272–279.

Peplau, H. E. (1980). The Peplau developmental model for nursing practice. In J. P. Riehl & C. Roy (Eds.), *Conceptual models for nursing practice* (2nd ed., pp. 53–75). New York: Appleton-Century-Crofts.

Roach, M. S. (1992). *The human act of caring: A blueprint for the health professions.* (Rev. ed.). Ottawa, Canada: Canadian Hospital Association Press.

Rogers, M. E. (1970). *An introduction to the theoretical basis of nursing.* Philadelphia: F. A. Davis.

Rogers, M. E. (1989). Nursing: A science of unitary human beings. In J. Riehl-Sisca (Ed.), *Conceptual models for nursing practice* (3rd ed., pp. 181–188). Norwalk, CT: Appleton and Lange.

Rogers, M. E. (1994, Spring). The science of unitary human beings: Current perspectives. *Nursing Science Quarterly, 7*(1), 33–35.

Roy, C. (1970, March). Adaptation: A conceptual framework in nursing. *Nursing Outlook, 18,* 42–45.

Roy, C. (1976). *Introduction to nursing: An adaptation model.* Upper Saddle River, NJ: Prentice Hall.

Roy, C. (1984). *Introduction to nursing: An adaptation model* (2nd ed.). Upper Saddle River, NJ: Prentice Hall.

Roy, C. (1997). Future of the Roy model: Challenge to redefine adaptation. *Nursing Science Quarterly, 10*(1), 42–48.

Roy, C., & Andrews, H. A. (1991). *The Roy adaptation model: The definitive statement.* Norwalk, CT: Appleton and Lange.

Roy, C., & Andrews, H. A. (1999). *The Roy adaptation model* (2nd ed.). Stamford, CT: Appleton and Lange.

Sarter, B. (1988). *The stream of becoming: A study of Martha Rogers' theory.* New York: National League for Nursing Press, Pub. No. 15–2205.

Tomey, A. M., & Alligood, M. R. (2002). *Nursing theorists and their work* (5th ed.). St. Louis: Mosby.

Tsai, P. (2003). A middle-range theory of caregiver stress. *Nursing Science Quarterly, 16*(2), 137–145.

Watson, J. (1979). *Nursing: The philosophy and science of caring.* Boston: Little, Brown.

Watson, J. (1985). *Nursing: Human science and human care. A theory of nursing.* Norwalk, CT: Appleton-Century-Crofts.

Watson, J. (1988). *Nursing: Human science and human care. A theory of nursing.* New York: National League for Nursing Press, Pub. No. 15–2236.

Watson, J. (1997). The theory of human caring: Retrospective and prospective. *Nursing Science Quarterly, 10*(1), 49–52.

Watson, J. (1999). *Nursing: Human science and human care. A theory of nursing.* Boulder, CO: University of Colorado Press.

Watson, J. (1999). *Postmodern nursing and beyond.* Edinburgh, Scotland, UK: Churchill-Livingstone: Harcourt-Brace.

Wesley, R. L. (1995). *Nursing theories and models* (2nd ed.). Springhouse, PA: Springhouse.

Unit II
Professional Nursing Roles

The Nurse as Health Promoter and Care Provider

Objectives

- Differentiate health preventive or protective care and health promotion.

- Discuss essential components of health promotion.

- Discuss the goals, focus areas, and leading health indicators of *Healthy People 2010*.

- Identify various types and sites of health-promotion programs.

- Compare three health-promotion models: those of Pender, Kulbock, and Neuman.

- Discuss Prochaska and DiClemente's five-stage model of behavior change.

- Analyze the nurse's role in health promotion.

M E D I A L I N K

Additional online resources for this chapter can be found on the companion Web site at http://www.prenhall.com/blais.

Health promotion is an important component of nursing practice. It is a way of thinking that revolves around a philosophy of wholeness, wellness, and well-being. In the past four decades, the public has become increasingly aware of and interested in health promotion. Many people are aware of the relationship between lifestyle and illness and are developing health-promoting habits, such as getting adequate exercise, rest, and relaxation; maintaining good nutrition; and controlling the use of tobacco, alcohol, drugs, and other substances that may be harmful to the body.

The vision of health promotion was expressed nationally in Canada in 1974 with the publication of the Lalonde Report, *A New Perspective on the Health of Canadians* (Lalonde, 1974), and in the United States in 1979 in the Surgeon General's report, *Healthy People* (U.S. Surgeon General, 1979). Both reports emphasized the role that individuals could play in modifying their lifestyle and personal behaviors to improve their health status. These reports also consider, to a lesser extent, environmental factors influencing health.

In 1980, the U.S. Public Health Service developed *Health Promotion/Disease Prevention: Objectives for the Nation* (U.S. Surgeon General, 1980). This report addressed more specifically the broad goals set forth in *Healthy People* by listing strategies to achieve each objective. These strategies included not only personal behavior changes but also the roles of institutions, legislation, and policy. In the mid-1980s, the Canadian government undertook a large restructuring of its approach to health care. This report, known as the Epp Report, emerged from a synthesis of the Lalonde Report and initiatives of the World Health Organization (1984, 1986). The Epp Report focused on achieving health for all citizens by reducing inequities between low- and high-income groups, increasing prevention, and enhancing coping (Epp, 1986). See Figure 7–1■.

In September 1990, *Healthy People 2000* was presented to the American public. This document encompassed 298 health-related objectives that provided a framework for a national health promotion, health protection, and preventive service strategy (U.S. Department of Health and Human Services [USDHHS], 1990). Individual nurses and 24 national nursing organizations were involved in the development of *Healthy People 2000* (Brown et al., 1992, p. 204).

Currently, *Healthy People 2010* (USDHHS, 2001, 2004) builds on the initiatives developed over the previous two decades. The major purpose of *Healthy People 2010* is to "promote health and prevent illness, disability, and premature death." It states national health objectives "designed to identify the most significant preventable threats to health and to establish national goals to reduce these threats." *Healthy People 2010* was developed through the Healthy People Consortium, an alliance consisting of 350 national organizations, including professional nursing and medical associations, and 250 state health, mental health, substance abuse, and environmental agencies. The public had the opportunity to be involved in the development of *Healthy People 2010* through an interactive Web site. Thus, *Healthy People 2010* is a collaborative effort of private, professional, and governmental agencies, with consumer input to determine the future health of the people of the United States. *Healthy People 2010* "is grounded in science, built through public consensus, and designed to measure progress" in achievement of its goals.

CHALLENGES AND OPPORTUNITIES

Health care and nursing have traditionally been more oriented toward curing and treating than preventing illness, injury, and disability. Shifting the focus toward maintaining and promoting health and wellness is a current challenge. Many forces in society, including

Figure 7–1

A Framework for Health Promotion

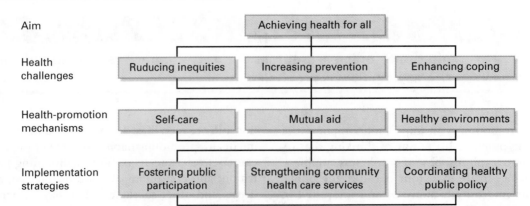

Source: From Achieving Health for All: A Framework for Health Promotion: Report of the Minister of National Health and Welfare, by J. Epp, November 1986, Ottawa, Canada: Government Printing Office.

cost containment and allocation of resources, have provided the impetus toward maintaining health rather than providing more resource-intensive care once health has been compromised. Nursing theories have been developed that focus on prevention and health promotion. The profession is challenged to use these theories and continue to develop its abilities to keep people healthy.

The role of health promoter provides the nurse with many opportunities to contribute to improved health. The nurse has an opportunity to educate individuals and groups in the community about prevention and maintaining health. Nurses practice in a variety of community settings, such as school-based clinics, primary care clinics, prenatal and well-baby clinics, and health departments, where they interact with healthy people and can provide guidance. However, the opportunities for health promotion can be found in more traditional health care settings as well. People with acute and chronic illnesses can learn ways of caring for themselves that will enhance health and increase well-being.

DEFINING HEALTH PROMOTION

Considerable differences appear in the literature regarding the use of the terms *health promotion, primary prevention, health protection,* and *illness prevention.* Maville and Huerta (2002, pp. 2–3) state that a "universally accepted definition of health promotion does not exist and that the phrase is often confused with or used synonymously for health education." Nurses practice health promotion through education of clients and their families and through community education programs. The nurse as educator will be discussed in Chapter 8 ⬤. Maville and Huerta state that there are "four major themes that provide for some unity" in understanding: "empowerment, lifestyles, health enhancement, and well-being (p. 3)." They define health promotion as "any endeavor directed at enhancing the quality of health and well-being of individuals, families, groups, communities, and/or nations through strategies involving supportive environments, coordination of resources, and respect for personal choice and values (p. 3)."

Leavell and Clark (1965, p. 21) defined three levels of prevention: primary, secondary, and tertiary. There are five steps that describe these levels: **Primary prevention** focuses on (1) health promotion and (2) protection against specific health problems. **Secondary prevention** focuses on (1) early identification of health problems and (2) prompt intervention to alleviate health problems. **Tertiary prevention** focuses on restoration and rehabilitation to an optimal level of functioning.

In the model used by Leavell and Clark, primary prevention precedes any disease symptoms. The purpose of primary prevention is to encourage optimal health and to increase the person's resistance to illness. Examples of primary prevention include health education concerning the hazards of smoking and specific protection against a particular disease, such as the vaccine against poliomyelitis.

The second level, secondary prevention, presumes the presence of a disease or illness. Screening procedures, such as a blood glucose test for a client with diabetes mellitus, and the Denver Developmental Screening Tests to assess developmental delays, are facets of secondary prevention. Screening procedures facilitate early discovery and allow treatment to begin before the illness progresses. Disability limitation, another step in secondary prevention, is also more effective in the early stages of a disease.

Tertiary prevention relates to situations in which a disability is already present. The goal of tertiary prevention is to restore individuals to their optimal level of functioning within the limitations imposed by their condition. A further discussion of the levels of prevention can be found in Chapter 17 ⬤.

Pender, Murdaugh, and Parsons describe the three levels of prevention (primary, secondary, and tertiary) as health protection. Health protection "is behavior motivated by a desire to actively avoid illness, detect it early, or maintain functioning within the constraints of illness (Pender, Murdaugh, & Parsons, 2002, p. 7)." In contrast, health promotion is "behavior motivated by a desire to increase well-being and actualize human health potential (p. 7)." In this instance, health promotion is considered to be an approach behavior, whereas primary prevention is considered avoidance behavior. Health promotion is not disease oriented; that is, no specific problem is being avoided. By contrast, primary prevention activities are geared toward avoiding specific problems.

Stachtchenko and Jenicek (1990, p. 53) support Pender's conceptual differences between the terms *health promotion* and *primary prevention* (or health protection). They describe health promotion as broad in scope, involving not only lifestyle changes but also the process of granting individuals and communities more control over determinants of health. Health prevention programs focus on risk reduction and are targeted toward specific populations.

Healthy People 2000 differentiated among health promotion, health protection, and preventive health services, outlining the following specific activities for each category:

- *Health promotion:* individual and community activities to promote healthful lifestyles. Examples of health-promotion activities include improving nutrition, preventing alcohol and drug misuse, restricting smoking, maintaining fitness, and exercising.
- *Health protection:* actions by government and industry to minimize environmental health threats. Health protection relates to activities such as maintaining occupational safety, controlling radiation and toxic agents, and preventing infectious diseases and accidents.
- *Preventive health services:* actions that health care providers take to prevent health problems. These services include control of high blood pressure, control of sexually transmitted diseases, immunization, family planning, and health care during pregnancy and infancy.

The difficulty in separating the terms *health promotion, disease prevention,* and *health protection* lies in the fact that an activity may be carried out for numerous reasons. For example, a 40-year-old male may begin a program of walking 3 miles each day. If the goal of his program is to "decrease the risk of heart disease," then the activity would be considered prevention or health protection. By contrast, if his walking regimen is instituted to "increase his overall health and feeling of well-being," then the activity would be considered health-promotion behavior.

A summary of essential concepts of health promotion proposed by Schultz (1995, p. 32) is shown in the

Concepts of Health Promotion

- Health promotion maintains and enhances health.
- Health promotion develops the resources and skills of the person or community.
- Health promotion alters personal or communal habits and the environment.
- Health promotion defines health as a continuum.
- Health promotion is self-directed.

Source: From "What Is Health Promotion?," by A. Schultz, 1995. *Canadian Nurse, 91*(7), 31–34.

accompanying box. These points are incorporated into her definition of health promotion:

> Health promotion facilitates an individual or a community in a process of self-determining a present health status, in order to actively choose ways of altering personal or communal health habits for improvement, and to develop resources and skills to alter the environment so that health is being maintained or a self-determined higher level of health can be achieved.

Reflect on...

- your personal definition of health promotion. How do your personal values and beliefs influence your definition of health promotion?
- how factors in society such as cultural beliefs, religious/spiritual beliefs, or political and economic factors influence health-promotion practices.
- whether you agree with Pender's conceptual differences between the terms *health promotion* and *primary prevention.*
- whether health promotion and/or health protection can be offered to all clients regardless of their age, health, and illness status.

HEALTHY PEOPLE 2010

Healthy People 2010 builds on prior *Healthy People* documents by identifying two overall goals:

1. Increase quality and years of healthy life.
2. Eliminate health disparities.

Increasing Quality and Years of Healthy Life

In 1995, Japan had the highest life expectancy in the world for nations with populations of more than 1 million: 82.9 years for women and 76.4 years for men; the United States ranked 19th for women (78.9) and 25th for men (72.5). (See Table 7–1.) Such data suggest the need for improvement in the United States as well as other nations. However, increasing the number of years is not sufficient if the quality of those years is not also improved. Quality of life is the general sense of well-being or satisfaction with one's life within one's environment. Quality of life embraces all aspects of life, including physical and mental health, recreation, culture, rights, values, beliefs, aspirations, and the conditions that support a life containing these elements (*Healthy People 2010*, USDHHS, 2001, 2004).

Table 7–1 Life Expectancy at Birth by Gender Ranked by Selected Countries, 1995

Female		Male	
Country	**Years of Life Expectancy**	**Country**	**Years of Life Expectancy**
Japan	82.9	Japan	76.4
France	82.6	Sweden	76.2
Switzerland	81.9	Israel	75.3
Sweden	81.6	Canada	75.2
Spain	81.5	Switzerland	75.1
Canada	81.2	Greece	75.1
Australia	80.9	Australia	75.0
Italy	80.8	Norway	74.9
Norway	80.7	Netherlands	74.6
Netherlands	80.4	Italy	74.4
Greece	80.3	England & Wales	74.3
Finland	80.3	France	74.2
Austria	80.1	Spain	74.2
Germany	79.8	Austria	73.5
Belgium	79.8	Singapore	73.4
England & Wales	79.6	Germany	73.3
Israel	79.3	New Zealand	73.3
Singapore	79.0	Northern Ireland	73.1
United States	78.9	Belgium	73.0
		Cuba	73.0
		Costa Rica	73.0
		Finland	72.8
		Denmark	72.8
		Ireland	72.5
		United States	72.5

Source: From *Healthy People 2010: A Systematic Approach to Health Improvement* (pp. 3–4), by U.S. Department of Health and Human Services, 2001, http://www.health.gov/healthypeople.

Eliminating Health Disparities

The focus of this goal is to eliminate health disparities among segments of the population. The principle of *Healthy People 2010* is that every person in the United States, "regardless of age, gender, race or ethnicity, income, education, geographic location, disability, and sexual orientation, deserves equal access to comprehensive, culturally competent, community-based health care systems that are committed to serving the needs of the individual and promoting community health" (USDHHS, 2001, p. 10).

Currently, there are many health disparities in the United States, including the following:

■ The infant death rate among African Americans is more than double that of Whites.

■ African Americans have higher death rates than Whites related to heart disease (40% higher), cancer (30% higher), HIV/AIDS (700%), and homicide (600%).

■ Hispanics living in the United States are more likely to die from diabetes than non-Hispanic Whites. They have higher rates of hypertension and obesity than non-Hispanic Whites.

■ Native Americans and Alaska natives have higher infant mortality rates, higher rates of diabetes, and higher death rates associated with unintentional injuries and suicide.

■ People with higher levels of education and income have a lower incidence of heart disease, diabetes, obesity, hypertension, and low birth weight.

■ People with disabilities report more anxiety, pain, sleeplessness, and days of depression than do those who do not have disabilities.

■ People in rural areas are more likely to have heart disease, cancer, and diabetes than those who live in urban areas.

These disparities are inconsistent with the constitutional philosophy of the equality of all people. *Healthy People 2010* urges that efforts be made to reduce these disparities.

To determine the nation's progress toward achieving the goals, 28 focus areas will be monitored via 467 objectives. (See the accompanying box.) The objectives focus on interventions designed to reduce or eliminate illness, disability, and premature death and to improve access to quality health care, strengthen public health services, and improve the availability and dissemination of health-related information. The focus areas relate to individual, group, and community efforts to achieve the overall goals.

Healthy People 2010 Focus Areas

- Access to quality health services
- Arthritis, osteoporosis, and chronic back conditions
- Cancer
- Chronic kidney disease
- Diabetes
- Disability and secondary conditions
- Educational and community-based programs
- Environmental health
- Family planning
- Food safety
- Health communication
- Heart disease and stroke
- HIV
- Immunization and infectious diseases

- Injury and violence prevention
- Maternal, infant, and child health
- Medical product safety
- Mental health and mental disorders
- Nutrition and overweight
- Occupational safety and health
- Oral health
- Physical activity and fitness
- Public health infrastructure
- Respiratory diseases
- Sexually transmitted diseases
- Substance abuse
- Tobacco use
- Vision and hearing

Source: From *Healthy People 2010: A Systematic Approach to Health Improvement,* by U.S. Department of Health and Human Services, 2001, http://www.health.gov/healthypeople.

Leading health indicators were developed reflecting the major public health concerns in the United States. (See the accompanying box.) They were chosen because they have the ability to motivate action, they can be measured by objective data to determine their progress, and they are relevant to broad public health issues. For each of the leading health indicators, specific objectives will be used to track progress. For example, for the leading health indicator physical activity, objectives include increasing the percentage of adolescents and adults who regularly engage in physical activity that promotes cardiovascular fitness (USDHHS, 2004). In tracking progress toward the goals, one needs to look at improvement in those populations with low rates of physical activity, such as women, people with lower incomes and less education, people from minority groups such as African Americans and Hispanics, and people with disabilities.

Reflect on...

■ yourself as a role model of healthy behaviors related to the achievement of the goals of *Healthy People 2010*. Do you smoke? Are you overweight? Do you engage in physical activity and exercise regularly? What are your own barriers in achieving the goals of *Healthy People 2010*? What are the factors that help you achieve healthy behaviors?

Leading Health Indicators

- Physical activity
- Overweight and obesity
- Tobacco use
- Substance abuse
- Responsible sexual behavior
- Mental health
- Injury and violence
- Environmental quality
- Immunization
- Access to health care

Source: From *Healthy People 2010: Leading Health Indicators,* by U.S. Department of Health and Human Services, 2001, http://www.health.gov/healthypeople.

HEALTH-PROMOTION ACTIVITIES

Health-promotion organizations, wellness centers, and traditional health care centers all offer a different approach to client care. Table 7–2 demonstrates these differences. Health-promotion activities can be carried

Table 7–2   Comparison of Three Foci of Health Care: Traditional, Health Promotion, and Wellness

	Traditional	Health Promotion	Wellness
Primary goal	Diagnosis and cure	Illness/injury prevention and risk reduction	Improved health and wellness
Focus of care	Disease/injury	Individuals, families, and communities	Individuals, families, and communities in cultural context
Intervention	Medical/surgical treatment	Health risk appraisal, health information, behavior change	Health information, nutritional counseling, exercise, stress management
Duration	Until problem is resolved	Length of program	Lifelong
Example	Treatment of client with acute myocardial infarction	Health risk appraisal for client with family history of heart disease and coaching for lifestyle change	Programs to prevent obesity in childhood, including developing lifelong nutrition and exercise habits

out on a governmental level (e.g., a national program to improve knowledge of nutrition) or on a personal level (e.g., an individual exercise program).

Health-promotion programs on an individual level can be active or passive. With passive strategies, the client is a recipient of the health-promotion effort. Many health professionals participate in national programs to define and institute these passive strategies. Examples of passive government strategies are maintaining the cleanliness of water and promoting a healthy environment by enforcing sewage regulations to decrease the spread of disease. Active strategies depend on individuals' commitment to and involvement in adopting a program directed toward their health promotion. Active strategies are important in that they encourage individuals to take control of their lives and assume the responsibility for their health. Examples of active strategies that involve changes in lifestyle are (1) a diet-management program to improve nutrition, (2) a self-help program to reduce stress related to parenting, (3) an exercise program to improve muscle strength and endurance, or (4) a combination diet and exercise regimen for weight reduction or control. For optimal health and well-being, a combination of both active and passive strategies is suggested.

Types of Health-Promotion Programs

A variety of programs can be used for the promotion of health, including (1) information dissemination, (2) health appraisal and wellness assessment, (3) lifestyle and behavior change, and (4) environmental control programs.

Information dissemination is the most basic type of health-promotion program. This method makes use of a variety of media to offer information to the public about the risk of particular lifestyle choices and personal behavior, as well as the benefits of changing that behavior and improving the quality of life. Billboards, posters, brochures, newspaper features, books, the Internet, and health fairs all offer opportunities for the dissemination of health-promotion information. Alcohol and drug abuse, driving under the influence of alcohol, hypertension, sexually transmitted diseases (including HIV/AIDS), and the need for immunizations are some of the topics frequently discussed. Information dissemination is a useful strategy for raising the level of knowledge and awareness of individuals and groups about health habits.

Health risk appraisal/wellness assessment programs are used to apprise individuals of the risk factors that are inherent in their lives in order to motivate them to reduce specific risks and develop positive health habits. Wellness assessment programs are focused on more positive methods of enhancement, in contrast to the risk factor approach used in the health appraisal. A variety of tools are available to facilitate these assessments. Some of these tools are computer based and can therefore be offered to educational institutions and industries at a reasonable cost.

Lifestyle- and behavior-change programs require the participation of the individual and are geared toward enhancing the quality of life and extending the life span. Individuals generally consider lifestyle changes after they have been informed of the need to change their health behavior and become aware of the potential benefits of the process. Many programs are available to the public, both on a group and individual basis, some of which address stress management, nutrition awareness, weight control, smoking cessation, and exercise.

Environmental-control programs have been developed in response to the recent growth in the number of contaminants of human origin that have been introduced into our environment. The amount of contaminants that are already present in the air, food, and water will affect the health of our descendants for several generations. The most common concerns of community groups are toxic and nuclear wastes, nuclear power plants, air and water pollution, and herbicide and pesticide spraying.

Sites for Health-Promotion Activities

Health-promotion programs are found in many settings. Programs and activities may be offered to individuals and families in the home or in the community setting, at schools, in hospitals, at worksites, or at shopping malls. Some individuals may feel more comfortable having the nurse, diet counselor, or fitness expert come to their home for teaching and follow-up on individual needs. This type of program, however, is not cost-effective for most individuals. Many people prefer the group approach, find it more motivating, and enjoy the socializing and group support. Most programs offered in the community are group oriented.

Community programs are frequently offered by cities and towns. The type of program depends on the current concerns and the expertise of the sponsoring department or group. Program offerings may include health promotion, specific protection, and screening for early detection of disease. The local health department may offer a community-wide immunization program or blood pressure screening. The fire department may disseminate fire-prevention information; the police may offer bicycle safety programs for children, safe-driving campaigns for young adults, or gun safety programs for all citizens. The recreation department may sponsor or provide facilities for group or individual sports programs for children and adults, such as youth baseball, football, and basketball programs or adult exercise programs.

Hospitals began the emphasis on health promotion and prevention by focusing on the health of their employees. Because of the stress involved in caring for the sick and the various shifts that nurses and other health care workers must work, the lifestyles and health habits of health care employees were given priority.

Programs offered by health care organizations initially began with the specific focus of prevention. Examples include infection control, fire prevention and fire drills, limiting exposure to X rays, and the prevention of back injuries. Gradually, issues related to the health and lifestyle of the employee were addressed with programs on topics such as smoking cessation, exercise and fitness, stress reduction, and time management. Increasingly, hospitals have offered a variety of these programs and others (e.g., women's health) to the community as well as to their employees. This community activity of the health care institution enhances the public image of the hospital, increases the health of the surrounding population, and generates some additional income.

School health-promotion programs may serve as a foundation for children of all ages to learn basic knowledge about personal hygiene and issues in the health sciences. Because school is the focus of a child's life for so many years, the school provides a cost-effective and convenient setting for health-focused programs. The school nurse may teach programs about basic nutrition, dental care, activity and play, drug and alcohol abuse, domestic violence, child abuse, and issues related to sexuality and pregnancy. Classroom teachers may include health-related topics in their lesson plans, for example, the way the normal heart functions or the need for clean air and water in the environment.

Worksite programs for health promotion have developed out of the need for businesses to control the rising cost of health care and employee absenteeism. Many industries feel that both employers and employees can benefit from healthy lifestyle behavior and have employed occupational health nurses as part of their human resources department to plan and provide health-promotion programs. The convenience of the worksite setting makes these programs particularly attractive to many adults who would otherwise not be aware of them or motivated to attend them. Health-promotion programs may be held in the company cafeteria so that employees can watch a film or have a discussion group during their lunch break. Worksite programs may include programs that address air-quality standards for the office, classroom, or plant; programs aimed at specific populations, such as accident prevention for the machine worker or back-saver programs for the individual involved in heavy lifting; programs to prevent repetitive stress injuries; programs to screen for high blood pressure; or health-enhancement programs, such as fitness information and relaxation techniques. Benefits to the worker may include an increased feeling of well-being, fitness, weight control, and decreased stress. Benefits to the employer may include an increase in employee motivation and productivity, an increase in employee morale, a decrease in absenteeism, and a lower rate of employee turnover, all of which may decrease business and health care costs.

Increasingly, health information is available on the World Wide Web. Internet sites such as WebMD offer information on prevention, screening, and management of many illnesses. It is important that health professionals inform patients and consumers of the reliability of information on the Internet. Although there are many reliable sources of health information on the Web, there are also Web sites that present opinions of the Web site developer, which may or may not be supported by scientific evidence. An example of health information disseminated on the Internet that must be viewed with caution are Web sites espousing various alternative medicine strategies.

Reflect on...

- the availability and accessibility of health-promotion and preventive care services to people of all ages and economic status in your community.
- the worksite wellness program at your place of employment. What services are provided? Do you participate in these services? How would you improve your current worksite wellness program?
- the effectiveness of environmental control programs in your community.
- health-promotion activities you would like to see implemented in your community if there were no limits in resources, such as time, expertise, and money.

Evidence for Practice

Callaghan, D. M. (2003). **Health-promoting self-care behaviors, self-care, self-efficacy, and self-care agency.** *Nursing Science Quarterly, 16*(3), 247–254.

The purpose of this study was to explore the relationships among health-promoting self-care behaviors, self-care self-efficacy, and self-care agency in an adult population. The conceptual frameworks for the study included Pender's health promotion model, Bandura's social cognitive theory, and Orem's self-care deficit theory. The sample consisted of 379 adults ranging in age from 18 to 65 who were responsible for self-care. Three instruments were used to determine the relationships between the concepts. The Health-Promoting Lifestyle Profile II (HPLPII) was used to measure the concept of health-promoting self-care behaviors. The Self-Rated Abilities for Health Practices (SRAHP) was used to measure four dimensions of health self-efficacy, including exercise, psychological well-being, nutrition, and health practices. The Exercise of Self-Care Agency (ESCA) was used to measure five dimensions of self-care agency, including attitude of responsibility for self, motivation to care for self, application of knowledge to self-care, the valuing of health priorities, and self-esteem. In this study, only the concept of spiritual growth indicated an influence on self-care agency. Based on this study, nurses should understand the importance of assisting clients to meet their spiritual needs as a component of health-promoting self-care practices.

HEALTH-PROMOTION MODELS

The health belief model (HBM) discussed in Chapter 17 ⊙⊙, Nursing in an Evolving Health Care Delivery System, focuses on a person's susceptibility to disease. According to Pender et al. (2002, p. 37), the HBM is considered appropriate for explaining health-protecting or preventive behaviors, but it is not considered an appropriate model for health-promoting behaviors. Discussion of three health-promotion models follows.

Pender's Health-Promotion Model

Nola Pender's Health-Promotion Model (Pender et al., 2002, pp. 60–79) was first published in the literature in the 1980s but has since been revised based on research using the model. It differs from the HBM in that it focuses on *health-promoting behaviors* rather than health-protecting or preventive behaviors (Figure 7–2■). The Health-Promotion Model is based on the following assumptions that "emphasize the active role of the client in shaping and maintaining health behaviors and in modifying the environmental context for health behaviors" (2002, p. 63):

1. Persons seek to create conditions of living through which they can express their unique human health potential.
2. Persons have the capacity for reflective self-awareness, including assessment of their own competencies.
3. Persons value growth in directions viewed as positive and attempt to achieve a personally acceptable balance between change and stability.
4. Individuals seek to actively regulate their own behavior.
5. Individuals in all their biopsychosocial complexity interact with the environment, progressively transforming the environment and being transformed over time.
6. Health professionals constitute a part of the interpersonal environment that exerts influence on persons throughout their life span.
7. Self-initiated reconfiguration of person-environment interactive patterns is essential to behavior change.

The components of the Health-Promotion Model are Individual Characteristics and Experiences, Behavior-Specific Cognitions and Affect, Commitment to a Plan of Action, Immediate Competing Demands and Preferences, and Behavior Outcome.

Individual Characteristics and Experiences

Individual characteristics and experiences are unique to each person and influence their subsequent behavior. This component includes Prior Related Behavior and Personal Factors. *Prior related behavior* includes previous experiences, knowledge, and skill in health-promoting actions. To explain the influence of prior related behavior, if a person has had positive prior experiences with health promotion and other health-

Figure 7–2

Health-Promotion Model

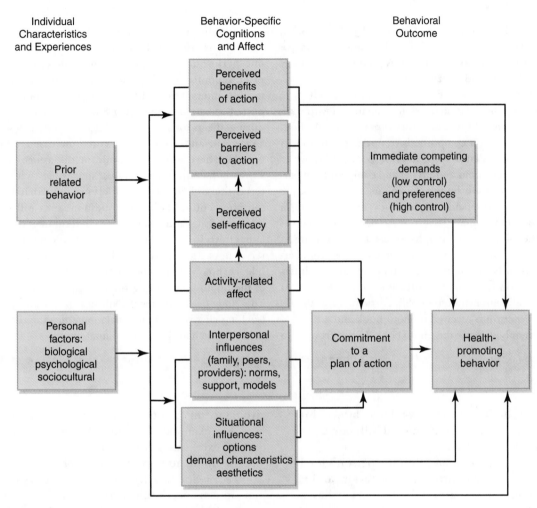

Source: From *Health Promotion in Nursing* (4th ed., p. 60), by N. J. Pender, C. L. Murdaugh, and M. A. Parsons, 2002, Upper Saddle River, NJ: Prentice Hall. Reprinted with permission.

related activities, they are more likely to maintain those activities than someone who has had negative prior experiences.

Personal factors include biologic, psychologic, and sociocultural factors. Biologic characteristics include factors such as age, gender, familial or hereditary risk for specific diseases such as cancer, strength, agility, balance, pubertal status, menopausal status, and percentage of body fat and total body weight. Psychologic factors include characteristics such as self-esteem, self-motivation, and perceptions of health status. Sociocultural factors include characteristics such as ethnicity,

race, education, income, and acculturation. Personal factors can also include cognitions, affect, and health behaviors.

Behavior-Specific Cognitions and Affect

Behavior-specific cognitions and affect are considered the "critical core for intervention because they are subject to modification through nursing actions" (Pender et al., 2002, p. 69). The components of behavior-specific cognitions and affect are perceived benefits of action, perceived barriers to action,

Evidence for Practice

Phelen, D. L., Oliveria, S. A., Christos, P. J., Dusza, S. W., & Halpern, A. C. (2003). Skin self-examination in patients at high risk for melanoma: A pilot study. *Oncology Nursing Forum, 30*(6), 1029–1036.

The purpose of this study was to compare the effect of providing patients at high risk for melanoma with standard educational brochures versus personalized photo books as part of a comprehensive nursing educational intervention on knowledge, awareness, and confidence with skin self-examination (SSE) and compliance in performing SSE. One hundred patients at high risk for melanoma participated in the study by completing a baseline questionnaire at two separate times, once before their initial photographs were taken and again at the end of a nurse-taught educational intervention. Participants in both groups received an educational intervention consisting of a short video on SSE and an individual demonstration of SSE. Participants in the intervention group received a photo book and a demonstration of how to use the photo book. In the group who received the nursing education intervention and the photo book, 10% of the participants reported at baseline performing SSE three or more times during the prior 4 months. In the group who received nursing education intervention without the photo book, 20% reported at baseline practicing SSE three or more times during the prior 4 months. Mean knowledge scores, awareness, and confidence scores increased in both groups. There were no significant differences in the scores between the two groups, suggesting that the intervention did not make a difference immediately after the intervention. Follow-up questionnaires will be administered at 4 and 18 months to determine if there is a later effect. Investigators concluded that educational interventions do increase knowledge, awareness, and confidence; however, they could not support the effectiveness of the photo book during the initial phase of the study. This study demonstrates the nurse's role as educator in teaching clients at risk for melanoma health-promoting behaviors such as skin self-examination.

perceived self-efficacy, activity-related affect, interpersonal influences, and situational influences. They are described as follows:

Perceived benefits of action affect the person's level of participation in health-promoting behaviors and may facilitate continued practice. If the person has had prior positive experiences with a health-promoting behavior or has observed someone else who has had a positive experience, the person is more likely to adopt or maintain the healthy behavior. For example, a person who starts losing excess weight by participating in a program of exercise is more likely to maintain the exercise program. Another example is a person who smokes sees a friend successfully stop smoking using a specific smoking-cessation technique is more likely to try the same smoking-cessation technique. Repetition of such behavior can strengthen and reinforce beliefs about benefits.

Perceived barriers to action include a person's perceptions about available time, expense, inconvenience, access to facilities, difficulty performing the activity, or other perceived negative consequences related to health-promotion activities. These barriers may be imagined or real. Barriers to action result in avoidance or a decrease in health-promoting behaviors. For example, a person who believes that she will put on excess weight if she tries to stop smoking may choose not to attempt stopping smoking.

Perceived self-efficacy refers to the conviction that a person can successfully carry out the behavior necessary to achieve a desired outcome, such as maintaining an exercise program to lose weight. Often people who have serious doubts about their capabilities decrease their efforts and give up, whereas those with a strong sense of efficacy exert greater effort to master problems or challenges.

Activity-related affect includes the subjective feelings that occur before, during, and following an activity. These feelings can influence whether a person begins a health-promotion activity or maintains the activity once it is begun. A person who has positive feelings about the activity is more likely to begin or maintain the activity. Individuals who have negative feelings about a health-promotion activity are less likely to begin or maintain an activity. For example, a person might experience muscle pain after starting an exercise program. The negative feelings associated with the pain may result in the person stopping the exercise program.

Interpersonal influences are the perceptions (real or unreal) of the health beliefs, behaviors, or attitudes of others. Family members, significant others, and health care providers are the primary sources of interpersonal influence on health-promoting behaviors. "Interpersonal influences include norms (expectations of significant others), social support (instrumental and emotional encouragement), and modeling (vicarious learning through observing others engaged in a particular behavior)" (Pender et al., 2002, p. 72). For example, an adult may maintain a dental hygiene program of brushing and flossing his teeth twice a day and visiting the dentist routinely for cleaning and screening because it is a habit that was established in childhood by his parents.

Situational influences include "perceptions of options available, demand characteristics, and aesthetic features of the environment in which a given behavior is proposed to take place" (Pender et al., 2002, p. 72). Situational influences may be direct or indirect. An environment that contains cues or triggers for health-promoting behaviors is a direct influence, for example, environments that prohibit smoking by posting "no smoking" signs and eliminating ashtrays.

Commitment to a Plan of Action

Commitment to a plan of action includes two underlying processes: (1) commitment to carry out a specific health-promotion activity at a given time and place and with specific persons or alone, and (2) identification of specific strategies for determining, initiating, and continuing the health-promotion behavior. It is important to determine the specific strategies so that the individual moves beyond the cognitive and emotional commitment to a realistic action plan that results in the initiation and maintenance of the desired health-promoting behavior.

Immediate Competing Demands and Preferences

Competing demands are those factors over which the individual has a low level of control such as family or work responsibilities. For example, a parent may commit to working out every other evening after work at a health club, but the parental responsibility to attend a child's sport activity competes for the same time. Failure to meet the competing demand, attending the child's sport activity, may result in negative consequences, such as the child being angry at the parent or thinking that the parent does not care. Competing preferences are those factors or behaviors over which

> ## Critical Thinking Exercise
>
> Ann Johnson is a 38-year-old female who is the married mother of three children, ages 16 (female), 12 (male), and 8 (female). Her husband is a 42-year-old airline pilot. She has a family history of breast cancer, and her husband has a family history of heart disease. At the present time all members of the family are healthy. Use Pender's Health-Promotion Model to analyze this family. What health-promotion and illness/injury prevention activities should the nurse assist this family to adopt? Consider the age and gender of all family members. What additional information about the family would help you develop a health promotion plan? Why is this additional information important? How would you as the nurse operationalize the various roles of the nurse, including care provider, health educator, research consumer, advocate, empowering agent, consultant, coordinator of care, proactive change agent, and role model in the care of this family?

the individual has a relatively high level of control. A competing preference may result in the person choosing a different or preferred behavior over the health-promoting behavior. For example, an individual on a low-fat diet (health-promoting behavior) may select a high-fat choice on a restaurant menu because of the taste (competing preference).

Behavioral Outcome

The behavioral outcome in the Health-Promotion Model is the adoption and integration of (a) health-promoting behavior(s) into the individual's lifestyle. Pender et al., (2002, p. 74) state that "health-promoting behaviors, particularly when integrated into a healthy lifestyle . . . should result in improved health, enhanced functional ability, and better quality of life . . . "

Kulbok's Resource Model of Preventive Health Behavior

The resource model of preventive health behavior developed by Kulbok (1985, pp. 67–81) proposes that people act in ways that maximize their "stock in health." It hypothesizes that the greater a person's social and health resources, the more frequently the person will perform preventive behaviors.

Social resources refer to education level and family income. *Health resources* refer to general psychological well-being; perceptions about health, health status, and energy level; the ability to take care of one's own health; participation in social groups; and number and closeness of friends and relatives. Preventive health behaviors relate to physical activity, diet, sleeping, smoking, drinking alcoholic beverages, drinking caffeinated beverages, dental hygiene, use of seat belts, use of professional health services for prevention of disease, and behavior to control high blood pressure.

Neuman Systems Model

In her health-promotion model, nurse theorist Betty Neuman (1995) includes levels of prevention (primary, secondary, and tertiary) and factors that strengthen a person's lines or barriers of defense. For additional information, see Chapter 6 ⚭, Theoretical Foundations of Professional Nursing, and the book *The Neuman Systems Model*.

Reflect on...

- ▪ determinants of health-promoting behaviors cited in Pender's and Kulbok's models that may influence your own health behavior.
- ▪ barriers that deter positive health-promoting behaviors in children, adolescents and young adults, middle-aged adults, and older adults. How can the nurse be a role model of health-promoting behaviors for these various age-groups?
- ▪ how demographic factors such as age, sex, race, ethnicity, education, and income influence health-promoting behaviors. What actions can the nurse take to help ensure access to health-promoting activities for people from all aspects of society?

STAGES OF HEALTH BEHAVIOR CHANGE

Health behavior change is a cyclic phenomenon in which people progress through several stages. In the first stage, the person does not think seriously about changing a behavior; by the time the person reaches the final stage, he or she is successfully maintaining the change in behavior. Several behavior change models have been proposed. The stage model proposed by Prochaska and DiClemente (1982, 1992) is discussed here. The stages are (1) precontemplation, (2) contemplation, (3) preparation, (4) action, and (5) maintenance. If the person does not succeed in changing behavior, relapse occurs.

In the *precontemplation stage*, the person does not think about changing behavior, nor is the person interested in information about the behavior. The negative aspects of making the change outweigh the benefits. Some people may believe the behavior is not under their control and may become defensive when confronted with information.

During the *contemplative stage*, the person seriously considers changing a specific behavior, actively gathers information, and verbalizes plans to change the behavior in the near future. Belief in the value of the change and self-confidence in the ability to change both increase in this phase. It is common for a person to feel some ambivalence when weighing the losses against the rewards of changing the behavior. Some people may stay in the contemplative stage for months or years.

The *preparation stage* occurs when the person undertakes cognitive and behavioral activities that prepare the person for change. At this stage, the person believes that the advantages of changing the behavior outweigh the disadvantages and makes specific plans to accomplish the change. Some people in this stage change small aspects of the behavior, such as cutting out sugar in their coffee.

The *action stage* occurs when the person actively implements behavioral and cognitive strategies to interrupt previous behavior patterns and adopt new ones. To prevent recurrences of previous behavior, the action stage needs to continue for several weeks or months.

During the *maintenance stage*, the person integrates newly adopted behavior patterns into his or her lifestyle. This stage lasts until the person no longer experiences temptation to return to previous unhealthy behaviors.

These five stages are cyclical; people generally move through one stage before progressing to the next. However, at any point in time a person may regress to any previous stage. Sudden or gradual relapses to previous behavior patterns may occur during the action or maintenance stages, for example. Individuals who relapse may return to the stage of precontemplation, contemplation, or preparation before their next attempt to change. To identify whether the client is in the precontemplative or contemplative stages, ask whether the client is thinking about changing a behavior in the next six months or a year. Those in precontemplation will answer no; those in contemplation or preparation will answer yes. Table 7–3 relates nursing strategies appropriate for each stage of health behavior change.

Table 7–3 Examples of Nursing Strategies for Each Stage of Health Behavior Change

Stage	Nursing Strategies
Precontemplation	• Raise the client's awareness of healthy behaviors, such as exercising, altering the diet, quitting smoking, using sunscreen, and undergoing regular mammography screening. • Provide personalized information about the benefits of specific health behaviors; for example, relate the client's cough to smoking or excessive fat intake to heart disease. • Explore the client's beliefs and feelings related to the health behavior. • Identify previous successful changes (e.g., previous weight loss) to increase the client's self-confidence, and offer positive feedback.
Contemplation	• Continue to provide the interventions cited in the previous stage. In addition, provide adequate and accurate information about available alternatives to encourage clients to make appropriate choices and actively participate in decision making. • Encourage the client to express ambivalent feelings. Include spouses, if appropriate (e.g., for dietary alterations). • Help the client further clarify values in relation to the health behavior, and encourage the client to consider how it would feel, for example, to be at an appropriate weight or to be an ex-smoker. • Help the client identify social pressures that encourage positive health behaviors, such as exercise facilities or bans on smoking at work.
Preparation	• Assist the client to make specific plans to implement the change; for example, discuss self-help groups and other available support persons or groups. • Help the client identify stimuli that trigger unhealthy behavior and consider ways to remove or minimize these stimuli (e.g., altering the environment or removing oneself from a troublesome area). • Teach the client to substitute activities to counteract the unhealthy behavior, such as relaxation exercises, internal dialogues, or thought stopping (suddenly saying "stop" loudly). • Plan appropriate rewards (e.g., a movie, dining out) for clients to give themselves for having achieved their goals.
Action	• Review plans and instructions discussed in the preparation phase. • Help the client set realistic goals. • Encourage positive self-talk that supports the behavior change. • Provide positive feedback, support, and encouragement for partial or complete achievement of goals.
Maintenance	• Encourage continuing use of support networks and open discussion of problems related to maintaining healthy behavior. • Identify and encourage strategies that support healthy behavior.

Sources: "Toward a More Integrative Model of Change," by J. Prochaska and C. DiClemente, 1982, *Psychotherapy: Theory, Research, and Practice, 19*, 276–288; "Stages of Change in the Modification of Problem Behaviors," 1992 by J. Prochaska and C. DiClemente, 1992, *Progress in Behavior Modification, 28,* 183–218; and "A Stage-Based Approach to Helping People Change Health Behaviors," by V. S. Conn, 1994, *Clinical Nurse Specialist , 8*(4), 187–193.

Critical Thinking Exercise

Identify a client under your care who is considering a health behavior change. At what stage of Prochaska and DiClemente's model is the client? What barriers exist in the client's experience that might interfere with the client reaching his goal? What activities or interventions would you suggest or do to help the client successfully make the health behavior change?

The Nurse's Role in Health Promotion

- Model healthy lifestyle behaviors and attitudes.
- Facilitate client involvement in the assessment, implementation, and evaluation of health goals.
- Teach clients self-care strategies to enhance fitness, improve nutrition, manage stress, and enhance relationships.
- Assist individuals, families, and communities to increase their levels of health.
- Educate clients to be effective health care consumers.
- Assist clients, families, and communities to develop and choose health-promoting options.
- Guide clients' development in effective problem solving and decision making.
- Reinforce clients' personal and family health-promoting behaviors.
- Advocate in the community for changes that promote a healthy environment.

Reflect on...

■ your own experience in changing an unhealthy behavior (e.g., quitting smoking, losing weight, maintaining proper nutrition, reducing stress). How did you progress through the stages of the Prochaska and DiClemente model? What barriers to health behavior change did you experience? How did you overcome the barriers and effect a successful health behavior change?

■ what barriers exist in your community that interfere with individual and family health behavior changes. What supports exist in your community to assist individuals and families in making health behavior changes? How might you promote and support health behavior changes in your community?

THE NURSE'S ROLE IN HEALTH PROMOTION

Individuals and communities who seek to increase their responsibility for personal health and self-care require health education. The trend toward health promotion has created the opportunity for nurses to strengthen the profession's influence on health promotion, disseminate information that promotes an educated public, and assist individuals and communities to change long-standing health behaviors. Health-promotion activities involve collaborative relationships with both clients and physicians. The role of the nurse is to work *with* people, not *for* them—that is, to act as a facilitator of the process of assessing, evaluating, and understanding health. Maville and Huerta (2002) identify the roles of the nurse in health promotion as advocate, educator, empowering agent, consultant, coordinator of care, members and leaders of the health

profession, proactive change agent, provider of care, research user, health-promotion models, researcher and role model. Many of these roles are further described in other chapters of this text. For examples of the nurse's role in health promotion, see the accompanying box.

In these roles, the nurse may work with individuals of all age-groups and diverse family units or concentrate on a specific population, such as new parents, school-age children, or older adults. In any case, the nursing process is a basic tool for the nurse in a health-promotion role. Although the process is the same, the nurse emphasizes teaching the client (who can be either an individual or a family unit) self-care responsibility. Adult clients decide the goals, determine the health-promotion plans, and take the responsibility for the success of the plans.

Reflect on...

■ types of health-promotion activities in which you have previously been involved. How easy or difficult was it to begin and maintain these activities? What were the

Critical Thinking Exercise

Identify health-promotion activities you would consider when planning care for the following clients in your community: an elderly client, an adolescent, a young adult, a school-age child, a newborn and her parents.

Critical Thinking Exercise

Identify health-promotion interventions that you would incorporate in the nursing care of the following clients with chronic illness: a 58-year-old white male with emphysema, a 76-year-old black female with diabetes mellitus, a 44-year-old white male with coronary artery disease, a 38-year-old black male with hypertension.

factors that contributed to your success in maintaining these activities? If you were unsuccessful, what were the factors that contributed to your lack of success? What have you learned from these experiences that might help you in assisting clients with health-promoting behaviors?

■ what personal responsibility means in relation to health and how that affects the nurse's role in health promotion.

EXPLORE MEDIALINK

Questions, critical thinking exercises, essay activities, and other interactive resources for this chapter can be found on the Web site at http://www.prenhall.com/blais. Click on Chapter 7 to select activities for this chapter.

Bookshelf

Edelman, C. L., & Mandle, C. L. (2002). *Health promotion throughout the lifespan* **(5th ed.). St. Louis: Mosby.**
This reference text is a must for nurses who work in settings that promote health. Units include "Foundations of Health Promotion," "Assessment for Health Promotion," "Interventions for Health Promotion," "Application of Health Promotion," and "Challenges as We Enter the New Millennium." Health-promotion activities for people from the prenatal period through older adults are presented from a developmental perspective.

Maville, J. A., & Huerta, C. G. (2002). *Health promotion in nursing.* **Albany, NY: Delmar Thomson Learning.**
This text provides a comprehensive overview of health promotion in nursing including sections on conceptual foundations and theoretical approaches to health promotion, factors related to health promotion, promoting health throughout the life cycle, health-promotion strategies and interventions, and health-promotion issues, including health care cost and quality issues, and ethical and legal issues.

Murray, R. B., & Zentner, J. P. (2001). *Health promotion strategies through the life span* **(7th ed.). Upper Saddle River, NJ: Prentice Hall.**
This text provides a comprehensive guide to health promotion and disease- and injury-prevention interventions for all age-groups. The authors use a holistic approach to the health care of individuals and families. The text offers guidelines for nursing assessment with suggested interventions and health-promotion strategies for each developmental stage from birth to death.

Pender, N. J., Murdaugh, C. L., & Parsons, M. A. (2002). *Health promotion in nursing practice* **(4th ed.). Upper Saddle River, NJ: Prentice Hall.**
This text provides comprehensive coverage of Pender's Health-Promotion Model. It describes the nurse's role in the promotion of healthy lifestyles. Units include an introduction to health promotion and disease prevention, the human quest for health, health promotion in diverse populations, planning for prevention and health promotion, interventions for prevention and health promotion, evaluating the effectiveness of health promotion, and approaches for promoting a healthier society.

SUMMARY

The goal of health promotion is to raise the level of health of an individual, family, or community. Health-promotion activities are directed toward developing client resources that maintain or enhance well-being. Health-protection activities are geared toward preventing specific diseases, such as obtaining immunizations to prevent measles.

Healthy People 2010 focuses on improving the health of individuals, families, communities, and the nation. The goals of *Healthy People 2010* are (1) to increase the quality and years of healthy life and (2) to eliminate health disparities.

Health-promotion strategies may be active or passive. With active strategies, the client participates in making lifestyle changes. With passive strategies, the client is the recipient of a health-promotion effort, such as maintaining an appropriate water supply. A variety of programs can be used for health promotion, including (1) information dissemination, (2) health appraisal and wellness assessment, (3) lifestyle and behavior change, and (4) environmental control programs. These programs are found in many settings—in the home, schools, community centers, hospitals, worksites, and shopping malls.

Three health-promotion models are described. Pender's Health-Promotion Model categorizes determinants of health-promoting behaviors as individual characteristics and experiences, behavior-specific cognitions and affect, immediate competing demands and preferences, commitment to a plan of action, and behavioral outcome. Pender differentiates health pro-

motion from health protection (prevention). The goal of health promotion is to increase well-being or to actualize human health potential; it is a health seeking behavior. The goal of health protection (prevention) is to avoid illness, detect it early, and maintain functioning within the constraints of illness or injury; it is a disease/injury avoidance behavior. It is the individual's motivation for health activities that determine whether the activities they pursue are health-promoting or health-protecting behaviors.

Kulbok's resource model of preventive health behavior hypothesizes that the greater the person's social and health resources, the more frequently the person will perform preventive behaviors.

The Neuman Systems Model includes dimensions of health promotion designed to strengthen a person's lines of defense and addresses primary, secondary, and tertiary levels of prevention.

Prochaska and DiClemente propose a five-stage model for health behavior change. The stages are (1) precontemplation, (2) contemplation, (3) preparation, (4) action, and (5) maintenance. If the person is not successful in changing behavior, relapse may occur during the action or maintenance stages. However, at any point in these stages, people may move to any previous stage. An understanding of these stages enables the nurse to provide appropriate nursing interventions.

The nurse's role in health promotion is to act as a facilitator of the process of assessing, evaluating, and understanding health.

REFERENCES

Brown, K. C., Mattson, A. H., Newman, K. D., & Sirles, A. T. (1992, Winter). A community health nursing curriculum and Healthy People 2000. *Clinical Nurse Specialist, 6*(4), 203–208.

Callaghan, D. M. (2003). Health-promoting self-care behaviors, self-care, self-efficacy, and self-care agency. *Nursing Science Quarterly 16*(3), 247–254.

Conn, V. S. (1994). A stage-based approach to helping people change health behaviors. *Clinical Nurse Specialist, 8,* 187–193.

Epp, J. (1986, November). *Achieving health for all: A framework for health promotion.* Report of the Minister of National Health and Welfare. Ottawa, Canada: Government Printing Office.

Kulbok, P. P. (1985, June). Social resources, health resources, and preventive behaviors: Patterns and predictions. *Public Health Nursing, 2,* 67–81.

Lalonde, M. (1974). *A new perspective on the health of Canadians.* Ottawa: Government of Canada.

Leavell, H. R., & Clark, E. G. (1965). *Preventive medicine for the doctor in the community* (3rd ed.). New York: McGraw-Hill.

Lewis, F. M. (1982, March/April). Experienced personal control and quality of life in late-stage cancer patients. *Nursing Research, 31,* 113–118.

Maville, J. A., & Huerta, C. G. (2002). *Health promotion in nursing.* Albany, NY: Delmar Thomson Learning.

Murray, R. B., & Zentner, J. P. (2001). *Health promotion strategies through the life span* (2nd ed.). Upper Saddle River, NJ: Prentice Hall.

Neuman, B. (1995). *The Neuman Systems Model* (3rd ed.). Norwalk, CT: Appleton and Lange.

Pender, N. J. (1996). *Health promotion in nursing practice* (3rd ed.). Stamford, CT: Appleton-Lange.

Pender, N. J., Murdaugh, C. L., & Parsons, M. A. (2002). *Health promotion in nursing practice* (4th ed.). Upper Saddle River, NJ: Prentice Hall.

Phelen, D. L., Oliveria, S. A., Christos, P. J., Dusza, S. W., & Halpern, A. C. (2003). Skin self-examination in patients at high risk for melanoma: A pilot study. *Oncology Nursing Forum, 30*(6), 1029–1036.

Prochaska, J., & DiClemente, C. (1982). Toward a more integrative model of change. *Psychotherapy: Theory, Research, and Practice, 19,* 276–288.

Prochaska, J., & DiClemente, C. (1992). Stages of change in the modification of problem behaviors. *Progress in Behavior Modification, 28,* 183–218.

Schultz, A. (1995, August). What is health promotion? *Canadian Nurse, 91,* 31–34.

Stachtchenko, S., & Jenicek, M. (1990, January—February). Conceptual differences between prevention and health promotion: Research implications for community health programs. *Canadian Journal of Public Health, 81,* 53–59.

United States Department of Health and Human Services. (1990, September). *Healthy people 2000: National health promotion and disease prevention objectives.* DHHS Pub. No. (PHS) 91-50212. Washington, DC: Government Printing Office.

United States Department of Health and Human Services. (2001). *Healthy people 2010.* Washington, DC: USDHHS. http://www.health.gov/healthypeople.

United States Department of Health and Human Services. (2004). *Healthy people 2010: Leading health indicators.* Washington, DC: USDHHS. http://www.health.gov/healthypeople.

U.S. Surgeon General. (1979). *Healthy people: The Surgeon General's report on health promotion and disease prevention.* DHHS Pub. No. 79-55071. Washington, DC: Government Printing Office.

U.S. Surgeon General. (1980). *Health promotion/disease prevention: Objectives for the nation.* Washington, DC: Department of Health and Human Services.

World Health Organization. (1984). *Report of the working group on the concept and principles of health promotion.* Copenhagen: WHO.

World Health Organization. (1986). *Framework for health promotion training.* Copenhagen: WHO.

CHAPTER 8

The Nurse as Learner and Teacher

Objectives

- Discuss selected learning theories.

- Explain the three domains of learning.

- Describe the various teaching roles of the nurse.

- Identify guidelines for effective teaching and learning.

- Develop a teaching plan.

- Identify strategies for teaching learners of different cultures.

M E D I A L I N K

Additional online resources for this chapter can be found on the companion Web site at http://www.prenhall.com/blais.

Nurses have both learning and teaching responsibilities. They must continue to learn so that they can maintain their knowledge and skills amid the many changes in health care. They teach clients and their families, other health care providers, and nursing assistants to whom they delegate care, and they share their expertise with other nurses and health professionals. Some teach their profession to others. Teaching and learning are not limited to classroom experiences and can occur in all settings for practice.

Learning is a complex process, and there are many theories about how learning occurs. These learning theories are generally based on assumptions about people, the nature of knowledge, and how people learn. The eclectic approach presumes that no one theory is more correct than another. More information is becoming available regarding people's learning styles.

There are also beliefs about how teaching can be most effective. These are commonly referred to as principles of teaching. Both learning and teaching are active and interactive processes. Currently, there is increasing focus on outcome-based teaching and evidence-based learning.

CHALLENGES AND OPPORTUNITIES

The challenges associated with teaching and learning in the current health care system are many. Federal and state regulations influence the content to be taught and the documentation required. Health care clients vary in age, ethnic diversity, socioeconomic status, primary language, and previous knowledge and experience. Information is constantly changing as new research becomes available. Today's resources are numerous and readily available through the World Wide Web (WWW). Providing clients with accurate, current information is a challenge for nurses. Teaching is a major role of nurses, and it is often performed without adequate preparation. Effective teaching is a challenge.

Nurses today must also keep up to date with theory and practice. Nursing education programs prepare the new practitioner with effective beginning nursing skills. Changes occur quickly and often in nursing and health care; consequently, nurses must continue learning to keep current. Many states require nurses to complete continuing education programs designed to increase knowledge and skill. Often employers provide programs at the work site for updating nurses' knowledge and skills. Sometimes nurses need to travel to specialized centers to gain advanced specialized skills. Many nurses return to school to obtain advanced degrees in nursing and other health-related disciplines.

The importance of the learning and teaching roles of nurses creates new opportunities for nurses as teachers of clients and their families, nursing assistants (e.g., patient care technicians) in the health care system, and peers and colleagues. Nurses can also influence the health of communities by participating in community health education programs. Nurses not only teach clients directly but also participate in the

development of health education literature and Internet-based health information.

NURSES AS LEARNERS

There are several ways in which the nurse may learn, including continued formal academic education, institution-based human resource development (HRD) programs, encouraged or legislatively mandated continuing education, or episodic individual-selected educational pursuits.

Continued formal academic education includes postbaccalaureate study at the master's or doctoral degree levels. Education at the graduate level requires critical thinking and knowledge of the research process. Graduate study may be in nursing or in other disciplines that enhance the nurses' practice. For example, nurses in administration may choose to pursue master's degrees in nursing administration, health care administration, or business administration. There are many factors the nurse must consider in choosing a graduate program. Chapter 23 ⬚, Advanced Nursing Education and Practice, provides guidelines for preparing for graduate study and selecting and applying to a graduate program.

Institution-based human resource development programs are administered by the employer. Swansburg (1995, p. 2) defines human resource development as "the process by which corporate management stimulates the motivation of employees to perform productively. HRD provides the stimuli that motivate nursing personnel to provide nursing care services to clients at quality and quantity standards that keep the health care entity reputable and financially solvent, the nurses satisfied with their professional accomplishments and quality of work life, and the clients treated successfully." Human resource development programs are designed to upgrade the knowledge and skills of employees. For example, an employer might offer programs to orient new staff members, to inform nurses about a new institutional policy, to familiarize nurses with a new piece of equipment or a new technique, to prepare nurses for certification at specialty or advanced levels of practice, or to implement a nurse theorist's conceptual framework as the guideline for nursing practice within the institution. Some HRD programs also offer nurses tuition benefits to enroll in work-related courses or to attend professional conferences. It is important for the nurse to remember that the primary intended benefit of HRD programs is for the institution; however, nurses who take advantage of institution-based programs can also benefit their own professional practice.

The term *continuing education* refers to formalized experiences designed to expand the knowledge or skills of nurses. Continuing education programs tend to be more specific and shorter than formal advanced academic degree study. Continuing education is the responsibility of each practicing nurse. Constant updating and growth are essential for the nurse to keep abreast of scientific and technologic change and changes within the nursing profession. Continuing education can be part of an employer's HRD program or may be offered by professional organizations or continuing education departments of colleges or universities. Continuing education may also be obtained through self-study programs offered through professional journals or through home study programs provided by private, public, and professional educational organizations.

Some states require nurses to obtain a certain number of continuing education (CE) credits to renew their professional licenses. In these states, required CE contact hours vary from 15 to 30 hours for every 2-year licensure period. Depending on the state, all, some, or none of these hours may be acquired through home study. Some states require specific content instruction as part of the legislated continuing education requirement, for example, current study in violence, HIV/AIDS, or medical errors. Nurses who hold licensure in several states must meet the continuing education requirements for each state.

Some professional organizations require continuing education to meet certification and recertification requirements for specialty practice. For example, to be certified as a pediatric nurse by the American Nurses Association, the nurse must have completed 30 contact hours of continuing education applicable to pediatric nursing within the previous 3 years (American Nurses Credentialing Center [ANCC], 2004). This continuing education requirement is in addition to other requirements.

Episodic learning activities are determined by the individual nurse. Episodic learning activities are those activities that are distinct and separate from formal or planned education. Subscribing to and reading professional journals and newsletters or commercial newspapers and magazines are examples of nurses' episodic educational activities. The learning the nurse gains through these activities can be just as important as formal educational pursuits. Through reading about the contemporary understanding of health care in professional or commercial literature, the nurse gains an awareness of how nurses can influence the health care system. Nurses can also gain knowledge of personal benefit, such as liability and malpractice issues, advanced practice and licensure issues, and portable pension plans and other retirement planning.

Reflect on...

- the various learning activities you have participated in during the last year. How many were episodic activities? How many were formal learning activities to obtain a degree or licensure as a registered nurse? How many were part of the human resource development program of your employer? How many were done to meet continuing education requirements for relicensure or recertification? How many were done for personal satisfaction?
- your personal goals related to professional learning activities. Are your learning activities directed toward becoming certified? To achieving an academic degree? For personal satisfaction?

THE LEARNING PROCESS

People, including clients, have a variety of learning needs. A learning need is evidenced by a desire or requirement to change behavior or to fill "a gap between the information an individual knows and the information necessary to perform a function or care for self" (Gessner, 1989, p. 593). **Learning** is a change in human disposition or capability that persists over a period of time and that cannot be solely accounted for by growth. Learning is represented by a change in behavior. See the accompanying box for attributes of learning.

Attributes of Learning

Learning is:

- An experience that occurs inside the learner
- The discovery of the personal meaning and relevance of ideas
- A consequence of experience
- A collaborative and cooperative process
- An evolutionary process
- A process that is both intellectual and emotional

An important aspect of learning is the individual's desire to learn and to act on the learning. This desire is best illustrated when the person recognizes and accepts the need to learn, willingly expends the energy required to learn, and then follows through with the appropriate behaviors that reflect the learning. For example, a person diagnosed as having diabetes willingly learns about the special diet needed and then plans and follows the learned diet.

Andragogy is "the art and science of helping adults learn" (Knowles, 1980, p. 43) in contrast to **pedagogy**, the discipline concerned with helping children learn. While nurses use pedagogic teaching strategies when teaching children, they also use the following andragogic concepts about learners as a guide for teaching adult clients (Knowles, 1984):

- As people mature, they move from dependence to independence.
- An adult's previous experiences can be used as a resource for learning.
- An adult's readiness to learn is often related to a developmental task or social role.
- An adult is more oriented to learning when the material is immediately useful, not useful sometime in the future.

Theories of Learning

Theories about how and why people learn can be traced back to the seventeenth century. Psychologists first focused on the mental phenomena. Today, there is more focus on the behaviors or activities of learning. There are a number of theories and numerous psychologists associated with theories of learning. Five contemporary theoretical constructs are behaviorism, cognitivism, humanism, constructivism, and multiple intelligence.

Behaviorism

Behaviorism was originally advanced by Edward Thorndike (1913), who believed that transfer of knowledge could occur if the new situation closely resembled the old situation. To Thorndike, the term *understanding* was used in the context of building connections. One of his major contributions applicable to teaching is that learning should be based on the learner's behavior. He is known for his "laws of learning." In addition to Thorndike, major behaviorist theorists include Pavlov and Skinner.

Behaviorists believe that the environment influences behavior and how a person controls it; moreover, they maintain that it is the essential factor determining human action. In the behaviorist school of thought, an act is called a response when it can be traced to the effects of a stimulus.

SKINNER'S OPERANT CONDITIONING THEORY Skinner (1953) postulates two types of conditioning (behavioral responses to a stimulus) that cause the response or behavior. The first type of conditioning, termed *classical conditioning,* is illustrated by Pavlov's well-known experiments with dogs. Pavlov (1849–1936) conditioned dogs to salivate in response to the sound of a tuning fork, a sound they heard when they received food. Classical conditioning is a procedure in which conditioned responses are established by the association of a new stimulus that is known to cause an unconditioned response. The resulting response is the conditioned response to the new (unrelated) stimulus.

The second type of conditioning is what Skinner refers to as *operant conditioning,* a process by which the frequency of a response can be increased or decreased depending on when, how, and to what extent it is reinforced. Skinner believes that humans, like animals, will always repeat actions that bring pleasure. He considers the consequences of an action, what he terms **reinforcement**, to be all-important. Positive consequences foster repetition of the action; negative consequences or the absence of consequences can cause the action to cease.

Extinction is the process in which a conditioned behavior is "unlearned" because the reinforcement has been removed. Greater effort, however, is required to extinguish a behavior than to condition it. The procedure involves removing the unconditional stimulus or the reward from the training situation. When the conditioning procedure is again instigated following complete extinction, it does not take the subject as long to show the conditioned response as it did in the original conditioning.

Studies of conditioning produced laws of learning that were thought to be universal; that is, they were thought to apply to all ages, all cultures, and all types of behavior—motor, cognitive, emotional, and social. Examples follow:

- The more quickly reinforcement follows a response, the more effective is the reinforcement.
- A response made in the presence of one stimulus generalizes to similar stimuli.
- Behavior that is reinforced only part of the time takes longer to extinguish than behavior that is reinforced continuously.

Social Learning Theory

Social learning theorists such as Bandura agree with Skinner that the environment exerts a great deal of control over overt behavior; however, they believe that the entire learning process involves the following three highly interdependent factors:

1. Characteristics of the person
2. The person's behavior
3. The environment

These factors influence and control each other through a process that Bandura calls **reciprocal determinism.** The major contribution of Bandura's reciprocal determinism is the concept that the child's behavior affects or "creates" that child's environment. This differs from Skinner's belief that the environment, viewed as a set of stimuli, controls behavior.

Bandura claims that most learning comes from observational learning and instruction rather than from overt trial-and-error behavior. **Observational learning** is the acquisition of new skills or the alteration of old behaviors simply by watching other children and adults. It is especially important for acquiring behavior in situations in which mistakes can be life-threatening or costly, for example, driving a car or medication administration.

Bandura's research focuses on **imitation**, the process by which individuals copy or reproduce what they have observed, and **modeling**, the process by which a person learns by observing the behavior of others. Imitation is regarded as one of the most powerful socialization forces. Various imitative behaviors are reinforced by a process of operant conditioning. For example, a boy may be praised for being "just like his father." The child may even self-reinforce the imitations by repeating an adult's words of praise. According to Bandura, models influence others mainly by providing information rather than by eliciting matching behavior, so that learning can occur without even once performing the model's behavior.

In recent years, Bandura's theory has become more cognitive, and he now calls his theory a "social cognitive theory." Learning is defined as "knowledge acquisition through cognitive processing information" (1971, p. xii). For example, television's effects on children depend on both cognitive and imitative processes. Whether the child can comprehend the story affects the child's perceptions of the model and the tendency to imitate the model. It is interesting to note that Bandura's research explored the concerns regarding the influence of televised violence.

Cognitivism

Cognitivism depicts learning as a complex cognitive activity. Major cognitive theorists include Piaget (1966), Lewin (1951), Gagne (1974), Bloom (1956), and Bruner (1966). Cognitivists view learning as the development of understandings and appreciation that help the individual function in a larger context. Learning is based on a change of perception, which itself is influenced by the senses and both internal and external variables. In other words, learning is largely a mental, intellectual, or thinking process. The learner structures and processes information based on his or her perceptions of the information. The learner's perceptions are influenced by their personal characteristics and their experiences. Cognitivists also emphasize the importance of social, emotional, and physical contexts in which learning occurs, such as the teacher-learner relationship and environment. Developmental readiness and individual readiness (expressed as motivation) are other key factors associated with cognitive approaches.

PIAGET'S PHASES OF COGNITIVE DEVELOPMENT   According to Piaget (1966), cognitive development is an orderly, sequential process in which a variety of new experiences (stimuli) must exist before intellectual abilities can develop. Piaget's cognitive developmental process is divided into four major phases: sensorimotor, preoperational, concrete operations, and formal operations. A person develops through each of these phases although not everyone achieves the formal operations phase. Each phase has unique characteristics.

The *sensorimotor* phase lasts from birth to about 2 years of age. It includes reflexive actions, perceptions of events centered on the body, objects as an extension of self, mental acknowledgment of the external environment, and discovery of new goals and ways to attain these goals. The *preoperational phase* occurs from about 2 to 7 years of age and includes an egocentric approach to accommodate the demands of the environment. Everything is significant and relates to "me." The child is able to think of one idea at a time, can use words to express thoughts, and includes others in the environment. The *concrete operations* phase (about 7 to 11 years old) involves a beginning understanding of relationships such as size, right and left, different viewpoints, and the ability to solve concrete problems. The *formal operations* phase may occur at about 11 to 15 years of age and includes the ability to use rational thinking and reasoning that is deductive and futuristic.

In each phase, the person uses three primary abilities: assimilation, accommodation, and adaptation. *Assimilation* is the process through which humans encounter and react to new situations by using the mechanisms they already possess. In this way, people acquire new knowledge and skills as well as insights into the world around them. *Accommodation* is the process of change whereby cognitive processes mature sufficiently to allow the person to solve problems that were unsolvable before. This adjustment is possible chiefly because new knowledge has been assimilated. Adaptation, or coping behavior, is the ability to handle the demands made by the environment.

LEWIN'S FIELD THEORY   Lewin's (1951) field theory involves theories of motivation and perception, which were considered precursors of the more recent cognitive theories. Lewin believed that learning involved four different types of changes: change in cognitive structure, change in motivation, change in one's sense of belonging to the group, and gain in voluntary muscle control. His well-known theory of change has three basic stages: unfreezing, moving, and refreezing. These stages are discussed in Chapter 14 ⬤⬤, Change Process.

GAGNE'S INFORMATION PROCESSING THEORY   Gagne (1974) postulates eight levels of intellectual skills: (1) signal; (2) stimulus-response; (3) chaining, which involves at least two stimulus-response connections; (4) verbal association, which involves assembling verbal chains from previous learning; (5) multiple discrimination involving differentiated responses to variable stimuli; (6) concept formation, which involves identifying and responding to a class of objects that serve as stimuli; (7) principle formation, which involves applying a principle that is made up of at least one chain of two or more concepts; and (8) problem solving, which involves processing at least two or more principles to produce a higher-level principle.

BLOOM'S DOMAINS OF LEARNING   Bloom (1956) identified three domains, or areas of learning: cognitive, affective, and psychomotor. The *cognitive domain* includes six intellectual skills including knowledge, comprehension, application, analysis, synthesis, and evaluation in order from simple to complex. The *affective domain* includes feelings, emotions, interests, attitudes, and appreciations. It involves five major categories: receiving, responding, valuing, organization, and characterization. The *psychomotor domain* includes motor skills such as playing a musical instrument or giving an injection. It includes seven categories: perception, set, guided response, mechanism, complex overt response, adaptation, and origination. See Table 8–1 for a further description of each of these categories. Nurses should include each of these three domains in client teaching plans. For example, teaching a client how to irrigate a colostomy is the psychomotor domain. An important part of such a teaching plan is to teach the client why a specific amount of fluid is used and when the irrigation should be carried out; this is the cognitive domain. Helping the client accept the colostomy and maintain self-esteem is in the affective domain. Each of these domains has a developed hierarchical classification system; that is, the behaviors in each category are arranged from the simplest to the most complex.

Critical Thinking Exercise

Consider how a nurse can employ Piaget's theory of cognitive development when developing teaching strategies for learners of different ages and developmental stages, for example, a toddler (egocentric and literal) or teenager (rational thinking). Identify appropriate teaching strategies for these stages.

Critical Thinking Exercise

Develop a teaching plan using each of the domains of learning (cognitive, affective, and psychomotor) for a new diabetic client who needs to learn how to self-inject insulin.

Table 8–1 Major Categories in Each Learning Domain

Category/Description	Client Learning Example
Cognitive Domain	
Knowledge Remembers previously learned material	A client lists the side effects of a medication 2 days after instruction.
Comprehension Understands the meaning of learned material	A client describes how the side effects of a medication can be recognized and what to do about them.
Application Applies newly learned material in new concrete situations	A client learns to take the medication after meals to minimize side effects.
Analysis Breaks learned material into component parts and separates important from unimportant material	A client describes which side effects are serious and when the physician is to be notified.
Synthesis Takes parts of learned material and puts them together to form new material	A client takes steps to prevent side effects of a medication.
Evaluation Judges the value of the learned material	A client describes how the knowledge of new material can help prevent accidents at work.
Affective Domain	
Receiving Willingness to attend to particular stimuli	A female client is willing to listen to a nurse's description of the preparation for mastectomy.
Responding Actively participates by listening and responding	The female client asks questions about the preparation for the scheduled surgery.
Valuing Attaches a value or worth to a particular object, phenomenon, or behavior	The female client refuses to look at the incision after her mastectomy.
Organization Develops a value system by bringing together different values and resolving conflicts	The client accepts changes brought about by the mastectomy.
Characterization Acts according to a value system	After surgery, the client returns to a lifestyle consistent with her value system.
Psychomotor Domain	
Perception Uses the senses to obtain cues to guide motor activity	A male client immediately calls a nurse when he sees another client fall from his bed.
Set Refers to readiness to take immediate action: includes mental, physical, and emotional sets	The client becomes ready to act when he sees the client who fell from his bed preparing to get out of his chair.
Guided Response Performs an act under the guidance of a nurse	A client moves himself from his bed to a wheelchair with a nurse's guidance.
Mechanism Performs a learned activity with confidence and proficiency	The client moves himself between his bed and a wheelchair quickly and competently.
Complex Overt Response Performs a motor skill competently, accurately, and smoothly	The client moves between the bed and the wheelchair, at the same time adjusting his intravenous line and his catheter.
Adaptation Performs skills and adapts them to special circumstances	The client stops transferring to the wheelchair and adjusts his intravenous line when it stops dripping.
Origination Creates new movement patterns to suit a particular problem	The client transfers from his bed to the wheelchair in a different way to avoid pull on the intravenous line.

Sources: Adapted from *Starting Objectives for Classroom Instruction* (3rd ed., pp. 34–40), by N. E. Gronlund, 1985, New York: Macmillan; and *Taxonomy of Educational Objectives. Vol. 1: Cognitive Domain* (pp. 18–24), by B. S. Bloom, (Ed.) 1956. New York: David McKay.

Humanism

Humanistic learning theory focuses on both cognitive and affective (feelings and attitudes) areas of the learner. It focuses on the whole person and therefore is pertinent to a holistic philosophy of care. Prominent members of this school of thought include Abraham Maslow (1970) and Carl Rogers (1961, 1969). According to humanistic theory, learning is believed to be self-motivated, self-initiated, and self-evaluated. Each individual is viewed as a unique composite of biologic, psychologic, social, cultural, and spiritual factors. Learning focuses on self-development and achieving full potential; it is best when it is relevant to the learner. Autonomy and self-determination are important; the learner identifies the learning needs and takes the initiative to meet these needs. The learner is thus an active participant and takes responsibility for meeting individual learning needs.

Maslow's hierarchy of needs suggests a way of prioritizing nursing interventions so that physiologic needs are met first, followed by safety and security needs, love and belonging needs, esteem and self-esteem needs, and ultimately growth needs. Carl Rogers was particularly concerned with personalized approaches. He emphasized that independence, creativity, and self-reliance are all facilitated when self-criticism and self-evaluation are of primary importance; evaluation by others is of secondary importance.

Categorization

According to Jerome Bruner (1966), perception, conceptualizing, learning, and decision making all depend on categorizing information. People interpret information in terms of the similarities and differences detected and arrange the information in related categories. For example, there are hundreds of bones in the body. By categorizing them into major bone types (e.g., long bones, flat bones) or areas of the body (e.g., bones of the head, bones of the hand, vertebrae), it is easier to learn them. This theory of cognitive learning emphasizes the formation of a coding system. These systems serve to facilitate transfer, enhance retention, and increase problem-solving motivation. Bruner advocates discovery-oriented learning to help students discover relationships between categories. Bruner's work is sometimes considered among the theories of the constructivists.

Constructivism

Constructivism is a relatively recent term. It represents a collection of theories with a common thread of individuals actively constructing knowledge to solve realistic problems, often in collaboration with others. The ideas of constructivism emerged with John Dewey and continued with Bruner (learning as discovery). The constructivist described learning as a change in meaning constructed from experience. Knowledge becomes an individual interpretation of experience; learning is the construction of new interpretations. Gagne, Bruner, and Ausubel, as well as the social development theorist Vygotsky and social learning theorist Bandura, are associated with the constructivists. Their focus is more on the learning, not the teaching, with language as a process. Constructivists encourage learning inquiry, acknowledge the critical role of experience in learning, and encourage cooperative learning. Constructivist theory is applicable to learning with technology.

Multiple Intelligence

Early psychologists gauged intelligence by the use of the intelligence quotient, or IQ. They felt that intelligence at too low a level inhibited individuals from participating in intellectually demanding learning situations and that intelligence at a higher level indicated a genius. Those in between were considered to be normal. Many individuals were incorrectly labeled and as a result were never encouraged to reach higher potential. Intelligence was thought to be fixed and unchangeable by training. Recent research studies suggest that this is not so. Today, new theories have emerged disputing IQ as the only indicator of intelligence. Intelligence has a number of dimensions. Howard Gardner, head of the Project of Human Potential at Harvard, has presented a theory of multiple intelligence. This was based on observations of how brain damage from a stroke might affect one area, such as language, while other areas of mental functioning remained intact. Gardner first cited seven intelligences: linguistic, musical/rhythmic (music), logical/mathematical, spatial (visual), body/kinesthetic/movement (body), personal, and symbols as intellectual strengths or ways of knowing (Gardner, 1983). He has since added naturalist as the eighth intelligence. Gardner offers a fresh perspective to learning.

Applying Learning Theories

The major attributes of *behaviorist* theories include the careful identification of what is to be taught and the immediate identification of and reward for correct responses. However, the theory is not easily applied to complex learning situations and is limiting in terms of the learner's role in the teaching process. Nurses applying behavioristic theory will do the following:

- Provide sufficient time for practice.
- Provide both immediate and repeat testing and redemonstration.
- Provide opportunities for learners to solve problems by trial and error.
- Select teaching strategies that avoid distracting information and evoke the desired response.
- Praise the learner for correct behavior and provide positive feedback at intervals throughout the learning experience.
- Provide role models of desired behavior.

The major attributes of *cognitive* theory are its recognition of developmental levels of learners, and acknowledgment of the learner's motivation and environment. However, some or many of the motivational and environmental factors may be beyond the teacher's control. Nurses applying cognitive theory will do the following:

- Assess a person's developmental and individual readiness to learn and adapt teaching strategies to the learner's developmental level.
- Provide a social, emotional, and physical environment conducive to learning.
- Encourage a positive teacher-learner relationship.
- Select multisensory teaching strategies because perception is influenced by the senses.
- Recognize that personal characteristics have an impact on how cues are perceived and develop appropriate teaching approaches to target different learning styles.
- Select behavioral objectives and strategies that encompass the cognitive, affective, and psychomotor domains of learning.

The major attributes of *humanism* are its focus on the feelings and attitudes of learners; on the importance of the individual in identifying learning needs and taking responsibility for them; and on the self-motivation of the learners to work toward self-reliance and independence. Nurses applying humanistic theory will do the following:

- Encourage learners to establish goals and promote self-directed learning.
- Encourage active learning by serving as a facilitator, mentor, or resource for the learner.
- Expose the learner to new relevant information and ask appropriate questions to encourage the learner to seek answers.

Cognitive Learning Processes

Learning involves three cognitive (mental) processes: acquiring information, processing the information, and using the information. These three processes can occur sequentially or simultaneously.

Acquiring Information

Acquiring information involves two processes: sensory reception and discrimination. Sensory reception is made possible by the neurosensory system. Stimuli in the environment signal the appropriate sense, such as sight, hearing, or smell. Impulses then travel by the nervous system to the brain. Sensory reception generally is continuous, but it is not always a conscious process.

The second aspect of acquiring information is discrimination. Discrimination is the ability to determine which stimuli are relevant in a particular situation. Stimuli can be objects, ideas, actions, or facts. They may be internal (i.e., inside the body) or external. Discrimination is the most difficult when there are multiple, complex stimuli.

Processing Information

Processing provides meaning to the information. Information is processed in three steps: association, generalization, and the formation of concepts. Association is the joining of two or more ideas. For example, a person may associate an object such as a needle with the word *needle* and/or with the experience of pain. *Generalization* is the perceiving of similarities among various stimuli, for example, the similarities between three different computers. *Concept formation* is the organization of stimuli that have some attributes in common. For example, a nurse who understands the concept of caring appreciates the characteristics associated with caring. The nurse can then help others to convey caring in the health care setting.

Using Information

Using information is the application of information in the cognitive, affective, and psychomotor areas. (See "Bloom's Domains of Learning," earlier in this chapter.) The ability to formulate and relate concepts is an essential critical thinking skill. In addition, relating concepts is essential for creative thinking and problem solving.

Factors Facilitating Learning

Learning is a complex phenomenon. It is an interactive process between the learner, the teacher, the environment, and many elements, including learning style and teaching style. Certain conditions or principles have been identified throughout years of research. When planning instruction, the nurse should consider the factors discussed in the following sections.

Motivation

Motivation to learn is the desire to learn. It greatly influences how quickly and how much a person learns. Motivation is generally greatest when a person recognizes a need and believes the need will be met through learning. It is not enough for the need to be identified and verbalized by the nurse; it must be experienced by the client. Often the nurse's task is to help the client work through the problem and identify the need. Sometimes clients or support persons need help identifying relevant situational elements before they can see a need. For example, clients with heart disease may need to know the effects of smoking before they recognize the need to stop smoking. Or adolescents may need to know the consequences of an untreated sexually transmitted disease before they see the need for treatment.

Readiness

Readiness to learn is the behavior that reflects motivation at a specific time. Readiness reflects a client's willingness and ability to learn. The nurse's role is to assess readiness to learn and often to encourage the development of readiness. Behaviors that might indicate readiness to learn include actively watching the nurse perform a procedure that the client might eventually have to do, or asking questions about a disease or procedure.

Active Involvement

Active involvement in the process makes learning more meaningful. If the learner actively participates in planning and discussion, learning is faster and retention is better. Passive learning, such as listening to a lecture or watching a film, does not foster optimal learning.

Once learners have been successful in accomplishing a task or understanding a concept, they gain self-confidence in their ability to learn. This reduces their anxiety about failure and can motivate continued learning. Successful learners have increased confidence with which to accept failure. People learn best when they believe they are accepted and will not be judged. The person who expects to be judged as a "poor" client will not learn as well as the person who feels no such threat.

Feedback

Feedback is information relating a person's performance to the desired goal. It has to be meaningful to the learner. Feedback that accompanies practice of psychomotor skills helps the person learn those skills. Support of desired behavior through praise, positively worded corrections, and suggestions of alternative methods are ways of providing positive feedback. Negative feedback such as ridicule, anger, or sarcasm can lead people to withdraw from learning. Such feedback, viewed as a type of punishment, may cause the client to avoid the teacher in order to avoid punishment.

Simple to Complex

Learning is facilitated by material that is logically organized and proceeds from the simple to the complex. Such organization enables the learner to comprehend new information, assimilate it with previous learning, and form new understandings. Of course, simple and complex are relative terms, depending on the level at which the person is learning. What is simple for one person may be complex for another.

Repetition

Repetition of key concepts and facts facilitates retention of newly learned material. Practice of psychomotor skills, particularly with feedback from the nurse, improves performance of those skills and facilitates their transfer to another setting. Also, when a person appreciates the relevance of specific material, learning is facilitated.

Timing

People retain information and psychomotor skills best when the *time between learning and use is short;* the longer the time interval, the more is forgotten. For example, a woman who is taught to administer her own insulin but is not permitted to do so until discharged from the hospital is unlikely to remember much of what she learned. However, if she is allowed to give her own injections while in the hospital, her learning will be enhanced and reinforced.

Timing can also include opportunity, sometimes referred to as a "teachable moment." When a nurse is caring for a patient's colostomy site, the patient may start asking questions about the procedure. Because the client has expressed interest in the procedure, the time, or opportunity, for learning is at that time. Learning occurs best when the learner is free from worry, fear, or pain. For example, it would be inappropriate to teach clients about lifestyle changes after surgery if they are still fearful about the outcome of the surgery.

Environment

An *optimal learning environment* facilitates learning by reducing distraction and providing physical and psychological comfort. It has adequate lighting that is free from glare, a comfortable room temperature, and good ventilation. Most students know what it is like to try to learn in a hot, stuffy room; the drowsiness that occurs in this situation interferes with concentration. Noise can also distract the student and interfere with listening and thinking. To facilitate learning in a hospital setting, nurses should choose a time when there are no visitors present and interruptions are unlikely. When possible, get the patient out of bed, because being in bed is associated with rest and sleep and not usually considered a place for learning. Some facilities have a patient education classroom, or the clinical nurse educator may provide patient teaching in her office. Privacy is essential for some learning. For example, when a client is learning to irrigate a colostomy, the presence of others can be embarrassing and thus interfere with learning. However, when a client is particularly anxious, having support persons present often gives the client confidence.

Reflect on...

■ your own learning experiences. What are the circumstances of your most effective learning experiences? What were the circumstances of your least effective learning experiences? What does this tell you about your learning style?

■ your experiences with teaching others. What were the circumstances of your most effective teaching experiences? What were the circumstances of your least effective teaching experiences? What is your teaching style?

Factors Inhibiting Learning

Many factors inhibit learning. Some of the most common are described next and in Table 8–2.

Table 8–2 Barriers to Learning

Barrier	Explanation	Nursing Implications
Acute illness	Client requires all resources and energy to cope with illness.	Defer teaching until client is less ill.
Pain	Pain decreases ability to concentrate.	Provide appropriate intervention for pain before teaching.
Age	Small children may not understand health teaching.	Include parents in teaching of small children. Use language that both parents and children can understand.
	Vision, hearing, and motor control can be impaired in the elderly.	Consider sensory and motor deficits in teaching plan.
Prognosis	Client can be preoccupied with illness and unable to concentrate on new information.	Defer teaching to a better time.
Biorhythms	Mental and physical performances have a circadian rhythm.	Adapt time of teaching to suit client.
Emotion (e.g., anxiety, denial, depression, grief)	Emotions require energy and distract from learning.	Deal with emotions first and possible misinformation.
Language and ethnic background	Client may not be fluent in the nurse's language.	Obtain services of an interpreter or nurse with appropriate language skills.
Iatrogenic barriers	The nurse may set up barriers by appearing condescending or hurried, ignoring client cues, or appearing incompetent or unsure.	Establish a helping relationship and be sensitive to the client's needs. Plan and prepare for teaching ahead of time with current information appropriate for the learner.

Emotions

A greatly elevated *anxiety* level can impede learning. Clients or families who are very worried may not hear spoken words or may retain only part of the communication. Extreme anxiety might be reduced by medications or by information that relieves uncertainty. By contrast, clients who appear disinterested and unconcerned may need to be cautioned about potential problems in order to enhance their motivation to learn.

Physiologic Factors

Learning can be inhibited by *physiologic factors* such as a critical illness, pain, or impaired hearing. Because the client cannot concentrate and apply energy to learning, the learning itself is impaired. The nurse should try to reduce physiologic barriers to learning as much as possible before teaching. Providing analgesics to relieve pain before teaching is usually helpful. However, if analgesics cause the client to feel drowsy, learning may be affected.

Cultural and Spiritual Barriers

There are also *cultural* and *spiritual barriers* to learning, such as language or values differences. Obviously, the client who does not understand the nurse's language will learn little. Western medicine may conflict with cultural or spiritual healing beliefs and practices. Nurses must deal directly with this conflict to be effective; otherwise the client may be partially or totally nonadherent to recommended treatments. Another impediment to learning is differing values held by the client and the health team. For example, a client who comes from a culture that does not value slimness may have difficulty learning about a reducing diet. See Chapters 21 ⌘ and 22 ⌘ for more information about cultural and spiritual factors affecting health care.

Critical Thinking Exercise

Consider a new mother who believes a fat baby is a healthy baby. She has grown up with this value and is told this repeatedly by her mother (the baby's grandmother). Develop a plan for teaching infant nutrition to this mother.

NURSES AS TEACHERS

Nurses have many teaching roles. They may teach individual learners, such as patients who need instruction about treatments, or they may teach groups of learners, such as prospective parents enrolled in a Lamaze class. They also teach different types of learners. They teach patients or clients and their families or caregivers. They teach health professionals, including other nurses and physicians. They teach health care assistants in various settings, including patient-care assistants, home health aides, and others. Nurses also teach in the community, providing instruction in disease and injury prevention and health promotion.

The primary teaching role of a nurse is in teaching patients and their families. Such instruction includes discharge teaching about how to perform self-care; about taking medications, including side effects; and how to perform prescribed treatments. Most teaching is done directly with patients. However, family members or caregivers also may be instructed in care of the patient. This is especially important for patients who have difficulty performing self-care. For example, parents who need to give medication to their children must be instructed in the proper administration of that medication. A diabetic client who has visual impairment may need assistance in administering insulin or in assessing his or her feet and lower extremities for skin breakdown. The caregiver or family member must be included in the diabetic patient's instruction. When diet teaching is done, it is important to include the person who purchases and prepares the food.

Nurses also teach other nurses and health professionals. Experienced nurses often act as preceptors, teaching new nurses the policies and procedures of the nursing unit. Nurses teach continuing education programs for other nurses. Continuing education programs may include specialty nursing courses such as intensive-care nursing or perioperative nursing, or they may be classes updating nurses' knowledge regarding new research, medications, or procedures, such as new information about care of people with HIV/AIDS. Nurses teach nursing students either informally when students are on the nursing unit or formally in the classroom. Nurses also teach other health care team members, including physicians. Nurse-educators often provide classes in the work setting about new policies, and the learners may include all those who are affected by the policy, such as when a new documentation system is implemented.

Nurses teach subordinate or ancillary staff. Patient-care assistants, volunteers, dietary aides, housekeeping personnel, and unit secretaries participate in patient care at various levels. Nurses may be responsible for teaching these staff members about their responsibilities.

Nurses also participate in community education activities. Nurses may teach high school students about sexually transmitted diseases, teenage pregnancy, and alcohol and drug abuse. They may teach senior citizens about self-medication or other self-care activities. They may teach community classes on hypertension, risk factors for heart disease, or other illnesses. To prevent illness or injury, the public must be provided with information. Nurses are respected by the public and are knowledgeable about health care matters. They are in a position to provide such information.

Reflect on...

■ the teaching activities you are involved in (in school, on the nursing unit, in your practice setting, in the community). What are your feelings about teaching others (fellow students, patients, nursing students, others nurses, other health care providers)?

THE ART OF TEACHING

Teaching is a system of activities intentionally designed to produce specific learning. It is a goal-directed activity that results in improved learning for the learner. Teaching is more than giving information; the art of teaching lies in providing the knowledge, skill, and desire within the learner to change some aspect of his or her life. Effective teaching requires knowledge of the subject matter, understanding of the learning process, judgment, and intuition.

The teaching/learning process involves dynamic interaction between teacher and learner. Each participant in the process communicates information, emotions, perceptions, and attitudes to the other.

The relationship between the teacher and the learner is essentially one of trust and respect. The learner trusts that the teacher has the knowledge and skill to teach, and the teacher respects the learner's ability to attain the recognized goals. Once a nurse starts to instruct a client and/or other learner, it is important that the teaching process continue until the participants achieve the mutually agreed upon learning goals, change the goals, or decide that the goals cannot be met.

Nurses have a responsibility to keep their clinical knowledge current. The American Nurses Association (ANA) lists two standards of clinical nursing practice that relate directly to learning and teaching. See the accompanying box.

American Nurses Association Standards of Professional Performance Related to Teaching and Learning

- *Standard 8. Education:* The nurse attains knowledge and competency that reflects current nursing practice. Measurement criteria include participating in educational activities related to appropriate knowledge bases and professional issues; demonstrating a commitment to lifelong learning through self-reflection and inquiry to identify personal learning needs; seeking experiences that reflect current practice in order to maintain skills and competence in clinical practice or role performance; acquiring knowledge and skills appropriate to the specialty area, practice setting, role, or situation; maintaining professional records that provide evidence of competency and lifelong learning; and seeking experiences and formal and independent learning activities to maintain and develop clinical and professional skills and knowledge.

- *Standard 10. Collegiality:* The nurse interacts with and contributes to the professional development of peers and other health providers as colleagues. Measurement criteria for this standard include sharing knowledge and skills with peers and colleagues; providing peers with feedback regarding their practice and/or role performance, and contributing to an environment that is conducive to the education of health care professionals.

Source: Adapted from *Nursing: Scope and Standards of Practice* (pp. 35, 37), by American Nurses Association, 2004, Washington, DC: ANA.

Guidelines for Learning and Teaching

The following guidelines for effective learning/teaching may be helpful to nurses:

■ Teaching activities should help a learner meet individual learning objectives. These objectives should be mutually determined by the client (learner) and the nurse (teacher). If certain activities do not assist the learner, these need to be reassessed; perhaps other activities can replace them. For example, explanation alone may not be sufficient to teach a client how to handle a syringe. Having the client handle the syringe may be more effective.

■ Rapport between teacher and learner is essential. A relationship that is both accepting and constructive will best assist learning. The nurse should take time to establish rapport before teaching.

■ The teacher who uses the client's previous learning in the present situation encourages the client and facilitates learning new skills. For example, a person who already knows how to cook can use this knowledge when learning to prepare food for a special diet.

■ The nurse-teacher must be able to communicate clearly and concisely. The words the nurse uses need to have the same meaning to the learner as to the teacher. For example, a client who is taught not to put water on an area of skin may think a wet washcloth is permissible for washing the area. In effect, the nurse needs to explain that no water or moisture should touch the area.

■ The nurse should have a knowledge of the learners and the factors that affect their learning before planning the teaching.

■ When the patient/client is involved in planning the instruction, learning is often enhanced.

■ Teaching that involves the learners' senses often enhances learning. For example, when learning about changing a surgical dressing, the nurse can tell the client about the procedure (hearing), show how to change the dressing (sight), and allow the learner to manipulate the equipment (touch).

■ The anticipated behavioral changes that indicate that learning has taken place must always be within the context of the client's lifestyle and resources. For example, it would probably not be reasonable to expect a woman to soak in a tub of hot water four times a day if she did not have a bathtub and had to heat water on a stove.

See the accompanying box for characteristics of effective teaching.

Assessing Learning Needs

The first step in teaching others is to assess their learning needs and the factors that may affect their learning. These factors include the learner's (1) age, (2) health beliefs and practices, (3) cultural factors, (4) economic factors, (5) learning styles, (6) readiness to learn, (7) motivation, and (8) reading level.

Age

Age provides information about the learner's developmental status that may indicate specific health teaching content and teaching approaches. Simple questions to

---

Characteristics of Effective Teaching

- Holds the learner's interest.
- Involves the learner in the learning process. Makes partners of the learner and the teacher.
- Fosters a positive self-concept in the learner; learner believes learning is possible and probable.
- Sets realistic goals.
- Is directed at helping the learner meet learner objectives.
- Supports the learner with positive reinforcement.
- Is accurate and current.
- Is appropriate for the learner's age, condition, and abilities.
- Is optimistic, positive, and nonthreatening.
- Uses several methods of teaching to accommodate a variety of learning styles; provides learning opportunities through hearing, seeing, and doing.
- Gathers information from reliable sources.
- Is cost-effective (cost of nurse's time spent teaching is less than the cost of treating health problems occurring when clients do not follow recommended treatments, fail to take medications correctly, or do not adapt lifestyle to changing health needs).

---

school-age children and adolescents will elicit information about what they know. Observing children in play provides information about their motor and intellectual development as well as relationships with other children. For the elderly person, conversation and questioning may reveal slow recall, limited psychomotor skills, diminished senses, or learning difficulties.

The age of learners also affects the duration of the instruction. Young children have a short attention span; therefore, instruction of children should be of shorter duration. Older adults may be uncomfortable sitting for long periods of time or may require more frequent bathroom breaks.

Health Beliefs and Practices

A learner's health beliefs and practices are important to consider in any teaching plan. However, even if a nurse is convinced that a particular learner's health beliefs should be changed, doing so may not be possible because so many factors are involved in a person's health beliefs. Information about the influence of cultural and spiritual influences on health beliefs can be found in Chapter 21 ∞, Nursing in a Culturally Diverse World and Chapter 22 ∞, Nursing in a Spiritually Diverse World.

Cultural Factors

Many cultural groups have their own beliefs and practices about health and healing: a number of them related to diet, health, illness, and lifestyle. It is therefore important to know how the practices and values held by learners impinge on their learning needs.

Folk beliefs of certain groups may also affect learning. Although the learner may readily understand the health care information being taught, this learning may not be implemented in the home, where folk healing practices prevail. More information about cultural beliefs and values can be found in Chapter 21 ∞, Nursing in a Culturally Diverse World.

Economic Factors

Economic factors can also affect learning. For example, a learner who cannot afford to obtain a new sterile syringe for each self-injection of insulin may find it difficult to learn to administer the insulin when the nurse teaches that a new syringe should be used each time.

Learning Style

Considerable research has been done on people's learning styles. The best way to learn varies with the individual. Some people are visual learners and learn best by watching. Other people do not visualize an activity well; they learn best by actually manipulating equipment and discovering how it works. Other people can learn well from reading things presented in an orderly fashion. Still other people learn best in groups relating to other people. For some, stressing the thinking part of a skill and the logic of something will promote learning. For other people, stressing the feeling part or interpersonal aspect motivates and promotes learning. When material is presented in more than one learning domain, the chances for learning and retaining information are greatly increased.

The nurse seldom has the time or skills to assess each learner, identify the person's particular learning style, and then adapt teaching accordingly. What the nurse can do, however, is to ask learners how they have learned things best in the past or how they like to learn. Many people know what helps them learn, and the nurse can use this information in planning the teaching. Using a variety of teaching techniques and varying activities during teaching are good ways to match learners with learning styles. One technique will be most effective for some learners, whereas other techniques will be suited to learners with different learning styles.

Readiness to Learn

People who are ready to learn often behave differently from those who are not. A learner who is ready may search out information, for instance, by asking questions, reading books or articles, talking to others, and generally showing interest. Today people have access to information with computers and the World Wide Web. The person who is not ready to learn is more likely to avoid the subject or situation. In addition, the unready learner may change the subject when the nurse brings it up.

In assessing readiness to learn, the nurse observes for the following:

- *Physical readiness:* Is the learner able to focus on things other than physical status; or are fatigue, pain, or disability using up all the learner's time and energy?
- *Emotional readiness:* Is the learner emotionally ready to learn? People who are extremely anxious, depressed, or grieving are not ready to learn.
- *Cognitive readiness:* Can the learner think clearly at this point? For example, a client who has an altered level of consciousness is not cognitively ready to learn.

Nurses can promote readiness to learn by providing physical and emotional support before and during learning activities.

Motivation

As discussed earlier, motivation relates to whether the learner wants to learn and is usually greatest when the learner is ready, the learning need is recognized, and the information being offered is meaningful to the learner. Nurses can increase a learner's motivation by doing the following:

- Relating content to something the learner values and helping the learner see the relevance of the content
- Making the learning situation pleasant and nonthreatening
- Encouraging self-direction and independence

Evidence for Practice

Suderman, E. M., Deatrich, J. V., Johnson, L. S., & Sawatzky-Dickson, D. M. (2000). Action research sets the stage to improve discharge preparation. *Pediatric Nursing, 26*(6), 571–576.

The purpose of this study was to determine parents' perspectives of the discharge process of their children from a hospital. The researchers interviewed 14 urban families and 6 rural families. The children were admitted for respiratory problems. Lewin's change theory served as the theoretical framework underpinning this study. Four major themes were identified in the analysis of data. These included the parent as learner, the content taught, the timing of discharge, and the continued impact of hospitalization after discharge. Results indicated the importance of the nurse as discharge planner and educator.

The implications are as follows: Obtaining the parents' perspective about the discharge planning process provides valuable information for the nurse-educator, who needs to consider the diversity of the parents as learners, the extent and depth of their knowledge of the health issue, the care required following discharge, and information about styles and home situations.

- Demonstrating a positive attitude about the learner's ability to learn
- Offering continuing support and encouragement as the learner attempts to learn (i.e., positive reinforcement)
- Creating a learning situation where the learner is likely to succeed
- Rewarding the learner for his or her success

Reading Level

The nurse should not assume that a learner's reading level is equal to the highest grade or level of formal education the learner has completed. Most patient education literature is written above the eighth grade level with the average level between the tenth and twelfth grades. However, the average reading level of adults is between the fifth and eighth grade (Bastable, 2003, p. 207). A variety of instruments exist to assess the readability of patient education ma-

Determining Readability Level of Written Materials Using the SMOG Formula

To determine the reading level of learning materials for clients, choose 30 sentences in the reading. Pick 10 from the beginning, 10 from the middle, and 10 from the end of the reading. Count all the words with 3 or more syllables; total these. Find the number in the list below, and read across to find the reading grade level.

Number of Words with 3 or More Syllables	Reading Grade Level
0–2	4
3–6	5
7–12	6
13–20	7
21–30	8
31–42	9
43–56	10
57–72	11
73–90	12

To decrease the reading level of and simplify the client educational material:

- Use smaller words.
- Avoid words with several syllables.
- Write shorter sentences.
- Explain terms that must be used.
- Use easy, common words.

Sources: Adapted from "Patient Educational Materials: Are They Readable?," by S. T. Stephens, January/February 1992, *Oncology Nursing Forum, 19,* 84; and "Self-Care Instructions: Do Patients Understand Educational Materials?" by M. Wong, February 1992, *Focus on Critical Care, 19,* 47–49.

terials, including the Flesch formula, the Fog formula, the Fry Readability Graph, and the SMOG formula. The SMOG formula is shown in the accompanying box.

Evidence for Practice

Singh, J. (2003). Reading grade level and readability of printed cancer education materials. *Oncology Nursing Forum, 30*(5), 867–870.

The purpose of this study was to examine cancer brochures to determine their reading level and their readability. Ten cancer brochures published by various cancer organizations were examined using the SMOG formula to estimate the reading grade level and the RAIN (Readability Assessment Instrument) to analyze 14 variables that affect comprehension. Based on the SMOG formula, the reading grade level of the brochures ranged from 9 to 15 (indicating ninth grade to junior year college level). The RAIN analysis showed that the number of variables incorporated across the ten brochures ranged from 12 to 14 and the number of variables reaching readability criteria ranged from 6 to 8. The authors concluded that the written levels of the cancer education materials may be too high for the average reader.

The implications of this study are that patient educational materials need to be written so that they match the reading levels of patients and the general public and they should incorporate more of the variables that affect comprehension so that readers can understand them easily. Nurses who use printed educational materials for patients can conduct a comprehensive analysis of these materials using SMOG and RAIN to determine their reading level and readability and revise the materials accordingly.

Planning Content and Teaching Strategies

Developing a teaching plan (see a sample teaching plan for wound care in the box on page 152) is accomplished in a series of steps. Involving the learner at this time promotes the formation of a meaningful plan and stimulates learner motivation. The learner who helps formulate the teaching plan is more likely to achieve the desired outcomes.

Determining Teaching Priorities

Learning needs must be ranked according to priority. The client and the nurse should do this together, with the client's priorities always being considered. Once a client's priorities have been addressed, the client is generally more motivated to concentrate on other identified learning needs. For example, a man who wants to know all about coronary artery disease may not be ready to learn how to change his lifestyle until he meets his own need to learn more about the disease. Nurses can also use theoretical frameworks, such as Maslow's hierarchy of needs, to establish priorities.

Setting Learning Objectives or Outcomes

Outcome-based learning is prevalent in education today. Learning objectives can be considered the same as outcome criteria for other nursing diagnoses. They are written in the same way. Like client outcomes, learning objectives do the following:

- State the learner behavior or performance, not nurse behavior. For example, "The learner will choose her own diet as instructed" (client behavior), not "To teach the client about his diet" (nurse behavior).
- Reflect an observable, measurable activity. The performance may be visible (e.g., walking) or invisible (e.g., adding a column of figures). However, it is necessary to be able to deduce whether an unobservable activity has been mastered from some performance that represents the activity. Therefore, the performance of an objective might be written: "Writes the total for a column of figures in the indicated space" (observable), not "Adds a column of figures" (unobservable). Avoid using words such as *knows, understands, believes,* and *appreciates;* they are neither observable nor measurable. Selected measurable verbs used for learning objectives are shown in the box on page 153.
- May add conditions or modifiers as required to clarify what, where, when, or how the behavior will be performed. Examples are "Walks to the end of the hall and back *without crutches*" (condition), "Irrigates his colostomy *independently* (condition) as taught," or "States *three* (condition) factors that affect blood glucose level."
- Include criteria specifying the time by which learning should have occurred. For example, "The client will state three things that affect blood glucose level *by the end of second diabetes class.*"

Teaching Plan: Wound Care

Assessment of Learner: A 24-year-old male college student suffered a 2.5-in. (7-cm) laceration on the left lower anterior leg during a hockey game. The laceration was cleansed, sutured, and bandaged. The client was given an appointment to return to the health clinic in 10 days for suture removal. The client states that he lives in the college dormitory and is able to care for wound if given instructions. The client is able to read and understand English.

Nursing Diagnosis: **Knowledge deficit** related to care of sutured wound.

Long-Term Goal: Client's wound will heal completely without infection or other complication.

Intermediate Goal: At clinic appointment, client's wound will be healing without signs of infection, loss of function, or other complication.

Short-Term Goal: Client will respond to questions regarding wound care and perform return demonstration of wound cleansing and bandaging.

Behavioral Objectives	Content Outline	Teaching Methods
Upon completion of the instructional session, the client will:		
1. Describe normal wound healing	I. Normal wound healing	Describe normal wound healing with the use of audiovisuals.
2. List signs and symptoms of wound infection	II. Infection Signs and symptoms include wound warm to touch, malalignment of wound edges, and purulent wound drainage. Signs of systemic infection include fever and malaise.	Discuss the mechanism of wound infection. Use audiovisuals to demonstrate infected wound appearance. Provide handout describing signs and symptoms of wound infection.
3. Correctly use equipment needed for wound care	III. Wound care equipment a. Cleansing solution as prescribed by physician (e.g., clear water, mild soap and water, antimicrobial solution, or hydrogen peroxide). b. Bandaging material: Telfa, gauze wrap, adhesive tape.	Provide handout listing equipment. Demonstrate equipment needed for cleansing and bandaging wound.
4. Demonstrate wound cleansing and bandaging	IV. Demonstration of wound cleansing and bandaging on the client's wound or a mannequin.	Demonstrate wound cleansing and bandaging on the client's wound or a mannequin. Provide handout describing procedure for cleansing and bandaging wound.
5. Develop a plan for appropriate client action if questions or complications arise	V. Resources available for client questions include health clinic, emergency department.	Discuss available resources. Provide handout listing available resources and follow-up treatment plan.
6. Identify date, time, and location of follow-up appointment for suture removal	VI. Follow-up treatment plan; where and when.	Provide written instructions.

Evaluation: The client will:

1. Respond to questions regarding self-care of wound
2. Return demonstration of wound cleansing and bandaging
3. State contact person and telephone number to obtain assistance
4. State date, time, and location of follow-up appointment

Selected Verbs for Behavior Learning Objectives

COGNITIVE	PSYCHOMOTOR	AFFECTIVE
Analyze	Arrange	Accept
Apply	Calibrate	Agree/Disagree
Calculate	Change	Attempt
Compute	Constructs	Attend
Defend	Demonstrate	Choose
Define	Dissect	Commit
Describe	Distinguish	Defend
Differentiate	Manipulate	Influence
Discuss	Mix	Qualify
Distinguish	Prepare	Value
Evaluate	Walk	
Explain		
Identify		
Outline		
Prioritizes		
Sorts		

Choosing Content

The content, or what is to be taught, is determined by learning objectives. For example, "Identify appropriate sites for insulin injection" means the nurse must include content about the body sites suitable for insulin injections. Nurses can select among many sources of information including books, nursing journals, and other nurses and physicians. Governmental agencies are excellent sources of free patient education materials. For example, the National Institute on Aging (NIA) provides large-print educational materials called Age Pages that are related to health topics appropriate for older adults. They can be downloaded free from the NIA Web site. Whatever sources the nurse chooses, content should be as follows:

- Accurate
- Current
- Based on learning objectives
- Adjusted for the learner's age, culture, language, and ability
- Consistent with information the nurse is teaching
- Selected with consideration for how much time and resources are available for teaching

Selecting Teaching Strategies

The method of teaching the nurse chooses should be suited to the individual, to the material to be learned, and to the teacher. For example, the person who cannot read needs material presented in other ways; a discussion is usually not the best strategy for teaching how to give an injection; and a teacher using group discussion for teaching should be a competent group leader. As stated earlier, some people are visually oriented and learn best through seeing; others learn best through hearing and having the skill explained. See Table 8–3 for selected teaching strategies.

Ordering Learning Experiences

To save nurses time in constructing their own teaching plans, some health agencies have developed standardized teaching guides for teaching sessions that nurses commonly give. These guides standardize content and teaching methods and make it easier for the nurse to plan and implement client teaching. Whether the nurse is implementing a plan devised by another or developing an individualized teaching plan, some guidelines can help the nurse order the learning experience.

- Start with something the learner is concerned about; for example, before learning how to administer insulin to himself, an adolescent wants to know how he can adjust his lifestyle and still play football.
- Begin with what the learner knows, and proceed to the unknown. This gives the learner confidence. Sometimes you will not know the client's knowledge or skill base and will need to elicit this information, either by asking questions or by having the client fill out a form, such as a pretest.
- Address first any area that is causing the learner anxiety. A high level of anxiety can impair concentration in other areas. For example, a woman highly anxious about turning her husband in bed might not be able to learn about bathing him until she has successfully learned to turn him.
- Teach the basics first, then proceed to the variations or adjustments. It is very confusing to learners to have to consider possible adjustments and variations before they master the basic concepts. For example, when teaching a female client how to insert a retention catheter, it is best to teach the basic procedure before teaching any adjustments that might be needed if the catheter stops draining after insertion.
- Schedule time for review of content and questions the learner(s) may have to clarify information.

Table 8–3 Selected Teaching Strategies

Strategy	Major Type of Learning	Characteristics
Explanation or description (e.g., lecture)	Cognitive	Teacher controls content and pace. Learner is passive; therefore, retains less information than when a participant. Feedback is determined by teacher. May be given to individual or group.
One-to-one discussion	Affective, cognitive	Encourages participation by learner. Permits reinforcement and repetition at learner's level. Permits introduction of sensitive subjects.
Answering questions	Cognitive	Teacher controls most of content and pace. Teacher must understand question and what it means to learner. Learner may need to overcome cultural perception that asking questions is impolite and may embarrass the teacher. Can be used with individuals and groups. Teacher sometimes needs to confirm whether question has been answered by asking learner, for example, "Does that answer your question?"
Demonstration	Psychomotor	Often used with explanation. Can be used with individuals, small or large groups. Does not permit use of equipment by learners; learner is passive.
Discovery	Cognitive, affective	Teacher guides problem-solving situation. Learner is active participant; therefore, retention of information is high.
Group discussions	Affective, cognitive	Learner can obtain assistance from supportive group. Group members learn from one another. Teacher needs to keep the discussion focused and prevent monopolization by one or two learners.
Practice	Psychomotor	Allows repetition and immediate feedback. Permits "hands-on" experience.
Printed and audiovisual materials	Cognitive	Forms include books, pamphlets, films, programmed instruction, and computer learning. Learners can proceed at their own speed. Nurse can act as resource person, need not be present during learning. Potentially ineffective if reading level is too high. Teacher needs to select language that meets learner needs if English is a second language.
Role playing	Affective, cognitive	Permits expression of attitudes, values, and emotions. Can assist in development of communication skills. Involves active participation by learner. Teacher must create supportive, safe environment for learners to minimize anxiety.
Modeling	Affective, psychomotor	Nurse sets example by attitude, psychomotor skill.
Computer-assisted learning programs	All types of learning	Learner is active. Learner controls pace. Provides immediate reinforcement and review. Use with individuals or groups.

Implementing a Teaching Plan

The nurse needs to be flexible in implementing any teaching plan because the plan may need revising. The learner may tire sooner than anticipated or be faced with too much information too quickly; the learner's needs may change; or external factors may intervene. For example, the nurse and the learner, Mr. Brown, have planned to irrigate his colostomy at 10 A.M., but when the time comes, Mr. Brown wants additional information before actually doing it himself. In this case, the nurse alters the teaching plan and discusses the desired information, provides written information, and defers teaching the psychomotor skill until the next day. It is also important for nurses to use teaching techniques that enhance learning and reduce or eliminate any barriers to learning such as pain or fatigue.

Guidelines for Teaching

When implementing a teaching plan, the nurse may find the following guidelines helpful:

1. The optimal time for each session depends largely on the learner. Some people, for example, learn best at the beginning of the day, when they are most rested; others prefer late afternoon, when no other activities are scheduled. Whenever possible, ask the prospective learner(s) for help in choosing the best time.

2. The pace of each teaching session also affects learning. Nurses should be sensitive to any signs that the pace is too fast or too slow. A learner who appears confused or does not comprehend material when questioned may be finding the pace too fast. When the learner appears bored and loses interest, the pace may be too slow, the learning period may be too long, or the learner may be tired.

3. An environment can detract from or assist learning; for example, noise or interruptions usually interfere with concentration, whereas a comfortable environment promotes learning.

4. Teaching aids can foster learning and help focus a learner's attention. To ensure the transfer of learning, the nurse should use the type of supplies or equipment the learner will eventually use. Before the teaching session, the nurse needs to assemble all equipment and visual aids and ensure that all audiovisual equipment is functioning properly.

5. Learning is more effective when learners discover the content for themselves. Ways to increase learning include stimulating motivation and self-direction, for example, by providing specific, realistic, achievable objectives; giving feedback; and helping the learner derive satisfaction from learning. The nurse may also encourage self-directed independent learning by encouraging the client to explore sources of information, such as the Internet.

6. Repetition helps reinforce learning. Summarizing content, rephrasing (using other words), and approaching the material from another point of view reinforces learning. For example, after discussing the kinds of foods that can be included in a diet, the nurse describes the foods again, but in the context of the three meals eaten during one day.

7. It is helpful to employ "organizers" to introduce material to be learned. Organizers provide a means of connecting unknown material to known material and generating logical relationships. For example: "You understand how urine flows down a catheter from the bladder. Now I will show you how to inject fluid so that it flows up the catheter into the bladder." The details that follow are then seen within its framework, and the details have added meaning.

8. Using a layperson's vocabulary enhances communication. Often nurses use terms and abbreviations that have meaning to other health professionals but make little sense to clients. Even words such as *urine* or *feces* may be unfamiliar to clients, and abbreviations such as RR (recovery room) or PAR (postanesthesia room) are often misunderstood.

9. Provide the learner with a handout that captures the key points of your instruction. Written material to which the learner can refer during and after the instruction provides security and reinforcement.

Evaluating Learning and Teaching
Evaluating Learning

Evaluating is both an ongoing (formative) and a final (summative) process in which the learner, the nurse, and, often, the support persons determine what has been learned. Learning is measured against the predetermined learning objectives selected in the planning phase of the teaching process. Thus, the objectives serve not only to direct the teaching plan but also to provide outcome criteria for evaluation. For example, the objective "Selects foods that are low in carbohydrates" can be evaluated by asking the learner to name such foods or to select low-carbohydrate foods from a list or a menu.

The best method for evaluating depends on the type of learning. In *cognitive learning*, the learner demonstrates acquisition of knowledge. Examples of the evaluation tools for cognitive learning include the following:

- Direct observation of behavior (e.g., observing the learner selecting the solution to a problem using the new knowledge).
- Written measurements (e.g., tests).
- Oral questioning (e.g., asking the learner to restate information or correct verbal responses to questions).
- Self-reports and self-monitoring. These can be useful during follow-up phone calls and home visits. Evaluating individual self-paced learning, as might occur with computer-assisted instruction; often incorporates self-monitoring.

The acquisition of psychomotor skills is best evaluated by observing how well the learner carries out a procedure, such as changing a dressing or self-administering insulin.

Affective learning is more difficult to evaluate. Whether attitudes or values have been learned may be inferred by listening to the learner's responses to questions, noting how the learner speaks about relevant subjects, and by observing the learner's behavior that expresses feelings and values. For example, do learners who state that they value health actually use condoms every time they have sex with a new partner? Have parents learned to value health sufficiently to have their children immunized? Often, the accomplishment of affective objectives is best measured some time later (e.g., Do the parents return to the clinic with their child for routine immunizations as appropriate?).

Following evaluation, the nurse may find it necessary to modify or repeat the teaching plan if the objectives have not been met or have been met only partially. For the hospitalized client, follow-up teaching in the home, in the clinic or doctor's office, or by phone may be needed.

Behavior change does not always take place immediately after learning. Often individuals accept change intellectually first and then change their behavior only periodically (e.g., Mrs. Green, who knows that she must lose weight, diets and exercises off and on). If the new behavior is to replace the old behavior, it must emerge gradually; otherwise, the old behavior may prevail. The nurse can assist learners with behavior change by allowing for vacillation and by providing encouragement.

Evaluating Teaching

It is important for nurses to evaluate their own teaching. Evaluation should include a consideration of all factors—the timing, the environment for learning, the teaching strategies, the amount of information, whether the teaching was helpful, and so on. The nurse may find, for example, that the learner was overwhelmed with too much information or was bored or in pain or the television and visitors were distracting.

Both the learner and the nurse should evaluate the learning experience. The learner may tell the nurse what was helpful, interesting, and so on. Feedback questionnaires and videotapes of the learning sessions also can be helpful.

The nurse should not feel ineffective as a teacher if the learner forgets some of what is taught. Forgetting is normal and should be anticipated. Having the learner write down information, repeating it during teaching, giving handouts on the information, and having the learner be active in the learning process all promote retention.

Special Teaching Strategies

There are a number of special teaching strategies that nurses can use: contracting, group teaching, computer-assisted instruction, multimedia presentations, discovery/problem solving, and behavior modification. Any strategy the nurse selects must be appropriate for the learner and the learning objectives.

Contracting

Contracting involves establishing a written agreement with a learner that specifies certain objectives and when they are to be met. The contract, drawn up and signed by the learner and the nurse, specifies not only the learning objectives but also the responsibilities of the learner and the nurse and the teaching plan. The agreement allows for freedom, mutual respect, and mutual responsibility.

Group Teaching

Group instruction is economical, and it provides members with an opportunity to share with and learn from others. A small group allows for discussion in which everyone can participate. A large group often necessitates a lecture technique or use of films, videos, slides, or role-playing by teachers.

It is important that all members involved in group instruction have a need in common (e.g., prenatal health or preoperative instruction). It is also important that sociocultural factors be considered in the formation of a group. Whereas middle-class Americans may value sharing experiences with others, people from a culture such as Japan may consider it inappropriate to reveal their thoughts and feelings.

Computer-Assisted Instruction

Computer-assisted instruction (CAI) has become popular. Initially, cognitive learning of facts was the primary use of computer educational methods. Now, however, computers also can be used to teach the following:

- Complex problem-solving skills
- Application of information
- Psychomotor skills

Programs can be used for instruction of the following:

- Individual health care professionals or learners using one computer.
- Small groups of three to five learners gathered around one computer taking turns running the program and answering questions together.
- Large groups, with the computer display screen projected onto an overhead screen and a teacher or one learner using the keyboard.

Individuals using a computer are able to set the pace that meets their learning needs. Small groups are less able to do this, and large groups progress through the program at a pace that may be too slow for some learners and too fast for others. It is therefore helpful to group learners of similar needs and abilities together. Whether using the computer alone or in large groups, learners read and view informational material, answer questions, and receive immediate feedback. The correct answer is usually indicated by the use of colors, flashing signs, or written praise. When the learner selects an incorrect answer, the computer responds with an explanation of why that was not the best answer and encouragement to try again. Many programs ask learners whether they want to review material on which the question and answer were based. Some computer programs feature simulated situations that allow learners to manipulate objects on the screen to learn psychomotor skills. When used to teach such skills, CAI must be followed up with practice on actual equipment supervised by the teacher.

Some learners may have a negative attitude about computers that could act as a barrier to learning. The nurse helps these learners by explaining the steps to

start and run the program, how to turn the computer on and off, and where and when to insert the computer disk so that the learner can use the program when the nurse is not present. Most media catalogs, professional journals, and health care libraries contain information about computer programs available to the nurse for client education. The media specialist or librarian in a health care facility or college is an excellent resource to help the nurse locate appropriate computer programs. Computer educational material is also available for learners with different language needs, for learners with special visual needs, and for learners at different developmental levels.

Multimedia Presentations

Multimedia presentations combine audio, film, video, and computers to stimulate many senses. This enhances learning and provides consistent instruction. Learners can stop the instruction and replay it as needed. Nurse-educators can use presentation software to create professional-looking lessons for clients. Storing the lessons on CD-ROM makes them transportable from one computer to another or programs can be networked to multiple computers.

Discovery/Problem Solving

In using the discovery/problem-solving technique, the nurse presents some initial information and then asks the learners a question or presents a situation related to the information. The learner applies the new information to the situation and decides what to do. Learners can work alone or in groups. This technique is well suited to family learning. The teacher guides the learners through the thinking process necessary to reach the best solution to the question or the best action to take in the situation. This may also be referred to as anticipatory problem solving. For example, the nurse-educator might present information on diabetes and blood glucose management. Then, the nurse might ask the learners how they think their insulin and/or diet should be adjusted if their morning glucose was too low. In this way, clients learn what critical components they need to consider to reach the best solution to the problem.

Behavior Modification

Behavior modification is an outgrowth of behavioral learning theory. Its basic assumptions include (1) human behaviors are learned and can be selectively

Critical Thinking Exercise

Using the teaching strategies described in Table 8–3,

1. Identify barriers that may influence the learning ability of older adults and children. What strategies would you employ to overcome these barriers? What teaching tools would you select for children? What teaching strategies would you select for older adults?

2. Describe strategies you would use to teach a 15-year-old diabetic about insulin injections. Include strategies for the cognitive, affective, and psychomotor domains.

3. Describe teaching strategies that would be more effective with individual learners, with groups of learners.

strengthened, weakened, eliminated, or replaced; and (2) a person's behavior is under conscious control. Under this system, desirable behavior is regarded and undesirable behavior is ignored. The learner's response is the key to behavior change. For example, learners trying to quit smoking are not criticized when they smoke, but they are praised or rewarded when they go without a cigarette for a certain period of time. For some people a learning contract is combined with behavior modification and includes the following pertinent features:

- Positive reinforcement (e.g., praise, reward) is used.
- The learner participates in the development of the learning plan.
- Undesirable behavior is ignored, not criticized.
- The expectation of the learner and the nurse is that the task will be mastered (i.e., the behavior will change).
- Success is maximized through positive reinforcement; failure and the threat of failure are minimized.

Reflect on...

- the teaching strategies you employ with clients in your clinical setting. Examining the strategies described in Table 8–3. Which do you find most effective in your teaching? Which do you find least effective in your teaching? Why?

Transcultural Client Teaching

The nurse and learners of different cultural and ethnic backgrounds have additional barriers to overcome in the teaching-learning process. These barriers include language and communication problems, differing concepts of time, conflicting cultural healing practices, beliefs that may positively or negatively influence compliance with health teaching, and unique high-risk or high-frequency health problems needing health-promotion instruction. See Chapter 7 ⚭, The Nurse as Health Promoter and Care Provider, and Chapter 21 ⚭, Nursing in a Culturally Diverse World, for detailed information. Nurses should consider the following guidelines when teaching learners from various ethnic backgrounds:

- Obtain teaching materials, pamphlets, and instructions in languages used by clients in the health care setting. Nurses who are unable to read the foreign language material for themselves can have a translator read the material to them. The nurse can then evaluate the quality of the information and update it with the translator's help as needed.
- Use visual aids, such as pictures, charts, diagrams, slides, or video to communicate meaning. Audiovisual material may be helpful if the English is spoken clearly and slowly. Even if understanding the verbal message is a problem for the learner, seeing a skill or procedure may be helpful. In some instances, a translator can be asked to clarify the printed materials. Alternatively, printed material and other audiovisual materials may be available in several languages, and the nurse can request the necessary version from the company.
- Use concrete rather than abstract words. Use simple language (short sentences, short words), and present only one idea at a time.
- Allow time for questions. This helps the learner mentally separate one idea or skill from another.
- Avoid the use of medical terminology or health care language, such as "taking your vital signs" or "apical pulse." Rather, nurses should say they are going to take a blood pressure or listen to the client's heart.

- If understanding another's pronunciation is a problem, validate information in writing. For example, during assessments, write down numbers, words, or phrases, and have the client read them to verify accuracy.
- Use humor very cautiously. Meaning can change in the translation process.
- Do not use slang words or colloquialisms. These may be interpreted literally.
- Do not assume that a learner who nods, uses eye contact, or smiles is indicating an understanding of what is being taught. These responses may simply be the learner's way of indicating respect. The learner may feel that asking the nurse questions or stating a lack of understanding is inappropriate because it might embarrass the nurse or cause the nurse to "lose face."
- Invite and encourage questions during teaching. Let learners know they are urged to ask questions and be involved in making information more clear. When asking questions to evaluate learner understanding, avoid asking negative questions. These can be interpreted differently by people for whom English is a second language. "Do you understand how far you can bend your hip after surgery?" is better than the negative question "You don't understand how far you can bend your hip after surgery, do you?" With particularly difficult information or skills teaching, the nurse might say, "Most people have some trouble with this. May I help you go through this one more time?" In some cultures, expressing a need is not appropriate, and expressing confusion or asking to be shown something again is considered rude.
- When explaining procedures or functioning related to personal areas of the body, it may be appropriate to have a nurse of the same sex do the teaching. Because of modesty concerns in many cultures and beliefs about what is considered appropriate and inappropriate male-female interaction, it is wise to have a female nurse teach female learners about personal care, birth control, sexually transmitted diseases (STDs), and other potentially sensitive areas. If a translator is needed during explanation of procedures or teaching, the translator should also be of the same gender.
- Include the family in planning and teaching. This promotes trust and mutual respect. Identify the authoritative family member and incorporate that person into the planning and teaching to promote adherence and support of health teaching. In some cultures, the male head of household is the critical family member to include in health teaching; in other cultures, it is the eldest female member.

DOCUMENTATION OF TEACHING

Documentation of the teaching process is essential when teaching clients in the clinical setting, because it provides a legal record that the teaching took place and communicates the teaching to other health professionals. If teaching is not documented, legally it did not occur. It is also important to document the response of the client and support persons. What did the client or support person say or do to indicate that learning occurred? The nurse records this in the client's chart as evidence of learning. The parts of the teaching process that should be documented in the client's chart include the following:

- Diagnosed learning needs
- Learning objectives
- Topics taught
- Client outcomes
- Need for additional teaching
- Resources provided

The written teaching plan that the nurse uses as a resource to guide future teaching sessions might also include the following elements. A copy may also be included in the patient's record.

- Actual information and skills taught
- Teaching strategies used
- Time framework and content for each class

Reflect on...

- the learning needs of clients in your specific practice setting. Is the instruction given by different health care providers consistent in its content? What problems might occur if there is inconsistency in instruction? How might you correct these inconsistencies?
- the specific health problems of your community (e.g., AIDS, teenage pregnancy, sexually transmitted disease, domestic violence). How might the nurse assist in solving community health problems through the teaching role?

EXPLORE MEDIALINK

Questions, critical thinking exercises, essay activities, and other interactive resources for this chapter can be found on the Web site at http://www.prenhall.com/blais. Click on Chapter 8 to select activities for this chapter.

Bookshelf

Bastable, S. B. (2003). *Nurse as educator: Principles of teaching and learning for nursing practice* **(2nd ed.). Boston: Jones and Bartlett.**

This text is an excellent reference for nurses who want to improve their teaching skills. Units include perspectives on teaching and learning, characteristics of the learner, and techniques and strategies for teaching and learning. Especially useful are discussions of literacy in adult patient groups, learning needs of special populations, and the use of technology in teaching.

Deck, M. (1995). *Instant teaching tools for health care educators.* **St. Louis, MO: Mosby.**

Deck, M. L. (1998). *More teaching tools for health care educators.* **St. Louis, MO: Mosby.**

These books are useful resources for health care educators. The first provides how-to teaching strategies for a variety of learning situations. The second provides exercises and tricks for teaching allied health professionals.

DeYoung, S. (2003). *Teaching strategies for nurse educators.* **Upper Saddle River, NJ: Prentice Hall.**

This text is a useful reference for nurses in developing their role as a patient educator. Foundational concepts of learning theory, types of learning, learning styles, and learner characteristics are discussed. More than half of the text is devoted to teaching strategies, including traditional teaching strategies and activity-based teaching strategies, computer teaching strategies, distance learning, teaching psychomotor skills, promoting and assessing critical thinking, clinical teaching, and assessing and evaluating learning.

Redman, B. K. (2001). *The practice of patient education* **(9th ed.). St. Louis: Mosby.**

This text provides foundational information on the role of the nurse in patient education. Unique to this text is the coverage of teaching in specific patient environments, including cancer patient education, cardiovascular and pulmonary patient education, diabetes self-management education, education for pregnancy and parenting, educating children, and patient self-management for rheumatic disease.

SUMMARY

Teaching clients, families, and other health professionals is a major nursing role. Learning is represented by a change in behavior.

Five main theories of learning are behaviorism, cognitivism, humanism, constructivism, and multiple intelligence. Behaviorism focuses on careful identification of what is to be taught and the immediate identification of a reward for correct responses. Cognitivism, which has a more holistic view of learning, emphasizes the importance of an integrated learning experience, one that develops understanding and appreciation that help the person function in a larger context. It also stresses the importance of social, emotional, and physical contexts in which learning occurs. The teacher-learner relationship is also an important factor in cognitive learning theory. Humanism focuses on the feelings and attitudes of the learner and stresses that individuals can become highly self-motivated learners. The learner identifies the learning needs and takes responsibility for meeting them. Constructivism is a collection of theories whereby the individual is actively involved in constructing knowledge. Learning is often collaborative. Multiple intelligence focuses on the many ways individuals are "smart."

Bloom has identified three learning domains: cognitive, affective, and psychomotor. The cognitive domain includes six intellectual skills: knowledge, comprehension, application, analysis, synthesis, and evaluation. The affective domain includes five categories: receiving, responding, valuing, organization, and characterization. The psychomotor domain includes seven categories: perception, set, guided response, mechanism, complex overt response, adaptation, and origination.

A number of factors facilitate learning, including motivation, readiness to learn, active involvement, success at learning, feedback, and moving from simple to complex. Factors such as extreme anxiety, certain physiologic processes such as pain, and cultural barriers impede learning.

Teaching is a system of activities intended to produce learning. Rapport between the teacher and the learner is essential for effective teaching. Teaching consists of five activities: assessing the learner, diagnosing learning needs, developing a teaching plan, implementing the plan, and evaluating learning outcomes and teaching effectiveness. Learning objectives guide the content of the teaching plan and are written in terms of client behavior. Teaching strategies should be suited to the client, the material to be learned, and the teacher. It should be adjusted to the client's developmental level and health status.

A teaching plan is a written plan consisting of learning objectives, content to teach, a time frame for teaching, and strategies to use in teaching the content. The plan must be revised when the client's needs change or the teaching strategies prove ineffective. Adaptations in teaching will facilitate learning for clients who are illiterate, elderly, or from non-Western cultural and ethnic backgrounds. Barriers to overcome when teaching clients of different cultures include language and communication problems, different concepts of time, and cultural beliefs and practices that conflict with those of Western medicine.

Evaluation of the teaching/learning process is both an ongoing and a final process. Documentation of client teaching is essential to communicate the teaching to other health professionals and to provide a record for legal purposes.

Nurses have the responsibility for personal life-long learning to maintain currency and proficiency in the knowledge and skills essential for safe and effective practice. Nurses can obtain learning through formal and informal instructional activities.

REFERENCES

American Nurses Association. (2004). *Nursing: Scope and standards of practice.* Washington, DC: ANA.

American Nurses Credentialing Center. (2004). *Specialty Nursing Practice Certifications.* Retrieved July 2, 2004, from http://www.ana.org/ancc/certification/cert/certs/specialty.html..

Bandura, A. (Ed.). (1971). Analysis of modeling processes. In *Psychological modeling.* Chicago: Aldine.

Bastable, S. B. (2003). *Nurse as educator: Principles of teaching and learning for nursing practice* (2nd ed.). Boston: Jones and Bartlett.

Bloom, B. S. (Ed.). (1956). *Taxonomy of educational objectives. Book 1, Cognitive domain.* New York: Longman.

Brooks, J. G., & Brooks, M. G. (1993). *In search of understanding: The case for constructivist classrooms.* Alexandria, VA: Association for Supervision and Curriculum Development.

Bruner, J. (1966). *Toward a theory of instruction.* Cambridge, MA: Harvard University Press.

DeYoung, S. (2003). *Teaching strategies for nurse educators.* Upper Saddle River, NJ: Prentice Hall.

Dick, W., Carey, L., & Carey, J. O. (2001). *The systematic design of instruction* (5th ed.). New York: Addison-Wesley Longman.

Driscoll, M. (2000). *Psychology of learning for instruction* (2nd ed.). New York: Allyn and Bacon.

Gagne, R. M. (1974). *Essentials of learning of instruction.* Hinsdale, IL: Dryden Press.

Gardner, H. (1983). *Frames of mind: The theory of multiple intelligences.* New York: Basic Books.

Gerty, C. (1997). *Learning with Bruner.* New York: Review of Books.

Gessner, B. A. (1989, September). Adult education: The cornerstone of patient teaching. *Nursing Clinics of North America, 24,* 589–595.

Gredler, M. E. (2001). *Learning and instruction: Theory into practice* (4th ed.). Columbus, OH: Merrill.

Gronlund, N. E. (1985). *Stating objectives for classroom instruction* (3rd ed.). New York: Macmillan.

Knowles, M. S. (1980). *The modern practice of adult education: From pedagogy to andragogy.* Chicago: Follet.

Knowles, M. S. (1984). *Andragogy in action.* San Francisco: Jossey-Bass.

Lewin, K. (1951). *Field theory in social science.* New York: Harper and Row.

Maslow, A. H. (1970). *Motivation and personality.* New York: Harper and Row.

Pavlov, I. P. (1927). *Conditioned reflexes* (trans. G. V. Anrep). London: Oxford University Press.

Piaget, J. (1966). *Origins of intelligence in children.* New York: Norton.

Redman, B. K. (2001). *The practice of patient education* (9th ed.). St. Louis: Mosby.

Rogers, C. R. (1961). *On becoming a person.* Boston: Houghton-Mifflin.

Rogers, C. R. (1969). *Freedom to learn.* Columbus, OH: Merrill.

Schoenly, L. (1994, September/October). Teaching in the affective domain. *Journal of Continuing Education in Nursing, 25,* 209–212.

Skinner, B. F. (1953). *Science and human behavior.* New York: Macmillan.

Stephens, S. T. (1992). Patient educational materials: Are they readable? *Oncology Nursing Forum, 19*(1), 84.

Suderman, E. M., Deatrich, J. V., Johnson, L. S., & Sawatzky-Dickson, D. M. (2000). Action research sets the stage to improve discharge preparation. *Pediatric Nursing, 26*(6), 571–576.

Swansburg, R. C. (1995). *Nursing staff development: A component of human resource development.* Boston: Jones and Bartlett.

Thorndike, E. L. (1913). *The psychology of learning.* New York: Teachers College.

Wong, M. (1992). Self-care instructions: Do patients understand educational materials? *Focus on Critical Care, 19*(2), 47–49.

The Nurse as Leader and Manager

Outline

Objectives

- Differentiate leadership from management.

- Compare and contrast the following leadership styles: charismatic, authoritarian, democratic, laissez-faire, situational, transactional, and transformational.

- Describe the management concepts of authority, accountability, planning, organizing, leading, controlling, and power.

- Compare and contrast the following nursing delivery models: total patient care, functional method, team nursing, primary nursing, case management, managed care, differentiated practice, and shared governance.

MEDIALINK

Additional online resource for this chapter can be found on the companion Web site at http://www.prenhall.com/blais.

Today's professional nurses assume leadership and management responsibilities regardless of the activity in which they are involved. Although leadership and management roles are different, they are frequently intertwined. Leadership is defined as "the ability to influence others" (Tappen, Weiss, & Whitehead, 2004, p. 5). Management involves not only leadership but also "coordination and integration of resources through planning, organizing, coordinating, directing, and controlling to accomplish specific institutional goals and

Table 9–1 Comparison of Leader and Manager Roles

Leaders	Managers
• Do not have delegated authority; power derives from other means, such as personal influence	• Have an assigned position in the formal organization
• Have a wider variety of roles	• Have a legitimate source of power because of the delegated authority that is part of their position
• May not be a part of the formal organization	• Are expected to carry out specific functions, duties, and responsibilities
• Focus on group process, information gathering, feedback, and empowering others	• Emphasize control, decision making, decision analysis, and results
• Emphasize interpersonal relationships	• Manipulate personnel, the environment, money, time, and other resources to achieve organizational goals
• Direct willing followers	• Have a greater formal responsibility and accountability
• Have goals that may or may not reflect those of the organization	• Direct willing and unwilling subordinates

Source: From *Leadership Roles and Management Function in Nursing* (3rd. ed.), by B. L. Marquis and C. J. Huston, 2000, Philadelphia: Lippincott.

objectives" (Huber, 2000). Leaders focus on people, whereas managers focus on systems and structures. See Table 9–1 for a comparison of leader and manager roles.

The ability to advocate for the client is linked to the nurse's leadership ability. The nurse may be a leader or manager in the care of the individual client, the client's family, groups of clients, or the community. Regardless of the setting, the nurse must demonstrate leadership and management skills in interacting with nursing colleagues, nursing students, physicians, and other health professionals.

CHALLENGES AND OPPORTUNITIES

Leadership challenges for nurses in the current U.S. health care system include limited access to health care services for many, especially the poor; limited resources for providing care; and the need to provide care for high numbers of uninsured or underinsured individuals and families. Nurse-managers and administrators are faced with the need to recruit and retain high-quality nurses who are capable of assuming new and rapidly changing nursing roles. These challenges must be met during a time of severe nursing shortage while there is an increasing need for nurses.

These challenges provide opportunities to develop innovative approaches to nursing care delivery and to redefine the roles of professional nurses. These innovations and changes provide opportunities to develop new recruitment and retention strategies that increase nursing satisfaction and commitment to the profession.

NURSING LEADERSHIP

Nurses may assume leadership roles in their work setting, their profession, and their community, whether or not they have designated positions of leadership. As leaders in the workplace, they may advocate for improvements in the quality of patient care. As leaders in the profession, nurses may advocate not only for improvements in client care, but also for improvements in the working environment of nurses and other health professionals. Because of their special knowledge and skill, nurses may also assume leadership roles in the community, advocating for changes that promote physical, psychologic, and social well-being in the society as a whole.

On a wider scope, nurses must apply leadership skills as they apply nursing knowledge to personal concerns. Nurses can demonstrate these leadership skills with their involvement in organizations such as Mothers Against Drunk Drivers (MADD), the American Cancer Society, and the American Heart Association. Nurses demonstrate leadership activities as they advocate for the homeless, older adults, persons living with AIDS, victims of violence, and environmental protection programs. In recent years, professional nurses have demonstrated a wide range of leadership and management skills to politicians and legislators in all parts of the country in their efforts to advocate and plan for a system of affordable health care for all residents of the United States through *Nursing's Agenda for Health Care Reform* (ANA, 1991).

Leadership occurs when someone influences others to act. Whereas managers are assigned their roles, leaders achieve their roles. One may be designated the manager and demonstrate no leadership skills, whereas another person may have no formal management title yet demonstrate excellent leadership skills.

Leadership Characteristics

What are the characteristics of successful leadership? Hellriegel and Slocum (1993, pp. 469–479) emphasize the following core leadership skills:

- *Empowerment.* Leaders who empower others share influence and control with group members in deciding how to achieve the organization's goals. Through empowerment, the leader gives others a sense of achievement, belonging, and self-esteem. One way in which the nursing leader can empower the staff is to discuss with them ideas about providing client care.
- *Intuition.* By using intuition, a leader can build trust with others, scan a situation, anticipate the need for change, and quickly move to institute appropriate change. Intuition involves having a "feel" for the environment and the needs and desires of others. Effective nurse leaders heighten their sense of intuition in order to keep abreast of the needs of clients and staff.
- *Self-understanding.* Self-understanding includes an ability to recognize one's strengths and weaknesses. Building on one's strengths and correcting or working on weaknesses are essential for effective leadership.
- *Vision.* Leaders with a vision imagine a different and better situation and identify ways of achieving it. Visionary leadership does not mean constantly imagining new and original goals; a vision may be as simple as incorporating caring and efficiency in meeting the needs of employees and clients.
- *Values congruence.* Values congruence is the ability to understand and accept the mission and objectives of the organization and the values of employees and to reconcile them. In this era of health reform and cost containment, values congruence is an important leadership characteristic.

Does the fact that effective leaders share certain characteristics imply that they all act the same? Not necessarily. Besides having the preceding characteristics,

Characteristics of Effective Leaders

- Use a leadership style that is natural to them
- Use a leadership style appropriate to the task and the members
- Assess the effects of their behavior on others and the effects of others' behavior on themselves
- Are sensitive to forces acting for and against change
- Express an optimistic view about human nature
- Are energetic
- Are open and encourage openness, so that real issues are confronted
- Facilitate personal relationships
- Plan and organize activities of the group
- Are consistent in behavior toward group members
- Delegate tasks and responsibilities to develop members' abilities, not merely to get tasks performed
- Involve members in all decisions
- Value and use group members' contributions
- Encourage creativity
- Encourage feedback about their leadership style

most effective leaders demonstrate the following: (1) achievement and ambition, (2) the ability to learn from adversity, (3) high dedication to the job, (4) sound analytic and problem-solving skills, (5) a high level of people skills, and (6) a high level of innovation.

Leadership Style

Leadership styles are defined "as different combinations of task and relationship behaviors used to influence others to accomplish goals" (Huber, 2000, p. 51). Several leadership styles have been described: charismatic leadership; authoritarian, or directive, leadership; democratic, or participative, leadership; laissez-faire, or nondirectional, leadership; situational leadership; transactional leadership; and transformational leadership.

Charismatic leadership is characterized by an emotional relationship between the leader and the group members in which the leader "inspires others by obtaining an emotional commitment from followers and by arousing strong feelings of loyalty and enthusiasm" (Marriner-Tomey, 2000, p. 139). A charismatic relationship exists when the leader can communicate a plan for change and the followers adhere to the plan because of their faith and belief in the leader's abilities. The followers of a charismatic leader may be able to overcome extreme hardship to achieve the goal because of their faith in the leader.

In **authoritarian leadership**, the leader makes the decisions for the group. This style of leadership has also been referred to as *directive* or *autocratic leadership*. Authoritarian leadership is likened to a dictatorship and presupposes that the group is incapable of making its own decisions. The leader determines policies, giving orders and directions to the group members. Authoritarian leadership generally has negative connotations and often makes group members dissatisfied. Because of the differences in status between the leader and group members, the degree of openness and trust between leader and group members is minimal or absent. Under this type of leadership, procedures are well defined, activities are predictable, and the group may feel secure. Although this is an efficient way to accomplish goals, group members' needs for creativity, autonomy, and self-motivation are not met (Tappen, 2001). Authoritarian leadership may, however, be most effective in situations requiring immediate decisions, such as cardiac arrest, fire on the unit, airplane crash, or other emergency, when one person must assume responsibility without being challenged by other team members. Similarly, when group members are unable or unwilling to participate in making a decision, the authoritarian style effects resolution of the problem and enables the individual or group to move on. This style can also be effective when a project must be completed quickly and efficiently.

In **democratic**, or **participative, leadership**, the leader acts as a catalyst or facilitator, actively guiding the group toward achieving the group goals. Providing constructive criticism, offering information, making suggestions, and asking questions become the focus of the participative leader. This type of leadership demands that the leader have faith in the group members to accomplish the goals. Democratic leadership is based on the following principles (Tappen, 2001, p. 26):

1. Every group member should participate in decision making.

2. Freedom of belief and action is allowed within reasonable bounds that are set by society and by the group.

3. Each individual is responsible for himself or herself and for the welfare of the group.

4. There should be concern and consideration for each group member as a unique individual.

Although democratic leadership has been shown to be less efficient and more cumbersome than authoritarian leadership, it allows for more self-motivation and more creativity among group members. Democratic leadership calls for a great deal of cooperation and coordination among group members. This style of leadership can be extremely effective in the health care setting (Tappen, 2001, p. 26).

The **laissez-faire**, or **nondirectional**, **leader** is described as inactive, passive, and permissive; offering few commands, questions, suggestions, or criticism (Tappen, 2001, p. 27). Although there are various degrees of nondirectional leadership, leadership participation is, in general, minimal. The group's members may act independently of each other and suffer from a lack of cooperation or coordination. Apathy, chaos, and frustration may arise. The laissez-faire approach works best when group members have both personal and professional maturity, so that once the group has made a decision, the members become committed to it and have the required expertise to implement it. Individual group members then perform tasks in their area of expertise, with the leader acting as a resource person. Table 9–2 compares the authoritarian, democratic, and laissez-faire leadership styles.

In **situational leadership**, levels of direction and support vary according to the level of maturity of the employees or group. The leader assumes one of four styles (Hellriegel, Jackson, & Slocum, 1999, pp. 514–515):

1. *Directive*. A leadership style characterized by the giving of clear instructions and specific direction to immature employees.

2. *Coaching*. A leadership style characterized by expanding two-way communication and helping maturing employees build confidence and motivation.

3. *Supporting*. A leadership style characterized by active two-way communication and support of mature employees' efforts to use their talents.

4. *Delegating*. A hands-off leadership style in which the highly mature employees are given responsibilities for carrying out plans and making task decisions.

Table 9–2 Comparison of Authoritarian, Democratic, and Laissez-Faire Leadership Styles

	Authoritarian	Democratic	Laissez-Faire
Degree of freedom	Little freedom	Moderate freedom	Much freedom
Degree of control	High control	Moderate control	No control
Decision making	By the leader	Leader and group together	By the group or by no one
Leader activity level	High	High	Minimal
Assumption of responsibility	Primarily the leader	Shared	Abdicated
Output of the group	High quantity, good quality	Creative, high quality	Variable, may be of poor quality
Efficiency	Very efficient	Less efficient than authoritarian	Inefficient

Source: From *Nursing Leadership and Management: Concepts and Practice* (4th ed., p. 26), by R. M. Tappen, 2001, Philadelphia: F. A. Davis. Reprinted with permission.

The situational leadership model poses some questions. First, can leaders actually choose one of these four leadership styles when faced with a new situation? Second, how do such factors as personality traits and the leaders' power base influence the leader's choice of style? Third, what should the leader choose for a group whose members are at different levels of maturity?

An important issue in situational leadership is the value placed on the accomplishment of tasks and on the interpersonal relationships between leader and group members and among group members. For example, the nurse-manager encourages input from staff members when planning daily work assignments so that the needs of both staff and clients are met. The nurse-manager may also solicit input from staff members when doing both short-range and long-range planning for the unit. However, when a new staff member is being oriented to the unit, the nurse-manager may be more directive in making assignments until the staff member develops experience and professional maturity. In emergency situations or situations in which the task needs to be completed quickly, the nurse-manager may be more authoritative in directing the actions of all staff members.

Transactional leadership represents the traditional manager focused on the day-to-day tasks of achieving organizational goals. The transactional leader understands and meets the needs of the group. Relationships with followers are based on an exchange (or transaction) for some resource valued by the follower. These incentives are used to promote loyalty and perfor-

mance. For example, to ensure adequate staffing on the night shift, the nurse-manager negotiates with a staff nurse to work the night shift in exchange for a weekend shift off.

In contrast, **transformational leadership** theory, which was developed in the 1980s, "reconsiders the characteristics of the leader-manager, reemphasizes the vision that the leader-manager shares with the group, and stresses the importance of preparing people for change" (Tappen, 2001, p. 44). This model combines elements of earlier theories and recognizes the influence of the leader, workers, tasks, and environment. Transformational leadership is characterized by four primary factors (p. 44):

1. *Charisma.* Charismatic leaders are highly respected and are viewed with reverence, dedication, and awe. They set high standards, challenging their staff to go beyond the expected level of effort.

2. *Inspirational motivation.* The leader shares visions with the staff that appeal to both their emotions and their ideals.

3. *Intellectual stimulation.* The leader stimulates followers to question the status quo: to question critically what they are doing and why.

4. *Contingent reward.* The leader recognizes mutually agreed-upon goals and rewards the employee's achievements.

It is expected that transformational leadership will become critically vital in the creation of a health care

Strategies for Putting Humanistic and Caring Leadership into Action

- Praise or positively recognize staff and colleagues.
- Always think good thoughts about yourself and others.
- Work on discovering group members' unique personal and professional needs.
- Always give before you get—give colleagues and staff a reason for doing whatever it is that you are asking of them.
- Smile often—it generates enthusiasm and goodwill.
- Recognize the expertise of others.
- Remember the names of the people you work with.
- Think, act, and look successful.
- Always greet others with a positive, affirmative statement.

- Foster an atmosphere of collegiality and mutual trust.
- Write informal appreciation notes; this shows appreciation and reinforces positive performance.
- Get out of the nurse's station or office; make a point of circulating among those who work in your circle of influence.
- Foster creativity, independence, and professional growth.
- Talk less and listen more; encourage communication and the sharing of ideas and information.
- Don't condemn, criticize, or complain; instead, work on ways to improve the situation or solve the problem.
- Accept responsibility.

Sources: Adapted from "Empowering Nurses through Enlightened Leadership," by T. K. Glennon, Spring 1992, *Revolution: The Journal of Nurse Empowerment, 2,* 40–44; and "Caring Leadership: Secret Path to Success," by M. A. Brandt, August 1994, *Nursing Management, 25,* 68–72.

system that embodies community well-being, basic care for all, cost-effectiveness, and holistic nursing care. The transformational leader is a myth-maker and storyteller, painting vivid descriptions of an inspiring, uplifting future everyone will build together. A survey of 2500 health care leaders identified six factors in transformational leadership that will effect these changes in the 21st century: (1) mastering change, (2) systems thinking, (3) shared vision, (4) continuous quality improvement, (5) an ability to redefine health care, and (6) a commitment to serving the public and community (Trofino, 1995, p. 45).

Caring leadership is a concept that is an extension of transformational leadership. The term *caring leadership* was introduced in 1991 by a Fortune 500 executive, who stated: "Good management is largely a matter of love. Or if you're uncomfortable with the word, call it caring, because proper management involves caring for people, not manipulating them" (Brandt, 1994, p. 68). Caring leadership recognizes the importance of caring in the practice of nursing, combining concepts from both caring and leadership theories.

Effective leadership is a learned process requiring an understanding of the needs and goals that motivate

people, the knowledge to apply the leadership skills, and the interpersonal skills to influence others. Much has been written about effective leadership and style; some descriptive statements about effective leaders are listed in the box on page 165. Humanistic leadership can serve as a means of creating an environment "that is stimulating, motivating, and empowering to the professional nurse" (Glennon, 1992, p. 41). Strategies for humanistic and caring leadership are identified in the accompanying box.

Reflect on...

- nursing leaders you admire. What characteristics of leadership do they have that you admire? Are there characteristics that you don't like? What leadership style or styles do they employ to influence others? Do they emphasize one style or several styles? Are the nursing leaders you admire well liked by other colleagues and health professionals?
- if you believe that it is important to be liked when you are a leader.
- your own leadership activities. What characteristics of leadership do you have? What leadership style or styles are you most comfortable with? How might you improve your abilities as a leader?

Evidence for Practice

Atsalos, C., & Greenwood, J. (2001). The lived experience of Clinical Development Unit (nursing) leadership in Western Sydney, Australia. *Journal of Advanced Nursing, 34*(3), 408–416.

The purpose of this qualitative study was to develop an understanding of the influence of stressors experienced by Clinical Development Unit (nursing) leadership. Clinical Development Units are designed to develop patient-focused care through the use of group process and action research based on principles of transformational leadership. Previous research had determined that the use of such units were successful in improving both patient and staff satisfaction; however, there was also evidence that nurse leaders on these units experienced significant stressors. A hermeneutic approach was used to identify how the leadership experience on these units changed over time. Participants were interviewed at 4 to 6 months after the start of the units and then again 12 months later. The study found a significant theme as the nursing leaders identified their own need for leadership "in order to sustain their confidence and motivation." Implications of the study suggest institutional support mechanisms must be available to nursing leaders to sustain them as they deal with unit stressors.

Critical Thinking Exercise

Think about nursing heroes past and present. Refer to Chapter 3 ⚭, Historical Foundations of Professional Nursing for a discussion of selected nursing leaders. What qualities of leadership do they share? How important is risk taking or sacrifice to effective leadership? How do nurses exhibit their leadership abilities in the various aspects of their lives?

NURSING MANAGEMENT

As a manager and provider of client care, the nurse coordinates various health care professionals and their services to help the client meet desired outcomes.

Theories of Management Style

Concern with management practices began in the latter part of the nineteenth century, as the United States began emerging as a leading industrial nation. Early management theory focused on how to get as much work as possible from each worker. The oldest and most widely accepted viewpoint on management is called the traditional, or classical, viewpoint.

The traditional style stresses the manager's role in a strict hierarchy and focuses on efficient and consistent job performance. Traditionalists are concerned with the formal relations among an organization's departments, tasks, and structural elements, and they stress the manager's role in a hierarchy. Superiors are assumed to have greater expertise and are therefore to be obeyed by subordinates. Time-and-motion studies and the development of early management principles were the work of the traditionalists. Characteristics of traditional management include adherence to routines and rules, impersonality, division of labor, hierarchy, financial motivation, and authority structure. The benefits of the traditional style include efficiency, consistency, clear structure, and an emphasis on productivity (Hellriegel et al., 1999, pp. 44–55). Although most traditionalists today recognize the emotional and humanistic components of management, the focus on efficient and effective job performance remains overriding. Many managers and health care organizations still use the traditional management style today.

The expansion of labor unions in the 1930s, the Great Depression, and World War II heralded another era in management theory. Against the backdrop of change and reform, managers were forced to focus on the humanistic side of managing organizations. *Behavioral theory* moves beyond the traditionalists' mechanical view of the work world and stresses the importance of group dynamics and the leadership style of the manager. The behavioral viewpoint includes the following four basic assumptions (Hellriegel et al., 1999, p. 60):

1. Workers are motivated by social needs and get a sense of identity through their associations with one another.

2. Workers are more responsive to the social forces exerted by their peers than to management's financial incentives and rules.

3. Workers respond to managers who can help them satisfy their needs.

4. Managers need to coordinate the work of their subordinates democratically in order to improve efficiency.

These assumptions really do not hold true for the workforce of the new century. Today's work world is more complex than the work world of the traditionalist and behaviorist. The post–World War II years brought a new management theory: systems theory. Just as the human body is a system consisting of organs, muscles, bones, and a circulatory system that links all the parts together, an organization is a system consisting of many departments that are linked by people working together. Systems theory approaches problems by looking at inputs, transformation processes, outputs, and feedback. Inputs are the physical, human, material, financial, and information resources that enter the system and leave as outputs. The technology used to convert the inputs are the transformation processes. Outputs are the original physical, human, material, financial, and information resources that are now in the form of goods and services. A vital part of systems theory is the feedback loops, which provide ongoing information about a system's status and performance. Another vital component of the systems theory is the interaction of the system with the environment. The manager who uses systems theory "makes decisions only after identifying and analyzing how other managers," units, clients, or others might be affected by the decisions (Hellriegel et al., 1999, p. 60).

Contingency theory emerged in the mid-1960s in response to managers' unsuccessful attempts to apply traditional, behavioral, and systems concepts to managerial problems. Contingency theory is a blend of these concepts. Using contingency theory, the manager is expected to determine which method or combination of methods will be most effective in a given situation. To apply the contingency viewpoint effectively, the manager must be able to diagnose and understand a situation thoroughly, determine the most useful approach, and recognize the impact of the external environment, technology, and the people involved before acting (Hellriegel et al., 1999, pp. 64–65).

The contingency theory of management moves the manager away from the "one size fits all" approach. Managers are encouraged to analyze and understand the differences in each situation, selecting the solution that best suits the organization and individual in each situation.

Management Competencies

Hellriegel et al. (1999, pp. 16–28) describe six competencies essential for successful managers: communication, planning and administration, teamwork, strategic action, global awareness, and self-management:

1. *Communication competency.* This competency is the most fundamental of managerial competencies. Effective managers are able to communicate so that the exchanged information is clearly understood by the managers and those with whom they communicate. Communication can involve information communication, formal communication, and negotiation. Communication is not only face-to-face discussion; it also includes effective use of the many means of communicating verbally and in writing, including telephone, individual or group conferences, written communications (such as memos and newsletters), electronic communications, and the effective use of body language. (See Chapter 13 ∞, Communication, for more information.)

2. *Planning and administration competency.* The effective manager must be able to decide which tasks need to be done, how they should be done, and what resources need to be allocated; then the manager must follow through to make sure that the tasks are accomplished. This competency includes information gathering and analysis, planning and organizing projects, time management, and budgeting and financial management.

3. *Teamwork competency.* Effective managers must be able to accomplish tasks through teams of people. This competency requires that managers be able to design work teams properly, create a supportive team environment, and manage team dynamics appropriately. Nurse-managers in the hospital or institutional environment have a team of registered nurses and other care providers who must work together to provide quality care to their patients. (See Chapter 15 ∞, Group Process, for information on working with groups.)

4. *Strategic action competency.* Managers must understand the overall mission and values of the organization. They must then ensure that their actions and those of the people they manage are consistent with the organization's mission and values. For nurses, the mission and values may reflect not only the organization where they work but also those of the nursing profession.

5. *Global awareness competency.* Contemporary nurse-managers must have an awareness of the multicul-

tural beliefs, values, and practices of their clients and their staff. In addition to cultural awareness, nurse-managers must be culturally sensitive and culturally competent in their interactions with clients and staff. (For more information on the influence of culture, see Chapter 21 ⊕, Nursing in a Culturally Diverse World.)

6. *Self-management competency.* Finally, effective nurse-managers must be able to take responsibility for their life at work and outside of work. This competency includes integrity and ethical conduct, personal drive and resilience, balancing life and work issues, and being aware of self and personal development needs.

The relative importance and skill mix at each level of management change as the nurse moves from a first-line manager position to middle and top management. Interpersonal and communication skills are of equal importance to all levels of management. The professional nurse may be promoted into a middle management position because of excellent technical nursing skills. These new managers often rely on their nursing expertise, unaware that they also need to develop other skills associated with business and finance. Duffield (1994, p. 64) explored the responsibilities of first-line managers. She found consensus that the first-line manager is required not only to maintain the technical skills associated with managing client care but also to master the technical skills of finance and business management, such as budget and finance, human resource management, and development of policies and procedures.

The higher a manager's position in the organization, the greater the need for conceptual and interpersonal skills. Many of the responsibilities of top nurse-managers, such as allocating resources and developing overall strategies, require a broad outlook and ability to see the "big picture." The ability to provide visionary leadership will become an even more highly valued managerial skill in the coming years. This means creating a vision with which people can identify and to which they can commit (Hellriegel et al., 1999, p. 521). Offering educational programs such as workshops, seminars, and mentor programs is one way the organization and profession can help new nurse-managers build on their nursing knowledge. Nurse-managers may also choose to take classes in budgeting and finance, human resource development, conflict management, informatics, organizational development, and other business-related areas.

Management Roles

Nurses function differently in various types of organizations. An autocratic organization confers primary knowledge and power to one person and places other persons in subordinate roles. Bureaucratic organizations exert control through policy, structured jobs, and compartmentalized actions. Other organizations decentralize control and emphasize self-direction and self-discipline of members. Still another type of organization is the component of a system that interacts interdependently with other components and adapts dynamically to change. This type of organization is particularly beneficial for the nurse who manages the care of individuals, families, and communities. On a larger scale, the nurse-manager must work in the organizational framework of the employing agency.

Authority is the official power given by the organization to direct the work of others. It is an integral component of managing. Authority is conveyed through leadership actions; it is determined largely by the situation, and it is always associated with responsibility and accountability.

Accountability is the ability and willingness to assume responsibility for one's actions and to accept the consequences of one's behavior. Accountability can be viewed within a hierarchic systems framework, starting at the individual level, through the institutional/professional level, and then to the societal level. At the individual or client level, accountability is reflected in the nurse's ethical integrity. At the institutional level, it is reflected in the statement of philosophy and objectives of the nursing department and nursing units. At the professional level, accountability is reflected in standards of practice developed by national or provincial nursing associations. At the societal level, it is reflected in legislated nurse practice acts.

To be successful, the nurse-manager must exert authority and assume accountability in implementing the managerial functions of planning, organizing, leading and delegating, and controlling. These functions help to achieve the goal of quality client care.

Planning

Planning is often considered the first and most basic management function. Planning is a process that includes the following steps (Hellriegel et al., 1999, pp. 218–222):

■ Choosing the organization's mission and vision. The mission describes the purpose or reason for the existence of the organization. The vision "expresses the organization's fundamental aspirations and purpose. A vision statement adds soul to the mission statement."

- Devising departmental goals. The nursing unit should reflect the more global goals of the nursing. department and the health care agency.
- Selecting strategies to achieve the goals. Strategies are the courses of action the unit staff will take in order to achieve the unit's goals.
- Deciding on the allocation of resources. Distribution of money, personnel, equipment, and physical space is included in resource allocation.

Nurse-managers must keep in mind that plans are the means, not the ends. Quick fixes may cause one to neglect the big picture. Planning can help the nurse-manager (1) identify future opportunities, (2) anticipate and avoid future problems, and (3) develop strategies and courses of action.

Organizing

Organizing is the formal system of working relationships. The nurse-manager is responsible for identifying particular tasks and assigning them to individuals or teams who have the training and expertise to carry them out. Along with organizing, the nurse-manager is responsible for coordinating activities to meet the unit's objectives. Health care reform, downsizing, restructuring, and the nursing shortage have all affected the management role of organizing.

Leading and Delegating

The beginning of this chapter discussed many of the elements of effective leadership. These elements, even when combined with the motivation to lead and basic leadership skills, will not necessarily make an effective leader; power is also an essential component of leading. Power is "that which enables one to accomplish goals" (Marquis & Huston, 2003, p. 184).

Power, in this context, is defined as "the ability to influence or control individual, departmental, team, or organizational decisions and goals" (Hellriegel et al., 1999, p. 275).

Another component of leading is delegating. *Delegation* is defined as "getting work done through others or as directing the performance of one or more people to accomplish organizational goals" (Marquis & Huston, 2003, p. 366). The function of delegation in the health care field is often complex because of the number and diversity of caregivers, the amount of different knowledge and skills needed to provide care, and the intricacy of the relationships among staff, client and family, and the environment (Tappen, 2001).

Delegation is a major tool in making the most efficient use of time. Delegation is a high-level implementation skill. To delegate effectively, the nurse must be aware of the needs and goals of the client and family, the nursing activities that can help the client meet the goals, and the skills and knowledge of various nursing and support personnel.

In delegating, the nurse must also determine how many and what type of personnel are needed. Decisions about delegation may be based on information from the client's records, the client, the charge nurse, other nursing personnel, and the nurse's own judgment.

After establishing that assistance is required, the nurse must identify what type of help is needed, how long help will be required, when it will be required, and what assistance is available. Before beginning the nursing activity, the nurse must arrange for assistance, usually by asking the appropriate person on the unit. Delegation does not require that the nurse have the personal knowledge and expertise to perform a specific nursing activity, but it does require that the nurse know who does have the knowledge and expertise and can recognize when it is needed. For example, a nurse may call a dietitian to assist a client in choosing foods from a menu or request a social worker to assist a client who needs financial assistance and homemaker services after discharge.

An important aspect of delegation is the development of the potential of nursing and support personnel. By knowing the background, experience, knowledge, skill, and strengths of each person, a nurse can delegate responsibilities that help develop each person's competence. Nursing personnel to whom aspects of care have been delegated need to be supervised and evaluated. The amount of supervision required is highly variable and depends on the knowledge and skills of each person. As the person who assigns the activity and observes the performance, the nurse contributes to the evaluation process. Because individual motivation varies, the nurse needs to realize that not all persons perform equally. Thus, the nurse must evaluate standards of performance against written job descriptions, rather than by comparing one person's performance to that of another. It is essential, too, for the nurse to realize that people require ongoing feedback about their performance and to give feedback, including both positive and negative input, in an objective manner. (More information about the legal basis for delegation can be found in Chapter 5 ⊂⊃, Legal Foundations of Professional Nursing.)

Controlling

Controlling is a method to ensure that behaviors and performances are consistent with the planning process. Control is not something managers do to employees, but rather with them. Formal, structured, bureaucratic controls, such as tightly written job descriptions, extensive rules and procedures, and top-down authority, are familiar control mechanisms. Increasingly in health care agencies, more flexible controls such as continuous quality improvement (CQI), shared governance, and team building help make control an easier and integral part of the management process.

The discussion of management roles would be incomplete without a few words on "the games people play" within the world of work. A lack of understanding of the politics of work can cause even the most competent and committed nurse to feel helpless and frustrated.

Many nurses feel that being politically astute is a genetic trait, that they have neither the ability nor desire to "get involved in the politics of the workplace." These nurses soon discover that power and politics are inevitable in today's workplace. First, there always will be those people who will do anything to obtain and hang on to power. Second, hard work is usually measured by the manager in charge, not by the rules and regulations in the policy and procedures manual. Menke and Ogborn (1993, pp. 35–37) describe the following behaviors that nurses should develop to negotiate the politics of the workplace.

1. *Read the environment.* Observe where the power lies in the organization. Historically, power has rested in those who bring in the money and those who supply the resources for those in power.

2. *Listen.* Listen to everyone, everywhere. Move slowly, and don't be anxious to exhibit everything you know.

3. *Read.* Read organizational charts, policies and procedure statements, and professional journals. Learn to identify what is acceptable and what is not.

4. *Detach.* Don't hook up with people who are on the losing side. Detach and stay independent until you know the political ropes.

5. *Analyze.* Identify your own unique characteristics that may be seen as being "different." For example, are you the only male, the only nurse with a baccalaureate degree, or the only newcomer? If so, you may have to work a little harder to achieve your goal.

6. *Create competence.* A firm handshake, introducing yourself, and basic courtesy never go out of style. Summarizing your project status with your manager while sharing credit for success when due keeps your manager aware of what is going on.

Characteristics of Effective Nurse-Managers

- Assume leadership of the group
- Actively engage in planning the current and future work of the group
- Provide direction to staff members regarding the way the work is to be done
- Monitor the work done by staff members to maintain quality and productivity
- Recognize and reward quality and productivity
- Foster the development of every staff member
- Represent both administration and staff members as needed in discussions and negotiations with others

Source: From *Nursing Leadership and Management: Concepts and Practice* (4th ed., pp. 221–222), by R. M. Tappen, 2001, Philadelphia: F. A. Davis. Reprinted with permission.

7. *Never gossip about the manager.* Keep the manager from being blindsided and embarrassed. Don't whine!

8. *Always roll with the punches.* Remain enthusiastic! The nurse may never like being in the political game, but being knowledgeable will make it easier to understand and survive it.

Characteristics of effective nurse-managers as described by Tappen (2001, pp. 221–222) are listed in the accompanying box.

Critical Thinking Exercise

Consider the organizational structure of your practice setting. How many levels of management are there? How many of these levels are managed by nurses? Identify advantages and disadvantages to having nurses in mid-level and high-management positions in health care organizations.

Reflect on...

■ the activities of nurse-managers at the unit level of your practice setting. What management activities do they perform? What management activities do staff nurses perform? What management activities do you perform? How do the management responsibilities of the staff nurse differ from those of the nurse-manager? What is the relationship between good unit management and effective client care?

■ the experience and educational background of nurse-managers at all levels of your organization. What are their clinical nursing experiences? What is their education? Do they have formal or informal education in management or business? Do the experience levels and educational backgrounds differ among nurse-managers at different levels of organizational or unit management? How could you best prepare yourself for the management responsibility?

NURSING DELIVERY MODELS

Common configurations for the delivery of nursing care include the case method, the functional method, team nursing, primary nursing, case management, managed care, differentiated practice, and shared governance.

Total Patient Care

Total patient care, also referred to as **case method**, is one of the earliest models of nursing care. This method was used by private-duty nurses in providing total care to the client. This method is client centered: one nurse is assigned to and is responsible for the comprehensive care of a client or group of clients during an 8- or 12-hour shift. For each client, the nurse assesses needs, makes nursing plans, formulates diagnoses, implements care, and evaluates the effectiveness of care. In this method, a client has consistent contact with one nurse during a shift but may have different nurses on other shifts. The case method, considered the precursor of primary nursing, continues to be used in a variety of practice settings, such as intensive care nursing. With the shortage of nursing personnel during World War II, the case method could no longer be the chief mode of care for clients. To meet staff shortages, managers hired personnel with less educational preparation than the professional nurse and developed on-the-job training programs for auxiliary helpers. The case method became unfeasible in such situations, and the functional method was developed in response.

Functional Method

The **functional nursing method**, which evolved from concepts of scientific management used in the field of business administration, focuses on the jobs to be completed. In this task-oriented approach, personnel with less preparation than the professional nurse perform less complex care tasks. The functional method is based on a production and efficiency model that gives authority and responsibility to the person assigning the work, for example, the nurse-manager. Clearly defined job descriptions, procedures, policies, and lines of communication are required. The functional approach to nursing is economical and efficient and permits centralized direction and control. Its disadvantages are fragmentation of care (the client receives care from several different categories of nursing personnel) and the possibility that nonquantifiable aspects of care, such as meeting the client's emotional needs, may be overlooked.

Team Nursing

In the early 1950s, Eleanor Lambertsen (1953) and her colleagues proposed a system of team nursing to overcome the fragmentation of care resulting from the task-oriented functional approach and to meet the increasing demands for professional nurses created by advances in the technologic aspects of care. **Team nursing** is the delivery of individualized nursing care to clients by a nursing team led by a professional nurse. A nursing team consists of registered nurses, licensed practical nurses, and, often, nursing assistants. This team is responsible for providing coordinated nursing care to a group of clients during an 8- or 12-hour shift. Compared to the functional system, team nursing emphasizes humanistic values and responds to the needs of both clients and employees. It emphasizes individualized client care on a personal level rather than task-oriented care on an impersonal level. The professional nurse leader motivates employees to learn and develop skills and instructs them, supervises them, and provides assignments that offer the potential for growth.

Primary Nursing

Primary nursing, a system in which one nurse is responsible for total care of a number of clients 24 hours a day, 7 days a week, was introduced at the Loeb Center for Nursing and Rehabilitation in the Bronx, New York. Primary nursing is a method of providing comprehensive, individualized, and consistent care.

Primary nursing uses the nurse's technical knowledge and management skills. The primary nurse assesses and prioritizes each client's needs, identifies nursing diagnoses, develops a plan of care with the client, and evaluates the effectiveness of care. Associates provide some care, but the primary nurse coordinates it and communicates information about the client's health to other nurses and health professionals. Primary nursing encompasses all aspects of the professional role, including teaching, advocacy, decision making, and continuity of care.

According to Tappen (2001, p. 247), "the primary nurse does all initial assessments and then develops care plans for assigned patients. They provide complex treatments, coordinate the nursing care plan with other disciplines, administer medications, prepare patients for discharge, provide needed education, and evaluate the efficacy of the interventions." The primary nurse may call upon other staff members to assist in the care of the assigned patients, but then he or she coordinates the work of the other staff members. Primary nursing has been implemented in various ways in different organizations to provide quality client care with the most effective use of personnel and other resources.

Case Management

Case management, a more recent model of nursing care delivery, was pioneered at the New England Medical Center in the 1980s. Initially, public health and psychiatric–mental health nurses served as case managers. Today, case management is used in insurance-based programs, employer-based health programs, worker's compensation programs, maternal-child health settings, mental health settings, and hospital-based practice. **Case management** is defined as "a collaborative process that assesses, plans, implements, coordinates, monitors, and evaluates options and services needed to meet a person's health needs" (Turner, 1999, p. 136). The American Nurses Credentialing Center (2001) further defines nursing case management as a "participative process to identify and facilitate options and services for meeting individuals' health needs, while decreasing fragmentation and duplication of care and enhancing quality, cost-effective clinical outcomes." Case managers assist clients through the complex health care system with the goal of increasing the quality of life in a cost-effective way. Case management enables patients, their families, and their health care providers to be actively involved in providing for ongoing care needs.

Nurse case managers combine their clinical knowledge, communication skills, and nursing process skills to assist clients in a variety of clinical settings. The activities of case management require the nurse to integrate a variety of disciplines and services in coordinating care throughout the client's span of illness. Collaboration, coordination, information processing, and information exchange are imperative in this role. The case manager must be familiar with eligibility criteria for the different services that the client requires. Effective case managers must have strong skills in critical thinking, communication, negotiation, and collaboration in addition to expert knowledge in clinical nursing. Case managers serve as patient advocates because they provide the link between the client, the health care provider, and the payer. Case managers also function as client advocates by providing for client education, wellness, and prevention services. They also work to obtain resources, improve access, and achieve a smooth transition for clients along the care continuum. Functions of nurse case managers can be seen in the box on page 176.

The American Nurses Credentialing Center (ANCC, 2001) recommends that case managers have a minimum educational preparation of a baccalaureate degree in nursing, have functioned as a registered nurse for 4000 hours, and have at least 2000 hours within the scope of practice during the last 2 years.

Shared Governance

Marquis and Huston (2003, p. 172) describe **shared governance** as organizational governance that is "shared among board members, nurses, physicians, and management." The focus of this model is to encourage nurses to participate in decision making at all levels of the organization, either at their own request or as part of their job criteria. More commonly, nurses participate through serving in decision-making groups, such as committees or task forces. The decisions they make may address employment conditions, cost-effectiveness, long-range planning, productivity, and wages and benefits. The underlying principle of shared governance is that employees will be more committed to an organization's goals if they have had input into planning and decision making. Marquis and Huston also state that "the number of health care organizations using shared governance models is increasing" (p. 173). In this model of delivery, the

Functions of Nurse Case Managers

ASSESSING AND ANALYZING

- Review client demographic data
- Administer assessment tools and risk screens
- Review client history and current health status
- Validate clinical data
- Identify client problems
- Identify educational needs of clients and readiness to learn
- Identify target populations in disease management programs

PLANNING

- Identify client health goals
- Identify available resources
- Plan and coordinate client care

IMPLEMENTING/INTERVENING

- Link clients to needed services
- Identify opportunities for health promotion and illness/injury prevention
- Advocate for client needs

EVALUATING

- Monitor adherence
- Identify barriers to availability, accessibility, and affordability of treatment
- Evaluate support systems (individual, family, significant other, and community)
- Monitor delivery of services
- Examine patterns of over- and/or underutilization of resources

nurse-manager becomes a consultant, teacher, and collaborator; he or she creates the environment for shared decision making between the nursing staff and administration. The nursing staff, in turn, must make a significant and long-term commitment to the organization.

Porter-O'Grady (1994, p. 187) sees shared governance as a tool that facilitates the maturing of the nursing professional: "It has facilitated the creation of a structure supportive of behaviors reflecting an adult, collaborative, and active decision-maker in any clinical partnership that will advance the integrative role of the nurse and the care of the patient."

Managed Care

Managed care is a method of organizing care delivery that emphasizes communication and coordination of care among health care team members. Managed care differs from case management in that it is unit based and designed to promote and support care at the client's bedside in the acute-care setting. Case management may be used as a cost-containment strategy in managed care. Managed care has gained popularity with the health care reform movement in the United States. "Managed care is a system that attempts to integrate efficiency of care, access, and cost of care" (Marquis & Huston, 2003, p. 137).

Both case management and managed care use critical pathways or care MAPS (multidisciplinary action plans) to track the client's progress. **Critical pathways** are "grids that outline the critical or key events expected to happen each day of a patient's hospitalization" (Yoder-Wise, 2003, p. 265). Care MAPS are a combination of the nursing care plan and the critical pathway. Other structured-care methodologies are algorithms, protocols, standards of care, order sets, and clinical practice guidelines. Critical pathways are used by all health care providers to plan the time and sequence of events for a diagnosis-specific episode of care delivery. Critical pathways often focus on high-cost, high-volume areas involving many physicians and specialties. They have become essential for the financial survival of a health delivery system within a managed-care environment.

Providing high-quality care within a highly regulated environment requires the identification and elimination of excessive or inefficient systems and a high degree of collaboration. The involvement of physicians, clinical nurse specialists, and a multidisciplinary staff are key to developing and implementing successful critical pathways.

More information about the impact of economics on health care can be found in Chapters 17 ⬥, Nursing in an Evolving Health Care Delivery System, and 18 ⬥, Health Care Economics.

Evidence for Practice

Stordeur, W., Vandenberghe, C., & D'hoore, W. (2000). Leadership styles across hierarchical levels in nursing departments. *Nursing Research, 49*(1), 37–43.

The purpose of this study was to examine the cascading effect of leadership styles across hierarchical levels, that is, how leadership styles of upper-level (e.g., chief nursing officers), mid-level (e.g., supervisors), and lower-level (e.g., nurse managers, charge nurses) administrators in an organization influence the leadership styles of their subordinates. The sample consisted of 464 respondents working on 41 nursing units in 12 divisions at 8 hospitals in Belgium. The study also examined whether the relationship between leader behavior and outcome variables is stronger at the upper levels of the organization. The Multifactor Leadership Questionnaire was used to measure leadership in the participants. The correlations between nurses' evaluation of their head nurse and the head nurses' evaluations of their associate directors showed no significant correlation between leadership behaviors across hierarchical levels. However, scores on transformational leadership and passive management by exception (MBEP) varied significantly (P > .0001). The study provides evidence for the impact of transformational components on nurses' satisfaction with their leader, extra effort, and perceived unit effectiveness. Transformational leaders provide a significant and positive influence on nurses' perceptions by encouraging nurses' autonomy, transforming staff into leaders, and providing a sense of mission and future vision. Leaders who use transformational leadership strategies may contribute to the quality of care beyond their clinical expertise.

Differentiated Practice

Differentiated nursing practice refers "to the sorting of the roles, functions, and work of registered nurses according to some identified criteria—usually education, experience, and competence—or some combination of these" (Huber, 2000, p. 584). Differentiated practice models recognize the broad domain of pro-fessional nursing, the multiple roles and responsibilities that nurses assume, and the contribution of all nursing personnel as valuable and unique. Differentiated practice can improve client care and contribute to client safety. Used effectively, differentiated practice models allow for the effective and efficient use of resources. Most important, if used properly, differentiated practice increases nurses' ability to provide safe, effective care based on their expertise and, in turn, increases their professional satisfaction (Koerner & Karpiuk, 1994, p. 10).

As early as 1967, a Harvard Business School research project identified the role of differentiated practice in nursing. Not only are technical tasks involved but also such factors as time frame, space, personal development, ethical action, interpersonal effectiveness, critical thinking, and commitment to lifelong learning. As the nursing paradigm changes, the areas of communication and critical thinking, rather than technical skills, expand. The American Hospital Association sees the need for differentiated practice in responding to change in the health care system, client acuity, payment systems, and reward systems (Allender, Egan, & Newman, 1995, p. 42). Differentiated practice models include nurses prepared at all educational levels: associate degree/diploma, baccalaureate degree, master's degree, and doctorate, recognizing the diversity of these roles.

The newer models of case management, managed care, differentiated practice, and shared governance may be the keys to meeting the demands of the future by (1) increasing demand for quality and excellence in service across the continuum of care; (2) facilitating the use of appropriate, efficient skill mix and delivery of client-centered care; (3) reducing health care costs; and (4) rewarding performance based on measured team outcomes, including the value of interdependent contributions (Wenzel, 1995, p. 62).

Reflect on...

- your own experience with the various nursing delivery models. Which models do you prefer, and why? Which models do you believe promote the value of the professional nurse? Are there models that you think tend to devalue the abilities of the professional nurse?
- key factors in determining the appropriateness of a specific nursing delivery model for a specific practice setting. Are there models of nursing delivery that are more appropriate for some practice settings and less appropriate for others?

Critical Thinking Exercise

You are the nurse manager on a 30-bed nursing unit. You and your staff have decided to analyze the effectiveness of your unit's current model of nursing care delivery and consider making a change to a different model. What are the advantages and disadvantages of your current model of nursing care delivery? Which alternative model might be more effective for your nursing unit? What factors will influence your decision about making a change to a different model of nursing care delivery? How would you go about implementing a different model of nursing delivery in your current practice setting?

MENTORS AND PRECEPTORS

Mentoring has been widely used as a strategy for career development in nursing during the last 20 years. Mentors are "competent, experienced professionals who develop a relationship with a novice for the purpose of providing advice, support, information, and feedback in order to encourage development of the individual" (Schutzenhofer, 1995, p. 487). Most nursing literature describes the nurse-mentor relationship as important for career development in nursing administration or nursing education. Through mentoring, the experienced nurse can also foster the professional growth of the new graduate, who may choose to mentor those who follow. Marriner-Tomey (2000, p. 313) describes three phases to the mentoring process:

1. *The invitational stage.* In this stage, the mentor must be willing to use time and energy to nurture an individual who is goal directed, willing to learn, and respectfully trusting of the mentor. The nurse-mentor invites the new nurse to share knowledge, skill, and personal experiences of professional growth.
2. *The questioning stage.* In this stage, the novice experiences self-doubt and fear of being unable to meet the goals. The mentor helps the protégé clarify goals and the strategies for achieving them, shares personal experiences, and serves as a sounding board and a source of support during times of doubt.
3. *The transitional stage.* In this stage, the mentor assists the protégé to become aware of the protégé's own strengths and uniqueness. The protégé now is able to mentor someone else.

Mentors provide support. Often, the mentor relationship is one of teacher-learner. The mentor instructs the protégé in the expected role, introduces the protégé to those who are important to the achievement of goals, listens to and helps the protégé evaluate ideas in light of institutional policy, and challenges the protégé to advance professional practice. Marriner-Tomey (2000, p. 313) describes a mentor as "a confidant who personalizes role modeling and serves as a sounding board for decisions."

Nurses who wish to improve and advance their professional practice, whether in education, administration, or clinical practice, should seek mentors to assist them. Mentors usually are of the same sex, 8 to 14 years older, and have a position of authority in the organization. Most are knowledgeable individuals who are willing to share their knowledge and experience. Mentors often choose protégés because of their leadership or managerial qualities. Mentoring is a process that can promote the personal and professional growth of both mentor and protégé.

A **preceptor** is "an experienced nurse who provides emotional support and is a strong clinical role model for the new nurse" (Marquis & Huston, 2003, p. 265). Preceptors are usually assigned to nurses who are new to the nursing unit to assist them in improving clinical nursing skill and judgment necessary for effective practice in their environment. They also assist new nurses in learning the routines, policies, and procedures of the unit. Preceptors must be patient and willing to teach new nurses, and they must be willing to answer questions and clarify the expectations of the nurse's role within the practice environment.

Although preceptors are usually assigned, mentors are more often sought out by the person being mentored. Mentors and preceptors are important for the successful development of a nurse from a beginning care provider to an expert practitioner and professional.

Reflect on...

- your own mentoring experiences. Were you mentored or did you seek out a mentor as a new graduate or as a new employee in a new practice setting? What qualities would you seek in a mentor? If you were mentored, how did your mentor assist you in your socialization to your work setting, the organization, the nursing profession?

- whether there are or should be differences between mentors and preceptors. If there are differences, what are they?

- your own ability to mentor a new graduate or new employee. What knowledge, attitudes, and skills do you have that would make you an effective mentor? What knowledge, attitudes, and skills do you need to become an effective mentor? How will you develop the knowledge, attitudes, and skills needed?

NETWORKING

To function effectively in all nursing roles, but especially in leadership and management roles, the nurse needs to network with other professionals. Kozier et al. (2004, p. 477) describe **networking** as "a process whereby professional links are established through which people can share ideas, knowledge, and information, offer support and direction to each other, and facilitate accomplishment of professional goals." Networking builds linkages with people throughout the profession, both within and outside the work environment. Getting to know people helps build a trust rela-tionship that can facilitate the achievement of professional goals. It is easier to access people one knows than it is to access strangers.

Networking is a long-term, deliberate process, a powerful tool for building relationships. Networking requires time, commitment, and follow-through. Networking is an opportunity for nurses to develop their careers, share information, organize for political action, and effectively promote change (Strader & Decker, 1995, p. 481). Active membership in professional organizations may be the nurse's most important networking tool. Other networking opportunities include (1) continuing education or university classes, (2) socializing with professional colleagues, and (3) keeping in touch with former professors and nursing associates.

Reflect on...

- the role of the professional nurse in a changing health care system. What new knowledge, attitudes, and skills do you need to be more effective in the changing health care system? How can you best prepare for changes in health and nursing care delivery?

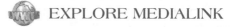 EXPLORE MEDIALINK

Questions, critical thinking exercises, essay activities, and other interactive resources for this chapter can be found on the Web site at http://prenhall.com/blais. Click on Chapter 9 to select activities for this chapter.

Bookshelf

Covey, S. R. (1989). *The 7 habits of highly effective people: Powerful lessons in personal change.* **New York: Simon and Schuster.**

This national best seller presents a paradigm of seven habits, starting with three self-mastery habits that move a person from dependence to independence (private victories) and followed by other habits that move a person toward effective interdependence (public victories). The seven habits become the basis of a person's character, "creating an empowering center of correct maps from which an individual can effectively solve problems, maximize opportunities, and continually learn and integrate other principles in an upward spiral of growth" (p. 52). Covey inspires readers to integrate personal, family, and professional responsibilities into their lives. He emphasizes the need to restore the "character" ethic in our society. The character ethic is based on the idea that there are principles that govern human effectiveness.

Ulrich, B. T. (1992). *Leadership and management according to Florence Nightingale.* **Norwalk, CT: Appleton-Lange.**

This pocket-sized book analyzes the writings of Florence Nightingale and points out the relevancy of her thoughts for nurses today. For example, it is still true today that "whoever is in charge keep this simple question in her head (not, how can I always do this right thing myself, but) how can I provide for this right thing to always be done?" (p. 38). It is a historical approach to the contemporary issue of delegation.

SUMMARY

Leadership and management are the responsibility of all professional nurses. Knowledge of the different, yet intertwined, roles of leader and manager are vital to nurses' ability to work within the health care system.

The ability of the professional nurse to advocate for clients is linked to leadership and management skills. As an individual, family, or community advocate, professional nurses may offer a wide variety of support and services.

Leadership styles include charismatic, authoritarian, democratic, laissez-faire, situational, transactional, and transformational. Effective leadership is a learned process involving understanding of the needs and goals that motivate others and interpersonal skills to influence others.

Management involves the basic functions of planning, organizing, leading, and delegating. The degree to which a nurse carries out these functions depends on the position the nurse holds in the organization. Regardless of degree, authority and accountability remain important to the process.

Nursing delivery models include the case method, the functional method, team nursing, primary nursing, case management, managed care, differentiated practice, and shared governance. Emphasis on efficiency, outcomes, cost-effectiveness, and client satisfaction have become buzzwords within the newer delivery models.

Mentors and preceptorships can have a positive impact. Mentoring and preceptorships can assist in the personal and professional growth of both the novice and professional nurse. Personal integrity, honesty, and a concern for human dignity should guide all the nurse's leadership and management decisions.

REFERENCES

Allender, C. D., Egan, E. C., & Newman, M. A. (1995). An instrument for measuring differentiated nursing practice. *Nursing Management, 26*(4), 42–45.

American Nurses Association. (1991). *Nursing's agenda for health care reform.* Washington, DC: ANA.

American Nurses Credentialing Center. (2001). *ANCC Board certification.* http://www.ana.org/ancc.

Atsalos, C., & Greenwood, J. (2001). The lived experience of Clinical Development Unit (nursing) leadership in Western Sydney, Australia. *Journal of Advanced Nursing, 34*(3), 408–416.

Bower, K. A. (1992). *Case management by nurses.* Washington, DC: American Nurses Association.

Brandt, M. A. (1994). Caring leadership: Secret and path to success. *Nursing Management, 25*(8), 68–72.

Christensen, P., & Bender, L. (1994). Models of nursing care in a changing environment: Current challenges and future directions. *Orthopaedic Nursing, 13*(2), 64–70.

Cohen, E. L., & Cesta, T. G. (1993). *Nursing case management: From concepts to evaluation.* St. Louis: Mosby-Year Book.

Duffield, C. (1994). Nursing unit managers: Defining a role. *Nursing Management, 25*(4), 63–67.

Glennon, T. K. (1992, Spring). Empowering nurses through enlightened leadership. *Revolution: The Journal of Nurse Empowerment, 2,* 40–44.

Hellriegel, D., & Slocum, J. W. (1993). *Management* (6th ed.). Reading, MA: Addison-Wesley.

Hellriegel, D., Jackson, S. E., & Slocum, J. W. (1999). *Management* (8th ed.). Cincinnati, OH: South-Western.

Huber, D. (2000). *Leadership and nursing care management* (2nd ed.). Philadelphia: W. B. Saunders.

Koerner, J. G., & Karpiuk, K. L. (1994). *Implementing differentiated nursing practice.* Gaithersburg, MD: Aspen.

Kozier, B., Erb, G., Berman, A., & Snyder, S. (2004). *Fundamentals of nursing: Concepts, process, and practice* (7th ed.). Upper Saddle River, NJ: Prentice Hall.

Lambertsen, E. C. (1953). *Nursing team: Organization and functioning.* Published for the Division of Nursing Education by the Bureau of Publications, Teachers College, Columbia University, New York, NY.

Lyon, J. C. (1993). Models of nursing care delivery and case management: Clarification of terms. *Nursing Economics, 11*(3), 163–169.

Marquis, B. L., & Huston, C. J. (2003). *Leadership roles and management functions in nursing: Theory and application* (4th ed.). Philadelphia: Lippincott.

Marriner-Tomey, A. (2000). *Guide to nursing management* (6th ed.). St. Louis: Mosby-Year Book.

Menke, K., & Ogborn, S. E. (1993). Politics and the nurse manager. *Nursing Management, 23*(12), 35–37.

Porter-O'Grady, T. (1994). Whole systems shared governance: Creating the seamless organization. *Nursing Economics, 12*(4), 187–195.

Schutzenhofer, K. K. (1995). Power, politics and influence. In P. S. Yoder-Wise, *Leading and managing in nursing.* St. Louis: Mosby-Year Book.

Simms, L. M., Price, S. A., & Ervin, N. E. (2000). *Professional practice of nursing administration* (3rd ed.). Albany, NY: Delmar.

Stordeur, S., Vandenberghe, C., & D'hoore, W. (2000). Leadership styles across hierarchical levels in nursing departments. *Nursing Research, 49*(1), 37–43.

Strader, M. K., & Decker, P. J. (1995). *Role transition to patient care management.* East Norwalk, CT: Appleton and Lange.

Tappen, R. M. (2001). *Nursing leadership and management: Concepts and practice* (4th ed.). Philadelphia: F. A. Davis.

Tappen, R. M., Weiss, S. A., & Whitehead, D. K. (2004). *Essentials of nursing leaderships and management* (3rd ed.). Philadelphia: F. A. Davis.

Trofino, J. (1995). Transformational leadership in health care. *Nursing Management, 26*(8), 42–47.

Turner, S. O. (1999). *The nurse's guide to managed care.* Gaithersburg, MD: Aspen.

Wenzel, K. (1995). Redesigning patient care delivery. *Nursing Management, 26*(8), 60–62.

Yoder-Wise, P. S. (2003). *Leading and managing in nursing* (3rd ed.). St. Louis: Mosby.

The Nurse as Research Consumer

Objectives

- Discuss the trend toward evidence-based practice in nursing.
- Describe the nurse's role in research.
- Analyze ethical concerns in nursing research.
- Differentiate approaches in nursing research.
- Identify the criteria for using research in nursing practice.
- Identify available resources for evidence-based practice in nursing.

M E D I A L I N K

Additional online resources for this chapter can be found on the companion Web site at http://www.prenhall.com/blais.

Nursing practice based on scientific evidence poses unique challenges for today's nursing care provider. It is a rather recent phenomenon. During the 1970s, research utilization became a buzzword and a focus for translating research findings into practice. This was slow to happen in part because there was a limited nursing research database from which to practice and also in part because nurses were not comfort-able enough with research to apply it to practice. Nurse researchers and nurses in practice were not interacting on a regular basis, and there was limited communication between them.

The term *evidence-based practice* has been applied to nursing in recent years. It brings together theory, clinical decision making and judgment, and knowledge of the research process; it incorporates them into the evaluation of research and scientific evidence. Resulting from this process is the application of clinically meaningful evidence to nursing practice and applying the best available research evidence to a specific clinical question. The evidence-based practice movement began in medicine during the 1970s but has developed within nursing since that time. In 1998 the journal *Evidence-Based Nursing* was established to advance evidence-based nursing practice, thus facilitating the highest quality of care and the best client outcomes.

CHALLENGES AND OPPORTUNITIES

Closing the gap between research and practice is a continuing challenge because nursing has more often based practice upon tradition, authority, or past experience. Looking to research to provide answers represents a change in thinking for many. Implementing practice changes based upon research is also a challenge.

Opportunities for providing high-quality care with accountability to clients and families are presented when practice decisions are based on scientific evidence and data. Confidence in that decision making can be founded upon information that has been tested and has demonstrated effectiveness in providing the best strategies to care for those needing nursing.

EVIDENCE-BASED PRACTICE

Nursing research represents a systematic search for the knowledge needed to provide high-quality care. It is one of the requirements for professionalism and supplies a foundation for accountability. A sound knowledge base is necessary for decision making in practice.

The knowledge base for practice in nursing has relied on information from a number of sources, representing varying degrees of rigor. Tradition as a source of knowledge has provided a substantial amount of the foundations for practice. Nursing has developed ways of doing things that have continued in practice simply because "that is the way it has always been done." One such example of this is the routine monitoring of vital signs at specified times during a shift, regardless of the client's condition. Another source of nursing knowledge is authority. Things are done a certain way because a physician or other person with a perceived higher level of knowledge has prescribed a particular way of providing care. Experience and trial and error have also provided an impetus for decision making and procedure development. As nurses become more grounded in a scientific rationale for practice, logical

reasoning and the application of research findings become the focus when care is planned.

Reflect on...

■ how nurses apply research in daily practice.
■ what happens when problems related to care are identified by nurses.
■ how solutions to problems are developed. What sources of information are used?

Empirical Nursing Knowledge

In Chapter 6 ⚭, Theoretical Foundations of Professional Nursing, the ways of knowing were discussed as they apply to nursing. Empirical knowledge comes from scientific evidence and is developed through research. It is a characteristic of the scientific approach that includes order and control and allows generalization of results. The purposes of scientific research are description, exploration, explanation, and prediction and control. The findings are then applied to practice.

One way for a nurse to access empirical knowledge is to learn about research methods and be able to assess strengths and weaknesses of studies when he or she reads them in professional journals. Another mechanism is to use systematic reviews that are conducted by expert groups for the purpose of critiquing studies and providing recommendations to guide practice. The Agency for Healthcare Research and Quality (formerly the Agency for Health Care Policy and Research) is a federal agency that provides evidence reports on numerous topics through its Evidence-Based Practice Centers. The evidence reports may be accessed online through the agency's Web site. As nurses move toward evidence-based care, they must be involved in clinical decision making and protocol development that strive to incorporate the best information available. Strategies for implementing evidence-based practice are presented in the box on page 185.

RESEARCH IN NURSING

Research is directed toward building a body of nursing knowledge about "human responses to actual or potential health problems" (ANA, 1980, p. 9) and to the effects of nursing action on human responses. The human responses may be (1) reactions of individuals, groups, or families to actual health problems, such as the caregiving burden on the family of an older individual with Alzheimer's disease; and (2) concerns of individuals and groups about potential health prob-

Strategies for Implementing Evidence-Based Practice (EBP)

1. Assess the extent to which your practice is evidenced based.

2. Review literature that provides evidence to strengthen your belief that EBP results in better patient outcomes.

3. Ask questions about your current practice strategies (e.g., Is use of distraction really effective in reducing children's distress during intrusive procedures? Does nonnutritive sucking alleviate pain in infants?).

4. Determine whether other colleagues at your practice site have an interest in the same clinical question so that you can form a collaboration to search for and review the evidence.

5. Conduct a search for studies or systematic reviews in the specific area of your clinical question. (Remember that randomized clinical trials are typically the gold standard for producing the best evidence.)

6. Critique the studies from your search to determine whether you have the "best evidence" to guide your practice.

7. Develop a practice guideline using the "best evidence."

8. Establish measurable outcomes that you can use to determine the effectiveness of your guideline.

9. Implement the practice guideline.

10. Measure the established outcomes.

11. Evaluate the effectiveness of the practice guideline and determine whether you should continue the practice guideline as established or whether there is a need for revision.

12. Develop a mechanism for routinely disseminating and discussing evidence-based literature upon which decisions can be made to improve practice at your clinical site (e.g., EBP rounds).

Source: From "Evidence-Based Practice: The Past, the Present, and Recommendations for the Millennium," by B. M. Melnyk, P. Stone, E. Fineout-Overhold, and M. Ackerman, 2000, *Pediatric Nursing, 26*(1), pp. 77–80. Used by permission.

lems, such as accident prevention or stress management in a factory or assembly plant.

- Nursing research also reflects the traditional nursing perspective. In this view, the client is seen as a whole person with physiologic, psychologic, spiritual, social, cultural, developmental, and economic aspects.

  For example, when a person has a head injury, the nurse needs to understand the body's processes for dealing with the increased pressure within the head and the changes this brings about in the patient's condition. At the same time, the nurse focuses on care that can maintain the person's cognitive (thinking and feeling) processes. A nurse would also examine the person's life patterns that could lead to other head injuries (Roy, 1985, pp. 2–3).

- In addition to reflecting the concern for the whole person, a nursing perspective implies 24-hour responsibility. Thus, this viewpoint encompasses all of the factors in a client's environment, such as fatigue, noise, sensory deprivation, nutrition, and positioning, that may influence coping patterns. Diers (1979, pp. 13–15) identifies the following three distinguishing properties of nursing research:

  1. The final focus of nursing research must be on a difference that matters for improving client care.

  2. Nursing research has the potential for contributing to developing theory and the body of scientific knowledge.

  3. A research problem becomes a nursing problem when nurses have access to and control over the phenomena being studied.

The information revolution that is transforming the present and shaping the future has made reading, understanding, and using nursing research as fundamental to professional practice as the knowledge of asepsis, application of the nursing process, and communication skills. Polit and Beck (2004) cite the following reasons why research is important in nursing:

1. Nurses are expected to adopt an evidence-based practice by using the best clinical evidence in making decisions related to patient care.

2. Nurses need to identify practices that improve health care outcomes and are cost-effective.

3. Research enables the nurse to describe situations about which little is known, explain phenomena, predict probable outcomes, control the occurrence of undesired outcomes, and initiate activities to promote desired client outcomes.

Roles in Research

According to the American Nurses Association *Position Statement on Education for Participation in Nursing Research* (1994), all nurses share a commitment to the advancement of nursing science. The responsibility for assuming various activities and roles is related to level of education. Research-based practice is seen as essential for effective and efficient patient care. The development and utilization of research depends upon the interaction between researchers and clinicians. Nurses in clinical practice identify the problems in need of investigation and collaborate with nurse-researchers, who design studies to address the problems identified and analyze the data. It is again up to the clinicians to determine the appropriate application of those findings to practice.

Nurses are sometimes employed on care units or in services where research is conducted by a variety of disciplines. It is the nurse's responsibility to support the research protocol and uphold the scientific rigor of the study by carefully maintaining the research protocol. At the same time, it is the right of the nurse to be informed of the purpose of the study and to understand the protocol. Likewise, the nurse has a right to know that human subjects are being protected, that the study has been reviewed by an Institutional Review Board (IRB), and that the researchers are qualified to do the research.

Preparation for these research roles begins at the undergraduate level as the student learns about research and develops practice that is based on the critical analysis of research findings. The preparation of nurse scientists who have primary responsibility for the conduct of research occurs in graduate education. It begins at the master's level and is concentrated at the doctoral and postdoctoral level. The accompanying box on page 187 lists the roles identified as appropriate for the varying levels of education.

With regard to the role of the nurse prepared at the baccalaureate level, the ANA makes this statement:

> . . . education for research prepares nurses to read research critically and to use existing standards to determine the readiness of research for utilization in clinical practice. Promoting understanding of the ethical principles of research, especially the protection of human subjects and other ethical responsibilities of investigators, is an essential objective of research preparation for baccalaureate students. (ANA, 1994)

During the curriculum of the BSN program, students will have a course in research that provides the tools needed for implementing the role in practice. It is not the purpose of this chapter to present research in that depth, but a brief overview will be given to provide a context for the discussion of evidence-based practice.

Historical Perspective

As early as 1854, Florence Nightingale demonstrated the importance of research in the delivery of nursing care. When Nightingale arrived in the Crimea in November of 1854, she found the military hospital barracks overcrowded, filthy, rat- and flea-infested, and lacking in food, drugs, and essential medical supplies. As a result of these conditions, men died from starvation and such diseases as dysentery, cholera, and typhus (Woodham-Smith, 1950, pp. 151–167). By systematically collecting, organizing, and reporting data, Nightingale was able to institute sanitary reforms and significantly reduce mortality rates from contagious disease.

Although the Nightingale tradition influenced the establishment of American nursing schools in 1873, the research approach did not take hold until the beginning of the twentieth century. Recognizing the need, nursing leader Isabel Stewart integrated research into the graduate nursing curriculum at Teachers College, Columbia University, and published the first research journal in nursing, the *Nursing Education Bulletin,* in the late 1920s. The journal *Nursing Research* was established in 1952 to serve as a vehicle to communicate nurses' research and scholarly productivity. The publication of many other nursing research journals followed, some dedicated to research and others combining clinical and research publications.

The National Institute of Nursing Research (NINR) was established as a Center at the National Institutes of Health (NIH) in 1986. In 1993, it was elevated to an Institute, placing it among the Institutes and Centers within NIH and adding a clinical and nursing perspective to the mainstream of the biomedical and behavioral research in the United States. According to its mission statement:

> The National Institute of Nursing Research supports clinical and basic research to establish a scientific basis for the care of individuals across the life span—from management of patients during illness and recovery to the reduction of risks for disease and disability, the promotion of healthy lifestyles, promot-

Research Roles at Various Levels of Nursing Education According to the ANA Position Statement on *Education for Participation in Nursing Research*

ASSOCIATE DEGREE IN NURSING

- Help to identify clinical problems in nursing practice
- Assist in the collection of data within a structured format
- In conjunction with nurses holding more advanced credentials, appropriately use research findings in clinical practice

BACCALAUREATE DEGREE IN NURSING

- Identify clinical problems requiring investigation
- Assist experienced investigators gain access to clinical sites
- Influence the selection of appropriate methods of data collection
- Collect data and implement nursing research findings

MASTER'S DEGREE IN NURSING

- Be active members of research teams
- Assume the role of clinical expert collaborating with experienced investigators in proposal de-

velopment, data collection, data analysis, and interpretation

- Appraise the clinical relevance of research findings
- Help create a climate that supports scholarly inquiry, scientific integrity, and scientific investigation of clinical nursing problems
- Provide leadership for integrating findings in clinical practice

DOCTORAL EDUCATION

- Conduct research aimed at theory generation or theory testing
- Design studies independently as well as collaborate with other clinicians and researchers
- Acquire funding for research
- Disseminate research findings

POSTDOCTORAL EDUCATION

- Develop a systematic program of research
- Become a sustaining member of the scientific community

Source: Based on the ANA Position Statement: *Education for Participation in Nursing Research,* originated by the Council of Nurse Researchers and Council of Nursing Practice and adopted by the ANA Board of Directors, April, 1994.

ing quality of life in those with chronic illness, and care for individuals at the end of life. This research may also include families within a community context. According to its broad mandate, the Institute seeks to understand and ease the symptoms of acute and chronic illness, to prevent or delay the onset of disease or disability or slow its progression, to find effective approaches to achieving and sustaining good health, and to improve the clinical settings in which care is provided. Nursing research involves clinical care in a variety of settings including the community and home in addition to more traditional health care sites. (NINR, 2000)

NINR has established the following goals for the 5-year period 2000–2004 (NINR, 2000):

1. Identify and support research opportunities that will achieve scientific distinction and produce significant contributions to health.

2. Identify and support future areas of opportunity to advance research on high-quality, cost-effective care and to contribute to the scientific base for nursing practice.

3. Communicate and disseminate research findings resulting from NINR-funded research, and

4. Enhance the development of nurse-researchers through training and career development opportunities.

The overall focus is to provide leadership in emphasizing the inclusion of cultural and ethnic considerations throughout the research, encompassing culturally sensitive interventions to decrease disparities among groups in health status and health care. In doing this, nurse-researchers will focus on health promotion and chronic illness–management strategies and an interdisciplinary and collaborative effort.

Sigma Theta Tau International is the honor society for nursing, and its mission is to provide leadership and scholarship in practice, education, and research to enhance the health of all people. *Strategic Plan 2005* contains a goal for research support to "advance the scientific base of nursing practice through the scholarship of research." According to the strategic plan:

> The scientific base of nursing practice is strengthened through the promotion of research studies and the dissemination of findings—particularly the findings that are readily integrated into practice. The diverse society membership has expressed a critical need for research support and innovations for clinical applications. The society is uniquely qualified to fill this need. Technological innovation, expansion of the Virginia Henderson International Nursing Library, development of systems to support evidence-based practice, and the provision of research funding are continued priorities of the society. (STTI, 2000)

Ethical Concerns

Because nursing research usually focuses on humans, a major nursing responsibility is to be aware of and to advocate on behalf of clients' rights. Participation must be voluntary, and all clients must be informed about the consequences of consenting to serve as research subjects. In other words, there must be informed consent to participate. The client needs to be able to assess whether an appropriate balance exists between the risks of participating in a study and the potential benefits, either to the client or to the development of knowledge.

Research ethics not only protect the rights of human subjects but also encompass a broader range of principles. Most of these principles are reflected in the ANA's *Human Rights Guidelines for Nurses in Clinical and Other Research* (1975). These guidelines are based on historic documents, such as the Nuremberg Code (1949) and the Declaration of Helsinki (adopted in 1964 by the World Medical Assembly and revised in 1975), and on United States federal regulations, all of which set standards governing the conduct of research involving human subjects. The notorious Tuskegee study in Alabama, begun in 1932 and ended in 1972, studied black men with syphilis without informed consent, violated confidentiality, and withheld treatment when it became available. It illustrates how subjects' human rights were violated for a period of 40 years while a research study was being conducted.

All nurses who practice in settings where research is being conducted with human subjects or who participate in such research as data collectors or collaborators play an important role in safeguarding the following rights.

Right Not to Be Harmed

The Department of Health and Human Services defines risk of harm to a research subject as exposure to the possibility of injury going beyond everyday situations. The risk can be physical, emotional, legal, financial, or social. For example, withholding standard care from a client in labor for the purpose of studying the course of natural childbirth clearly poses a potential physical danger. Risks can be less overt and involve psychologic factors, such as exposure to stress or anxiety, or social factors, such as loss of confidentiality or loss of privacy.

Right to Full Disclosure

Even though it may be possible to collect data about a client as part of everyday care without the client's particular knowledge or consent, to do so is considered unethical. **Full disclosure** is a basic right. It means that deception, either by withholding information about a client's participation in a study or by giving the client false or misleading information about what participating in the study will involve, violates ethical principles.

Right of Self-Determination

Many clients in dependent positions, such as people in nursing homes, feel pressured to participate in studies. They feel that they must please the doctors and nurses who are responsible for their treatment and care. The **right of self-determination** means that subjects should feel free from constraints, coercion, or any undue influence to participate in a study. Masked inducements, such as suggesting to potential participants that by taking part in the study they might become famous, make an important contribution to science, or receive special attention, must be strictly avoided. Nurses must be assertive in advocating for this essential right.

Right of Privacy and Confidentiality

Privacy enables a client to participate without worrying about later embarrassment. There should be either anonymity or confidentiality depending upon the nature of the study. Anonymity of a study participant is ensured when even the investigator cannot link a specific person to the information reported. **Confidentiality** means that any information collected in a study will not be made public or available to others without the person's consent. Investigators must inform research subjects about the measures that provide for these rights. Such measures may include the use of pseudonyms or code numbers or reporting only aggregate or group data in published research.

Approaches in Nursing Research

There are two major approaches to investigating phenomena in nursing research. These approaches originate from different philosophical perspectives and use different methods for collection and analysis of data.

Quantitative research uses precise measurement for data collection and analyzes numerical data. The design is rigorously controlled, and statistical analysis is used to summarize and describe findings or to test relationships among variables. The quantitative approach is most frequently associated with a philosophical doctrine called *logical positivism,* which asserts that scientific knowledge is the only kind of factual knowledge. It is viewed by some as "hard" science and tends to use deductive reasoning and emphasize measurable aspects of the human experience. The following are examples of research questions that lend themselves to a quantitative approach:

- What are the differential effects of continuous versus intermittent application of negative pressure on tracheal tissue during endotracheal suctioning?
- Is the use of therapeutic touch effective in reducing pain perception postoperatively?

- Are there differences in skin breakdown between premature infants bathed with plain water and those bathed with bacteriostatic soap?

Qualitative research investigates phenomena through narrative data that describe the phenomena in an in-depth and holistic fashion. The research design is typically more flexible and less controlled than quantitative designs. The data may be the transcription of an unstructured interview, and the analysis looks for patterns and themes that come from the narrative data by using an inductive approach. This allows exploration of the subjective experiences of human beings and can provide nursing with a better understanding of phenomena from the client's perspective. The qualitative approach is appropriate for the following types of questions:

- What is the nature of the bereavement process in spouses of clients with terminal cancer?
- What is the nature of coping and adjustment after a radical prostatectomy?
- What is the process of family caregiving for older family relatives with Alzheimer's dementia as experienced by the caregiver?

There are several important steps in the conduct of research, and each of these requires decision making by the researcher. The first step is identification of the problem. Ideally, this is the step at which the nurse in clinical practice makes known the information needs. Once the problem is clearly identified and a statement is formulated, the next step is a search of existing literature, especially related research. Before the researcher designs a study to answer the question, the state of the art of current knowledge should be known.

A literature review will identify other studies related to the topic, and this can serve several purposes. It can provide an answer or partial answer to the question and may even eliminate the need to conduct further research, or it may change the problem focus. Gaps in the literature will support the need for the research. In performing a literature review, the focus should be on primary rather than secondary sources. A **primary source** is a publication authored by the person who conducted the research. A secondary source is a description of a study or studies prepared by someone other than the person who conducted the research. Review articles describing a number of studies on a particular topic are considered secondary sources. The **secondary sources** are helpful in identifying studies that are related to the topic of interest, but a researcher needs to rely on primary sources when designing a study.

One of the challenges in conducting a literature review is identifying the sources to be included. Electronic databases and computer searches have become the mainstay of literature searches. The *Cumulative Index of Nursing and Allied Health* (CINAHL) is one of the most common databases accessed by nurses. Medline also references nursing journals. Hard copies or CD-ROM indexes are also available in most libraries and include such sources as the *Cumulative Index to Nursing and Allied Health, International Nursing Index,* and *Cumulative Index Medicus.* These sources give bibliographical references. Other databases provide abstracts for review; some of these are *Annual Review of Nursing Research, Dissertation Abstracts International,* and *Nursing Research Abstract.*

Once the researcher has identified the problem, reviewed the literature, and identified specific research questions or hypotheses, an appropriate study can be designed to answer the questions or test the hypotheses. Decisions need to be made regarding who should be included in the study. The researcher needs to select a sample that is representative of the population of interest so that findings from the study are applicable or generalizable to that group. Data-collection methods will determine the quality of the data being analyzed in the study. The researcher will have to decide on a reasonable way to either observe or measure the concepts in the study; this is referred to as **operational definition of the variable.** Data collection can be done according to three categories: **biophysiologic measures, observation,** and **self-report by the study participants or subjects.** Decisions need to be made about the amount of control over outside influences (extraneous variables) and timing of data collection. The tools selected for data collection need to be evaluated for reliability and validity, that is, how well they measure what they claim to measure and how consistently they do so. A procedure or protocol must be developed, clearly spelled out, and consistently adhered to during the study. An appropriate method of data analysis must be selected, whether the study is quantitative (descriptive or inferential statistics) or qualitative (content analysis). Once the data are analyzed and results are known, the researcher must be very careful about the interpretation of those results and be certain that any conclusions are supported by the study data. It is at this point that the practicing nurse is again a valuable team member. The utilization of research in practice and the development of evidence-based practice need a close partnership between the nurse-scientist and the nurse in clinical practice.

USING RESEARCH IN PRACTICE

Critiquing Research Reports

If professional nurses are to use research, they must first learn to conduct a critical appraisal of research reports published in the literature. A research critique enables the nurse as a research consumer to evaluate the scientific merit of the study and decide how the results may be useful in practice. Critiquing involves intensive scrutiny of a study, including its strengths and weaknesses, statistical and clinical significance, as well as the generalizability of the results.

Polit and Beck (2004) proposed that the following elements be considered in conducting a research critique: substantive and theoretical dimensions, methodologic dimensions, ethical dimensions, interpretive dimensions, and presentation and stylistic dimensions.

- *Substantive and theoretical dimensions.* For these dimensions, the nurse needs to evaluate the significance of the research problem, the appropriateness of the conceptualizations and the theoretical framework of the study, and the congruence between the research question and the methods used to address it.
- *Methodologic dimensions.* The methodologic dimensions pertain to the appropriateness of the research design, the size and representativeness of the study sample as well as the sampling design, validity and reliability of the instruments, adequacy of the research procedures, and the appropriateness of data analytic techniques used in the study.
- *Ethical dimensions.* The nurse must determine whether the rights of human subjects were protected during the course of the study and whether any ethical problems compromised the scientific merit of the study or the well-being of the subjects.
- *Interpretive dimensions.* For these dimensions, the nurse needs to ascertain the accuracy of the discussion, conclusions, and implications of the study results. The findings must be related back to the original hypotheses and the conceptual framework of the study. The implications and limitations of the study should be reviewed, together with the potential for replication or generalizability of the findings to similar populations.
- *Presentation and stylistic dimensions.* The manner in which the research plan and results are communicated refers to the presentation and stylistic dimensions. The research report must be detailed, logically organized, concise, and well written. Research that is poorly presented or poorly communicated is of little value to nurses in practice.

Reflect on...

■   resources (libraries, colleges and universities, schools of nursing, and so on) that are available in your practice setting and in your community to assist you in researching nursing practice problems.

■   nursing problems encountered in your nursing practice setting. What nursing problems might be solved through research?

Research Utilization

Research utilization is the process in which study findings are used to initiate and support innovations in the delivery of nursing care. In the 1970s, the lag between publication of research and the transfer of findings into actual practice was recognized. This gap was demonstrated in Ketefian's study (1975, p. 91), in which she found that despite widely published research about the optimal placement time for oral glass thermometers (9 min.), only 1 of 87 nurses surveyed was aware of the correct placement time.

The Western Interstate Commission for Higher Education (WICHEN) and the Conduct and Utilization of Research in Nursing (CURN) projects were developed to promote the dissemination and utilization of nursing research (Horsley, Crane, & Bingle, 1978; Krueger, Nelson, & Wolanin, 1978). As a result, research-utilization training programs and research-based innovations were implemented.

Research on the process of adoption of research-based innovations has used Rogers' theory of diffusion of innovation (1983). According to this theory, a nurse passes through four stages before adopting research-based ideas or practices:

1. *Knowledge stage*—when a nurse learns about an innovation
2. *Persuasion stage*—when a nurse develops a positive or negative attitude about the innovation
3. *Decision stage*—when a nurse determines whether to adopt or reject the innovation
4. *Implementation stage*—when the nurse uses the innovation regularly

Inhibitors and Facilitators of Research Utilization

Factors that inhibit and facilitate the process of using research in clinical settings have been identified. The availability of research findings and nurses' attitudes toward research are related to research utilization. The factors inhibiting the use of research in practice are the nurses' perceived lack of authority to change client care procedures; insufficient time to implement new ideas; lack of support and cooperation from physicians, administrators, and other staff; inadequate facilities for implementation; and lack of time to read research. Other inhibitors are characteristics of the research reports; these reports are perceived as difficult to read and understand, particularly when statistical information is reported. Often nurses are not aware of research that has been done (Champion & Leach, 1989; Funk et al., 1991; McCleary & Brown, 2003).

Evidence for Practice

Retsas, A. (2000). Barriers to using research evidence in nursing practice. *Journal of Advanced Nursing, 31*(3), 599–606.

The purpose of this study was to (1) establish the extent to which research use and research expertise existed at a particular medical center in Melbourne, Australia; (2) identify barriers the nursing staff believe interfere with their ability to use research findings in clinical practice; and (3) establish the extent to which nursing staff perceived that they were supported in these efforts. A self-administered questionnaire was used to collect data on demographics, education background, and research access habits of the full-time nursing staff. The questionnaire incorporated items from the Barriers to Research Utilization Scale (Funk et al., 1991) and qualitative questions about what helps in the use of research.

Two thirds of the 400 participants read a journal monthly or more frequently. Barriers were classified by four factors: accessibility of research findings, anticipated outcomes of using research, organizational support to use research, and support from others to use research. The most outstanding finding was considered to be the significance participants gave to the need for organizational support to use research. The most significant barrier to using research evidence was having insufficient time to implement new ideas on the job and insufficient time to read research.

The researcher concluded that staff nurses have a high level of research readiness and value the contribution that research can make to improve practice. The organizational change that needs to occur is increasing the time available for nurses to achieve this goal.

Evidence for Practice

Kajermo, K. N., Nordstrom, G., Krusebrant, A., & Bjorvell, H. (2000). Perceptions of research utilization: Comparisons between health care professionals, nursing students and a reference group of nurse clinicians. *Journal of Advanced Nursing, 31*(1), 99–109.

This study, conducted in Sweden, was done to investigate perceptions of barriers to and facilitators of nurses' use of research findings in clinical practice. Five comparison groups were surveyed with a Barriers Scale and a demographic questionnaire; the five groups were (1) teachers of nursing, (2) nursing students, (3) nursing administrators, (4) physicians, and (5) registered nurses in clinical practice.

The organization and communication of research were seen as barriers by all of the groups except the physicians. Education to increase the nurses' knowledge of research and to develop their competence to evaluate research results, increased resources for education, more staff, support from the administration, and research presented in a user-friendly way were the most frequently suggested facilitators. The nurses' isolation from knowledgeable colleagues with whom to discuss the research was seen as a barrier by the majority of the participants.

These findings among the Swedish population were similar to findings in the United States and other countries.

Evidence for Practice

McCaughan, D., Thompson, C., Cullum, N., Sheldon, T., & Thompson, D. (2002). Acute care nurses' perceptions of barriers to using research information in clinical decision-making. *Journal of Advanced Nursing, 39*(1), 46–60.

Acute-care nurses' perception of barriers to using research in clinical decision making was investigated using interviews, observation, document audit, and Q method at three large hospitals on Northern England. Four perspectives were drawn from this qualitative data. They related to the individual nurse, the organization employing the nurse, the nature of research reports, and the work environment. These four perspectives were:

1. It was difficult to interpret and use research because it was seen as complex, "academic," and overly statistical.

2. Nurses who felt confident with research-based information perceived the significant barrier as the lack of organizational support for research utilization.

3. The research and researchers were seen as lacking in clinical credibility and failed to offer real direction to care.

4. Some nurses lacked the skills and motivation to use research in their practice. They preferred to have the information presented to them by a third party rather than be directly involved.

The researchers conclude that more work is needed to foster the promotion of research use in nurses' clinical decisions. They suggest that nurse educators need to teach more about epidemiology and statistics. Researchers need to present findings more clearly and in an easily understood format. Managers need to promote dissemination of research findings by fostering guidelines and protocols that are research based.

The factors facilitating research utilization are those that provide nurses with information about research developments. These factors include monthly research newsletters, research meetings, continuing education programs, computer networks, and research study guides (Caramanica et al., 2002; Tsai, 2003).

To be able to integrate research as part of day-to-day practice, nurses must work to overcome the inhibitors and perpetuate the facilitators of research utilization. Key strategies for success follow:

- Nurses must develop a positive attitude toward research utilization, viewing it as a tool to attain clinical excellence.

- Nursing administrators need to provide time, facilities, equipment, and support personnel needed for research utilization activities.

- Administrators of hospitals and clinical agencies must create an environment that is conducive to research-based innovation.

Criteria for Research Utilization

If a nurse reads in a research journal that teaching guided imagery to clients was found to be effective in enabling clients to manage postoperative pain, should the nurse utilize the intervention in his or her own clients? How would a nurse know that the research he or she reads is ready for use in practice?

Haller, Reynolds, and Horsley (1979) formulated criteria for utilization of research in nursing practice, based on the CURN project. These criteria are replication, scientific merit, risk, clinical merit, clinical control, feasibility, cost, and potential for clinical evaluation.

REPLICATION The criterion of replication requires that the results of a study be replicated a number of times before its findings are accepted as credible and applicable to practice. A change in current practice or procedure ordinarily should not be based solely on one study. Establishing a research base of three or more studies confirms the likelihood that the findings are true and prevents nurses from committing a type I error. A type I error is concluding that the intervention was effective when in reality it was not; in other words, it is a false positive.

SCIENTIFIC MERIT The scientific merit of a study is probably the single most important criterion in judging its readiness for application in practice. Scientific rigor is evident in all steps of the research project—the clarity of the research problem; adequacy of the literature review; and the appropriateness of the design, sampling, data collection procedures, and data analytic techniques. The validity and reliability of the instruments used must also be evaluated.

Internal validity and external validity are key concerns. Internal validity is the degree to which the independent variable influences the dependent variable. A classic monograph by Campbell and Stanley (1963) discussed factors that threaten internal validity. An example is selection bias if subjects in a study are not randomly assigned to the experimental or control groups. If a statistically significant difference is found, it would be difficult to conclude whether the change in the dependent variable is truly attributable to the independent variable (the intervention) or whether it is related to some preexisting differences between the groups.

External validity pertains to the degree to which the findings of the study can be generalized to similar settings and populations. Even if statistically significant differences are demonstrated, findings can be generalized to other settings or populations only if these settings and populations are similar to those of the study.

RISK The degree of risk involved in using the findings of a study is another criterion to be considered. Nursing interventions that have been found effective through research may be readily implemented if they carry little risk. According to Haller et al. (1979), risk must be evaluated along with scientific merit. If a protocol entails serious risks, then the evaluation of scientific merit must be applied more stringently.

CLINICAL MERIT The criterion of clinical merit evaluates the degree to which research findings have the potential to solve an existing problem in the clinical setting. Nurses working in a neonatal nursery may be concerned about the pain that infants experience during blood drawing for laboratory tests or during surgical procedures. For nurses working in this unit, a published study by Campos (1994) that reported the effects of rocking and pacifiers on relieving heelstick pain in infants would be rated high for clinical merit.

CLINICAL CONTROL Clinical control refers to the degree to which nurses are in control of the circumstances related to the implementation and evaluation of the research-based innovation. Nurses may not be able to exert clinical control if a research-based protocol requires collaboration or decision making by a team of health professionals. There may also be instruments or methods documented to be effective in research but unavailable to nurses in certain settings.

FEASIBILITY The criterion of feasibility is defined as the degree to which resources—time, personnel, expertise, equipment—are available to implement the innovation. For example, the introduction of a new intervention may require the ordering and purchasing of equipment or supplies and in-service training for nursing staff.

COST In this era of downsizing and restructuring, cost is always a vital consideration. Cost is closely related to feasibility. A cost-benefit analysis would be important in order to weigh the costs against the benefits of implementing a new intervention. Benefits may include improved client outcomes or improved staff satisfaction.

Critical Thinking Exercise

Select a research article from one of the nursing research journals. Apply the criteria for research utilization found on pages 193 to 194. Decide whether you are comfortable applying the research findings to practice or whether you feel more research should be done before implementing a research-based protocol.

POTENTIAL FOR CLINICAL EVALUATION

Potential for clinical evaluation pertains to the degree to which the variables in the original research base can be evaluated by nurses in the clinical setting. Specifically, this criterion requires that nurses have control over the variables in the protocol and that they possess the knowledge and skills needed to measure the outcome of the innovation.

What began in nursing as research utilization or the process of transforming research knowledge into practice has expanded into evidence-based practice (EBP). EBP is broader than research utilization and recognizes other sources of evidence, including the "value of the intuitive aspects of nursing practice" (Caramanica et al., 2002). Other sources of evidence include reliable data from quality improvement programs, evaluation projects, consensus of experts, and clinical experience.

Recently one of the models of research utilization developed by Marram and Stetler (1994) has been updated to include EBP. The model includes five phases: Preparation, Validation, Comparative Evaluation/Decision Making, Translation/Application, and Evaluation. Table 10–1 depicts processes at each phase. The model can be used by individuals for making judgments at the level of the individual practitioner or of groups making EBP decisions.

Mechanisms for Application of Research to Practice

Research utilization in the clinical setting may occur through several mechanisms. There are situations in which research utilization takes place through individual action by nurses. In other cases, research-based protocols are developed by groups of nurses for a unit or hospital and may require changes in existing hospital or agency procedure.

Table 10–1 Phases of Stetler Model Applied to Evidence-Based Practice

Preparation	Validation	Comparative Evaluation	Translation/Application	Evaluation
This phase requires that there be clarity of purpose and potential significance. The nurse is reminded to consider external factors that influence application and to consider internal factors (personal) that may influence objectivity. Relevant information should be identified.	Utilization-focused critique is used. The findings are appraised rather than the study itself. Critical thinking is applied.	This involves synthesis from multiple studies. The nurse identifies, organizes, and integrates information across multiple studies. The utilization decision will be to use, to consider use, or to not use. The decision to consider use might result in modification.	This phase focuses on how to implement the synthesized findings. This may include development of plans for formal organizational change. It will include evidence-based strategies for dissemination of translated findings and facilitation of behavioral change in the users.	Evaluation of the application is done. There is a deliberate, systematic, and continuous evaluation process with feedback to users and refinement in the implementation.

INDIVIDUAL ACTION According to the ANA Standards of Clinical Nursing Practice, nurses are expected to integrate research findings into practice. See the accompanying box. Low-risk, low-cost interventions that have potential to improve client outcomes may be readily implemented by individual nurses. One example is an innovation listed in the Coyle and Sokop (1990, p. 177) study—internal rotation of the femur during dorsogluteal intramuscular injection to reduce client discomfort.

RESEARCH-BASED PROTOCOLS AND PROCE-DURES Many hospitals and clinical agencies follow a compendium of policies, procedures, and protocols in specific client care situations. For example, there are procedures to be followed when irrigating a Foley catheter, administering nasogastric tube-feeding, or performing wound care. Current research literature must be the basis for developing or revising these procedures or protocols.

EXPLORE MEDIALINK

Questions, critical thinking exercises, essay activities, and other interactive resources for this chapter can be found on the Web site at http://www.prenhall.com/blais. Click on Chapter 10 to select activities for this chapter.

American Nurses Association's Standard of Professional Performance Pertaining to Research

Standard 13. Research
THE REGISTERED NURSE INTEGRATES RESEARCH FINDINGS INTO PRACTICE.
Measurement Criteria
The registered nurse:

1. Utilizes the best available evidence, including research findings, to guide practice decisions.

2. Actively participates in research activities at various levels appropriate to the nurse's level of education and position. Such activities may include:

   - Identifying clinical problems specific to nursing research (patient care and nursing practice).

   - Participating in data collection (surveys, pilot projects, formal studies).

   - Participating in a formal committee or program.

   - Sharing research activities and/or findings with peers and others.

   - Conducting research.

   - Critically analyzing and interpreting research for application to practice.

- Using research findings in the development of policies, procedures, and standards of practice in patient care.

- Incorporating research as a basis for learning.

Additional Measurement Criteria for the Advanced Practice Registered Nurse:
The advanced practice registered nurse:

1. Contributes to nursing knowledge by conducting or synthesizing research that discovers, examines, and evaluates knowledge, theories, criteria, and creative approaches to improve health care practice.

2. Formally disseminates research findings through activities, such as presentations, publications, consultation, and journal clubs.

Additional Measurement Criteria for the Nursing Role Specialty:
The registered nurse in a nursing role specialty:

1. Contributes to nursing knowledge by conducting or synthesizing research that discovers, examines, and evaluates knowledge, theories, criteria, and creative approaches to improve health care.

2. Formally disseminates research findings through activities, such as presentations, publications, consultation, and journal clubs.

Source: From *Nursing: Scope and Standards of Practice,* by American Nurses Association, 2004, Washington, DC: ANA. Used by permission.

Bookshelf

Laurence, L., & Weinhouse, B. (1994). *Outrageous practices.* **New York: Fawcett Columbine.**

This book focuses on the lack of research studies related to women's health issues, such as hormone-replacement therapy, breast cancer, heart disease in women, menopause, premenstrual syndrome (PMS), and other disease processes that have a higher incidence in women than men. In many cases, research has been done on exclusively male populations, and women have been purposely excluded because of female-specific hormone changes, physiological differences, and the potential for pregnancy during the study. The authors also discuss how women are treated differently from men in the health care system. These differences in treatment are grounded in assumptions by both physicians and researchers about women—assumptions based on studies that have been done exclusively in men.

Moore, T. J. (1995). *Deadly medicine.* **New York: Simon and Shuster.**

This book chronicles the history of multiple studies over approximately 10 years in the effectiveness of cardiac arrhythmia suppressant therapy (CAST) in the treatment of clients diagnosed with cardiac dysrythmias. It points out how inaccurate assumptions and errors in study design can cause errors in conclusions that can have fatal results in client populations.

Palmer, M. (1998). *Miracle cure.* **New York: Bantam Doubleday.**

The political pressures in biomedical research form the backdrop for this novel presenting the story of the phase II clinical trial and FDA decisions about a drug under investigation as a cure for cardiovascular disease.

SUMMARY

Nursing research refers to research directed toward building a body of nursing knowledge about human responses to actual or potential health problems. Research is important in nursing to expand the scientific body of knowledge, to maintain specific accountability to the public, to document nursing contribution to health care delivery, and to provide the bases for sound clinical decision making in client care.

The information revolution that is transforming the present and shaping the future has made reading, understanding, and using nursing research as fundamental to professional practice as are knowledge of asepsis, application of the nursing process, and communication skills. The *Cumulative Index to Nursing and Allied Health Literature*, the *International Nursing Index*, and the *Cumulative Index Medicus* are excellent resources for locating published research on a phenomenon of interest.

The quantitative and qualitative approaches are both valid approaches to investigations of nursing phenomena, although they proceed from different philosophic perspectives and use different methods of data collection and analysis.

If nursing is to develop evidence-based practice, the clinical nurse must know the process and language of research, be sensitive to protecting the rights of human subjects, participate in identifying significant researchable problems, and be a discriminating consumer of research findings.

All nurses who practice in settings where research is conducted with human subjects or who participate in research as data collectors or collaborators play an important role in safeguarding the rights of human subjects.

REFERENCES

American Nurses Association. (1975). *Human rights guidelines for nurses in clinical and other research.* Kansas City, MO: ANA.

American Nurses Association. (1980). *Nursing: A social policy statement.* Kansas City, MO: ANA.

American Nurses Association, Council of Nurse Researchers and Council of Nursing Practice. (1994). *Position statement on education for participation in nursing research.* Washington, DC: ANA.

American Nurses Association. (2004). *Nursing: Scope and standards of practice.* Washington, D.C.: ANA.

Beckstrand, J., & McBride, A. B. (1990). How to form a research interest group. *Nursing Outlook, 38*(4), 168–171.

Brett, J. L. L. (1987). Use of nursing practice research findings. *Nursing Research, 36*(6), 344–349.

Brink, P. J., & Wood, M. J. (1988). *Basic steps in planning nursing research* (3rd ed.). Boston: Jones and Bartlett.

Campbell, D. T., & Stanley, J. C. (1963). *Experimental and quasi-experimental designs for research.* Boston: Houghton Miflin.

Campos, R. G. (1994). Rocking and pacifiers: Two comforting interventions for heelstick pain. *Research in Nursing and Health, 17*(5), 321–331.

Caplan, A. L. (1992). When evil intrudes. *Hastings Center Report, 22*(6), 29–32.

Caramanica, L., Maljanian, R., McDonald, D., Taylor S., MacRae, J. B., & Beland, D. K. (2002). Evidence-based nursing practice, Part 1: A hospital and university collaborative. *Journal of Nursing Administration, 32*(1), 27–30.

Carlson, D. S., & Rouse, C. L. (1999). Staff nurses: Using research in everyday practice. *Journal of Emergency Nursing, 25*(6), 564–568.

Carper, B. A. (1978). Fundamental patterns of knowing in nursing. *Advances in Nursing Science, 1*(1), 13–23.

Champion, V. L., & Leach, A. (1989). Variables related to research utilization in nursing: An empirical investigation. *Journal of Advanced Nursing, 14*(9), 705–710.

Cohen, I. B. (1984). Florence Nightingale. *Scientific American, 250*(3), 128–137.

Coyle, L. A., & Sokop, A. G. (1990). Innovation adoption behavior among nurses. *Nursing Research, 39*(3), 176–180.

Coyne, C., Baier, W., Perra, B., & Sherer, B. K. (1994). Controlled trial of backrest elevation after coronary angiography. *American Journal of Critical Care, 3*(4), 282–288.

Diers, D. (1979). *Research in nursing practice.* Philadelphia: Lippincott.

Ellis, R. (1970). Values and vicissitudes of the scientist nurse. *Nursing Research, 19*(5), 440–445.

Fawcett, J., & Downs, F. (1992). *The relationship of theory and research.* Norwalk, CT: Appleton-Century-Crofts.

Funk, S. G., Champagne, M. T., Wiese, R. A., & Tornquist, E. (1991). Barriers: The barriers to research utilization scale. *Applied Nursing Research, 4*(1), 39–45.

Good, M. (1995). A comparison of the effects of jaw relaxation and music on postoperative pain. *Nursing Research, 44*(1), 52–57.

Gortner, S. (2000). Knowledge development in nursing: Our historical roots and future opportunities. *Nursing Outlook, 48*(2), 60–67.

Grossman, D. G. S., Jorda, M. L., & Farr, L. A. (1994). Blood pressure rhythms in early school-age children of normotensive and hypertensive parents: A replication study. *Nursing Research, 43*(4), 232–237.

Haller, K. B., Reynolds, M. A., & Horsley, J. A. (1979). Developing research-based innovation protocols: Process, criteria, and issues. *Research in Nursing and Health, 2*(2), 45–51.

Horsley, J. A., Crane, J., & Bingle, J. D. (1978). Research utilization as an organizational process. *Journal of Nursing Administration, 8*(7), 4–6.

Janken, J. K., Rudisill, P., & Benfield, L. (1992). Product evaluation as a research utilization strategy. *Applied Nursing Research, 5*(4), 188–193.

Ketefian, S. (1975). Application of selected nursing research findings into nursing practice. *Nursing Research, 24*(2), 89–92.

Krueger, J. C., Nelson, A. H., & Wolanin, M. O. (1978). *Nursing research: Development, collaboration, and utilization.* Germantown, MD: Aspen Systems.

McCaughan, D., Thompson, C., Cullum, N., Sheldon, T., & Thompson, D. (2002). Acute care nurses' perceptions of barriers to using research information in clinical decision-making. *Journal of Advanced Nursing, 39*(1),46–60.

McCleary, L., & Brown, T. (2003). Barriers to pediatric nurses' research utilization. *Journal of Advanced Nursing, 42*(4), 364–372.

Melnyk, B. M., Stone, P., Fineout-Overholt, E., & Ackerman, M. (2000). Evidence-based practice: The past, the present, and recommendations for the millennium. *Pediatric Nursing, 26*(1), 77–80.

Munro, B. H., Visintainer, M. A., & Page, E. B. (1986). *Statistical methods for health care research.* Philadelphia: Lippincott.

National Institute of Nursing Research. (2000). *Mission statement and strategic planning for the 21st century.* http://www.nih.gov/ninr/a_mission.html.

Nativio, D. G. (2000). Guidelines for evidence-based clinical practice. *Nursing Outlook, 48*(2), 58–59.

Orem, D. E. (1971). *Nursing: Concepts of practice.* New York: McGraw-Hill.

Pettengill, M. M., Gillies, D. A., & Clark, C. C. (1994). Factors encouraging and discouraging the use of nursing research findings. *Image: Journal of Nursing Scholarship, 26*(2), 143–147.

Polit, D. F., & Beck, C. (2004). *Nursing research: Principles and methods* (7th ed.). Philadelphia: Lippincott.

Retsas, A. (2000). Barriers to using research evidence in nursing practice. *Journal of Advanced Nursing, 31*(3), 599–606.

Rogers, E. (1983). *Diffusion of innovations* (3rd ed.). New York: Free Press.

Roy, C. (1985). Nursing research makes a difference. *Nurses' Educational Funds Newsletter, 4*(1), 2–3.

Sigma Theta Tau International. (1995). Listing of doctoral programs in the United States. *Reflections, 21*(3), 18–19, 22–23.

Sigma Theta Tau International. (2000). *Strategic Plan 2005.* http://www.nursingsociety.org/stratplan/man.html.

Stetler C. (1994). Refinement of the Stetler-Marram Model for Application of Research Findings to Practice. *Nursing Outlook, 42,* 15–25.

Stetler, C. B. (2001). Updating the Stetler model of research utilization to facilitate evidence-based practice. *Nursing Outlook, 49*(6), 272–279.

Stetler, C. B., & DiMaggio, G. (1991). Research utilization among clinical nurse specialists. *Clinical Nurse Specialist, 5*(3), 151–155.

Stetler, C. B. & Marram, G. (1976). Evaluating research findings for applicability in practice. *Nursing Outlook, 24*(9), 559–563.

Titler, M. G., Kleiber, C., Steelman, V., Goode, C., Rakel, B., Barry-Walker, J., Small, S., & Buckwalter, K. (1995). Infusing research into practice to promote quality care. *Nursing Research, 43*(5), 307–313.

Tsai, S. (2003). The effects of a research utilization inservice program on nurses. *International Journal of Nursing Studies, 40,* 105–113.

Woodham-Smith, C. (1950). *Florence Nightingale.* London: Constable & Co.

Youngblut, J. M., & Brooten, D. (2000). Moving research into practice: A new partner. *Nursing Outlook, 48*(2), 55–56.

The Nurse as Political Advocate

Objectives

- Discuss the role that power plays in nursing practice.
- Discuss the relevance of political action to nursing.
- Explain various strategies used to influence political decision making.
- Identify skills that are essential to political action.
- Identify ways in which nurses can participate in the political arena.

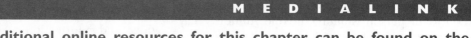

M E D I A L I N K

Additional online resources for this chapter can be found on the companion Web site at http://www.prenhall.com/blais.

Nurses are actively participating in political processes to promote change within the profession and to influence policymaking regarding nursing and health care policy issues. The realities of the health care scene, such as more government regulation and increasingly scarce resources, demand that nurses become knowledgeable about and capable of influencing the development of health care policy and the delivery of care to clients.

Although political action is ordinarily associated with governmental concerns, Mason, Leavitt, and Chaffee (2002) identify four spheres of political action.

These spheres are interconnected and overlapping; they include the workplace, government, professional organizations, and community. In the workplace, policies and procedures may be the focus of political action, and government and professional organizations as well as the community may influence these workplace policies. Professional organizations play a key role in influencing the practice of nursing through standards of practice, lobbying, and collective action. Nursing has become increasingly focused on the community, particularly through the American Nurses Association's agenda for health care reform. (See Chapter 17 ⚭, Nursing in an Evolving Health Care Delivery System.)

CHALLENGES AND OPPORTUNITIES

Political power is a concept that has not been traditionally associated with nursing. In fact, nursing has been seen as powerless with regard to decisions about clinical practice, stemming from the fact that nurses are predominantly female, working in a male-dominated setting. Nursing is challenged to change that perception and assume more power over its own practice.

In recent years, more nurses have been appointed to senior administrative positions and elected to public office, and the image is changing. These changes create opportunities for nurses to influence policy and assume power commensurate with their knowledge and expertise as care providers.

POWER

Power is described as one of the most difficult concepts to define and measure (Mason & Leavitt, 1998). One definition is "power is the potential capacity to influence events, cause change, initiate action, and control outcomes" (Lee, 2000, p. 26). Often, the terms *power, influence,* and *authority* are used interchangeably, but they need to be differentiated. Power is the potential ability to influence action and the capacity to produce or prevent change. Influence is the use of power, but it is more subtle than power. Authority is based on one's position within an organization that assigns power to the person assuming the role. Authority may be delegated for certain tasks.

Empowerment

The concept of empowerment has been applied since the 1970s to promote the rights of ethnic and sexual minorities in training and education programs and organizational development (Kuokkanen & Leino-Kilpi, 2000). It is associated with attempts to increase power and influence of oppressed groups. Recently the concept has been more broadly applied to varying groups and the individual. The basic element of empowerment is taking action to generate positive results at both the individual and organizational level.

A useful theoretical framework for application of empowerment to practice is Kanter's (1993) theory of organizational empowerment. Assumptions of this theory are that people react rationally to their situations and that situations structured to support employees' feelings of empowerment result in benefit to the organization in effectiveness and employee attitude. The organizational structures that benefit the growth of empowerment are (1) having access to information, (2) receiving support, (3) having access to resources necessary to do the job, and (4) having the opportunity to learn and grow. Management should create conditions for work effectiveness by ensuring that employees have the access they need to information, support, and resources in order to do their job and that they have opportunity for employee development. This results in employees being more productive and effective in meeting the organization's goals. A model of Kanter's theory is shown in Figure 11–1■.

Conger and Kanungo (1988) pose additions to the Kanter model by arguing that managers or leaders need to eliminate situations fostering powerlessness and use motivation strategies. They further pose that task accomplishment builds a sense of competence and self-determination. Attempts at empowerment without consideration of employee capability may not result in empowerment of people who are incapable or overwhelmed or unmotivated.

Sources of Power

Power theorists describe a variety of sources from which a person derives power. Understanding these sources of power is prerequisite to formulating a plan for developing one's own power and recognizing it in others. French and Raven (1960, pp. 607–623) identified five sources of power: legitimate, reward, coercive, referent, and expert powers. Hershey, Blanchard, and Johnson (2001) added two more: connection (association) and information powers. Most leaders use all types of power at different times, depending on the particular situation.

- *Legitimate (or positional) power* derives from one's formal position or title in an organization. It is associated with the authority that the position gives its holder to make and enforce decisions. The title "vice president for nursing" implies that the holder has power by virtue of the position, regardless of who holds that position or how effective that person is.
- *Reward power* is derived from the perception of one's abilities to bestow rewards or favors on others.
- *Coercive power,* by contrast, arises from the perception of one's ability to threaten, harm, or punish others.
- *Information power* is associated with persons who are perceived to control key information. Reward, coercive, and informational power all relate to the degree an individual can control the distribution of resources.

Figure 11–1

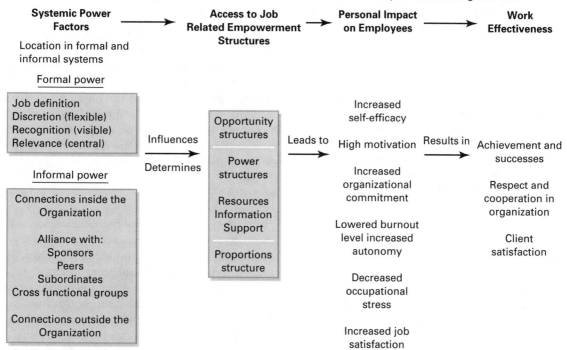

Relationship of Concepts in Rosabeth Kanter's (1979) Structural Theory of Power in Organizations

Source: From "Organizational trust and empowerment in restructured healthcare settings: Effects on staff nurse commitment," by H. K. S. Laschinger, J. Finegan, J. Shamian, and S. Casier, 2000, *Journal of Nursing Administration, 30*(9), 415. Used by permission.

Evidence for Practice

Laschinger, H. K. S., Almost, J., & Tuer-Hodes, D. (2003). Workplace empowerment and magnet hospital characteristics. *Journal of Nursing Administration, 33*(7/8), 410–422. Data from three studies were combined for secondary analysis testing a model linking nurses' perception of workplace empowerment, magnet hospital characteristics, and job satisfaction. Two of the studies were conducted with staff nurses and one with acute-care nurse practitioners working in Ontario, Canada. Hypotheses were:

1. Higher levels of workplace empowerment are positively related to perceptions of autonomy, control over practice environments, and collaboration with physicians within the work setting.

2. Higher levels of empowerment and magnet hospital characteristics in nursing work settings are positively related to nurses' job satisfaction.

Data were collected by survey using three instruments: Conditions of Work Effectiveness II, Nursing Work Index-R, and a job satisfaction questionnaire.

Nurse practitioner's ratings of work empowerment were higher than those of the staff nurses. Both hypotheses were supported. Empowerment strongly correlated to the score on the Nursing Work Index. The combination of empowerment and magnet hospital characteristics were significant predictors of job satisfaction. Access to resources was strongly related to magnet hospital characteristics for all three samples but was particularly important for empowerment of the staff nurses; this included adequate staffing.

Key findings of the study are that greater access to workplace empowerment was associated with higher perceptions of autonomy, increased control over the practice environment, and better nurse-physician relationships. Access to resources and support had the greatest impact over autonomy and control over practice, and informal power had the strongest impact on nurse-physician relationships. Empowerment increased perceptions of magnet hospital characteristics in the workplace and increased job satisfaction.

Nursing administrators can use the research to examine the workplace for barriers to nurse empowerment factors that support professional practice.

■ *Referent (charismatic or personal) power* is derived from an individual's own vision, sense of self, and ability to communicate these so that others regard the person with admiration and are motivated to follow.

■ *Connection (associative) power* derives from the perception that one has important contacts or relationships with others. These connections can be an aspect of both formal and informal networks.

■ *Expert (or knowledge) power* is derived from one's expertise, talents, and skills. One can include in this category Benner's (1984) vision of power, that is, the positive power the nurse brings to the nurse-client relationship. This power enables the nurse to transform the client's life through advocacy and other means of caring.

The box on page 203 provides guidelines for the use of each source of power.

Some feminist scholars believe this framework of power to be based on masculine norms. They prefer to see sources of power available to women as based on structural, individual, organizational, interpersonal, and symbolic factors (Kelly & Duerst-Lahti, 1995). Women tend to be more comfortable with power sharing and view models of power as being less hierarchical (Mason, Leavitt, & Chaffee, 2002).

Caring Types of Power

Benner (1984), in her classic work on clinical nursing excellence, describes six types of power that nurses can use when dealing with clients and significant others. These are powers that are associated with caring: transformative, integrative, advocacy, healing, participative/affirmative, and problem-solving powers.

Transformative Power

Transformative power represents the ability of the nurse to assist clients to change their views of reality or their own self-images. Nurses display this type of power in caring for clients who have long-term illness. Providing compassionate care to clients who are unable to perform their normal hygienic care can help transform their self-image from one of worthlessness to one of value.

Integrative Power

Integrative power is the nurse's ability to assist a client to return to a normal life. In this process, the nurse helps clients integrate any disabilities into their lives and assists them back into the family and society.

Advocacy Power

Advocacy power enables the nurse to help a client and significant others deal with a health care bureaucracy. The nurse can explain to the client what services are available. In addition, the nurse can act as an "interpreter" between the client and physician. For example, a client may hesitate to express a concern to a busy physician. Recognizing that the physician may be able to ease the client's mind, the nurse may act as a liaison between the two.

Healing Power

Nurses can establish a healing relationship and a healing climate with a client. According to Benner, nurses can do this by mobilizing hope in themselves, the staff, and the client; finding an interpretation or understanding of a specific situation; and assisting the client to use social, emotional, and/or spiritual support. Benner writes that an affirming and caring nurse-client relationship provides a basis for healing. A healing relationship empowers the client by bringing hope, confidence, and trust (1984, p. 213).

Participative/Affirmative Power

Participative/affirmative power is the nurse's ability to draw strength by investing it in others. Benner disputes the more traditional view that nurses have only so much emotional strength to draw on and suggests that involvement and caring permit nurses to obtain strength (1984, p. 214).

Problem Solving

A committed person is more sensitive to cues than a less committed person; thus, a caring and involved nurse is able to solve problems at a higher level than a less involved nurse. Commitment and caring enhance the nurse's receptivity to cues and enables the nurse to recognize solutions that are not obvious. These abilities are due partly to intuition and feeling.

Laws of Power

Berle describes power as a "universal experience and human attribute of man with five discernable natural laws" (1969, p. 32).

Law 1: Power invariably fills any vacuum. People generally prefer peace and order and are usually willing to

Guidelines for the Use of Power in Organizations

USING AUTHORITY

1. Make polite requests, not arrogant demands.
2. Make requests in clear, simple language; check for staff understanding.
3. Explain reasons for requests.
4. Follow up to check for compliance.

USING REWARDS

1. Don't overemphasize incentives; staff will expect rewards for every request. Emphasize mutual loyalty and teamwork.
2. Rewards are unlikely to produce commitment.
3. Reinforce past behavior; don't bribe for future performance.
4. The size of rewards should reflect total performance.
5. Money is not the only (and is often the least effective) reward.
6. Avoid appearing manipulative at all costs.

USING COERCIVE POWER

1. Avoid coercion and punishment except when absolutely necessary.
2. Punish only to deter extremely detrimental behavior.
3. Try to determine genuine responsibility or liability before taking corrective action.
4. Discipline promptly and consistently without favoritism. Fit the punishment to the seriousness of the infraction.
5. State consequences without hostility; remain calm and express desire to help subordinate comply with requirements and avoid discipline.
6. Invite subordinate to share in responsibility for correcting disciplinary problems; set improvement goals and develop improvement plans.
7. Warn before punishing; don't issue idle or exaggerated warnings you are not prepared to carry out.

USING EXPERT POWER

1. Preserve credibility by avoiding careless statements and rash decisions.
2. Keep informed about technical developments affecting the group's work.
3. In a crisis, remain calm; act confidently and decisively.
4. Avoid arrogance or talking down to staff; show respect for staff ideas and suggestions and incorporate them whenever feasible.
5. Do not threaten subordinates' self-esteem.
6. Recognize subordinates' concerns; explain why a proposed plan of action is best and what steps will be taken to minimize risk to them.

USING REFERENT POWER

1. Be considerate, show concern for staff needs and feelings, treat them fairly, and defend their interests to superiors and outsiders.
2. Avoid expressing hostility, distrust, rejection, or indifference toward subordinates. Actions speak louder than words.
3. Explain the personal importance of requests and your reliance on staff support and cooperation.
4. Don't make requests too often; make requests reasonable.
5. Be a good role model.

USING CONNECTION POWER

1. Consider carefully the appropriate use of the connection or relationship.
2. Avoid name dropping.
3. Provide sound rationale for using the relationship.
4. Recognize the likelihood of being expected to reciprocate in return for favors provided in a relationship.
5. Recognize the reasonable limits of the connection. Don't overuse or exploit.

Source: From *Effective Leadership and Management in Nursing* (5th ed., p. 46), by E. J. Sullivan, and P. J. Decker, 2001, Upper Saddle River, NJ: Prentice Hall. Used by permission.

Evidence for Practice

Laschinger, H. K. S., Finegan, J., Shamian, J., & Casier, S. (2000). Organizational trust and empowerment in restructured healthcare settings. *Journal of Nursing Administration, 30*(9), 413–425.

A predictive, nonexperimental design was used to test Kanter's theory linking staff-nurse work empowerment to organizational trust and organizational commitment. A random sample of 412 Canadian staff nurses was surveyed, with five self-report scales used to measure work empowerment. The overall work-empowerment score suggests that nurses perceived only moderate empowerment in their work settings. They did not believe that they had a high degree of formal power in their jobs but did perceive a moderate amount of informal power. The nurses reported higher confidence and trust in their peers than in management. The results of the study support the proposition that staff nurses' empowerment affects their trust in management and ultimately influences affective commitment. Staff nurses believed that their sense of workplace empowerment strongly affected their trust in management and subsequently their belief and acceptance of organizational goals and values, their willingness to exert effort in the workplace, and their desire to stay in the organization (affective commitment). The strongest relationships were found between trust in management and perceived access to information and support. The authors believe that the findings stress the importance of creating environments that provide access to structures that empower nurses to accomplish their work.

give power to someone who will restore order and thereby reduce their discomfort. When a problem arises, an individual will usually show the initiative to handle the problem and thus will exert power. Nurses should be aware that these are opportunities to assume power.

Law 2: Power is invariably personal. In many instances, people who effect change find common ground and come together committed to that change. To be successful, nurses must develop personal power, that is, the power one develops in oneself: self-esteem, self-respect, and self-confidence. Through their pro-

Evidence for Practice

Ellefsen, B., & Hamilton, G. (2000). Empowered nurses? Nurses in Norway and the USA compared. *International Nursing Review, 47,* 106–120.

This comparative study investigated the degree to which nurses from two major university hospitals in two different countries experienced empowerment. Five hundred ninety Norwegian nurses and 135 North American nurses responded to five self-report questionnaires based upon Kanter's theory of empowerment. Formal power explained 51% of the variance in the overall empowerment score, and the combination of formal and informal power explained 65%. The Norwegian nurses experienced slightly more informal power, whereas the North American nurses experienced more formal power. The small difference in reported experience of the nurses in two different countries is an interesting finding.

Rules for Using Power

1. Use the least amount of power you can to be effective in your interactions with others.
2. Use power appropriate to the situation.
3. Learn when not to use power.
4. Focus on the problem, not the person.
5. Make polite requests, never arrogant demands.
6. Use coercion only when other methods don't work.
7. Keep informed to retain your credibility when using your expert power.
8. Understand you may owe a return favor when you use your connection power.

Source: From *Becoming Influential: A Guide for Nurses* (p. 35), by E. J. Sullivan, 2004, Upper Saddle River, NJ: Prentice Hall. Used by permission.

fessional organizations, nurses can then exert personal power in the health care field.

Law 3: Power is based on a system of ideas and philosophy. When people demonstrate behaviors that indicate power, they reflect a personal belief or philosophy. It is this belief or philosophic system that gains followers and their respect. Nurses, however, have traditionally been comfortable "taking orders" and accommodating a hospital hierarchy rather than taking the initiative in such spheres as clients' rights and preventive care. Current problems in the health care system, such as increasing technology and cost, offer nurses an opportunity to fill a vacuum for change in the health care system and thereby offer solutions to these problems.

Law 4: Power is exercised through and depends on organizations. Individuals can feel powerless and unable to deal with many situations in a hospital, community agency, government agency, or other institution. By banding together with others through a state or provincial nursing organization, nurses can magnify their power and support changes in health care.

Law 5: Power is invariably confronted with, and acts in the presence of, a field of responsibility. Nurses in power positions act on behalf of other nurses or clients. Power is communicated to people observing the situation and is reinforced by positive responses. If group members believe that their beliefs or ideals are not represented, the vacuum will be filled by another person who can carry out the role and is supported by the organization.

Reflect on...

- sources of power available to you as a clinical nurse. How can you enhance your expert power, your advocacy power, your healing power, your connection power, and your participative/affirmative power?
- how a nurse's self-image can affect that nurse's referent power.
- how expert power can enhance legitimate power.

POLITICS

Politics can also be defined as "influencing—specifically, influencing the allocation of scarce resources" (Mason et al., 2002, p. 9). Defined in this way, the word denotes more than action in the governmental arena; it is also applicable to every sphere of life where resources are limited and more than one person or group competes for them. It is altering the outcome in decisions about how to divide resources among competing people or groups. *Resources* may refer not only to money but also to any number of cherished assets that are limited, such as personnel, programs, time, status, and power.

The allocation of scarce resources involves everyone in some way. The following are examples of situations of scarce resources:

- A student applying for a college loan or competing with other students for his or her fair share of a teacher's time and attention.
- A client advocate competing for hospital education funds in order to provide more preoperative teaching.
- A citizen lobbying against the school board's proposal to divide one RN's time between two large schools.
- A member of a professional association seeking association action on a practice issue, such as care of clients with acquired immune deficiency syndrome (AIDS).

Nurses have long been involved in politics. For example, the founder of modern nursing, Florence Nightingale, used her contacts with powerful men in government to obtain needed personnel and supplies for wounded soldiers in the Crimea. Subsequent nursing leaders such as Lavinia Dock, Lillian Wald, Harriet Tubman, and Margaret Sanger—who were all skilled politicians and made significant contributions to the profession and society—may have been influenced by these wise words of Nightingale:

> When I entered service here, I determined that, happen what would, I never would intrigue among the Committee. Now I perceive that I do all my business by intrigue. I propose in private to A, B, or C the resolution I think A, B, or C most capable of carrying in Committee, and then leave it to them, and I always win. (Huxley, 1975, p. 53)

Political action refers to action by a group of individuals that is designed to attain a purpose through the use of political power or through the established political process. Policy is shaped by politics and has been defined as the principles that govern actions directed toward given ends; policy statements outline a plan, direction, or goal for action. **Policy** encompasses the choices that a society, segment of society, or organization make regarding its goals and priorities and how it will allocate its resources. Governmental bodies form public policy. Social policy pertains to directives that promote the welfare of the public. Institutional policies govern the workplace. Organizational policies govern professional organizations. Policies may be laws, guidelines, or regulations that govern behavior in government, workplaces, organizations, and committees.

Guidelines for Negotiation

- Obtain all of the essential facts of the issue beforehand.
- Explore the other party's viewpoint. If the other party is a legislator, for example, obtain information about his or her views from news media and congressional records.
- Consider the consequences of the issue and how you can deflect those consequences to support your viewpoint.
- Verify the strength of your own viewpoint and ways to strengthen it further; then consider ways to counteract or weaken the other party's viewpoint.
- Determine any limitations surrounding your viewpoint, such as time constraints or other resources.
- Consider other groups that support your viewpoint or that of the other party.

Strategies to Influence Political Decisions

Many of the strategies used to influence political decisions will serve the nurse well in everyday professional activities.

Negotiating

Negotiation is a give-and-take process between individuals and groups to work out differences of opinion regarding the best solution to an issue. Two basic forms of negotiation are problem-solving negotiation and trade-off negotiation. In *problem-solving negotiation,* both parties confer to resolve a complex situation together. In *trade-off negotiation,* one party gives some concessions, or "points," to the other party in exchange for other concessions, or points. Negotiating demands good communication skills of all participants. Before beginning negotiation, the nurse needs to know all the essential facts of the issue and conduct research to support a particular viewpoint. A familiar example of the negotiating process for nurses is the collective bargaining (contract negotiations) process between employees and employers. Guidelines for negotiation are found in the accompanying box.

Networking

Networking refers to a process in which people with similar interests and goals communicate, share ideas and information, and offer support and direction to each other. Network development builds linkages with people throughout the profession, both within and outside the work environment. Getting to know people helps build a trust relationship that can facilitate

the achievement of professional goals: It is easier to access people one knows than it is to access strangers.

Nurses can develop networks by (1) attending local, regional, and national conferences; (2) taking classes for continuing education or toward an academic degree; (3) joining alumni associations and attending alumni meetings; (4) joining and participating in professional organizations; (5) keeping in touch with former teachers and coworkers; and (6) socializing with professional colleagues.

Political networks generally have three functions: (1) to provide information about legislative activities

Critical Thinking Exercise

Using the Guidelines for Negotiation found in the accompanying box, plan a strategy for the following situations:

1. Your institution has money available for a 6% salary increase for RNs. Administration wants to give it all on the basis of merit (reward). You and several of your colleagues believe there should be an across the board cost of living raise for all RNs.

2. Your state legislature or provincial government is considering whether mandatory CEUs should be a condition of relicensure. You can assume the position of advocating either for or against mandatory continuing education.

on particular issues, (2) to increase political action and awareness, and (3) to promote issues through the legislative process. These networks may be formal, with signed agreements and fee structures, or informal, requiring minimal monetary contributions.

Preparing Resolutions

Resolutions are formal statements expressing the opinion, will, or intent of an individual or group. Most nurses will be familiar with the specific format used to present resolutions at annual association meetings or conventions about nursing and health care concerns. Resolutions are an effective means of writing concise reasons and proposed recommendations for action, particularly for areas where services are inadequate. Nurses who present resolutions must, however, be well informed about the data presented, be prepared to offer additional data others might request, and be willing to consider amendments to the recommendations.

Establishing Political Action Committees

Political action committees (PACs) endorse candidates for public office, such as the senate and the house of representatives. Because tax laws limit nonprofit professional organizations from participating in various types of political activities, PACs provide an avenue for professional political action activities. Groups such as nursing organizations, women's groups, church groups, and civic groups may form PACs. Members of a PAC provide additional donations or pay dues to support the organization's activities because general membership fees in any nonprofit organization cannot be used to support such activity. Because they are used for political purposes, donations made to a PAC are not tax deductible.

The American Nurses Association (ANA) Political Action Committee (ANA-PAC) is a political organization formed by the ANA. Many state nursing organizations also have political action organizations that serve similar functions on the state level as ANA-PAC does on the national level. PACs support legislative candidates based on their stands on key issues. For example, ANA-PAC would consider a candidate's stand on such specific health and nursing issues as national health insurance, third-party reimbursement for nurses, funding for biomedical and nursing research, elder abuse, and so on. Although nursing PACs have not created power equal to that of such groups as labor, education, and medicine, nurses are becoming more sophisticated in the political process and are gaining increased power.

Communicating with Legislators

Nurses can communicate with legislators through telephone calls, telegrams, face-to-face meetings, e-mail, fax, and written letters. For each method, the nurse needs to identify clearly the issue and the bill (by number if possible), explain reasons for interest in the issue, and provide constructive information and ideas. Telephone calls are usually received by a legislative assistant who keeps a record of all calls and the positions of the callers. In many regions, a toll-free number is available during the legislative session.

For visits to legislative officials, the nurse first needs to contact the local offices, which will provide assistance in arranging the visit and may additionally arrange other activities, such as tours of the legislature, attendance at committee hearings, and visits to a legislative session. Before the visit, the nurse should obtain information about the legislators's background, such as the legislator's occupation, previous professional and civic activities, political affiliation, voting record, and interests. Because only a few minutes may be allotted to the visit, the nurse should be prepared to be succinct in presenting personal ideas and facts, allow time for the legislator to answer questions, and leave a summary of facts and recommendations with the legislator to emphasize your perspective of the visit.

Letters are probably the most common mode of communicating with elected officials. Personal letters that reflect thoughtful and informed comments about an issue often receive more attention from legislators than form letters or postcards. When writing to legislators, the nurse should use a professional letterhead and address the public official appropriately. For example, in written communication, the president, vice president, senators, and state representatives are cited as The Honorable (full name) followed by their position (e.g., President of the United States) and the specific address. Salutations in letters are written as Dear Mr. (or Madame) President/Vice President or Dear Senator (full name), or Dear Representative (last name). When communicating in person it is appropriate to say the following: Mr. or Madame President/ Vice President or President (last name); Senator (last name); and Representative or Mr./Ms. (last name). Elements to include in the letter follow:

- A statement of the request in the first sentence (e.g., "I request that you support Bill XY604") and a brief summary of the issue.
- A brief rationale for the request (e.g., "The bill is vital to improving . . ." or "the bill will adversely affect . . .").

■ Factual data that support your viewpoint.

■ A closing statement thanking the legislator for his or her concern and continuing support or attention.

■ Appropriate closing. For a letter to the president of the United States, the appropriate closing is "Very respectfully yours"; for all other letters, "Sincerely yours."

In general, e-mail messages and faxed copies are useful when time constraints exist, but they tend to have less impact.

Building Coalitions

Coalitions are alliances that distinct bodies, persons, or states form to achieve a common purpose. Coalitions are like networks in function but differ in that the members of the coalition represent groups with numerous purposes and issues. The groups negotiate, compromise, and merge to achieve specific goals. Groups or organizations may be in coalition on one issue but adversaries on another. Building coalitions is a strategy to empower oneself; thus, nurses solicit organizations whose power is greater than their own. Groups with whom nurses may form coalitions are as diverse as the topics that are of concern to nurses; women's issues, child care, and the environment are only a few examples.

Professional specialty organizations frequently form coalitions for areas of common interest. For example, the American Association of Critical Care Nurses is building coalitions with the American Nurses Association, the Emergency Nurses Association, and the American Hospital Association in order to advocate for common interests of those groups.

Lobbying

Lobbying is a process in which individuals or groups attempt to influence legislators to support or oppose particular legislation. Lobbyists monitor legislative activities and communicate the group's position to members of the legislature. Groups from various sources may employ professional lobbyists: public relations firms, management relation firms, legal firms, legislative consultants, and independent lobbyists, many of whom are former legislators. Which source is used depends on the issue. Law firms, for example, can provide legal advice as well as lobbying; public relations firms generally provide media resources for campaigns. Individuals and groups can lobby independently, but such efforts require considerable time, personnel, and funding. Lobbyists must follow various legal guidelines. Lobbying techniques include negoti-

ating, media and letter-writing campaigns, testifying, endorsements, and donations.

Testifying

Decisions related to health care and nursing are often made by committees and commissions of various levels of government. These committees frequently conduct hearings to obtain information before making a decision. Hearings generally include people or groups with opposing views. **Testifying** refers to the presentation of information at a committee hearing, usually about controversial aspects of a proposed bill. Nurses may testify either as independent individuals or as official representatives of an organization. Opportunities to testify may be found in professional publications or newspapers. Guidelines for testifying are shown in the box on page 209. Most committees will accept written testimony if the individual cannot be present.

Developing Political Astuteness and Skill

By contributing to political activities in various ways, nurses can develop their political astuteness and skills. All nurses, as citizens and employees, can join and participate in organizations and participate in election processes. However, nurses who are employed by a governmental agency, such as the Veterans Administration or a public health department, must follow restrictions defined in the Hatch Act regarding their political activity. These restrictions do not apply to the general public and include serving as an officer or spokesperson of a particular political party. The major objective of the Hatch Act initiated in the 1930s was to prevent government workers from being forced to support political activities. Although these restrictions remain controversial, attempts to modify and repeal the Hatch Act have failed. Because each state has its own version of this act, nurses who are employed by state governmental agencies are advised to investigate specific limitations in their state of employment.

A statement of three key assumptions must precede a discussion of when and where to engage in political action:

1. *Individuals who are deeply concerned about a particular issue or cause are most likely to identify ways to take action.* Before becoming politically involved, an individual must make choices, including the conscious decision to set aside the necessary resources. For

Guidelines for Testifying

- Confirm the time to register. In some instances, registration occurs at the meeting place on the day of testifying; in others, you must notify the committee of your visit to testify at a specified time before the hearing.

- Prepare your testimony concisely and clearly in advance. Avoid the use of professional terminology that may not be understood by the legislators, or explain any technical terms used.

- Dress appropriately to convey your professional status, and introduce yourself. Make your position clear so that legislators know whether you are representing an organization. Some places may have a dress code; for example, men may be required to wear a suit and tie when testifying before a legislative body. The dress code may be stated or inferred. It is always a good idea to ask if you are unsure.

- Maintain a courteous, professional composure throughout the hearing. Adhere to the rules of the proceedings.

- Verify any time limits to your presentation so that you can present essential facts and arguments first.

- Provide copies of your written testimony, including any graphs or other illustrations, to each committee member.

- Present your material without reading it to make the presentation more interesting for the listeners. Summarize the main ideas. Convey knowledge of the subject.

- Answer any questions completely. Be prepared to support any facts and figures you present with appropriate sources.

- Thank the committee for allowing your testimony.

example, a student who wants her or his school to offer evening or weekend clinical practice hours may decide to seek election to the student council to work for this change from within.

2. *Political action in any sphere is best carried out by a group.* Individual activism is laudable, but group action is much more effective. It provides change agents with the collegiality and support necessary to sustain a vision for change and fosters creative thinking and planning.

3. *Successful political action requires the thoughtful application of change theory.* Before embarking on a project, the politically astute nurse will review the principles of change theory. Achieving goals for change requires thoughtful planning. Effective political activists plan strategy, much as nurses use the nursing process to evaluate clients' needs for care.

Seeking Opportunities for Political Action

Workplace

The workplace for nurses may be a public or a private (for-profit or nonprofit) organization and that can influence who sets policies and the values underlying the

policies. These can have a profound influence on a nurse's professional life, and it is therefore important to examine ways to influence those policies. It is up to nurses to see that a nursing perspective is available, listened to, and incorporated into decisions about the administration of the organization (Mason et al., 2002). Nurses can exert expert, position, and economic power by negotiating the presence of nurse members on standing committees and the board of trustees and by becoming involved in the collective bargaining process.

In most hospitals, nursing homes, and public health agencies, a system of committees exists to deal with specific issues. For example, a nursing department has an equipment evaluation committee that selects and evaluates client care products used by the nursing staff. A pharmacy committee in the same hospital has representatives from nursing, medicine, and the pharmacy. In addition to formal standing committees, ad hoc committees or task forces can be appointed to deal with particular issues or problems. For example, a task force on a nursing unit might examine the best way to initiate a case management program and critical pathways.

Nurses who have an idea or problem they want addressed are advised to look for existing committees that might already be dealing with the concern or are likely to do so. For example, nurses concerned about staff safety in the parking lot may find that a hospital security committee is already looking into the problem.

Another way to generate interest in an issue is to write an article for the hospital or nursing department newsletter. Nurses who are present at nursing grand rounds also have the opportunity to inform their colleagues of an issue of mutual concern and enlist their aid in dealing with it. If there are no newsletters or grand rounds, a nurse can form a task force of concerned nurses and, using a model for change, plan a strategy to establish ways of helping nurses communicate with one another through a newsletter, grand rounds, or possibly a support group.

Nurses need certain knowledge and skills to increase their political astuteness and activity (Ellis & Hartley, 2001, p. 83–89; Skaggs, 1994, p. 239), as follows:

- *Keeping informed about health care issues.* Obtain information from sources such as the daily newspaper; television and radio news reports; professional journals (space about current legislative issues is routinely provided in national, state, and provincial nursing journals); open meetings of nursing organizations or other health-related organizations, which often sponsor speakers who are knowledgeable about the issue.
- *Ability to analyze an issue.* Identify all the relevant facts about the issue, look at the issue from all angles, and recognize how the issue fits into the larger picture.
- *Ability to speak out and voice an opinion.* Obtain knowledge of both the issue and the best person to whom to voice the opinion. After studying the dynamics of the organization, the nurse may choose a head nurse or supervisor who is a good listener and is concerned about the issue.
- *Ability to participate constructively.* Be a team player who encourages creative brainstorming and offers positive feasible alternative solutions to an issue, rather than offering only criticism.
- *Ability to use power bases.* Through discussion with colleagues and other professional experiences, identify people who influence decision making. It is important to remember that power does not always follow the hierarchical lines on the organizational chart and that the source of information is sometimes considered as powerful as the information itself. The nurse who uses many different channels of information gains power to choose among them.

The politics of client care impinge on the practice of every nurse. For example, the prospective payment system has drastically shortened hospital stays in efforts to reduce hospital costs. Preparing clients for earlier discharge has brought about the need for nurses to be "faster and smarter" in delivering client care and client education.

How can nurses ensure that cost-containment measures do not impair the quality of nursing care? One way is for nurses to collaborate with each other and other providers to delegate nonnursing tasks, such as answering the telephone, emptying the garbage, and transporting nonacute clients. Developing a demonstration project that compares cost and quality of care issues under different hospital unit structures can provide the necessary data and generate support from other providers and administrators for changing the role of staff nurses. This sort of "proactive" planning can empower nurses to take charge of nursing practice in ways that benefit clients and health professionals while conserving scarce resources such as money, time, and supplies.

Nursing Organizations

Powerful and influential professional associations, such as the American Nurses Association and Canadian Nurses Association and their affiliated state/ province and district associations, provide a collective voice for promoting nursing and quality health care. As such, these associations exert influence on the individual nurse as well as in the spheres of government, the workplace, the community, and the profession. Associations monitor and influence laws and regulations affecting nursing and health care. Their role in workplace matters ranges from studying practice issues to acting as the collective bargaining agent for nurses. Additionally, the professional nursing organization is often a visible presence in the community because it presents the nursing perspective on health care issues.

Professional organizations—including the ANA, CNA, NLN, and NSNA—publish articles on legislative matters and encourage nurses to take action on behalf of health care consumers and the nursing profession. Nursing lobbyists at the state and national level work to influence the development of health policy and legislation, but their success depends on the active support of nurses who back up these paid lobbyists by doing personal lobbying among their own elected officials.

The collective efforts of nurses influence the federal government through the political action committees such as the American Nurses Association Political Action Committee (ANA-PAC). ANA-PAC also counts on nurses at the grassroots level to work for these candidates and to serve as congressional district coordinators (CDCs). CDCs are responsible for organizing nurses in their congressional districts for lobbying and campaigning. This effort has provided a mechanism for nurses to influence governmental politics collectively at the federal level.

Individual nurses can become politically active in local, state or provincial, and national organizations by participating in the activities of their professional associations, by serving as delegates at conventions, by becoming members of commissions, and by supporting national association efforts such as the ANA's Nursing Agenda for Health Care Reform. Student nurses can benefit from participation in the National Student Nurses Association (NSNA) by learning about the politics of professional associations.

Community

The community in which the nurse lives and works can include the local neighborhood, the corporate world, the nation, and the international community. The community encompasses the workplace, professional organizations, and government. Many nurses, including Lillian Wald, founder of the Henry Street Settlement and modern public health nursing, view the community as more than a practice setting. Nurses who live in the community where they work can understand and influence the complex interplay among individuals and groups that compete for scarce resources.

Many communities depend on expert nurses to help with a wide variety of health and social policy decisions, such as environmental pollution and health care for the homeless. For example, a nurse who serves as an elected member of the community school board can influence decisions that affect the health and health care of students, such as the hiring of nurses for the school system. Nurses' opinions on matters of public health are frequently sought, and the enterprising nurse looks for opportunities to promote a positive image of nursing while serving the community.

Political involvement in the community often arises out of one's own interest in living and working in a community that is supportive of the health and well-being of its citizens. For example, a nurse may become involved with an ad hoc committee to stop unlawful dumping of hazardous wastes in the neighborhood. As a member of such a group, the nurse wears two hats, as a concerned citizen and as an expert on health issues.

At the same time, the nurse's position in the group enables the nurse to extend networks and expand a support base for nursing.

As the self-help movement continues to expand, nurses are realizing how influential consumer groups can be. In many instances, such groups are founded by nurses who realize the need for a self-help group for their clients. Sometimes nurses who have been clients themselves start postmastectomy support groups or similar groups. Nurses contribute their leadership skills to many organizations, including the National Alliance for the Mentally Ill (NAMI). The personally devastating experience of having a child with schizophrenia can be a powerful motivating force toward working on behalf of others through a group such as NAMI. The political power of groups with particular health concerns—including the Gray Panthers, the American Association of Retired Persons, and the Juvenile Diabetes Association—can generate extraordinary political influence on elected and appointed officials. Such groups offer nurses a variety of ways to learn about grassroots political activism. These groups can also provide a community support base for nursing.

A variety of other opportunities for community involvement exist for nurses. Since many nurses are also parents, they can work on health issues through their school board. Those who ultimately run for government office have frequently begun their careers by running for the school board. Other nurses volunteer for community action groups, such as a community planning board or a fund-raising committee for the city's art museum. Or, a nurse may get involved in the tenant's organization in her or his apartment building. Regardless of the issue, the same opportunity to organize and plan for change exists in the community as it does in the workplace, government, or professional association.

The Government

Numerous ways to influence governments personally are open to nurses. Of course, the most basic step is registering to vote. Voter-registration drives are sponsored by a variety of organizations, including NSNA, which has developed a kit for nursing students to hold such drives. By voting, responsible citizens convey their opinions to elected and appointed officials on matters of concern.

The laws and regulations of local, state, and federal governments greatly influence nursing practice and health care. For example, federal laws and regulations establish funding of health care for the elderly, poor, and disabled (Medicare and Medicaid); authorize care services for special groups (including Native Americans, migrant workers, and veterans); set policies and formulas for reimbursement of health care services (as with prospective payment); and appropriate funding for special health care and social services (such as community health centers, the food stamp program, and the school lunch program).

State and provincial laws are responsible for defining and regulating nursing practice. Nurse practice acts in some states prohibit nurses from providing a broad range of services and can effectively limit nurses' ability to compete with other health care professionals in providing primary care services.

Nurses can become involved with political parties and local political clubs, work with elected officials, and accept political appointments as a means to influence health policy as well as nursing practice. Involvement in political parties and local political clubs enables the nurse to have some influence over affairs in the community and to develop a nonnursing support base for nursing and health care issues.

Nurses can also actively participate in campaigns of politicians who support nursing and health care, can become candidates for legislative offices, and act as information sources for legislative representatives. The accompanying box lists ways to influence the legislative process for nursing and become politically active.

Reflect on...

■ ways in which you have participated in political activities in the past—in the work setting, in professional organizations, in the community, and in government.

■ how you would like to increase your participation in political activities.

■ whether you believe nurses have an obligation to be politically active. Why or why not?

How to Influence Legislative and Regulatory Processes

• Become informed about the public policy and health policy issues that are currently under consideration at the local, state, and federal levels of government.

• Become acquainted with the public officials and elected officials that represent you in the legislative arena at the local, state, and federal levels of government. Communicate with them regularly to share your expertise and perspective on health care and nursing issues.

• Call, write, or send a fax or e-mail message to your legislator, stating briefly the position you wish him or her to take on a particular issue. Always remember to mention that you are a registered nurse and that you live and vote in the legislator's district.

• Request that legislation be introduced or a regulatory change made. Offer your expertise to assist in developing new legislation or in modifying existing legislation/rules.

• Become active in your professional association and work to activate a strong grassroots network of members who are prepared to contact their elected representatives on key health care issues.

• Attend a public hearing on a bill or regulation to show support for an issue, or actually testify yourself.

• Build your own political résumé—become active in local politics in your area.

• Volunteer to work on the campaigns of candidates who are knowledgeable and supportive of nursing's perspective on health care issues.

• Seek appointment to a government task force or commission and have the opportunity to make legislative, regulatory, and public policy changes.

• Seek election to public office or employment in an administrative or executive agency.

• Explore opportunities to be involved with the policy and legislative process through internships, fellowships, and volunteer experiences at the local, state, and federal levels.

Source: From *Policy and Politics in Nursing and Health Care* (4th ed., p. 461), by D. J. Mason, J. K. Leavitt, and M. Chaffee, 2002, Philadelphia: W. B. Saunders. Used by permission.

Critical Thinking Exercise

Select a political issue affecting nursing, such as one of the following:

   a. Reimbursement of nursing services

   b. Equal pay for work of comparable value

   c. National health insurance

   d. Health care reform

Applying the information from the box on page 212, How to Influence Legislative and Regulatory Processes, plan a strategy to bring about change you believe is needed.

 EXPLORE MEDIALINK

Questions, critical thinking exercises, essay activities, and other interactive resources for this chapter can be found on the Web site at http://www.prenhall.com/blais. Click on Chapter 11 to select activities for this chapter.

Bookshelf

Byham, W. C., & Cox, J. (1997). *Zapp! The lightning of empowerment: How to improve quality, productivity, and employee satisfaction.* **New York: Random House.** This book discusses helping workers take ownership of their jobs and manage their own performance improvement. Specific empowerment strategies are presented.

Keller, E. B., & Berry J. L. (2003). *The influentials: One American in ten tells the other nine how to vote, where to eat, and what to buy.* **New York: Simon and Schuster.** Addresses the question, Who are the most influential Americans? This book discusses ways in which these people become influential and how they influence others.

Loeb, P. R. (1999). *Soul of a citizen: Living with conviction in a cynical time.* **New York: St. Martin's Press.** This book presents an alternative to powerlessness and cynicism. It tells stories of ordinary Americans providing lessons about moving from passivity to participation.

SUMMARY

Power is an invaluable instrument, the effects of which can be positive or negative depending on the way it is used and the ends to which it is applied. Power is assumed by a person; it is a skill that can be learned and effectively practiced. Sources or bases of power are described as reward, coercive, legitimate, referent, expert, connection, and information powers. An understanding of these sources helps nurses formulate a plan to develop their own power and to recognize it in others. Benner describes six types of power that nurses use when caring for clients: transformative power, integrative power, advocacy power, healing power, participative/affirmative power, and problem-solving power. Empowerment enables individuals and groups to participate in actions and decision making in a context that supports an equitable distribution of power.

Politics is the process of influencing the allocation of scarce resources in the spheres of government,

workplace, organizations, and community. Political action in one sphere often affects other spheres. Strategies to influence political decisions include negotiating, networking, establishing political action committees, communicating with legislators, building coalitions, lobbying, and testifying.

As citizens, parents, and members of the nursing profession, all nurses can contribute to political activities in numerous ways—by voting, joining organizations, becoming members of committees, supporting deserving candidates, and so on. To make any effective contribution, nurses must keep themselves informed about health care and nursing issues, be able to analyze an issue, voice an opinion, participate constructively, use power bases, and communicate clearly. Nurses who value the nursing perspective on health issues recognize that a powerful voice for nurses is a powerful voice for health care consumers, the profession, and the nation.

REFERENCES

Benner, P. (1984). *From novice to expert: Excellence and power in clinical nursing practice.* Menlo Park, CA: Addision-Wesley Nursing.

Berle, A. A. (1969). *Power.* New York: Harcourt, Brace, and World.

Boykin, A. (Ed.) (1995). *Power, politics and public policy: A matter of caring.* New York: National League for Nursing. Pub. no. 14–2684.

Conger, J. A., & Kanungo, R. N. (1988). The empowerment process: Integrating theory and practice. *Academic Management Review, 13*(3), 471–482.

Ellefsen, B., & Hamilton, G. (2000). Empowered nurses? Nurses in Norway and the USA compared. - *International Nursing Review, 47,* 106–120.

Ellis, J. R., & Hartley, C. L. (2001). *Nursing in today's world: Challenges, issues, and trends* (7th ed.). Philadelphia: Lippincott.

French, J. R., & Raven, B. H. (1960). The bases of social power. In D. Cartwright & A. Zanders (Eds.), *Group dynamics: Research and theory* (2nd ed.). New York: Harper and Row.

Hershey, P., Blanchard, K., & Johnson, D. (2001). *Management of organizational behavior: Utilizing human resources* (8th ed.). Upper Saddle River, NJ: Prentice Hall.

Huxley, E. (1975). *Florence Nightingale.* New York: Putnam.

Kanter, R. M. (1993). *Men and women of the corporation,* (2nd ed.). New York: Basic Books.

Kelly, R. M., & Duerst-Lahti, G. (1995). The study of gender power and its link to governance and leadership. In G. Duerst-Lahti & R. N. Kelly (Eds.), *Gender power, leadership and governance* (pp. 39–64). Ann Arbor: University of Michigan Press.

Kuokkanen, L., & Leino-Kilpi, H. (2000). Power and empowerment in nursing: Three theoretical approaches. *Journal of Advanced Nursing, 31*(1), 235–241.

Laschinger, H. K. S., Almost, J., & Tuer-Hodes, D. (2003). Workplace empowerment and magnet hospital characteristics. *Journal of Nursing Administration, 33*(7/8), 410–422.

Laschinger, H. K. S., Finegan, J., Shamian, J., & Casier, S. (2000). Organizational trust and empowerment in restructured healthcare settings: Effects on staff nurse commitment. *Journal of Nursing Administration, 30*(9), 413–425.

Lee, L. (2000, October). Buzzwords with a basis. *Nursing Management, 10,* 25–27.

Mason, D. J., & Leavitt, J. K. (1998). *Policy and politics in nursing and health care* (3rd ed.). Philadelphia: W. B. Saunders.

Mason, D. J., Leavitt, J. K., & Chaffee, M. (2002). *Policy and politics in nursing and health care* (4th ed.). Philadelphia: W. B. Saunders.

Skaggs, B. (1994). Political action in nursing. In J. Zerwekh & J. C. Claborn, *Nursing today: Transitions and trends* (pp. 236–256). Philadelphia: W. B. Saunders.

Sullivan, E. (2004). *Becoming influential: A guide for nurses.* Upper Saddle River, NJ: Prentice Hall.

Sullivan, E., & Decker, P. (2001). *Effective leadership and management in nursing.* Upper Saddle River, NJ: Prentice Hall.

The Nurse as Colleague and Collaborator

Objectives

- Explain the essential aspects of collaborative health care.
- Discuss the nurse's collaborative role.
- Describe the competencies in collaborative practice.
- Analyze factors that affect collaboration in health care.

M E D I A L I N K

Additional online resources for this chapter can be found on the companion Web site at http://www.prenhall.com/blais.

Changing models of health care have created a need for modification of traditional roles. Nurses and physicians have been especially affected by these changes and work more collaboratively as colleagues. According to the American Nurses Association (ANA) (1995):

The boundaries of each health care professional are constantly changing, and members of various professions cooperate by exchanging knowledge and ideas about how to deliver high-quality health care. Collaboration among health care professionals involves recognition of the expertise of others within and outside one's profession and referral to those providers when appropriate. Collaboration also involves some shared functions and common focus on the same overall mission.

Traditionally, models of health care have shown a one-sided distribution of power in provider-client relationships. The system has been physician dominated and has focused on cure of illness. Recently, however, the health care system has moved toward more collaborative efforts and initiatives in which providers and clients become partners in care. Many advance the idea that care is client centered and client directed and involves collaboration between provider and client.

With the restructuring of health care, the old systems and practices have changed health jobs in ways designed to improve care and control costs. This restructuring has changed roles and created new ways of interacting among the members of the health care team.

CHALLENGES AND OPPORTUNITIES

Resistance to change is inevitable when the traditional ways of providing care have been so drastically disrupted by the changes in health care that were outside the control of those affected by the change. Changes in power structure are particularly difficult to manage. Nurses need to develop the ability to assume a new place in health care and work with those members of the team who are not fully accepting of the new structure.

Opportunities to create new practice models and redefine relationships are now abundantly available to nurses. The time is ripe for a reshaping of practice under the direction of those willing to assume leadership.

COLLABORATIVE HEALTH CARE

During the early years, the nurse was seen as providing assistance to the physician in caring for patients. The term *handmaiden* has been used to describe the role. However, during wars and times of crisis, nurses worked in a more collegial and autonomous manner. As early as the American Civil War, there is documentation of a more independent practice (ANA, 1998). The emergence of advanced practice nursing roles provided impetus to the emerging concerns about collegiality and collaboration. In 1992, the ANA held a Congress on Nursing Practice and adopted the following operational definition of collaboration:

Collaboration means a collegial working relationship with another health care provider in the provision of (to supply) patient care. Collaborative practice requires (may include) the discussion of patient diagnosis and cooperation in the management and delivery of care. Each collaborator is available to the other for consultation either in person or by communication device, but need not be physically present on the premises at the time the actions are performed. The patient-designated health care provider is responsible for the overall direction and management of patient care. (ANA, 1992)

Virginia Henderson (1991, p. 44), one of the pioneers of nursing, defines collaborative care as "a partnership relationship between doctors, nurses, and other health care providers with patients and their families." It is a process by which health care professionals work together with clients to achieve quality health care outcomes. Mutual respect and a true sharing of both power and control are essential elements. Ideally, collaboration becomes a dynamic, interactive process in which clients (individuals, groups, or communities) confer with physicians, nurses, and other health care providers to meet their health objectives. Effective collaboration requires cooperation and coordination between client(s) and various health care providers across the continuum of care. See the box on page 217.

More recently, a published executive summary from the ANA (1998) released in *Nursing Trends and Issues* described collaboration as intrinsic to nursing, as follows:

■ Nurses and physicians working together and independently assessing, diagnosing, and caring for consumers by preparing patient histories, conducting physical and psychosocial assessments, and reviewing and discussing their cases with other health professionals to determine the changing health status of each client.

■ To provide effective and comprehensive care, nurses, physicians, and other health care professionals must collaborate with each other. No group can claim total authority over the other.

■ The different areas of professional competence exhibited by each profession, when combined, provide a continuum of care that the consumer has come to expect.

The ANA *Nursing: Scope and Standards of Practice* (2004) include collaboration by the registered nurse with clients and families as well as other health care providers. See the box on page 217.

Characteristics and Beliefs Basic to Collaborative Health Care

- Clients have a right to self-determination: that is, the right to choose to participate or not to participate in health care decision making.

- Clients and health care professionals interact in a reciprocal relationship. Instead of making decisions about the client's health care, health care professionals foster joint decision making. Client dependence and professional dominance are minimized; client participation in the health care process is maximized.

- Equality among human beings is desired in health care relationships. The ideas of both clients and health care professionals receive an equal hearing.

- Responsibility for health falls on the client rather than on health care professionals.

- Each individual's concept of health is important and legitimate for that individual. Although clients lack expert knowledge, they have their own ideas about health and illness. Health care professionals need to understand these ideas to be able to effectively help the client.

- Collaboration involves negotiation and consensus seeking rather than questioning and ordering.

ANA Standard of Professional Nursing Performance

Standard 11. Collaboration
THE REGISTERED NURSE COLLABORATES WITH PATIENT, FAMILY, AND OTHERS IN THE CONDUCT OF NURSING PRACTICE.

Measurement Criteria
The registered nurse:

- Communicates with the patient, family, and other health care providers regarding patient care and the nurse's role in the provision of that care.

- Collaboration in creating a documented plan, focused on outcomes and decisions related to care and delivery of services, that indicates communication with patients, families, and others.

- Partners with others to effect change and generate positive outcomes through knowledge of the patient or situation.

- Documents referrals, including provisions for continuity of care.

Additional Measurement Criteria for the Advanced Practice Registered Nurse:
The advanced practice registered nurse:

- Partners with other disciplines to enhance patient care through interdisciplinary activities, such as education, consultation, management, technological development, or research opportunities.

- Facilitates an interdisciplinary process with other members of the health care team.

- Documents plan of care communications, rationales for plan of care changes, and collaborative discussions to improve patient care.

Additional Measurement Criteria for Nursing Role Specialty:
The registered nurse in a nursing role specialty:

- Partners with others to enhance health care and, ultimately, patient care through interdisciplinary activities, such as education, consultation, management, technological development, or research opportunities.

- Documents plans, communications, rationales for plan changes, and collaborative discussions.

Source: From *Nursing: Scope and standards practice,* by American Nurses Association, 2004, Washington, DC: ANA. Used by Permission.

A Practice Exemplar of Collaboration

The Heart Center of Excellence of the North Broward Hospital District has developed a practice model based on collaboration, problem solving, and reevaluation, referred to as CPR techniques. Using this model has resulted in drastically reducing postoperative intubation time and the out-of-bed interval following extubation. Same-day admissions, first-day postoperative transfers, and length of stay following cardiac surgery also declined.

The key players in the team included medical staff, nursing, respiratory therapists, perfusionists, radiology technicians, exercise physiologists, case managers/social services, and pharmacy personnel. Collaboration was considered an essential component of success in the team effort.

As the model was implemented, some barriers to collaboration emerged, including the perspectives of the multiple disciplines. A second was the multicultural nature of this diverse staff group; cultural influences were apparent in practice and communication. Beliefs and traditional practices were challenged, which created tension. To build a collaborative team, cultural awareness and education were approached with a variety of techniques, including role-playing, cross-cultural experiences, exploration of personal beliefs and values, and evaluating communication styles.

Self-directed work teams (SDWT) were implemented and made accountable for outcomes. This improved the teamwork and resulted in increased resilience, with a direct effect on patient outcomes. It provided for a best-practice model for successfully improving outcomes in heart centers.

Collaborative Practice

The overall objectives of collaborative initiatives are high-quality client care and client satisfaction. In addition, many health care professionals believe that a multidisciplinary, collaborative framework can limit costs as well as enhance quality. Collaborative practice models propose to achieve the following objectives:

- Provide client-directed and client-centered care using a multidisciplinary, integrated, participative framework.
- Enhance continuity across the continuum of care, from wellness and prevention, prehospitalization through an acute episode of illness, to transfer or discharge and recovery or rehabilitation.
- Improve client(s) and family satisfaction with care.
- Provide quality, cost-effective, research-based care that is outcome driven.
- Promote mutual respect, communication, and understanding between client(s) and members of the health care team.
- Create a synergy among clients and providers, in which the sum of their efforts is greater than the parts.
- Provide opportunities to address and solve system-related issues and problems.
- Develop interdependent relationships and understanding among providers and clients.

Collaborative practice can include nurse-physician interaction in joint practice, nurse-physician collaboration in caregiving, or interdisciplinary teams or committees.

Collaborative health care teams provide comprehensive care by providing a full range of expertise. They can manage care with less redundancy, more efficiency, and fewer omissions (Patel, Cytryn, Shortliffe, & Safran, 2000). These interdisciplinary health care teams have been particularly effective in outpatient services where patients are seen by a primary care physician or by a nurse practitioner and consultations are implemented as needed. The teams deal with specific patient-related problems as well as moving patients through the clinic and hospital efficiently.

The ability to collaborate becomes particularly important when nurses implement advanced-practice roles; it has been designated as a core competency for advanced-practice nurses. The drivers for this have been health care reform, leading to group practice and managed care as well as certification and practice standards. A continuum of collaboration begins with parallel communication, whereby everyone is communicating with the client independently and asking the same questions. Parallel functioning may have more coordinated communication, but each professional

Evidence for Practice

Hojat, M., Nasca, T., Cohen, M., Fields, S., Rattner, S., Griffiths, M., Ibarra, D., de Gonzalez, A., Torres-Ruiz, A., Ibarra, G., & Garcia, A. (2001). Attitudes toward physician-nurse collaboration: A cross-cultural study of male and female physicians and nurses in the United States and Mexico. *Nursing Research, 50*(2), 123–128.

The purpose of this study was to test three hypotheses about attitudes toward collaboration across genders, disciplines, and cultures.

1. U.S. physicians and nurses would both express more positive attitudes toward physician-nurse collaboration than their Mexican counterparts.

2. Nurses would express more positive attitudes toward physician-nurse collaboration than physicians regardless of the country in which they practice.

3. Female physicians would express more positive attitudes toward physician-nurse collaboration than their male counterparts.

An attitude scale was administered to a total of 639 physicians and nurses working in the United States and Mexico. A three-way analysis of variance confirmed the first two hypotheses and did not confirm the third. Based upon these findings, the researchers recommend that medical and nursing schools in both countries include interprofessional education in their curricula to facilitate an understanding of the complementary nature of the roles and to encourage an interdependent relationship. This collaborative education is needed to promote positive attitudes toward collaborative practice.

Figure 12–1

Continuum of Collaboration

Highest Level

- Referral
- Co-management
- Consultation
- Coordination
- Information exchange
- Parallel functioning
- Parallel communication

Lowest Level

are directed to other providers when the problem is beyond their expertise. Figure 12–1■ illustrates this continuum.

Characteristics of effective collaboration include the following:

1. Common purpose and goals identified at the outset
2. Clinical competence of each provider
3. Interpersonal competence
4. Humor
5. Trust
6. Valuing and respecting diverse, complementary knowledge

Processes associated with these characteristics include recurring interactions among the providers of health care that bridge professional boundaries and develop connections. Interpersonal skills and respect for the competence of collaborators are essential to the outcome. Successful consultation comes about when there is recognition of the unique contribution that each person can make so that a unified plan can be implemented.

The Nurse as a Collaborator

Nurses collaborate with clients, peers, and other health care professionals. They frequently collaborate about client care but may also be involved, for example, in collaborating on bioethical issues, on legislation, on health-related research, and with professional

has separate interventions and a separate plan of care. Information exchange involves planned communication, but decision making is unilateral, involving little, if any, collegiality. Coordination and consultation represent midrange levels of collaboration seeking to maximize the efficiency of resources. Co-management and referral represent the upper levels of collaboration, where providers retain responsibility and accountability for their own aspects of care and patients

Evidence for Practice

Sommers, L., Marton, K., Barbaccia, J., & Randolph, J. (2000). Physician, nurse, and social worker collaboration in primary care for chronically ill seniors. *Archives of Internal Medicine, 160*(12), 1825–1833.
An interdisciplinary, collaborative practice intervention for community-dwelling seniors with a chronic illness included a primary care physician, a nurse, and a social worker. A cohort study of 543 patients in 18 private offices was conducted, with half the group receiving care from the collaborative practice team and the other half receiving care from the primary care physician only. Before the start of the study, both groups were determined to be equivalent in service use and self-reported health status. During the study the control group (physician only) increased their hospitalization rate while the intervention group stayed at baseline. Readmission in the intervention group decreased over a year and the control group readmission rate increased. Visits to the physician increased in the control group and decreased in the intervention group. Further, the seniors in the intervention group reported that they engaged in an increased number of social activities compared to the control group. This model of primary care collaborative practice supports the effectiveness in reducing utilization of service and maintaining health status for seniors with chronic illness.

The Nurse as a Collaborator

With Clients:

- Acknowledges, supports, and encourages clients' active involvement in health care decisions.
- Encourages a sense of client autonomy and an equal position with other members of the health care team.
- Helps clients set mutually agreed-upon goals and objectives for health care.
- Provides client consultation in a collaborative fashion.

With Peers:

- Shares personal expertise with other nurses and elicits the expertise of others to ensure quality client care.
- Develops a sense of trust and mutual respect with peers that recognizes their unique contributions.

With Other Health Care Professionals:

- Recognizes the contribution that each member of the interdisciplinary team can make by virtue of his or her expertise and view of the situation.
- Listens to each individual's views.
- Shares health care responsibilities in exploring options, setting goals, and making decisions with clients and families.
- Participates in collaborative interdisciplinary research to increase knowledge of a clinical problem or situation.

With Professional Nursing Organizations:

- Seeks out opportunities to collaborate with and within professional organizations.
- Serves on committees in state (or provincial), national, and international nursing organizations or specialty groups.
- Supports professional organizations in political action to create solutions for professional and health care concerns.

With Legislators:

- Offers expert opinions on legislative initiatives related to health care.
- Collaborates with other health care providers and consumers on health care legislation to best serve the needs of the public.

organizations. The accompanying box outlines selected aspects of the nurse's role as a collaborator.

Collaboration is important in professional nursing practice as a way to improve client outcomes. To fulfill a collaborative role, nurses need to assume accountability and increased authority in practice areas. Education is integral to ensuring that the members of each professional group understand the collaborative nature of their roles, specific contributions, and the importance of working together. Each professional needs to understand how an integrated delivery system centers on the client's health care needs rather than on the particular care given by one group.

Collaboration is not limited to health care professionals. Collaboration with clients is essential. Kim's theory of collaborative decision making in nursing practice (1983, 1987) describes and explains collaborative interactions between clients and nurses in making health care decisions and the effect on outcomes. Dalton (2003) expanded the theory to include the client, nurse, and family caregiver. In this theory, all three enter into the collaboration from their own context of role expectations and attitudes, knowledge, personal traits, and definition of the situation. The three combine to form a coalition with opportunities for collaboration within the context of the situation. The level of collaboration achieved and the nature of the decision are the primary outcomes leading to secondary outcomes of goal attainment, autonomy, and satisfaction. The level of collaboration can range from complete domination of the decision making by the nurse to equal influence on a joint decision by all three.

Benefits of Collaborative Care

A collaborative approach to health care ideally benefits clients, professionals, and the health care delivery system. Care becomes client centered and, most important, client directed. Clients become informed consumers and actively participate with the health care team in the decision-making process. When clients are empowered to participate actively and professionals share mutually set goals with clients, everyone—including the organization and health care system—ultimately benefits. When quality improves, adherence to therapeutic regimens increases, lengths of stay decrease, and overall costs to the system decline. When professional interdependence develops, collegial relationships emerge and overall satisfaction increases. The work environment becomes more supportive and acknowledges the contributions of each team member. "Because authority is shared, this effort results in more integrated and comprehensive care, as well as shared control of costs and liability" (Miccolo & Spanier, 1993, p. 447).

COMPETENCIES BASIC TO COLLABORATION

Key features necessary for collaboration include effective communication skills, mutual respect, trust, giving and receiving feedback, decision making, and conflict management.

Communication Skills

Collaborating to solve complex problems requires effective communication skills. Initially, the health care team needs to define collaboration clearly, establish its goals and objectives, and specify role expectations.

Effective communication can occur only if the involved parties are committed to understanding each other's professional roles and appreciating each other as individuals. Additionally, they must be sensitive to differences among communication styles. Instead of focusing on distinctions, each professional group needs to center on their common ground: the client's needs.

Communication styles are especially important to successful collaboration. Norton's theory of communicator style (1983) defines style as the manner in which one communicates and includes the way in which one interacts. Therefore, what is said and how it is said are both important. This theory describes nine specific communicator styles that are commonly used and influence the nature of the relationship between communicants. Three of these communicator styles (dominant, contentious, and attentive) have been used in a nursing study of collaboration styles as they relate to degree of collaboration and improved quality of care (Van Ess Coeling & Cukr, 2000). Using attentive style and avoiding contentious and dominant styles made a significant difference in nurse-physician collaboration, positive patient outcomes, and nurse satisfaction. The researchers assert that attentive style can be taught by modeling the behavior of obvious listening, such as making eye contact while communicating and refraining from participating in other activities that interrupt communication while someone is trying to communicate. Verbal feedback and repeating back offers the opportunity to reflect on what was said and to correct misunderstanding. Questioning provides an opportunity to share concerns and initiate dialogue. Developing a noncontentious style means developing judgment in recognizing when it is necessary to stop a conversation and insist on clarification because it is an important point and when it is better to ignore a comment that is disagreed with because it is not essential to the goal. Developing a nondominant style involves controlling one's behavior of monopolizing the conversation or speaking so forcefully that others feel pushed back and unwilling to respond. Role-playing followed by discussion and role modeling have been identified as effective strategies for developing positive communicator styles.

Mutual Respect and Trust

Mutual respect occurs when two or more people show or feel honor or esteem toward one another. Trust occurs when a person is confident in the actions of another person. Both mutual respect and trust imply a mutual process and outcome. They must be expressed both verbally and nonverbally. Sometimes professionals may verbalize respect or trust of others but demonstrate by their actions a lack of trust and respect. The health care system itself has not always created an environment that promotes respect or trust of the various health care providers. Although progress has been made toward creating more collegial relationships, past attitudes may continue to impede efforts toward collaborative practice.

Giving and Receiving Feedback

One of the most difficult challenges for professionals is giving and receiving timely, relevant, and helpful **feedback** to and from each other and their clients. When professionals work closely together, it may be appropriate to address attitudes or actions that affect the collaborative relationship. Feedback may be affected by each person's perceptions, personal space, roles, relationships, self-esteem, confidence, beliefs, emotions, environment, and time.

Negative feedback implies not negative content but rather a negative communication style, such as an attitude of condescension; positive feedback is characterized by a communication style that is warm, caring, and respectful. A review of basic communication skills and an opportunity to practice listening and giving and receiving feedback can enhance any professional's ability to communicate effectively (Ferguson, Howell, & Batalden, 1993, p. 5). Giving and receiving feedback helps individuals acquire self-awareness, while assisting the collaborative team to develop an understanding and effective working relationship.

Decision Making

The decision-making process at the team level involves shared responsibility for the outcome. Obviously, to create a solution, the team must follow each step of the decision-making process, beginning with a clear definition of the problem. Team decision making must be directed at the objectives of the specific effort. Factors that enhance the process include mutual respect and constructive and timely feedback (Mariano, 1989, p. 287).

Decision making at the team level requires full consideration and respect of diverse viewpoints. Members must be able to verbalize their perspectives in a nonthreatening environment. Group members effectively use communication skills and give and re-

ceive feedback in the decision-making process. Interdependent relationships are actualized as members focus on client care issues (Velianoff, Neely, & Hall, 1993, p. 28).

An important aspect of decision making is the interdisciplinary team focusing on the client's priority needs and organizing interventions accordingly. The discipline best able to address the client's needs is given priority in planning and is responsible for providing its interventions in a timely manner. For example, a social worker may first direct attention to a client's social needs when these needs interfere with the client's ability to respond to therapy. Nurses, by the nature of their holistic practice, are often able to help the team identify priorities and areas requiring further attention.

Conflict Management

Role conflict can occur in any situation where individuals work together. **Role conflict** arises when people are called on to carry out roles that have opposing or incompatible expectations. In an interpersonal conflict, different people have different expectations about a particular role. Interrole conflict exists when the expectations of a person or group differ from the expectations of another person or group. Any one of these types of conflict can affect interdisciplinary collaboration.

To reduce role conflict, team members can also conduct interdisciplinary conferences, take part in interdisciplinary education in basic programs, and, most important, accept personal responsibility for teamwork (Benson & Ducanis, 1995). Ongoing research exploring how professionals relate and how teams function will help professionals better understand ways to reduce role conflict when they collaborate with others.

Reflect on...

- what barriers to collaborative care you experience in your practice setting.
- what characteristics support collaborative practice in your practice setting.
- how your values, beliefs, and work experiences influence your abilities to be a collaborative member of a health care team.

It has been suggested that the failure of professionals to collaborate is due not to intent but rather to lack of necessary skills (Van Ess Coeling & Cukr, 2000). Expertise in collaboration and education in collaborative skills have been overlooked. Historically, nursing has been interested in identifying and valuing "nursing" as a unique entity and concentrating on nursing theory, nursing research, and nursing practice. Now the attention is shifting toward interdisciplinary collaboration and recognition of alternative perspectives. This requires not only the ability to articulate one's own perspective, but also the ability to engage in mutual give and take in order to determine the best approach to the specific situation.

Organizational structure can contribute to the success of interdisciplinary collaboration. Structures that maintain a hierarchical authoritarian structure do not support interdisciplinary collaboration. The organization can be particularly effective in the promotion of collaboration between physicians and nurses by intervening where the tradition of an authority figure has been particularly strong. The relationship among participants must be one of trust and respect. The failure on anyone's part to either assume or yield power appropriately can block collaboration.

Conflict is inevitable in organizations, and that conflict can be functional, serving to generate positive changes, or dysfunctional, serving to choke the organization's efforts. There are five stages, or levels, of conflict. Latent conflict is always present when there is a complex organization or when roles are differentiated and may come into conflict. Perceived conflict is when awareness begins. The conflict may or may not progress beyond a latent or perceived level. When it does progress, felt conflict occurs, and hostilities, anxieties, and stress erupt. Overt conflict results when the conflict is acted out and battle lines are drawn. Conflict aftermath comes about with a resolution, and it may or not be optimal. The results may range from full cooperation to active or passive resistance. Although the conflict is resolved, the behaviors may still be affected. There may be difficulty "letting go" once there is resolution.

The conflicts may be interpersonal between or among individuals, or the conflicts may involve groups. Intergroup conflicts may occur between nurses and laboratory personnel or between nurses and physicians, for example. Intragroup conflicts may occur within a group, such as when nurses on a care unit disagree about policies governing practice, such as a plan or policy for floating to another unit.

Whatever the conflict, resolution strategies are important to success. *Problem solving* or *confrontation* can be applied through open discussion and a thorough investigation of the dimensions of the conflict. When the goal is a win-win outcome in which each side is satisfied with the outcome, success is more likely. *Negotiating,* or *bargaining,* entails identifying one's bottom line as well as one's optimal result and then making trade-offs to get a final agreement that is as close as possible to one's optimal position. For this approach to be successful, both parties must be sincere in the desire to negotiate. Negotiation can be either cooperative or competitive; characteristics of each are found in Table 12–1. *Smoothing over* is a short-term resolution focused on minimizing the felt conflict without resolving it. With this approach, the felt conflict is likely to reemerge. *Avoidance* may be used when one side makes the decision to cease discussion and withdraw. *Forcing* uses power or influence to impose a preference; this often involves "going over someone's head" and using a higher authority to enforce the resolution.

Table 12–1 Characteristics of Negotiation

Cooperative Negotiation	Competitive Negotiation
The tangible goals of the negotiation are seen as fair and reasonable to each side.	The tangible goals are for each side to get as much as possible.
There are sufficient resources for a win-win resolution.	There are insufficient resources for each side to attain the desired goal.
Each side believes they can attain their desired goal.	Each side believes it is not possible for each side to attain the desired goal.
The sides work together to maximize joint outcomes.	The goal is to win against the other side.

Critical Thinking Exercise

Recall a time when you engaged in shared decision making. This could be a clinical situation or a personal one. Using Figure 12–1, decide where this collaborative effort fell on the continuum. Applying the competencies basic to collaboration (communication skills, mutual respect and trust, giving and receiving feedback, decision making, and conflict management), plan a strategy that would improve the level of collaboration in that situation.

Critical Thinking Exercise

Nurses working in an outpatient surgical unit want to plan the on-call schedule at monthly staff meetings with their nurse manager. Currently, the staffing office for the entire surgical service plans that schedule. The nurses will need to negotiate the change and are planning a meeting to discuss strategy. Using the information in Table 12–1, describe the application of competitive and cooperative negotiation and how they would differ. Which is more likely to be successful and why?

FACTORS LEADING TO THE NEED FOR INCREASED COLLEGIALITY AND COLLABORATION

Collaboration is necessary to effectively meet the current problems facing the health care system. Among those problems are unmet health care needs of the older adult, the increased number of people who have chronic illnesses, and poverty and homelessness. These health problems are complex and involve diverse needs requiring expertise across disciplines.

Worldwide, there are a number of significant influences on health and health care that will require international collaboration. The World Health Organization (WHO) set an objective that they hoped all persons would achieve by the year 2000, a level of health that would permit them to lead socially and economically productive lives. The report *Healthy People 2000* (U.S. Department of Health and Human Services [USDHHS]) focused on national health promotion and disease prevention goals for U.S. citizens. *Healthy People 2010* (USDHHS, 2000) continues the objective of improving health and well-being worldwide.

Increasingly, governments and society are striving to reduce health risks, minimize the incidence of chronic illness, and improve the health and quality of life for all. The overall goal is to provide health care for all individuals, but health and health care are not guaranteed. Today, the most pressing question for the health care system remains how to pro-

vide quality health care that is in line with the socioeconomic realities of society. A number of factors influence the provision of health care; they are described here.

Consumer Wants and Needs

Although the diagnosis and treatment of illness are still necessities, the focus of health care is changing. Health care consumers are demanding comprehensive, holistic, and compassionate health care that is also affordable. Clients expect that health care providers will view each person as a biopsychosocial whole and respond to his or her individual needs. They want wellness-related care that focuses on the quality of life. They want expert, humanistic care that integrates that available technology and provides information and services related to health promotion and illness prevention.

Today's health care consumers have greater knowledge about their health than in previous years and they are increasingly influencing health care delivery. Formerly, people expected a physician to make decisions about their care; today, however, consumers expect to be involved in making any decisions.

Consumers have also become aware of how lifestyle affects health. As a result, they desire more information and services related to health promotion and illness prevention.

Increasingly, people are actively assuming responsibility for their level of health and are willing to participate in health-promoting activities. They are beginning to view health care professionals as a resource to guide these activities. Many health plans already provide participants with memberships to physical fitness clubs and nutrition classes or offer free attendance at smoking-cessation classes.

Self-Help Initiatives

Responsibility for the self is a major belief underlying holistic health that recognizes the interdependency of body, mind, and spirit. Increasingly, people are adopting the view that the self is empowered with the ability to create or maintain health or disease.

Today many individuals seek answers for acute and chronic health problems through nontraditional approaches to health care. Alternative medicine and support groups are among two of the most popular self-help choices. Each year, more adults are using alternative or unconventional therapies to treat numerous health problems. The most commonly used therapies include relaxation techniques, chiropractic treatments, massage, imagery, spiritual healing, weight-loss programs, and herbal medicine. Back problems, fibromyalgia, cancer, allergies, arthritis, insomnia, chronic fatigue syndrome, strains or sprains, headache, high blood pressure, digestive problems, anxiety, and depression are common conditions for which individuals seek unconventional therapy.

In addition to alternative therapies, many adults participate in one or more self-help groups during their lifetime. In North America, there are more than 500 different mutual support or self-help groups that focus on nearly every major health problem or life crisis people experience. These groups developed, in part, because people felt such organizations could meet needs not addressed by the traditional health care system. Alcoholics Anonymous (AA), which formed in 1935, serves as a model for many of these groups. The National Self-Help Clearinghouse in the United States provides information on current support groups and guidelines about how to start a self-help group. Groups vary in effectiveness, but most provide education to encourage self-care as well as offering social and emotional support.

Changing Demographics and Epidemiology

It is predicted that by the year 2020, there will be more than 50 million adults over the age of 65 years living in the United States (Abrams, Beers, & Berkow, 2000). The growing number of older adults, combined with the fact that the average older adult has three or more chronic health conditions, will greatly influence the health care system and insurers in the future.

Closely related is the major epidemiological influence posed by chronic illness. One of these is HIV/AIDS, a problem that is growing each year. The Centers for Disease Control and Prevention report that a total of 886,575 Americans have been diagnosed with AIDS through 2002 and the estimated number of deaths is 501,669. Worldwide, it is estimated that 37 million adults and 2.5 million children are living with HIV/AIDS as of the end of 2003 (Centers for Disease Control and Prevention, 2004).

According to the National Coalition for the Homeless (2002a), homelessness and poverty are inextricably linked. Limited resources result in difficult choices when trying to pay for housing, food, childcare, health care, and so on. The number of poor in the United States has remained fairly stable in recent years; however, the number of people living in extreme poverty has increased. Limited access to health care services significantly impacts the health of the poor and the homeless.

Health Care Access

The lack of affordable health care is a problem for many. An estimated 15.2% of the population were without insurance coverage in 2002; this represents an increase from 14.6% in 2001. There are no accurate data about how many individuals are underinsured (U.S. Bureau of the Census, 2003).

The health care system in the United States is thought to be in financial distress. For example, since its inception, Medicare has repeatedly increased monthly premiums, deductibles, and related taxes.

Several alternative health delivery systems have been implemented to control costs. These include health maintenance organizations (HMOs), preferred provider organizations (PPOs), physician/hospital organizations (PHOs), and so on. Additionally, the development of prospective payment systems significantly influenced the health care system. Concerns remain, however, about ways to further reduce health care costs and at the same time achieve the desired goal of improving the quality of health care delivery.

Employers, legislators, insurers, and health care providers continue to collaborate in efforts to resolve these concerns. Ethical issues such as rationing of health care, access to health care, the use of health care technology and extraordinary interventions, and organ transplantation can be resolved only through collaboration.

Technological Advances

Technology has had a major influence on health care costs and services. In fact, available technology often influences decisions about the level of care and intervention. With advances in medicine and technology, an individual's life span can in many cases be extended. However, that same technology may result in fragmentation of care and acceleration of health care costs. New medical devices, technological advances, and new medications frequently are introduced with limited consideration to the associated costs or the efficacy of their use. For example, the vital functions of circulation and breathing of a client who has no measurable brain activity can be maintained through advanced life support. In the United States, it is estimated that more than 25% of Medicare dollars are expended for the last year of life (Abrams et al., 2000). At the societal level, the difficult questions of when and how life should be extended through use of technology have not been answered.

EXPLORE MEDIALINK

Questions, critical thinking exercises, essay activities, and other interactive resources for this chapter can be found on the Web site at http://www.prenhall.com/

blais. Click on Chapter 12 to select activities for this chapter.

Bookshelf

Linden, R. M. (2002). *Working across boundaries: Making collaboration work in government and nonprofit organization.* New York: **John Wiley and Sons.**
A practical guide regarding techniques and strategies of successful collaboration. It includes case studies that illustrate overcoming differences.
Schrage, M. (1995). *No more teams! Mastering the dynamics of creative collaboration.* New York: **Currency Doubleday.**
In this follow-up book to *Shared Minds,* the author discusses communication in organizations and the optimum use of modern technology.
Schrage, M. (1990). *Shared minds: The new technologies of collaboration.* New York: **Random House.**
This book discusses business management with a focus on communication using new technologies.

SUMMARY

Collaborative health care is a concept that addresses many existing problems in the health care system. Its multidisciplinary, integrated, and participative approach focuses on client-centered and client-directed care. Collaborative care involves mutual goal setting and care planning between the client, physicians, nurses, and other involved health care providers.

Key competencies necessary for collaborative practice include effective communication skills, mutual respect and trust, giving and receiving feedback, decision-making ability, and conflict management. In addition, each health team member needs knowledge about the roles, views, and unique contributions of the other team members.

Several factors are currently influencing health care delivery. These include (1) the World Health Organization's objective for all people to achieve by the year 2000 a level of health that will permit them to lead socially and economically productive lives;

(2) consumers of health care, who are insisting on comprehensive, holistic, compassionate, and affordable health care that includes services related to health promotion and illness prevention; (3) increasing recognition by consumers of self-help initiatives such as alternative or nontraditional health care and self-help groups; (4) changing demographics, such as an increase in the older, homeless, and AIDS populations; (5) economic issues related to health care, in particular, the exorbitant costs of health care and inequities in people covered by insurance in the United States; and (6) technological advances.

Health care systems remain challenged to provide cost-efficient care and, at the same time, to ensure quality care to all. Nursing's Agenda for Health Care Reform emphasizes a basic "core" of essential health care services for everyone and a restructuring of the health care system to focus on consumers and their health needs.

REFERENCES

Abrams, W. B., Beers, M. H., & Berkow, R. (Eds.). (2000). *The Merck manual of geriatrics* (3rd ed.). Whitehouse Station, NJ: Merck.

American Nurses Association. (1992). *House of delegates report: 1992 convention, Las Vegas, Nevada.* Kansas City, MO: ANA, 104–120.

American Nurses Association. (1995). *Nursing's policy statement.* Washington, DC: ANA.

American Nurses Association. (1998). Collaboration and independent practice: Ongoing issues for nursing. *Nursing Trends and Issues, 3*(5).

American Nurses Association. (2004). *Nursing: Scope and standards of practice.* Washington, DC: ANA.

Benson, L., & Ducanis, A. (1995). Nurses' perceptions of their role and role conflicts. *Rehabilitation Nursing, 20,* 204–211.

Centers for Disease Control and Prevention. (2004). *Basic statistics.* Division of HIV/AIDS Prevention. http://www.hivmail@cdc.gov.

Dalton, J. M. (2003). Development and testing of the theory of collaborative decision-making in nursing practice for triads. *Journal of Advanced Nursing, 41*(1), 22–33.

Ferguson, S., Howell, T., & Batalden, P. (1993). Knowledge and skills needed for collaborative work. *Quality Management in Health Care, 1,* 1–11.

Foley, B. J., Minick, P., & Kee, C. (2000). Nursing advocacy during a military operation. *Western Journal of Nursing Research, 22*(4), 492–507.

Hamric, A. B. (2000). What is happening to advocacy? *Nursing Outlook, 48*(3), 103–104.

Henderson, V. A. (1991). *The nature of nursing: Reflections after 25 years.* New York: National League for Nursing.

Kim, H. S. (1983). Collaborative decision-making in nursing practice: A theoretical framework. In P. L. Chinn, (Ed.), *Advances in nursing theory development* (pp. 271–283). Rockville, MD: Aspen.

Kim, H. S. (1987). Collaborative decision-making with clients. In K. Hannah, M. Reimer, W. Mills, & S. Letourneau (Eds.), *Clinical judgment and decision making: The future with nursing diagnosis* (pp. 58–62). New York: Wiley.

Mariano, C. (1989). The case for interdisciplinary collaboration. *Nursing Outlook, 37,* 285–288.

Miccolo, M. A., & Spanier, A. H. (1993). Critical care management in the 1990s. *Critical Care Unit Management, 9*(3), 443–453.

National Coalition for the Homeless. (2002a). *NCH fact sheet #1: Why are people homeless?* Washington, DC: NCH.

National Coalition for the Homeless. (2002b). *NCH fact sheet #2: How many people experience homelessness?* Washington, DC: NCH.

Norton, R. W. (1983). *Communicator style: Theory, applications, and measures.* Beverly Hills, CA: Sage Publications.

Patel, V. L., Cytryn, K. N., Shortliffe, E. H., & Safran, C. (2000). The collaborative health care team: The role of individual and group expertise. *Teaching and Learning in Medicine, 12*(3), 117–132.

Smith-Love, J., & Carter, C. (1999, Fall). Collaboration, problem-solving reevaluation: Foundation for the Heart Center of Excellence. *Progress in Cardiovascular Nursing,* 143–149.

U.S. Bureau of the Census. (2003). *Health insurance coverage in the United States: 2002.* Washington, DC: Current Population Reports.

U.S. Department of Health and Human Services, Public Health Service. (1990). *Healthy People 2000: National Health Promotion and Disease Prevention Objectives.* DHHS Pub no. (PHS) 91–50212. Washington, DC: U.S. Government Printing Office.

U.S. Department of Health and Human Services, Public Health Service. (2000). *Healthy People 2010 Goals.* http://www.health.gov/healthy people.

Van Ess Coeling, H., & Cukr, P. L. (2000). Communication styles that promote perceptions of collaboration, quality, and nurse satisfaction. *Journal of Nursing Care Quality, 14*(2), 63–74.

Velianoff, G. D., Neely, C., & Hall, S. (1993). Development levels of interdisciplinary collaborative practice committees. *Journal of Nursing Administration, 23,* 26–29.

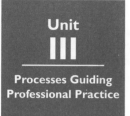

Unit
III
Processes Guiding
Professional Practice

C H A P T E R 1 3

Communication

Outline

Objectives

- Define communication.
- Describe the four components of the communication process.
- Analyze factors influencing the communication process.
- Discuss the types of communication and their characteristics.
- Differentiate between therapeutic and nontherapeutic communication.
- Identify barriers to effective communication.
- Differentiate between nursing documentation and other forms of written communication.
- Discuss technology as a form of communication.

M E D I A L I N K

Additional online resources for this chapter can be found on the companion Web site at http://www.prenhall.com/blais.

Nursing is an interaction between nurses and clients, nurses and other health professionals, and nurses and the community. The process of human interaction occurs through communication: verbal and nonverbal, written and unwritten, planned and unplanned. Communication between people conveys thoughts, ideas, feelings, and information. For nurses to be effective in their interactions, they must have good communication skills. They must be aware of what their words and body language are saying to others. As nurses assume leadership roles they must be effective in both verbal and written communication skills. And as nurses practice in the 21st century, they must have effective computer and other electronic communication skills.

CHALLENGES AND OPPORTUNITIES

Clear and appropriate communication is essential for providing effective nursing care, and this is a unique challenge in the current health care environment. Overcoming barriers to communication is necessary in a society in which many languages are spoken and the population is multicultural. Individual nurses cannot be fluent in each language that will be encountered, nor can they be fully informed of the cultural contexts of words and phrases that may have multiple meanings. Nonverbal communication also has cultural meaning. Not only is this a challenge in providing care to clients, it is also a challenge in working with colleagues when there is diversity of cultures and languages. Clear communication about care and about client information is equally important, whether it is in the form of verbal interactions with co-workers, written records, or publications in professional journals. A challenge for nurses in the 21st century is to become proficient in communicating via technology, including telephone communication such as telephone triage and communication using computers such as nursing-documentation systems, personal data information systems, and e-mail.

Finding effective ways to overcome communication barriers provides the opportunity for nurses to bridge cultural gaps in delivering health care. Nurses who can use available resources and solve problems when there are communication difficulties will be better able to assist clients and families to access care and benefit from health care services. Clear communication will help the health care team provide effective care. It is essential in interdisciplinary teams. When nurses are able to communicate well in verbal and written form, the quality of professional publications benefits and nurses can provide better resources to the profession. Nurses can use technology to enhance communication with clients and other health care providers, to improve access to care for people in remote areas, and to increase their own knowledge using the information resources available on the Internet.

DEFINITIONS OF COMMUNICATION

Communication can be defined as the giving or exchanging of information through verbal or written means. Kozier, Erb, Berman, and Snyder (2004, p. 420) expand on earlier definitions of communication to include "any means of exchanging information or feelings between two or more people." This suggests a broader concept of communication that goes beyond the simple transfer of information to the establishment of a relationship between people. Such relationships are founded upon effective communication skills.

Most definitions of communication suggest that it is a process between two or more individuals, or interpersonal communication. However, people can communicate within themselves—intrapersonal communication—as they reflect upon their own knowledge, ideas, and feelings.

Nurses who communicate effectively are better able to establish successful relationships between themselves and others, including clients and their families, other nurses and health care professionals, health care administrators, and the lay public. Effective communication can also prevent many of the errors that lead to legal incidents associated with nursing practice.

THE COMMUNICATION PROCESS

The communication process involves a sender, message, channel, receiver, and response or feedback. (See Figure 13–1■.) In its simplest form, communication involves the sending and receiving of a message between two people. The sender defines the original message and transmits it to the receiver through a selected channel. The receiver then interprets the message and provides a response to the sender. This enables the sender to determine if the receiver understood or interpreted the message correctly. If the message was not interpreted correctly or if additional information is needed, the process starts again. Therefore, communication is an ongoing process, in which the roles of sender and receiver transact as each transmits new information or understandings to the other.

Communication also can be an exchange of information between an individual and a group of people (e.g., by giving a lecture or teaching a class) or an ex-

Figure 13–1

The Communication Process

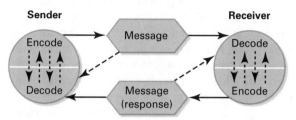

The dashed arrows indicate intrapersonal communication (self-talk). The solid lines indicate interpersonal communication.

Source: From *Fundamentals of Nursing: Concepts, Processes, and Practice* (7th ed., p. 422), by B. Kozier, G. Erb, A. J. Berman, and S. Snyder, 2004, Upper Saddle River, NJ: Prentice Hall Health. Reprinted with permission.

change of information between several people (e.g., a change-of-shift report or a group meeting). The components of the communication process are sender, message, channel, receiver, and feedback.

Sender

The **sender** is the person or group who wishes to transmit a message to another. Another term for sender is *source encoder.* This means that the originator of the message, or source, has a purpose for the message and determines its content. The content of the message must be put in a form that is understandable to the receiver, called encoding. Encoding involves "the selection of specific signs or symbols (codes) to transmit the message" (Kozier et al., 2004, p. 421). Encoding includes the choice of specific words and the language of the message. It also includes the speech inflection and body language used to accompany the message. For example, when nurses are communicating with other nurses about a client's condition, they may use medical terminology (e.g., hypertension); however, when they are talking with the client or family, they may use lay terminology (e.g., high blood pressure).

Message

The second part of the communication process is the encoded message itself—the information or feelings to be transmitted and the content and context of the message. Messages between nurses and clients include verbal and written discharge instructions, interactions of support and caring, and information gathering.

Channel

The **channel** is the method selected to convey the message, including whether the message is spoken or written, the choice of words or language, and the choice of accompanying body language. A change-of-shift report between nurses may be verbal in a face-to-face interaction or it may be recorded on audiotape. Client-discharge instructions may be written or verbal. Communications with physicians may be face to face, via telephone, or through the client record. The channel can be visual, auditory, or through touch. Some of the most effective communication interactions use more than one sensory channel.

Receiver

The **receiver**, also called the *decoder,* is the one who receives the message, interprets (decodes) it, and makes a decision about how to respond. If the message is aural, the receiver must be able to hear or attend to the message and the sender. If the message is written or visual, the receiver must be able to see and read. The receiver decodes or interprets the message in relation to his or her past experiences, knowledge, and personal characteristics. If the receiver interprets the message congruently with the intent of the sender, then communication has been effective. Ineffective communication occurs when the message is not understood or is interpreted inaccurately. For example, a nurse may instruct the client to take his medication three times a day with meals. The client, however, eats only twice a day. This difference could result in the client not taking the medication as required. Feedback, or response, from the client is essential to validate interpretation and understanding of the message.

Response

The receiver's **response** is the feedback that enables the sender to know if the message was received and interpreted correctly. Feedback is the message that the receiver returns to the sender. Failure to obtain a response or feedback can result in ineffective communication. Feedback also can be verbal or nonverbal. Feedback may be verbal clarification or acceptance or rejection of the information or feelings. It may also be nonverbal. Examples of nonverbal feedback are nodding of the head, a facial expression of confusion or understanding, or signs of boredom, such as yawning. It is important to use verbal feedback to be sure that nonverbal language has not been misinterpreted. For example, clients may nod their head indicating understanding, but further questioning might show that they misunderstood the message.

The response is the message back to the sender. The receiver has changed roles and becomes the sender. And so the process continues until the communication is ended.

FACTORS INFLUENCING THE COMMUNICATION PROCESS

Many factors influence the communication process. These include the developmental stage, gender, roles and relationships, sociocultural characteristics, values and perceptions, space and territoriality, environment, congruence, and interpersonal attitudes.

Developmental Stage

As individuals grow and develop, language and communication skills develop through various stages. It is important for a nurse to understand the developmental processes related to speech, language, and communication skills. Knowledge of the client's developmental stage enables the nurse to select appropriate communication strategies. For example, when communicating with infants and toddlers whose language skills are not well developed, the nurse may rely more on the child's nonverbal communications to assess comfort and pain. The nurse may hold the child and use touch to provide comfort and demonstrate caring. For older children, nurses may use pictures as an adjunct to verbal language to communicate. For adolescents and adults, nurses are more able to rely on verbal language for communication. With older adults, physical changes associated with the aging process may affect communication. For example, it may be more effective to use visual communication methods for clients who are hearing impaired or aural communication methods for clients who are visually impaired. Also, intellectual processes develop across the life span as people acquire knowledge and experience. The knowledge and experiences that people have influence their understanding and acceptance of transmitted information and feelings.

Gender

Males and females tend to communicate differently. They may give different meanings to transmitted information or feelings. This may be the result of differences during psychosocial development, because boys use communication to establish independence and ne-

---

Evidence for Practice

Sudia-Robinson, T. M., & Freeman, S. B. (2000). Communication patterns and decision making: Parents and health care providers in the neonatal intensive care unit—A case study. *Heart and Lung: The Journal of Acute and Critical Care, 29*(2), 143–148.

The purpose of this study was to examine patterns of communication and decision making among NICU health care providers and the parents of a premature infant who required neonatal intensive care. A descriptive design was used for data collection to answer the question: What patterns of communication and decision making are evident in the interactions of parents of an infant in the NICU and the NICU professionals providing care? A parent-professional conference was videotaped, and audiotapes were used for interviews with the parents and the professionals directly involved in care (two nurses, a neonatologist, a resident, and a social worker). The parents and the professionals reviewed the videotape individually, and each was interviewed about feelings, impressions, and concerns.

The audiotapes of the interviews were transcribed and analyzed by content analysis. The parents were found to have four areas of concern regarding their infant's routine care: parental visitation, change of shift, the infant's transfer to the IMCU, and administration of immunizations. The parents indicated a desire to be involved in daily decisions and expressed a need for more information. They expressed a desire to have adequate time to establish a trusting relationship with the new set of caregivers at shift change. They felt they needed an opportunity to engage in additional conversation with the professionals before the transfer of the infant. Misinterpretation of information from the professionals was evident. Therapeutic communication techniques and spending time and sharing perceptions with parents were recommended.

gotiate status within a group, whereas girls use communication to seek confirmation, minimize differences, and establish or reinforce intimacy. It is important that nurses, when working with clients or colleagues of the opposite gender, be aware that the same communication may be interpreted differently by a man and a woman.

Roles and Relationships

The roles and relationships between the sender and the receiver can influence communication. Roles such as nurse and client, nurse and colleague, nurse and physician, and nurse and administrator/supervisor can affect the content and response in communication. Roles may influence choice of message content, communication vehicle, tone of voice, and body language. For example, nurses may choose face-to-face communication for interaction with clients or health providers on the nursing unit, whereas they may use e-mails or telephones to communicate with physicians or administrators. Nurses may choose a more informal or comfortable stance when communicating with clients or colleagues and a more formal stance when communicating with physicians or administrators. The length of the relationship may also affect communication. For example, nurses may use more formal language and a more formal stance when meeting clients or colleagues for the first time but use a more relaxed stance when interacting with clients or colleagues with whom they have an established relationship.

Sociocultural Characteristics

Sociocultural characteristics such as culture, education, or economic level can influence communication. Nonverbal communication characteristics such as body language, eye contact, and touch are influenced by cultural beliefs about appropriate communication behavior. Some cultures may believe direct eye contact is disrespectful, whereas other cultures believe that direct eye contact shows trustworthiness. In some cultures, touch would be appropriate to communicate caring and concern, but in other cultures physical touch would be offensive. Verbal communication may be difficult for the receiver whose primary language is not that of the sender. More information about the influence of culture on communication can be found in Chapter 21 ⚭, Nursing in a Culturally Diverse World.

People's level of education may affect the extent of their vocabulary or their ability to read written

---

Evidence for Practice

Frank, D. I. (2003). Elderly client's perceptions of communication with their health care provider and its relation to health deviation self-care behaviors. *Self-Care, Dependent-Care, and Nursing, 11*(2), 1–10.

The purpose of this qualitative study was to explore the nature of communication that elderly clients experienced with their health care providers, the barriers to communication that they experienced, and how these communications influenced their health deviation self-care behavior. Orem's self-care model was the theoretical foundation for the study. Four focus groups consisting of 6 to 8 individuals over 60 years of age who were retired or unemployed, lived independently, and were under a physician's care were conducted by registered nurses. Attributes of effective health care provider communication included (1) respect for the client and their family, (2) honesty, (3) friendliness and warmth, (4) appreciation for the client's home life and situation, (4) being nonjudgmental about the client's appearance/behavior, (5) conveying time to listen, and (6) a sense of humor. Nursing implications: Benefits of effective communication for older clients include the client's being able to maintain independence, maintain their optimal level of health, and having the best possible quality of life. A further benefit is the potential for reducing health care costs by promoting independence and decreasing costly health care utilization.

---

communication. Economic level may affect a person's ability to access written communication. Today, when many people are using e-mail to communicate or the Internet to obtain health information, people who cannot afford a computer or who do not have access to one will not be able to communicate using that means.

Values and Perceptions

Communication is influenced by the values people hold about themselves, others, and the world in which they live. Because all people have values and perceptions based on their own experiences and characteristics, people who hold different values may send, receive, and interpret messages differently. For example, a client who values stoicism in managing his or her pain may not tell the nurse about the pain and may be offended when the nurse inquires about pain or offers pain medication.

Space and Territoriality

Space involves the distance at which an interaction takes place. Territoriality involves the space and contents of the space that the individual considers belonging to him or her.

Hall (1969) describes four distances at which interactions take place: *intimate distance, personal distance, social distance,* and *public distance. Intimate distance* ranges from physical contact to 1½ feet. Nurses interact with clients within the intimate range when they assess and provide some direct care activities for clients. Taking blood pressure, listening to body sounds with a stethoscope, assessing pulse, changing a dressing, or giving an injection are all performed with physical contact. The manner in which the tasks are performed and the conversation during these activities communicate to the client in various ways. If the nurse is brusque when changing a dressing, the client may interpret the nurse's behavior as uncaring. If the nurse is gentle and shows concern, the client may perceive that the nurse is caring and feel comforted. Clients may feel uncomfortable when others enter their intimate space, especially if a trusting relationship has not been established. Nurses can alleviate this discomfort by telling the client before moving into the intimate distance range.

Personal distance ranges from 1½ to 4 feet. Most one-to-one communication takes place within this range. Nurses interact with clients in the personal distance range when they sit with a client to obtain a health history or when they teach clients self-care. Nurses also interact with colleagues in the range of personal distance when they exchange information with a nursing colleague or physician.

Social distance ranges from 4 to 12 feet. Interactions with clients and family members or groups of clients are more likely to occur in the range of social distance. This is also the range of distance within which nurses interact with groups of colleagues, such as during a group change-of-shift report. It is important to note that usually the voice is louder when communicating in this range; therefore, a nurse must be aware of issues of client confidentiality. Communication with a client who is in a semiprivate room may be compromised if the nurse asks personal questions at this range while in the presence of other clients or caregivers.

Public distance starts at 12 feet and goes beyond that distance. This is the distance at which interactions with larger groups take place. There is less individual interaction or awareness of individual needs when communicating at this distance. Nurses communicate in public distance when they conduct community health education classes.

It is human nature to establish a boundary or territory that is considered to be one's own. Whether clients are being cared for in their own home, their own room in a long-term care facility, or in a hospital room, they create a personal environment that gives them comfort. They may have photographs, religious materials, or other personal items on a nearby table or bed tray. If the nurse attempts to change or rearrange furniture or objects in the client's environment, the client may perceive this as not caring or devaluing. Similarly, nurses who have their own desk or locker often have personal objects that create their personal work territory or environment.

Environment

The nature of the environment can also affect communication. Communication occurs best in an environment that supports the exchange of information, ideas, or feelings. Loud noises, poor lighting, noxious odors, or an uncomfortable temperature can all interfere with effective communication. The arrangement of furniture can affect communication. For example, communicating across a desk conveys a more formal interaction than when the nurse sits in a chair next to the client. When interacting with clients, their families, or others, nurses should try to create an environment that is conducive to effective communication and minimizes environmental distractions.

Congruence

When communication is congruent, the nonverbal behaviors match the verbal message. Nurses may state that they want clients to call if they have any questions or need anything. However, if a nurse appears to be rushed or distracted, a client may be unsure about calling the nurse when he or she has a question or is experiencing pain.

Interpersonal Attitudes

Positive attitudes of respect, acceptance, trust, and caring facilitate communication, whereas negative attitudes of mistrust, rejection, and condescension in-

Evidence for Practice

Ahrens, T., Yancey, V., & Kollef, M. (2003). Improving family communications at the end of life: Implications for length of stay in the intensive care unit and resource use. *American Journal of Critical Care, 12*(4), 317–323.

The purpose of this study was to evaluate the effect of a communication team consisting of a physician and a clinical nurse specialist on length of stay and costs for patients near the end of life in the intensive care unit. Over a 1-year period, 151 patients who were judged to be at high risk for death were divided into two groups: 43 patients who were cared for by the communication team and 108 patients who were provided standard care by an attending physician. Findings showed that patients who were cared for by the communication team had significantly shorter stays in both the intensive care unit and the hospital, and had lower fixed and variable costs. Nursing implications: Physician/clinical nurse specialist teams focused on improving communication with patients and their families can reduce lengths of stay and health care costs.

hibit effective communication. When one person is interacting with another, attitudes are conveyed by facial expression, tone of voice, the choice of words, and other body language. It is important to convey a nonjudgmental attitude during interactions. If the client feels that the nurse disapproves of some aspect of his or her lifestyle (e.g., smoking, promiscuity, addiction to drugs or alcohol), the client might not share the information.

TYPES OF COMMUNICATION

There are two types of communication, verbal and nonverbal. Verbal communication may be spoken or written and involves words. Verbal communication is mainly conscious because people choose the words they use. Verbal communication depends on language mastery. Language mastery includes vocabulary and grammar and is dependent on one's culture, educational level, socioeconomic background, and age. Because of these factors, information can be given, ideas discussed, and feelings exchanged using many different words and word configurations. Nonverbal communication uses other forms such as facial expression, gestures, touch, or other types of body language. Nonverbal communication also includes the use of pictures to communicate. Although both verbal and nonverbal communication occur simultaneously, the majority of communication during face-to-face interactions is nonverbal.

Oral Communication

Oral communication is a spoken exchange of information, ideas, or feelings using words. Words can have different meanings for different people. Wilson and Kneisl (1996) describe four concepts related to word meanings: (1) denotative meaning, (2) connotative meaning, (3) private meaning, and (4) shared meaning. Denotative meaning is the way in which the word is generally used by people who share a common language. Connotative meaning is the meaning of a word that derives from one's personal experiences; for example, the word love may have different meanings when used with a parent, a child, a spouse, or a lover or to describe one's favorite flavor of ice cream. Private meanings are those held by the individual. Shared meanings are the mutual understanding of the word or words between people who are trying to communicate effectively.

Kozier et al. (2004) state that when choosing words for oral communication, nurses must consider (1) pace and intonation, (2) simplicity, (3) clarity and brevity, (4) timing and relevance, (5) adaptability, (6) credibility, and (7) humor.

1. *Pace and intonation.* Pace is the speed or rapidity of speech. Intonation is the tone, accent, or inflection used when speaking. Pace and intonation can express a variety of states, including interest, happiness, anxiety, boredom, anger, fear, or depression. For example, when people speak in a monotone, not changing the pace or tone of their speech, they may be expressing boredom or apathy.

2. *Simplicity.* Simplicity in communication is the choice of commonly understood words. Nurses must remember to use language that is clearly understood when communicating with clients. This may mean avoiding complex medical terminology when discussing a client's illness or injury. It also means that the nurse must clarify that the client understands the word meanings in the same way that the nurse does.

3. *Clarity and brevity.* Clarity means choosing words that say unmistakably what is meant. Brevity is using the fewest words necessary to convey a message. It is important to communicate clearly so that the message is understood.

4. *Timing and relevance.* Timing is an important aspect of effective communication. If the client is experiencing pain or is otherwise distracted, it is not an appropriate time to give complex instructions in self-care. Communication must also be relevant to the receiver. If the receiver is not interested in the information at the time it is being given, he or she may be less attentive.

5. *Adaptability.* When speaking with clients and others, nurses must be cognizant of verbal and nonverbal cues from the receiver and adapt their communication accordingly. If the receiver appears confused after instructions have been given, the nurse must clarify understanding by restating or rephrasing the instructions.

6. *Credibility.* Credibility means being believable and trustworthy. To be credible when communicating, nurses must be consistent, dependable, and honest. Nurses must give accurate information and be willing to say when they don't know something or don't have information. It is more credible to state, "I don't know, but I'll find out for you" than to give inaccurate information that must be corrected later. Consistency is important when communicating to avoid confusion or misunderstanding. When a nurse is consistent and accurate in communicating, he or she is more believable or credible.

7. *Humor.* Humor can be effective in communication when used appropriately. It can help people adjust to difficult situations and decrease tension. Laughter can release endorphins that promote a sense of well-being. However, one must be careful in using humor, especially when communicating with people whose primary language is different or who are from a different culture. For example, jokes may seem funny only when used within a particular culture; they may be offensive to or not understood by people of a different culture.

Paralanguage or paralinguistic sounds are the sounds that accompany verbal language and add to the message being given by the spoken word. Fontaine and Fletcher (2003) and Frisch and Frisch (2002) include the tone and volume of the voice, the rate of speech, hesitation, and the emotions expressed that accompany speech as paralanguage. Emotions that accom-

pany speech may include anger, laughter, crying, fear, anxiety, or nervousness. Because these sounds accompany speech they influence the message that is received by the listener so that the same words accompanied by different paralinguistic cues may be interpreted differently. It is important, however, to consider these sounds in the context of the culture of the client because they may have different meanings in different cultures.

Nonverbal Communication

Nonverbal communication is also referred to as body language. It is the way in which one uses one's body to reinforce or contradict verbal, specifically oral, communication. Nonverbal communication includes (1) eye contact, (2) facial expressions, (3) body movements, (4) gestures, (5) touch, and (6) physical appearance.

1. *Eye contact.* Eye contact may initiate interaction and communication. Often when a person is trying to get another's attention, he or she does so by trying to make eye contact. However, before making judgments about the importance of eye contact, the nurse must know the meaning of eye contact within the client's culture. In many Western cultures, eye contact is interpreted as attentiveness, interest, understanding, or trustworthiness. In some cultures, however, direct eye contact is considered disrespectful. Knowing the cultural meaning of eye contact can help a nurse assess its meaning in a specific interaction.

2. *Facial expression.* Facial expressions provide the emotion or feeling underlying the verbal communication. The face can express feelings of surprise, fear, concern, disgust, happiness, anger, confusion, and sadness. As with eye contact, facial expression can have a cultural meaning. Some cultures are more expressive than others. It is important that one's facial expression is congruent with the verbal message. An expression of concern when inquiring about a client's pain is congruent, whereas an expression of boredom or anger would be incongruent and could lead the client to believe that the nurse does not care.

3. *Body movements.* The way in which people stand, sit, or move their bodies also communicates to others. Posture and gait can communicate one's feelings about self, one's mood, and one's current state of health. When interacting with a client, a nurse demonstrates interest and concern by leaning to-

ward the client or by reaching out his or her hands and arms toward the client. Leaning away from the client or crossing his or her arms and legs may indicate distance or withdrawal. Standing over a client during interaction may be intimidating to the client. Agitated movements may convey fear or anxiety. Lack of movement may indicate pain, discomfort, or depression.

4. *Gestures.* Hand and body movements may emphasize or clarify verbal communication, such as when separating fingers or hands to indicate the size of something or to point to a part of the body where one has pain. When the client is asked to describe chest pain, a different meaning could be attributed to the gesture of a clenched fist in the center of the chest as opposed to an open hand waived vaguely in front of the chest. Some people use their hands as part of their verbal speech and may find difficulty in expressing themselves if they are unable to use their hands. For people who are hearing impaired or unable to speak, sign language may be their primary means of communicating.

5. *Touch.* Physical touch can convey concern, comfort, and caring or it can convey anger or agitation. Like eye contact, touch has cultural meaning. In some cultures, touch is inappropriate between people of the opposite gender or between people of different classes. It is important that the nurse determine the meaning of touch in the client's culture. When touch is inappropriate, clients may withdraw if a nurse reaches out toward them.

6. *Appearance.* How people present themselves, their dress, and their grooming can convey information about them. People who are physically or mentally ill may not be as attentive to their dress and grooming. Dress may indicate a person's position or status. For example, physicians, some nurses, and therapists may wear lab coats over business clothes; administrators may wear suits; and nursing assistants and dietary personnel may wear required uniforms or smocks. Jewelry may provide information about a person. Religious jewelry provides important information about a client or colleague. Nurses often wear pins or other insignia that indicate their position or accomplishments, such as their school of nursing pin or a pin indicating they are a member of Sigma Theta Tau, the nursing honor society.

It is important that nurses be aware of their verbal and nonverbal communication patterns and characteristics. How they speak, their mannerisms, and their gestures may be effective tools for communication or they may impede communication.

Reflect on...

- your speech patterns when communicating verbally with others, such as colleagues, clients, and friends. What feedback do you receive?
- mannerisms and gestures you use when communicating nonverbally with others. What feedback do you receive?

Therapeutic Communication

Therapeutic communication is defined as "an interactive process between nurse and client that helps the client overcome temporary stress, to get along with other people, to adjust to the unalterable, and to overcome psychological blocks which stand in the way of self-realizations" (Kozier et al., 2004, p. 1467). Therapeutic communication differs from social communication in that there is always a specific purpose or direction to the communication; therefore, therapeutic communication is planned communication. Communication is most therapeutic when the nurse demonstrates an attitude of trust and caring for the client (Frisch & Frisch, 2002). There are specific verbal and nonverbal techniques of communication that express such an attitude.

Presence, or an attitude of being wholly there for the client, is part of therapeutic communication. A nurse cannot appear to be distracted; rather, a client must feel that he or she is the primary focus of the nurse during the interaction. Being there for a client is conveyed by presenting an open and relaxed posture and leaning toward the client. The nurse faces the client directly and maintains eye contact.

Listening, sometimes referred to as attentive listening, is active listening. Frisch and Frisch (2002) and Kozier et al. (2004) describe listening as the most important communication technique. To be therapeutic, listening must be active and involve all the senses rather than passively involving only the ear. Silence is a part of attentive listening. Nurses need to become comfortable with silence. Silence allows clients to think about or reflect upon what has been said. Sometimes silence can communicate more than words; it can enable the expression of feelings or emotions.

Therapeutic communication techniques facilitate effective communication and enhance the nurse-client interaction. This communication focuses on the client's thoughts and concerns. Therapeutic communication techniques are described in Table 13–1.

Table 13–1 Therapeutic Communication Techniques

Technique	Description	Examples
Using silence	Accepting pauses or silences that may extend for several seconds or minutes without interjecting any verbal response.	Sitting quietly (or walking with the client) and waiting attentively until the client is able to put thoughts and feelings into words.
Providing general leads	Using statements or questions that (a) encourage the client to verbalize, (b) choose a topic of conversation, and (c) facilitate continued verbalization.	"Perhaps you would like to talk about . . ." "Would it help to discuss your feelings?" "Where would you like to begin?" "And then what?" "I follow what you are saying."
Being specific and tentative	Making statements that are specific rather than general, and tentative rather than absolute.	"You scratched my arm." (specific statement) "You are as clumsy as an ox." (general statement) "You seem unconcerned about Mary." (tentative statement) "You don't give a damn about Mary and you never will." (absolute statement)
Using open-ended questions	Asking broad questions that lead or invite the client to explore (elaborate, clarify, describe, compare, or illustrate) thoughts or feelings. Open-ended questions specify only the topic to be discussed and invite answers that are longer than one or two words.	"I'd like to hear more about that." "Tell be about . . ." "How have you been feeling lately?" "What brought you to the hospital?" "What is your opinion?" "You said you were frightened yesterday. How do you feel now?"
Using touch	Providing appropriate forms of touch to reinforce caring feelings. Because tactile contacts vary considerably among individuals, families, and cultures, the nurse must be sensitive to the differences in attitudes and practices of clients and self.	Putting an arm over the client's shoulder. Placing your hand over the client's hand.
Restating or paraphrasing	Actively listening for the client's basic message and then repeating those thoughts and/or feelings in similar words. This conveys that the nurse has listened and understood the client's basic message and also offers clients a clearer idea of what they have said.	Client: "I couldn't manage to eat any dinner last night—not even the dessert." Nurse: "You had difficulty eating yesterday." Client: "Yes, I was very upset after my family left." Client: "I have trouble talking to strangers." Nurse: "You find it difficult talking to people you do not know?"
Seeking clarification	A method of making the client's broad overall meaning of the message more understandable. It is used when paraphrasing is difficult or when the communication is rambling or garbled. To clarify the message, the nurse can restate the basic message or confess confusion and ask the client to repeat or restate the message.	"I'm puzzled." "I'm not sure I understand that." "Would you please say that again?" "Would you tell me more?"
	Nurses can also clarify their own message with statements.	"I meant this rather than that." "I guess I didn't make that clear—I'll go over it again."

Table 13–1 Therapeutic Communication Techniques (Cont.)

Technique	Description	Examples
Perception checking or seeking consensual validation	A method similar to clarifying that verifies the meaning of specific words rather than the overall meaning of a message.	*Client:* "My husband *never* gives me any presents." *Nurse:* "You mean he has *never* given you a present for your birthday or Christmas?" *Client:* "Well—not *never*. He does get me something for my birthday and Christmas, but he never thinks of giving me anything at any other time."
Offering self	Suggesting one's presence, interest, or wish to understand the client without making any demands or attaching conditions that the client must comply with to receive the nurse's attention.	"I'll stay with you until your daughter arrives." "We can sit here quietly for a while; we don't need to talk unless you would like to." "I'll help you to dress to go home."
Giving information	Providing, in a simple and direct manner, specific factual information the client may or may not request. When information is not known, the nurse states this and indicates who has it or when the nurse will obtain it.	"Your surgery is scheduled for 11 A.M. tomorrow." "You will feel a pulling sensation when the tube is removed from your abdomen." "I do not know the answer to that, but I will find out from Mrs. King, the nurse in charge."
Acknowledging	Giving recognition, in a nonjudgmental way, of a change in behavior, an effort the client has made, or a contribution to a communication. Acknowledgment may be with or without understanding, verbal or nonverbal.	"You trimmed your beard and mustache and washed your hair." "I notice you keep squinting your eyes. Are you having difficulty seeing?" "You walked twice as far today with your walker."
Clarifying time or sequence	Helping the client clarify an event, situation, or happening in relationship to time.	*Client:* "I vomited this morning." *Nurse:* "Was that after breakfast?" *Client:* "I feel that I have been asleep for weeks." *Nurse:* "You had your operation Monday, and today is Tuesday."
Presenting reality	Helping the client to differentiate the real from the unreal.	"That telephone ring came from the program on television." "That's not a dead mouse in the corner; it is a discarded washcloth." "Your magazine is here in the drawer. It has not been stolen."
Focusing	Helping the client expand on and develop a topic of importance. It is important for the nurse to wait until the client finishes stating the main concerns before attempting to focus. The focus may be an idea or a feeling; however, the nurse often emphasizes a feeling to help the client recognize an emotion disguised behind words.	*Client:* "My wife says she will look after me, but I don't think she can, what with the children to take care of, and they're always after her about something—clothes, homework, what's for dinner that night." *Nurse:* "You are worried about how well she can manage."
Reflecting	Directing ideas, feelings, questions, or content back to clients to enable them to explore their own ideas and feelings about a situation.	*Client:* "What can I do?" *Nurse:* "What do you think would be helpful?" *Client:* "Do you think I should tell my husband?" *Nurse:* "You seem unsure about telling your husband."

Table 13-1 Therapeutic Communication Techniques (Cont.)

Technique	Description	Examples
Summarizing and planning	Stating the main points of a discussion to clarify the relevant points discussed. This technique is useful at the end of an interview or to review a health teaching session. It often acts as an introduction to future care planning.	"During the past half hour we have talked about . . ." "Tomorrow afternoon we may explore this further." "In a few days I'll review what you have learned about the actions and effects of your insulin."

Source: From *Fundamentals of Nursing: Concepts, Processes and Practice* (7th ed.), by B. Kozier, G. Erb, A. J. Berman, and S. Snyder, 2004, Upper Saddle River, NJ: Prentice Hall Health. Reprinted with permission.

WRITTEN COMMUNICATION

Nurses have many requirements as well as opportunities for written communication. The most common form of written communication in nursing are the notes made in the medical record about a client's status. Nurses also write discharge instructions for clients and their families, memos to nursing colleagues and other health professionals, and client educational materials. Nurse-managers write employee evaluations, policies and procedures, and other communications to administrators, colleagues, and nursing staff. Nurse-educators write educational handouts and course syllabi. An important consideration in written communication is that decoding often occurs when the writer is not present and may occur long after the document is written. Therefore, clarity is important because it may not be possible to ask questions or clarify areas of confusion.

Characteristics of Effective Written Communication

In addition to simplicity, brevity, clarity, relevance, credibility, and humor (characteristics of effective oral communication), written communication must contain (1) appropriate language and terminology; (2) correct grammar, spelling, and punctuation; (3) logical organization; and (4) appropriate use and citation of resources.

1. *Appropriate language and terminology.* Language and terminology must be appropriate for the age, education and reading level, and culture of the reader. Health education materials written for children should be different than materials written for adults. For people whose primary language is other than English, it may be more effective to have written materials translated into their primary language by a professional translator. Appropriate lay terminology may be substituted for medical terminology; for example, high blood pressure may be used instead of hypertension. See Chapter 8 ∞, The Nurse as Learner and Teacher, for more information about reading level of written materials.

2. *Correct grammar, spelling, and punctuation.* Using correct grammar, spelling, and punctuation provides clarity for the reader. Misspelled words, misplaced punctuation, or incorrect grammar can change the intended meaning and lead to confusion on the part of the reader. Most computer word-processing programs have spelling- and grammar-checking features that assist writers in improving their writing.

3. *Logical organization.* Written materials are well organized when they are logical and easy for readers to follow. Consider what the reader needs to know first. Simple and foundational information is usually provided first, followed by more complex information. Using examples can also assist readers.

4. *Appropriate use and citation of resources.* Information taken from other sources must always be credited to the original source. Failure to reference work taken from another writer is called plagiarism, is considered unethical, and may violate copyright laws. There are various styles of referencing, including the Modern Language Association (MLA) and the American Psychological Association (APA). Another benefit of citing references is that readers who want additional information have other references to read.

Reflect on...

■ your professional activities other than charting on client records that require written communication. What professional activities of you and your colleagues require written communication?

Critical Thinking Exercise

Choose a nursing topic to discuss with one or more colleagues or classmates. After the discussion ask the participants to analyze your verbal and nonverbal communication using the information in Table 13–1, Therapeutic Communication Techniques, and Table 13–2, Barriers to Communication. Are there words or phrases that you use that distract from your communication, for example, excessive use of the phrase "you know." Are there nonverbal mannerisms that detract from the communication, for example, frequent looking at your watch, interrupting, not making eye contact, and so on. What strategies will you implement to improve your communication?

Critical Thinking Exercise

Videotape an interaction with a colleague or client. (You must first obtain permission to videotape.) Analyze the videotape to identify inconsistencies between your verbal and nonverbal communication. In what ways would you improve your verbal and nonverbal communication behaviors?

■ your own comfort and ability at written communication. What strategies would you implement to improve your ability at written communication? How would you assist your colleagues to improve their written communication?

BARRIERS TO COMMUNICATION

Just as there are characteristics of effective communication, there are identified barriers to effective communication. Nurses need to be cognizant of these barriers and avoid them. Nurses also need to recognize them when they occur so that they can change to more effective communication. Kozier et al. (2004, p. 429) state "failure to listen, improperly decoding the client's intended message, and placing the nurse's needs above the client's needs are major barriers to communication." Additional barriers to effective communication are given in Table 13–2.

NURSING DOCUMENTATION

Documentation of clients' care and their responses to that care is essential for effective communication of clients' status between health care providers. When such documentation is complete, accurate, and clearly understood by all health care professionals involved in providing the care, the quality of clients' care is improved. Although the primary purpose of documenting care in clients records is for communication

between health care providers so that they can plan appropriate care, there are other uses of the information provided in clients' records: (1) auditing for quality assurance, (2) research, (3) education, (4) reimbursement, (5) legal documentation, and (6) health care analysis (Kozier et al., 2004).

■ *Auditing for quality assurance.* The client record is used by accrediting organizations such as JCAHO to review and evaluate the quality of care given in health care institutions.

■ *Research.* Information in a client record can be used as a source of data for health care research. Data gathered from the medical records of numerous clients with the same health problem may yield information about (1) the effectiveness of specific treatment methods, (2) the effectiveness of specific nursing interventions, or (3) specific client characteristics that enhance or impede the effectiveness of a specific treatment or intervention.

■ *Education.* Client records are used by students in the health professions as educational tools. Although textbooks provide generalized information about pathophysiology, signs and symptoms, usual treatment, and outcomes of a specific health problem, client records provide a comprehensive view of specific clients, their health problems, their medical treatments and nursing interventions, and their responses to the treatment and interventions. A client record provides a case study of the unique experience of one client with a specific health problem. This helps students understand the individual experience of the client with the health problem.

■ *Reimbursement.* Documentation of care helps the health care organization receive reimbursement from third-party payers, including private insurance companies and governmental sources of reimbursement such as Medicare and Medicaid. Medicare requires that the client record must contain the correct diagnosis-related group (DRG) codes and document that the appropriate care was given for the health care provider to receive payment.

Table 13–2 Barriers to Communication

Technique	Description	Examples
Stereotyping	Offering generalized and oversimplified beliefs about groups of people that are based on experiences too limited to be valid. These responses categorize clients and negate their uniqueness as individuals.	"Two-year-olds are brats." "Women are complainers." "Men don't cry." "Most people don't have any pain after this type of surgery."
Agreeing and disagreeing	Similar to judgmental responses, agreeing and disagreeing imply that the client is either right or wrong and that the nurse is in a position to judge this. These responses deter clients from thinking through their position and may cause a client to become defensive.	*Client:* "I don't think Dr. Smith is a very good doctor. He doesn't seem interested in his patients." *Nurse:* "Dr. Smith is head of the Department of Surgery and is an excellent surgeon."
Being defensive	Attempting to protect a person or health care services from negative comments. These responses prevent the client from expressing true concerns. The nurse is saying, "You have no right to complain." Defensive responses protect the nurse from admitting weaknesses in the health care services, including personal weaknesses.	*Client:* "Those night nurses must just sit around and talk all night. They didn't answer my light for over an hour." *Nurse:* "I'll have you know we literally run around on nights. You're not the only client, you know."
Challenging	Giving a response that makes clients prove their statement or point of view. These responses indicate that the nurse is failing to consider the client's feelings, making the client feel it necessary to defend a position.	*Client:* "I felt nauseated after that red pill." *Nurse:* "Surely you don't think I gave you the wrong pill?" *Client:* "I feel as if I am dying." *Nurse:* "How can you feel that way when your pulse is 60?" *Client:* "I believe my husband doesn't love me." *Nurse:* "You can't say that; why, he visits you every day."
Probing	Asking for information chiefly out of curiosity rather than with the intent to assist the client. These responses are considered prying and violate the client's privacy. Asking "why" is often probing and places the client in a defensive position.	*Client:* "I was speeding along the street and didn't see the stop sign." *Nurse:* "Why were you speeding?" *Client:* "I didn't ask the doctor when he was here." *Nurse:* "Why didn't you?"
Testing	Asking questions that make the client admit to something. These responses permit the client only limited answers and often meet the nurse's need rather than the client's.	"Who do you think you are?" (forces people to admit their status is only that of client) "Do you think I am not busy?" (forces the client to admit that the nurse really *is* busy)
Rejecting	Refusing to discuss certain topics with the client. These responses often make clients feel that the nurse is rejecting not only their communication but also the clients themselves.	"I don't want to discuss that. Let's talk about . . ." "Let's discuss other areas of interest to you rather than the two problems you keep mentioning." "I can't talk now. I'm on my way for coffee break."

Table 13–2 Barriers to Communication (Cont.)

Technique	Description	Examples
Changing topics and subjects	Directing the communication into areas of self-interest rather than considering the client's concerns is often a self-protective response to a topic that causes anxiety. These responses imply that what the nurse considers important will be discussed and that clients should not discuss certain topics.	*Client:* "I'm separated from my wife. Do you think I should have sexual relations with another woman?" *Nurse:* "I see that you're 36 and that you like gardening. This sunshine is good for my roses. I have a beautiful rose garden."
Unwarranted reassurance	Using clichés or comforting statements of advice as a means to reassure the client. These responses block the fears, feelings, and other thoughts of the client.	"You'll feel better soon." "I'm sure everything will turn out all right." "Don't worry."
Passing judgment	Giving opinions and approving or disapproving responses, moralizing, or implying one's own values. These responses imply that the client must think as the nurse thinks, fostering client dependence.	"That's good (bad)." "You shouldn't do that." "That's not good enough." "What you did was wrong (right)."
Giving common advice	Telling the client what to do. These responses deny the client's right to be an equal partner. Note that giving expert rather than common advice is therapeutic.	*Client:* "Should I move from my home to a nursing home?" *Nurse:* "If I were you, I'd go to a nursing home, where you'll get your meals cooked for you."

Source: From *Fundamentals of Nursing: Concepts, Processes and Practice* (7th ed.), by B. Kozier, G. Erb, A. J. Berman, and S. Snyder, 2004, Upper Saddle River, NJ: Prentice Hall Health. Reprinted with permission.

■ *Legal documentation.* The client's record is considered a legal document that can be used as evidence in a legal action. Such a record is a major source of information about the care that a client received when there is an accusation of negligence or malpractice against a health care provider.

■ *Health care analysis.* In addition to being used by accrediting organizations to review the quality of care in a health care agency, client records can also help the health care agency analyze and plan the agency's needs. For example, analysis of client records can help the agency identify services that are underutilized or overutilized such as specific diagnostic studies or medications. This analysis can help the agency determine which services generate revenue and which cost the agency money.

Methods of Documentation

There are several methods of organizing the client record, including the traditional source-oriented narrative record, problem-oriented medical record, focus charting, charting by exception (CBE), and CORE documentation. Table 13–3 provides a brief description of the various methods of documentation and their advantages and disadvantages.

Critical Thinking Exercise

What nursing documentation systems are used in your health care agency? What computer programs are used for documenting care? What forms, flowsheets, or other paper documents are used to document care? What are the advantages and disadvantages of the documentation systems used in your health care agency? Are there areas that need improvement? How would you go about making needed changes?

Table 13–3 Methods of Documentation

Method	Organization	Advantages	Disadvantages
Source-oriented narrative record	Each provider documents in a separate section or sections of the client's record (e.g., Progress Notes, Nurse's Notes, etc.). Information is written in chronological order in the appropriate section.	Each discipline can easily locate the forms on which to document their data. Easy-to-follow information specific to one's discipline.	Information scattered throughout the record. Difficult to find chronological information.
Problem-oriented medical record (POMR) or problem-oriented record (POR) S —Subjective data O—Objective data A—Assessment P —Plan I —Interventions E —Evaluation R —Revision	Consists of baseline data, a problem list at the front of the record, a plan of care for each problem, and progress notes written in SOAP, SOAPIE, SOAPIER, or PIE format. Data are organized according to the client problems identified.	Encourages collaboration between health care providers. The problem list in front alerts caregivers to client's needs. Easier to track the status of each problem.	Caregivers differ in their ability to use the required format. Requires constant vigilance to maintain up-to-date problem list. Inefficient because assessments and interventions that apply to more than one problem must be repeated.
Focus charting	Client concerns and strengths are the focus of care. Data are organized according to data (D), nursing action (A), and client response (R); often uses flowsheets.	Allows charting on any significant area, not just problems. Flexible.	Not multidisciplinary. Difficult to identify chronological order. Notes may not relate to care plan.
CORE	Focuses on nursing process— the core of documentation. Consists of database (D), plan of action (A), and evaluation (E).	Incorporates the entire nursing process in one system. Groups nursing diagnoses and functional status assessments together. Promotes concise documentation with minimal repetition.	Does not always present information chronologically. Notes may not always relate to the plan of care.
Charting by exception (CBE)	Only significant findings or exceptions to norms are recorded.	Efficient—uses flowsheets. Rapid detection of changes. Can take place of plan of care.	Expensive to institute. Not prevention focused.

Table 13–3 Methods of Documentation (Cont.)

Method	Organization	Advantages	Disadvantages
FACT	Incorporates elements of charging by exception (CBE). Consists of: F—Flowsheets for specific services. A—Assessment. C—Concise, integrated progress notes and flowsheets. T—Timely entries recorded when care is given.	Computer ready. Eliminates duplication. Encourages consistent language and structure. Outcome oriented. Permits immediate recording of current data. Readily accessible at the client's bedside. Eliminates the need for different forms.	Narrative notes may be too brief. Nurse's perspective may be overlooked. Nursing process framework may be difficult to identify.

Sources: Adapted from *Mastering Documentation,* 1995, Springhouse, PA: Springhouse Corporation; and *Fundamentals of Nursing: Concepts, Process, and Practice,* (7th ed.), by B. Kozier, G. Erb, A. J. Berman, and S. Snyder, 2004, Upper Saddle River, NJ: Prentice Hall Health.

COMMUNICATION THROUGH TECHNOLOGY

Nurses are increasingly using computers to enhance their communication. Nurses use e-mail to communicate with other nurses, other departments in their employment setting, and resources outside the employment setting. Nurses can use computers to access health information through Web sites and literature databases.

Many health care agencies are implementing computer programs for client record systems. Computers may be found at nurses' stations, the clients' bedsides, or as hand-held models in nurses' pockets. Computers at the bedside enable nurses to check orders immediately before administering a treatment or medication. Data from bedside monitors can be incorporated readily into clients' records through bedside computers. Computerized client information can be transmitted rapidly from one health care setting to another to facilitate consultation with other health care providers. Computer documentation systems decrease the time spent in charting and increase the legibility and accuracy of information. More information about the use of computers and technology is provided in Chapter 16 ⊕, Technology and Informatics.

EXPLORE MEDIALINK

Questions, critical thinking exercises, essay activities, and other interactive resources for this chapter can be found on the Web site at http://www.prenhall.com/blais. Click on Chapter 13 to select activities for this chapter.

SUMMARY

For nurses to be effective in their interactions with clients, they must have effective communication skills. They must be aware of what their words and body language are saying to others. Professional nurses must be effective in both verbal and written communication, and they need to possess good computer skills in order

Bookshelf

Arnold, E. N., & Boggs, K. U. (1999). *Interpersonal relationships: Professional communication skills for nurses* **(3rd ed.). Philadelphia: W. B. Saunders.**
This text covers all aspects of nursing interaction and communication, including communication with clients, families, and colleagues.

Luckmann, J. (1999). *Transcultural communication in nursing.* **New York: Delmar.**
This text provides a resource for better communication with clients, interpreters, and colleagues whose primary language is other than English. It also provides resources of books, novels, videos and other media that demonstrate communication between cultures.

Springhouse. (1999). *Mastering documentation* **(2rd ed.). Springhouse, PA: Springhouse Publishing.**
This text covers all aspects of documentation in nursing, including documentation in acute care, long-term care, and home-care settings. A significant amount of content focuses on the legal and ethical aspects of nursing documentation.

to communicate with clients and other health care providers and to increase their knowledge through Internet resources.

Communication involves the sending and receiving of messages between two or more people. The communication process involves a sender, message, channel, receiver, and response, or feedback. The sender defines the original message and transmits it to the receiver through the channel or method of communication. The receiver then interprets the message and provides a response to the sender. By responding, the receiver becomes the sender of a new message. Thus, communication is an ongoing process, where the roles of sender and receiver are exchanged as each transmits new information or understandings to the other.

There are many factors that influence the communication process. These include developmental stage, gender, roles and relationships, values and perceptions, sociocultural characteristics, space and territoriality, environment, congruence, and interpersonal attitudes.

Types of communication include verbal and nonverbal. Verbal communication includes both spoken and written words. Nonverbal communication uses facial expression, gestures, touch, or other types of body language. Therapeutic communication is an interactive process between the nurse and the client that helps the client overcome temporary stress, to get along with other people, to adjust to the unalterable, and to overcome psychological blocks that stand in the way of self-realizations.

Documentation of clients' care and their responses to that care is essential for effective communication of the clients' status between health care providers. Additional uses of nursing documentation are in auditing for quality assurance, research, education, reimbursement, legal documentation, and health care analysis.

Nurses are increasingly using computers to enhance their communication. They use e-mail to communicate with other nurses, other departments in their employment setting, and resources outside the employment setting. Nurses can use computers to access health information through Web sites and literature databases.

REFERENCES

Ahrens, T., Yancey, V., & Kollef, M. (2003). Improving family communications at the end of life: Implications for length of stay in the intensive care unit and resource use. *American Journal of Critical Care, 12*(4), 317–323.

Fontaine, K. L., & Fletcher, J. S. (2003). *Mental health nursing* (5th ed.). Upper Saddle River, NJ: Prentice Hall.

Frank, D. I. (2003). Elderly client's perceptions of communication with their health care provider and its relation to health deviation self-care behaviors. *Self-Care, Dependent-Care, and Nursing, 11*(2).

Frisch, N. C., & Frisch, L. E. (2002). *Psychiatric mental health nursing* (2nd ed.). Albany, NY: Delmar.

Hall, E. T. (1969). *The hidden dimension.* Garden City, NJ: Doubleday (Classic).

Kozier, B., Erb, G., Berman, A. J., & Snyder, S. (2004). *Fundamentals of nursing: Concepts, process, and practice* (7th ed.). Upper Saddle River, NJ: Prentice Hall Health.

Springhouse. (1995). *Mastering documentation.* Springhouse, PA: Springhouse Corporation.

Sudia-Robinson, T. M., & Freeman, S. B. (2000). Communication patterns and decision making: Parents and health care providers in the neonatal intensive care unit—A case study. *Heart and Lung: The Journal of Acute and Critical Care, 29*(2), 143–148.

Wilson, H. S., & Kneisl, C. R. (1996). *Psychiatric nursing* (5th ed.). Menlo Park, CA: Addison-Wesley.

Change Process

Objectives

- Differentiate spontaneous, developmental, and planned change.
- Explain the empirical-rational, normative-reeducative, and power-coercive approaches to change.
- Compare the change process models of Lewin, Lippitt, Havelock, and Rogers.
- Discuss types and characteristics of change agents.
- Identify ways to manage change by enhancing motivating forces and decreasing resistive forces.
- Identify steps in the change process.

MEDIALINK

Additional online resources for this chapter can be found on the companion Web site at http://www.prenhall.com/blais.

To be effective and influential in today's world, nurses need to understand change theory and apply its precepts in the workplace, in government and professional organizations, and in the community. Change is a part of everyone's life; it is the way in which people grow, develop, and adapt. Change can be positive or negative, planned or unplanned.

Even though change is inevitable, it is not always welcome because it produces anxiety and fear even when it is planned. There is a sense of loss of the familiar, and a grief reaction may occur. The intensity can be worse when the change is unplanned. In the words of Tiffany and Lutjens (1998, p. 3), "Change is difficult. It helps. It hurts. It helps and hurts at the same time. Change is inevitable. We ignore change at our own peril."

The process of change is integral to many areas of nursing, such as teaching, client care, and health promotion. It involves individual clients, families, communities, organizations, nursing as a profession, and the entire health care–delivery system. Change can involve gaining knowledge, obtaining new skills, or adapting current knowledge in the light of new information. It can be particularly difficult when presenting challenges to one's values and beliefs, ways of thinking, or ways of relating.

CHALLENGES AND OPPORTUNITIES

The experience of change always presents some level of challenge to the person who must adapt. The rapidity and amount of change experienced in recent decades in health care has been particularly challenging for the nursing profession. New administrative structures, new technology, new professional roles, and new ways of providing care have been incorporated. Assisting clients to make changes in lifestyle to enhance their health and well-being is likewise a challenge for nurses.

With these challenges come opportunities to adapt to the new demands in a positive way. There are opportunities to incorporate the demands of change into improved ways of providing care. Nursing can meet the challenges of changing times with resistance and hang on to what is familiar or with acceptance and help create improved environments of care and improved ways of delivering health care. There is an opportunity for nursing to be proactive and manage planned change, thus emerging as a more autonomous and recognized profession.

MEANINGS AND TYPES OF CHANGE

Change is the process of making something different from what it was (Sullivan & Decker, 2001, p. 249). Change disrupts equilibrium, and it involves endings, transitions, and beginnings. People grieve when they lose something or are threatened with the loss of something. If they go through the steps of grieving, they may come to acceptance. Those who do not reach acceptance may experience disengagement or withdrawal, disidentification, with sadness and worry, disorientation and confusion, or disenchantment, accompanied by anger. Disengaged workers quit or retire in place doing only the bare minimum. People with disidentification are vulnerable, and they tend to sulk and dwell in the past and resist new tasks. Disoriented workers no longer know where they fit in the organization and often do in-

correct things because they do not know the new priorities. Disenchanted people become angry and negative and engage in destructive behavior (Tomey, 2000).

Changes are disturbing to those affected, and resistance often develops. Change is most threatening in the presence of insecurity. Causes of resistance to change include threats to self-interest, embarrassment, insecurity, habit, complacency, loss of power, and objective disagreement. Careful planning, appropriate timing of communication, adequate feedback, and employee confidence can reduce resistance to change. Informing personnel of reasons for change can help reduce resistance. Helping them cope and recognizing their contributions also minimize resistance (Tomey, 2000).

The noun and verb forms of the word *change* have different meanings. The noun form denotes substitution of one thing for another, an alteration in the state or quality of a thing, or permutations constituting varied arrangements of a set or series of things. Used as a verb, *change* means to make a thing other than it was (outward directed change) or to become different, to undergo alterations, or to vary (inward directed change). Synonyms for the verb *change* include *alter, transform, convert,* and *vary.* All these terms suggest that a fundamental difference or substitution is the outcome of change.

Change is not always the result of rational decision making. It generally occurs in response to three different activities: (a) spontaneous reactions, (b) developmental activities, and (c) consciously planned activities. Both individuals and organizations can undergo change.

Spontaneous Change

Spontaneous change is also referred to as reactive or unplanned change because it is not fully anticipated, it cannot be avoided, and there is little or no time to plan response strategies. Examples of spontaneous change affecting an individual include an acute viral infection, a spinal cord injury, and the unsolicited offer of a new position.

On a larger scale, spontaneous change can be either short term or long term. Examples of short-term spontaneous change include an earthquake or other natural disaster, a major airplane crash that is near a small hospital, or a wildcat strike that closes a tertiary health care facility. The impact of human immunodeficiency virus (HIV) on the policies and practices of health care facilities is an example of change with long-term consequences.

Responses to spontaneous change can be either positive or negative. For example, the cold virus may create only minor inconveniences for one person but may lead to life-threatening illness in another. Likewise, an organization may respond successfully to the injuries resulting from a natural event if a well-developed disaster plan is in place; conversely, without such a plan the organization may experience disorganization, confusion, and major difficulties. The result of spontaneous change can be unpredictable. To ensure a successful response, spontaneous change demands flexibility and cohesiveness.

Developmental Change

Developmental change refers to physiopsychologic changes that occur during an individual's life cycle or to the growth of an organization as it becomes more complex. Examples of developmental change of individuals include the increasing size and complexity of a human embryo and fetus and the decreasing physical capability of an older person. These changes are not consciously planned; they just happen. However, the individual may make plans for dealing with the changes. For example, an older person may make plans for dealing with the physical changes, such as moving to a smaller, one-floor residence that is easier to care for and in which it is easier to move around.

Organizations often grow and develop in unpredictable ways. A once-successful small health organization may no longer meet the increasing demands and needs of a community. As the organization evolves into a larger, more complex entity, it may undergo such unwanted change as overwork, task changes, less personalized service, and more formalized staff communication patterns. Such unavoidable changes necessitate development of organizational charts, revised job descriptions, and, often, formal staff meetings to meet the defined needs.

Planned Change

According to Lippitt (1973), **planned change** is an intended, purposive attempt by an individual, group, organization, or larger social system to influence the status quo of itself, another organism, or a situation. Problem-solving skills, decision-making skills, and interpersonal skills are important factors in planned change. An example of planned change is an individual who decides to improve his or her health status by attending a smoking-cessation program or carrying out an exercise program. Organizations are continually involved in planned changes. In health care agencies changes are made in policies, in methods of care delivery, in staffing, and so on. Bringing about planned change is a major part of any nurse-manager's role.

From a personal perspective, Alfaro-LeFevre (1999, p. 1) addresses four ways people change. See the accompanying box.

Four Ways We Change

1. Pendulum change: "I was wrong before, but now I'm right."
2. Change by exception: "I'm right, except for . . . "
3. Incremental change: "I was almost right before, but now I'm right."
4. Paradigm change: "What I knew before was partially right. What I know now is more right, but only part of what I'll know tomorrow."

PARADIGM CHANGE IS TRANSFORMATIONAL
Paradigm change combines what's useful about old ways with what's useful about new ways and keeps us open to looking for even better ways.

We realize

- Our previous views were only part of the picture.
- What we now know is only part of what we'll know later.
- Change is no longer threatening: It enlarges and enriches.
- The unknown can then be friendly and interesting.
- Each insight smoothes the road, making the change process easier.

Sources: From *Aquarian Conspiracy: Personal and Social Transformation in Our Time,* by M. Ferguson, 1980, New York: Putnam; *Critical Thinking in Nursing: A Practical Approach* (2nd ed., p. 1), by R. Alfaro-LeFevre, 1999, Philadelphia: W. B. Saunders. Reprinted with permission.

Reflect on...

■ spontaneous changes that have occurred in your personal and professional life. How did those changes affect you or your organization? What personal or professional strategies helped you or your organization adjust to the spontaneous changes?

■ planned changes that have occurred in your personal or professional life during the last year. Do planned professional changes result in planned personal changes? Is it possible that planned professional changes might result in spontaneous personal changes?

■ developmental changes that might be identified in the clients seen in your practice setting. Do the policies, procedures, and plans of care accommodate the identified developmental changes that are routinely occurring in your clients?

■ developmental changes that are occurring in your organization. What are the staff reactions to these changes? How might the professional nurse cope with or assist colleagues to cope with organization change?

CHANGE THEORY

Approaches to Planned Change

Three broad strategies or approaches to planned change have been identified; they represent a continuum of least coercive (empirical-rational) through middle ground (normative-reeducative) to the most obtrusive (power-coercive). They are compared in Table 14–1. Each is appropriate in different situations and at different times. It is important to carefully select the appropriate strategy.

Empirical-Rational

The *empirical-rational approach* is based on two beliefs: that people are rational and that they will change if it is in their self-interest. Therefore, change will be adopted if the change can be rationally justified and shown to be advantageous to the people involved (Bennis, Benne, & Chinn, 1985). An example of this would be convincing nurses that the implementation of a new bar coding procedures for medication administration is needed because it protects them from medication errors and provides greater safety for patients. The nurses would then be educated about the procedure so that they become comfortable with it.

However, people do not always act rationally, and therein can be the shortcoming. This strategy is most effective when there is little resistance to the change and the change is perceived as reasonable. Staff development in this strategy is through education and systems analysis (Tomey, 2000). The power ingredient is knowledge, and the flow of influence is from

Table 14–1 Change Approaches

Approach	Characteristics
Power-coercive	• Based on the application of power from a legitimate source. • Power is often economic or is political. • Minimal participation by target members. • Resistance may occur and morale may decrease. • Feelings and values of opposing forces are not a factor. • Model is nonparticipative and undemocratic.
Empirical-rational	• Knowledge is power. • Influence moves from those with knowledge to those without. • Once members of the target group have knowledge, they will accept or reject the idea. • Is a noncoercive model. • Appropriate for new technology. • Works well when the target group is discontented. • Fully participative and democratic.
Normative-reeducative	• Recognizes that change must deal with feelings, values, and needs. • Recognizes that not all responses of people to change are rational. • Information and rational arguments are often insufficient to bring about change. • Model is partially participative and democratic.

those who know to those who do not know. The style can be compared to marketing. Once people are informed, they will accept or reject the idea based upon its merits and consequences (Sullivan & Decker, 2001, p. 257).

Normative-Reeducative

The *normative-reeducative approach* is based on the assumption that human motivation depends on the sociocultural norms and the individual's commitment to these norms. The sociocultural norms are supported by the attitudes and value systems of the individuals. In this instance, change occurs if the people involved develop new attitudes and values by acquiring new information. In this approach, knowledge is the power for change, but it may be a lengthy process because attitudes and values are difficult to change. People's roles and relationships, perceptual orientations, attitudes, and feelings will influence their acceptance of change. In this approach, getting nurses to accept a new bar coding procedure for medication administration might center on showing the successful use of the procedure at a prestigious institution and convincing them that they are out of step by not using it.

The communication is participative and two-way (Baird, 1998). Staff development is through more individual means, such as personal counseling, small groups, and experiential learning. People participate in their own reeducation. The change agents are usually internal to the organization, and their relationship to other personnel is important (Tomey, 2000). The power ingredient is interpersonal relationships, and the change agent uses collaboration.

This approach can be effective in reducing resistance and stimulating creativity. It is well suited to nursing because nurses are well versed in behavioral science and communication skills (Sullivan & Decker, 2001, p. 258).

Power-Coercive

With the *power-coercive approach*, power lies with one or more persons of influence. The influence may come through political power, wealth, status, or ability. This approach does not deny the intelligence or rationality of people or the importance of their attitudes or values, but it recognizes the need to use power to attain change. It is a command and control approach in which positions of authority enforce the change. As a strategy, it can provoke resistance. The communication style is telling people what to do (Baird, 1998). A new procedure for bar coding medications would be presented to the staff and they would be told that it is now policy for the institution and that they must use it.

This approach is sometimes appropriate in large-scale changes or when consensus is unlikely to be achieved, time is short, resistance is anticipated, and the change is critical for the organization's survival. It tends to be better received when combined with the other two approaches. Strikes, sit-ins, and conflict resolutions are sometimes employed. These strategies should be used cautiously if there is a desire to foster a climate of openness to change (Sullivan & Decker, 2001, p. 257).

Change Strategies

Tiffany and Lutjens (1998) have identified seven change strategies that fit on a continuum from most neutral to most coercive.

1. *Educational.* This strategy provides a relatively unbiased presentation of fact that is intended to serve as a rational justification for the planned action.
2. *Facilitative.* This strategy provides resources critical to change. It assumes that people are willing to change but need the resources to bring it about.
3. *Technostructural.* This strategy alters the technology to access the social structure in groups or alters the social structure to get at technology. It assumes a relationship among technology, space, and structure. The use of space might be altered to affect the social structure. An example is the introduction of e-mail communication.
4. *Data-based.* This strategy collects and uses data to make social change. Data are used to find the best innovation to solve the problems at hand.
5. *Communication.* Communication strategies spread information over time through channels in a social system.
6. *Persuasive.* The use of reasoning, arguing, and inducement are employed to bring about a change.
7. *Coercive.* There is an obligatory relationship between planners and adopters. Power is used to bring about change.

Frameworks for Change

Frameworks such as those of Lewin, Lippitt, Rogers, and Havelock follow the normative-reeducative approach. They are compared in Table 14–2.

Table 14–2 Comparison of Change Models

Lewin	Lippitt	Havelock	Rogers
1. Unfreezing	1. Diagnose problem 2. Assess motivation 3. Assess change agent's motivations and resources	1. Building a relationship 2. Diagnosing the problem 3. Acquiring resources	1. Knowledge 2. Persuasion 3. Decision
2. Moving	4. Select progressive change objects 5. Choose change agent role	4. Choosing the solution 5. Gaining acceptance	4. Implementation
3. Refreezing	6. Maintain change 7. Terminate helping relationship	6. Stabilization	5. Confirmation

Lewin

Kurt Lewin (1948) originated change theory within the physical sciences based on his belief that change is a result of forces within a field or environment. He later expanded the theory to psychology and included all the psychologic activity confronting a person. The result was his Force Field Analysis Model, in which two forces affect the change process: driving forces that attempt to move action and static or restraining forces that attempt to maintain the status quo. For change to be successful the driving forces must be stronger; this can come about by strengthening the driving forces or weakening the restraining forces. Lewin presented three basic steps or stages: unfreezing, moving, and refreezing.

During the *unfreezing* stage, the motivation to establish some sort of change occurs. The individual becomes aware of the need for change. This stage is a cognitive process in which the person becomes aware of a problem or of a better method of accomplishing a task and hence of the need for change. Having identified this need, the individual must also identify restraining and driving forces. For example, a nurse who is instructing an adolescent client and his mother in dietary management of type I diabetes may see the client's mother as a driving force and the client's father and siblings, who don't want to change their sugar-loaded diet, as restraining forces.

In the second stage, *moving*, the actual change is planned in detail and then started. Information is gathered from one or several sources. At this stage, it is important that the people involved agree that the status quo is undesirable. In this example, the nurse needs to help the family understand the importance of dietary management for diabetics and to enlist their support for the client. The nurse could ask the dietitian to meet with the client and his family to demonstrate how a diabetic diet can be nutritious and tasty. The nurse might also provide printed food exchange lists, sample menus, and recipes, as well as resources for diabetic information. As change agent, the nurse should work with the family to create an environment that is conducive to the change, including, perhaps, rewards to reinforce desired behaviors.

In the third stage, *refreezing*, the changes are integrated and stabilized. Those involved in the change integrate the idea into their own value system. Thus, in the example, the client and his family would come to value the importance of family involvement in dietary management of their diabetic son and sibling. The family may develop their own strategies for assisting their loved one to comply with the plan.

These three stages are described in Lewin's *force field theory*. Lewin recommended that before a change is begun, the forces operating for and against the change be analyzed. The forces for change are the *driving forces*, and the forces against change are *restraining forces*. When the driving forces predominate, change occurs; when restraining forces predominate, change does not occur. It then becomes the responsibility of the change agent to use strategies to reduce the restraining forces and increase the driving forces. Reducing restraining forces usually is more effective than increasing the driving forces. This unfreezing is directed at the target system, that is, the individual, family, or group. See Figures 14–1■ and 14–2■.

Figure 14–1

Process of Change

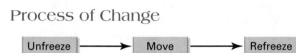

Lippitt

Gordon Lippitt and his colleagues described planned change as having seven phases, as shown in Table 14–2 (Lippitt, Watson, & Westley, 1958). This extended Lewin's theory and focused more on what the change

Figure 14–2

Status Quo

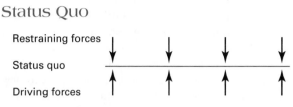

agent must do rather than on the evolution of the change. These seven phases begin with the recognized need for change. The manager can stimulate awareness and present the idea that a more desirable state is possible. Assessment can be made of the motivation and capacity to change as well as the resources for change. In Lewin's theory, this would be comparable to unfreezing.

For the process to move, a helping relationship must begin. The success or failure of the planned change will often depend upon the quality and workability of the client and change agent relationship.

Evidence for Practice

Bennett, M. (2003). Implementing new clinical guidelines: The manager as agent of change. *Nursing Management, 10*(7), 20–23.
Change management for the implementation of new clinical guidelines on sedation in a pediatric intensive care unit (PICU) applied Lewin's field theory in planning the change. Unfreezing involved the identification of a need for change on the unit. Current policy was believed to be at least partially responsible for critically ill children experiencing drug withdrawal symptoms that could affect recovery and hospital length of stay. A literature review indicated a gap in current practice from evidence in the literature. The staff wanted to improve practice, and they were provided with information they understood and a plan for supportive training. They were involved in drafting the new guidelines.

The new guidelines were implemented after they were clear and user-friendly. Staff was trained. Potential barriers were identified as the perception that assessing sedation is time-consuming and a low priority when a child is critically ill. Another was the additional responsibility. These were countered with driving forces of increased understanding of the benefits to the child, the development of a user-friendly assessment tool, and interpersonal skills of the manager in giving and interpreting feedback.

The final stage of refreezing was implemented by providing positive feedback and reinforcement from the change agents. Plans were implemented to evaluate the new policy's effectiveness through peer review and audit (identifying gaps in practice).

Common Driving and Restraining Forces

MOTIVATING FORCES

- Perception that the change is challenging
- Economic gain
- Perception that the change will improve the situation
- Visualization of the future impact of change
- Potential for self-growth, recognition, achievement, and improved relationships.

RESTRAINING FORCES

- Fear that something of personal value will be lost (e.g., threat to job security or self-esteem)
- Misunderstanding of the change and its implications
- Low tolerance for change related to intellectual or emotional insecurity
- Perception that the change will not achieve goals; failure to see the big picture
- Lack of time or energy

Problems must be identified and analyzed, alternative possibilities must be examined, and goals and objectives must be planned. Resources will be examined and strategies developed. This corresponds to moving in Lewin's theory.

Generalization and stabilization correspond to Lewin's refreezing process. These are necessary to prevent slipping back into old ways. The change needs to spread and stabilize. A change in momentum, positive evaluation of the change, reward for change, and procedural and structural change are each important factors (Tomey, 2000).

Havelock

Ronald Havelock (1973) modified Lewin's theory regarding planned change by emphasizing planning the change process. He described the six-step process shown in Table 14–2. More attention is paid to the unfreezing stage, which he defines as building a relationship, diagnosing the problem, and acquiring resources. In the moving stage, the solution is chosen and acceptance is gained. Refreezing is referred to as stabilization and self-renewal.

Rogers

Everett Rogers developed a *diffusion-innovation theory* rather than a planned change theory. He defines *diffusion* as the process by which an innovation is communicated through certain channels over time among the members of a social system. Diffusion that involves innovation becomes social change when the diffusion of new ideas results in widespread consequences. His framework, diffusion of innovation, emphasizes the reversible nature of change. Participants may initially adopt a proposal and later discontinue it, or they may initially reject it and adopt it at a later time. Rogers thus introduced the idea that an adopted change is not necessarily permanent. Rogers' three phases in the diffusion of innovation follow (Rogers & Shoemaker, 1971; Rogers, 1995):

1. *Invention.* Collecting information about the proposed change. Data are collected and analyzed.
2. *Diffusion.* Communicating information or the idea to others. It includes disseminating information and estimating the case or difficulty of diffusing the new idea or information.
3. *Consequences.* The dissemination of information may result in the adoption or rejection of the change.

Rogers wrote that the factors associated with successful planned change are relativity, advantage, compatibility, complexity, divisibility, and communicability. His five steps to the diffusion of innovations, referred to as the *innovation-decision process,* follow:

1. *Knowledge.* The individual, called the decision-making unit, is introduced to change and begins to comprehend it.
2. *Persuasion.* The individual develops a favorable or unfavorable attitude toward the change.
3. *Decision.* The person makes a choice to adopt or not to adopt the change.
4. *Implementation.* The person acts on the choice. At this time, alterations may take place.
5. *Confirmation.* The individual looks for confirmation that the choice was right. If the person encounters mixed messages, the choice may be changed.

Rogers emphasized that for change to succeed, the people involved must be interested in the change and committed to implementing it. His theory is particularly useful for individuals who wish to track the adoption of technologic innovations (Tiffany & Lutjens, 1998).

MANAGING CHANGE

There are internal and external forces that affect change. Internal forces originate inside the organization, but they may be due to external forces. There may be an internal force for changing the organization of health care delivery related to low staffing levels, but these low staffing levels may be caused by external forces such as the shortage of nurses or changing health care economics.

The change manager must be able to identify the source of the problem, assess motivations and capacity for change, determine and examine alternatives, and then determine and implement a helping relationship. Havelock (1973) believes change agents facilitate planned change by being a catalyst, solution giver, process helper, and resource linker. In using Lewin's theory, change agents identify the restraining and driving forces and assess the relative strengths of each. Driving forces could include desire to please authority figures or a desire to improve a situation. Restraining forces could include such things as conformity or threats to prestige. Strategies are then planned to reduce the restraining forces and strengthen the driving forces.

Evidence for Practice

Barr, B. J. (2002). Managing change during an information systems transition. *AORN Online,* **75(6), 1085–1088, 1090–1092.**

Innovation-diffusion theory was applied to implementing a computerized system of perioperative patient documentation. Application of the model involved examining the process by which innovation is communicated using social channels in particular groups. The first phase of diffusion began with the acquiring of initial knowledge and exposure to the change. This was followed by persuasion when the nurses began to integrate the information to form a perception of the change. This was followed by a decision to accept or reject the innovation. When the decision was made to accept the change, the implantation phase began with practice using the technology and finally seeking validation to support their choice during the final or conformation phase.

Five adopter groups were identified in the groups; these were:

- Risk-takers
- Early adopters
- Early majority (not leaders but willing to adopt change)
- Late majority (in need of intense encouragement)
- Laggards (experiencing resistance)

Frequent and effective communication was a key factor in facilitating successful change.

Cognitive dissonance is believed to be a powerful motivator for change. It assumes four concepts:

- People like consistency in their thoughts, beliefs, attitudes, values, and actions.
- Dissonance is a result of psychological inconsistency which is experienced as discomfort.
- Dissonance drives people to action.
- Dissonance stimulates people to attain consistency and reduce inconsistency.

The degree of dissonance experienced is directly related to the importance of the issue. To reduce these feelings of imbalance, people often change attitudes or behavior to regain that feeling of consistency (Gruber, 2003).

Change Agent

A **change agent** is one who works to bring about a change (Sullivan & Decker, 2001, p. 249). The change agent is the person or group who initiates, motivates, and implements the change. Change agents are leaders. The nurse uses critical thinking and knowledge of change theory to act as an effective change agent in a variety of health care settings.

An effective change agent must be highly skilled. As the nurse moves through the process of change with clients, families, groups, communities, or institutions, the nurse assumes a variety of roles, depending on the type of change and the needs of the individuals involved in the change. It is also important for the change agent to be accessible to all people involved in the change process. The change agent should be honest and straightforward about goals and problems. The box on page 258 describes effective change agent skills.

A key element in the change process is trust. The change agent must trust the participants in the change, and they in turn must trust the change agent. One of the greatest risks of change is that it can disrupt the system or even render it nonfunctional. For example, changing the method of nurse assignments could result in gaps and missed care for some clients. To

Critical Thinking Exercise

Identify a nursing situation in which a client is presented with the need to change a behavior in order to better manage a health problem, such as obesity. Apply one of the frameworks discussed and identify how a nurse might assist with this change.

Identify a need for change you have observed in your community, such as improved trash pickup. Apply one of these frameworks and identify steps you could take to facilitate this change.

Change Agent Skills

- The ability to combine ideas from unconnected sources
- The ability to energize others by keeping the interest level up and demonstrating a high personal energy level
- Skill in human relations; well-developed interpersonal communication, group management, and problem-solving skills
- Integrative thinking; the ability to retain a "big picture" focus while dealing with each part of the system
- Sufficient flexibility to modify ideas when modifications will improve the change, but persistent enough to resist nonproductive tampering with the planned change
- Confidence and the tendency not to be easily discouraged
- Realistic thinking
- Trustworthiness; a track record of integrity and success with other changes
- Ability to articulate a "vision" through insights and versatile thinking
- Ability to handle resistance

Source: From *Effective Management in Nursing* (5th ed., p. 258), by E. J. Sullivan and P. J. Decker, 2001, Upper Saddle River, NJ: Prentice Hall. Reprinted with permission.

avoid this problem, the change agent must closely observe the situation during the change process.

A change agent may be formally or informally designated. A formally designated change agent is one who has the role and responsibility for change, such as a clinical nurse-specialist expected to make changes beneficial to specified clients. This person has the authority to plan and implement change. An informally designated change agent does not have the authority to make change by virtue of a position but does have the leadership skills and respect of others and therefore can serve an important function in the change process. A change agent who has formal status carries authority, whereas an informal change agent can operate only through persuasion (Ehrenfeld, Bergman, & Ziv, 1992, p. 23).

Change agents may also be internal or external. An *internal change agent* is a person who is part of the situa-

tion or system, for example, a charge nurse on a hospital unit or a public health nurse providing school health services to a specific school or within a school system. Internal change agents are familiar with the situation and the organization. However, they may have vested interests in the present system as well as biases. An *external change agent* comes to the situation from the "outside," for example, a nursing administrator from another hospital, a nurse-specialist from another health care facility, or a nurse-educator from a local college. External change agents are able to view the problem and the situation objectively and usually have no biases; they are often viewed as experts and are called consultants. However, they may not have personal knowledge of the situation and the problems. They may not be viewed as openly as an "insider"; therefore, they must develop a cooperative working relationship with the people involved in the change. A third option is to pair the external agent with the internal person to serve together as change agents. There are advantages and disadvantages to each of these options, and it is important for any change agent to be aware of both in each situation.

Coping with Change

The pace of change has accelerated in the past decades because of factors such as the changes in technology and communication. Individuals vary in their ability to tolerate change, yet today's work environment demands that people be able to manage change skillfully. Organizations also differ in their ability to absorb change. The questions in the box on page 259 can help assess the organization's "hardiness for change."

Reflect on...

- the questions in the box on organizational hardiness to change. How would you answer those for your current workplace?

Although change is inevitable and necessary for growth, it is not always welcome and often produces anxiety. Even when change is well planned, it can be threatening because the process renders something different from the status quo. Change evokes emotional reactions, consumes considerable internal resources and energy, and often is associated with feelings of loss, grief, and pain. Various models have been proposed to explain the psychologic problems associated with change. Seven stages of change are identified and can be used as a framework for navigating transitions (Manion, 1998). These seven stages were introduced in Chapter 1 ⏳ and are depicted in Figure 14–3■.

Questions Reflecting the Organization's Hardiness to Change

- How often does major organizational change occur in my organization?

- How many changes are made within a month in my patient care unit?

- For how many of these changes were we alerted beforehand?

- How readily do people in my organization accept change?

- Who decides on what changes are going to take place?

- How many people must approve an idea?

- Do people view change as an opportunity or necessary evil?

- How are people who think differently viewed in my organization?

- If I had an interesting new way to change some aspect of patient care, what would the response of my colleagues be? My supervisor?

- Are the following phrases often heard?
  - When we get done with all of the changes . . .
  - Why can't we leave well enough alone?
  - What's wrong with how we've always done it?

Source: From "Creating Change in the Workplace" by J. Disch, and K. Taranto. In D. Mason, J. Leavitt, and M. Chaffee, *Policy and Politics in Nursing and Health Care* (4th ed., p. 335), St. Louis: W. B. Saunders.

Stage 1: Losing focus. Confusion and disorientation occur and decisions are difficult. On the positive side, this stage is usually short and may not require specific interventions.

Stage 2: Minimizing the impact. Some denial is used to reduce the significance and portray the event as no big deal. Often the person feels the need to "put on a good face." If it is prolonged, productivity and commitment can disintegrate.

Stage 3: The pit. This represents the lowest point on the mood curve shown in Figure 14–3. There is anger, discouragement, resentment, and resistance. Morale suffers, and people often have difficulty dealing with the emotions in this stage.

Stage 4: Letting go of the past. This is a more positive stage; energy starts to return and people begin to see the end of the change process. There are two main tasks during this stage: letting go of the past and looking ahead. People begin to prepare for the future. There is optimism and renewed energy. It is not unusual to be dragged back to the pit from this stage, because things do not always unfold in a perfectly linear fashion, but the time is usually much shorter.

Figure 14–3

The Seven Stages of Change

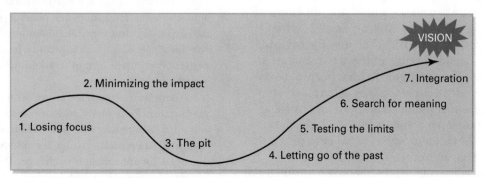

Source: From "Understanding the Seven Stages of Change," by J. Manion, 1998. In E. C. Hein, *Contemporary Leadership Behavior Selected Readings* (5th ed., p. 237), Philadelphia: Lippincott. Used by permission.

Stage 5: Testing the limits. Optimism is more energizing; people try new coping skills and deal with the situation in more creative ways.

Stage 6: Search for meaning. At this stage, there is an ability to look back and realize that even though the change was painful, meaning can be seen in the experience. There is a newly found confidence and freedom and sometimes a desire to reach out to others who are still experiencing difficulty.

Stage 7: Integration. By this stage, the transition is complete. The change has been integrated into life, and people are oriented toward the future.

Unfortunately, people often are called upon to deal with another change before they have reached full integration of a previous change. In today's rapidly changing health care environment, coping with change may be one of the biggest challenges. It calls for resilience, adaptability, and flexibility. The box on page 261 shows some tips for getting through each of the seven stages of change.

Resistance to Change

Resistance to change is not merely lack of acceptance but rather behavior intended to maintain the status quo—that is, to prevent the change. The change agent should anticipate some resistance to change, no matter how beneficial the change may seem. Resistance to change is often greatest when the idea is not concurrent with existing trends, such as trying to change from primary nursing to functional nursing when primary nursing is the current trend. Resistance is also usually great when a proposed change would alter a situation with which people are comfortable.

Accepting change often takes time, particularly when it does not fit into a person's attitudinal frame of reference; in such a case, change may not occur at all. For example, stopping smoking may not be accepted as a desirable change by a person who enjoys smoking and does not believe that it is harmful. Optimally, this belief changes before the person tries to change the behavior.

A change agent should anticipate resistance to change. It is important to listen to what people are saying and under what circumstances. There are often nonverbal signs of resistance and perhaps passive aggression, including poor work habits and lack of effort in assigned tasks. Open resisters are easier to deal with than the more passive resisters.

Resistance to change is not always a bad thing; it can prevent the unexpected and provide a barrier to change that may not be desirable for the institution.

Some degree of resistance to change is a natural response. Resistance may help people adapt to the proposed change as they try to understand the meaning on a personal level, establish a thread of continuity, and then accept and grow with the change. It forces the change agent to be clear and convincing about the need and to provide motivation. On the other hand, persistent resistance can wear down supporters and use up energy that could be directed to implementation. Morale can suffer. It then becomes necessary for the change agent to minimize the resistance.

To manage resistance, the leader (change agent) can analyze the field forces operating in the change (see the discussion on Lewin). After the analysis, three kinds of tactics can be used to "unfreeze" the system: (1) create discomfort, (2) induce guilt or anxiety, (3) provide psychological safety (Tappen, 2001, p. 207). To create discomfort, the change agent can confront the target system with conflicting evidence that challenges the

Evidence for Practice

Ingersoll, G. L., Fisher, M., Ross, B., Soja, M., & Kidd, N. (2001). Employee response to major organizational redesign. *Applied Nursing Research, 41*(1), 18–28.

Semistructured focus group interviews were conducted in two acute-care hospitals undergoing major organizational change to introduce a patient-focused model. The interviews were conducted on all shifts and focused on staff nurse perceptions of the redesign process and its effect on the work environment. Several themes emerged from the interview data. Considerable distress was evident along with feelings of loss, anger, despair, and abandonment. Staff morale was low, and there was mistrust of administration. The groups described periods of crying, irritability, and physical exhaustion. There was role ambiguity with the change and a loss of unit cohesiveness and peer group relationships. Resource availability was a concern.

There were a number of implications for administrators. Particularly evident was the need for administration to take into consideration the effect upon staff when such a change is implemented and the need for information exchange. Planned debriefing sessions were recommended.

Tips for Getting Through the Stages of Change

1. Losing focus
   - Expect some forgetfulness.
   - Use to-do lists.
   - Ask for clarification of expectations and temporary lines of authority.

2. Minimizing the impact
   - Tell yourself the truth about what's happening. List the gains and losses associated with the change. Be honest about what you're losing or giving up.
   - If others offer help but you're not ready to accept it, respond in a way that leaves the door open for their support at a later date.
   - Take one step at a time.
   - Don't stay in this stage too long–but don't try to end it precipitously either. Start gathering your courage for the next stage, which is the most difficult.

3. The pit
   - Expect to feel angry, discouraged, and resentful. If you know what's happening inside you, you're more likely to keep your equilibrium.
   - Let yourself experience the feelings. Suppressing or denying them will make it more difficult for you to deal with change in the future.
   - Find a safe place to express your feelings, preferably with someone who can listen comfortably without taking them on or trying to talk you out of them.
   - Develop a positive vision of what things will be like when you've finished this transition, then think of it often. People with a clear vision have an easier time getting through the pit.

4. Letting go of the past
   - Say good-bye to the past, either formally or informally. You might do this with a "letting-go" ritual. An example of such a ritual would be to review what was positive about the past, recount good memories, and then bury it. Or it may be more appropriate to have a graduation party.
   - Allow some sadness and longing for the way things used to be.
   - As you look ahead, think of what you'll need to adjust to the change—new skills and new approaches, for example. Consider specific ways to obtain them.
   - Take care of yourself. Celebrate the small successes.

5. Testing the limits
   - Seek new experiences and ways to use the skills you've gained.
   - Spend time with people who have experienced the same change or loss.
   - Talk about the past only with those who will listen and not become impatient.
   - Associate with people who are encouraging and supportive.

6. Search for meaning
   - Spend time reflecting on your experiences since the change occurred. Sort through your feelings. Ask yourself: "What have I learned that I didn't know before?"
   - Look back to how you handled the different emotional stages. Notice which were particularly difficult and give yourself a pat on the back for getting through them.
   - Find others going through the same experience. Listen carefully to see if you can offer any support.

7. Integration
   - Appreciate reaching this final stage. (It doesn't always happen.)
   - Recognize how far you've come and the skills you've learned along the way.

Source: From "Understanding the Seven Stages of Change," by J. Manion, 1998. In E. C. Hein, *Contemporary Leadership Behavior: Selected Readings* (5th ed., p. 239), Philadelphia: Lippincott. Used by permission.

Managing Resistance

1. Communicate with those who oppose the change. Get to the root of their reasons for opposition.

2. Clarify information and provide accurate feedback.

3. Be open to revisions but clear about what must remain.

4. Present the negative consequences of resistance (threats to organizational survival, compromised client care, and so on).

5. Emphasize the positive consequences of the change and how the individual or group will benefit. However, do not spend too much energy on rational analysis of why the change is good and why the arguments against it do not hold up. People's resistance frequently flows from feelings that are not rational.

6. Keep resisters involved in face-to-face contact with supporters. Encourage proponents to empathize with opponents, recognize valid objections, and relieve unnecessary fears.

7. Maintain a climate of trust, support, and confidence.

8. Divert attention by creating a different "disturbance." Energy can shift to a "more important" problem inside the system, thereby redirecting resistance. Alternatively, attention can be brought to an external threat to create a "bully phenomenon." When members perceive a greater environmental threat (such as competition or restrictive governmental policies), they tend to unify internally.

9. Follow the "politics of change."

Source: From *Effective Management in Nursing* (5th ed., p. 259), by E. J. Sullivan and P. J. Decker, 2001, Upper Saddle River, NJ: Prentice Hall. Reprinted with permission.

status quo. Often the change agent meets with defensive responses that attempt to protect the individuals. By inducing guilt—for example, by pointing out that accepted goals are not being met—the change agent often upsets the balance of the driving and restraining forces. Then, by providing psychologic safety, the change agent can help the target system feel more comfortable and less threatened about the change.

The change agent needs to be aware of the sources of power that can energize change. This often means being politically astute within an organization. The following four political strategies may be helpful:

1. Analyze the organizational chart and be aware of the formal and informal lines of authority.

2. Identify the key people affected by the change. In an organizational hierarchy, the people immedi-

Table 14–3   Examples to Unfreeze a Target System

Producing discomfort	• Meet with small groups of nurses (target system) to discuss the inadequacies of the system of concern (e.g., staffing).
Inducing guilt and anxiety	• Demonstrate how the system is not meeting clients' needs for care.
	• Explain that the administration wants the new system.
	• Provide examples of how the old system has endangered client safety.
Providing psychological safety	• Assure nurses (target system) that adequate numbers of nurses will be provided.
	• Point out that sufficient time will be provided to implement the new system.
	• Express confidence in the nurses' abilities to implement the change.
	• Assure the nurses that there will be regular meetings to discuss progress.

ately above and below those directly affected should be given attention.

3. Find out as much as possible about what makes these key people tick. It is important to know their likes and dislikes and with whom they usually align on decisions.

4. Begin to build a coalition of support before the change begins by identifying those individuals who are most likely to support the effort and those most likely to be persuaded easily. Their counsel on costs and benefits and objections can be used to make modifications that make the innovation more appealing (Sullivan & Decker, 2001, p. 259).

The successful change agent has a good sense of timing and can effectively adapt a timetable to facilitate the process and gain support. Unfreezing can best be accomplished during coalition building when interest is high and resistance has not yet consolidated. For behavioral change to occur, some kind of evidence is useful in building the case for change. This evidence can come from research, quality management data, patient satisfaction data, or someone else's experience, for example. As the change is implemented, some feedback loop is desirable so that people can see any improvement that may be resulting from the change. Incentives may be needed for moving and maintaining the change; the incentives might include commendations, access to prized resources, money, and so on. But the incentives should be in alignment with the individual's motivation and the organization's goals (Mason, Leavitt, & Chaffee, 2002).

If resistance continues for a prolonged time, the change agent must consider two possibilities. One is that the change is not workable and must therefore be modified and compromise is necessary to meet the strongest objections. The other possibility is that the change is appropriate and the plan is sufficiently developed but must proceed through more coercive means so resistance can be overcome.

Evidence for Practice

Ingersoll, G. L., Kirsch, J. C., Merk, S. E., & Lightfoot, J. (2000). Relationship of organizational culture and readiness for change to employee commitment to the organization. *Journal of Nursing Administration, 30*(1), 11–20.

This study was done to determine the influence of organizational culture and organizational readiness on employee commitment to the work of the institution. A longitudinal survey design was used, and questionnaires were distributed through the hospital's internal mailing system. Subjects were selected from all nursing, administrative, and ancillary support personnel using a systematic, stratified sample-selection plan. Two questionnaires were used for data collection, the Organizational Culture Inventory and the Pasmore Sociotechnical Systems Assessment Survey. Two tertiary hospitals undergoing the implementation of a patient-focused redesign were the sites of the study. The focus of the redesign was on bringing services closer to the patient, reducing the number of persons interacting with patients and families, and improving the efficiency and quality of services to consumers. Data were collected approximately 6 months after planning began and immediately before implementation. A sample size of 684 was analyzed by multiple regression. Organizational readiness was the strongest predictor of commitment. The researchers conclude that organizations in which change is seen as a positive characteristic of the environment and employees are reinforced for their contribution are more likely to develop work groups committed to the work of the institution.

Critical Thinking Exercise

Identify a change that is needed in policy at your workplace, such as staffing ratios. What are the different driving and restraining forces involved in the proposed change? What strategies might you implement to reduce the restraining forces? What strategies might you implement to enhance the driving forces? How might you obtain the assistance of formal and informal change agents in your practice setting to facilitate the change?

Examples of Change

It is exciting to realize how effective nurses can be when they determine the need for change and plan strategies to bring it about. The following examples outline changes initiated by nurses who have identified a need to "do something" in each of four spheres of influence: the workplace, organizations, government, and the community.

THE WORKPLACE   At each of three staff meetings Jane Hawkins, nurse-manager, listened to nurses complain about problems with getting clients' laboratory work done and reported to the unit in a timely manner. She conferred with other nurse-managers and with the attending and resident physicians on her unit. It appeared that similar complaints were widespread.

At the next management meeting, Jane described the problem. The group appointed a task force, with Nurse Hawkins as chair, and asked it to present a plan to solve the problem at the next meeting. After gathering more data, the task force invited representatives from the attending and resident staff and the laboratory director to meet with them to review the data, consider alternative solutions, and select a plan to solve the problem.

By the next management meeting, a preliminary plan to alter the system of laboratory reporting had been devised, and all concerned were working cooperatively to implement the plan.

THE PROFESSIONAL ORGANIZATION   Nurses on the Education Committee of a district nurses' association recognized the need to make a public policy statement concerning the care of clients with AIDS. The board of directors had recently expressed interest in promulgating such policy statements, so the committee sensed the timing was right and that the board would welcome its draft despite the controversial subject matter.

Members of the committee researched and drafted a statement. The full committee offered a critique and selected an articulate spokesperson to present the statement to the association president and seek support before asking to have the statement presented to the board. Once the president had approved the statement, it was placed on the agenda for the next board meeting.

After making minor additions, the board approved it for distribution to the lay and nursing press and asked the education committee to suggest a nurse to present the statement at a local hearing of the city council health committee.

THE GOVERNMENT   Although the pressure to contain health care costs escalated through the first half of the 1980s, a coalition representing the shared interests of the ANA, the National League for Nursing (NLN), and the American Association of Colleges of Nursing (AACN) mounted a campaign to convince Congress of the cost-effectiveness of a center for nursing research within the National Institutes of Health (NIH). Despite incredible odds, including a presidential veto and opposition from the American Medical Association, the American Association of Medical Colleges, and the NIH administrations, the proposal was passed by Congress in the fall of 1985. The success of this effort demonstrates the effectiveness of carefully planned change, including the collaboration of nursing organizations. It also illustrates the clout organized nurses can wield on any level and in any sphere.

THE COMMUNITY   Every nurse plays several roles besides that of registered nurse. Each resides in a community, and many are parents. Some serve on school boards, belong to the League of Women Voters, or participate in religious, club, or scouting activities. There are numerous opportunities for nurses to contribute to the health and welfare of the communities in which they live. A group of nursing students recognized a health problem within their community and developed a plan to intervene. Many of the students were parents of children in local elementary schools where a high percentage of children were being sent home daily with head lice. Because of previously enacted budget cuts, the district's school nurses were each responsible for between three and five schools. The students volunteered to work with the district nurses to provide screening and health teaching at each of the elementary schools, thereby helping to resolve the community's problem.

All nurses are affected by change; nobody can avoid it. Knowledgeable nurses make rational plans to deal with both opportunities to initiate and guide needed change and to respond to change that affects them in the workplace, government, organizations, and the community. To recognize these opportunities for change and respond to the factors that influence nursing from outside the profession, it is helpful to consider the history of nursing, current trends in nursing, and present political, social, technologic, and economic issues.

Reflect on...

■ what changes are needed in your professional skills and abilities to help you to become a more effective change agent. How will you approach these changes?

EXPLORE MEDIALINK

Questions, critical thinking exercises, essay activities, and other interactive resources for this chapter can be found on the Web site at http://www.prenhall.com/blais. Click on Chapter 14 to select activities for this chapter.

Bookshelf

Driegel, R. J., & Brandt, D. (1997). *Sacred cows make the best burgers: Developing change-ready people and organizations.* **New York: Warner Books.**

Outdated and costly practices exist in every organization, and they slow down innovative ideas. This book provides a guide to why people hold on to the old and how to inspire them to bring on the new.

Johnson, S., & Blanchard, K. (1998). *Who moved my cheese? An amazing way to deal with change in your work and in your life.* **New York: Putnam Publishing.**

This book presents a parable of four not-so-blind mice who learn to accept and adapt to change to get what they need. They live in a maze and look for cheese but are faced with an unexpected change. One of them

learns to deal with it successfully and writes what he has learned on the maze walls.

Sills, J. (2004). *The comfort trap (or, what if you're riding a dead horse?)* **New York: Viking Penguin Press.**

The book is about change and how to get over the hump when leaving one's comfort zone. Advice is given with warmth and humor.

Vance, M., & Deacon, D. (1997). *Think out of the box.* **New York: Career Press.**

Written by the former dean of Disney University, this book uses a nine-dot matrix to plot the nine necessary points of a creative culture: people, place, product, involving, informing, inspiring, cooperation, and creativity.

SUMMARY

To be effective and influential in current and future health care delivery systems, nurses need to understand and apply change theory. Change generally occurs in response to three different activities: spontaneous reactions or events, developmental activities, and consciously planned activities. These three types of change can occur on an individual or organizational level.

The three most commonly used approaches to change are the empirical-rational approach, the power-coercive approach, and the normative-reeducative approach. In reality, all three of these approaches may operate in a situation of change simultaneously.

Lewin's theory of change has three stages: unfreezing, moving, and refreezing. His force field analysis is a means of examining the driving forces for change and the restraining forces that would limit change. The analysis of the opposing forces is done in

the unfreezing stage. Reducing restraining forces is usually more effective in accomplishing change than is increasing the driving forces.

Lippitt proposed a seven-stage process beginning with diagnosing the problem and ending with terminating the helping relationship. Havelock modified Lewin's theory to emphasize the planning stage of the change process. His six-stage theory begins with building a relationship and ends with stabilization and generating self-renewal. Rogers introduced the idea that adopted change is not necessarily permanent. He developed a five-step diffusion-innovation process.

A change agent seeks to facilitate the processes of change. An effective change agent uses an understanding of the change process to plan and implement any change. To be effective change agents, nurses require excellent skills of communication, problem solving, decision making, and teaching and must be able to project expertise, know how to use available resources, be able to inspire trust in themselves and others, and have a good sense of timing. A change agent may be formally or informally designated, internal or external. Nurses frequently act as formal or informal change agents in relation to clients, families, work settings, and communities. The change agent works to alter the driving and restraining forces and facilitates the acceptance of change by encouraging the participation of all involved in the change process. Effective communication is vital to the success of planned change.

Change is stressful, and the individuals experiencing change need to be supported and empowered. The stress is often associated with emotional reactions of denial, anger, feelings of loss, grief, and pain. An understanding of these responses enables both change agents and those experiencing the change to minimize the trauma associated with it. Managing change requires adaptability, flexibility, and resilience.

REFERENCES

Alfaro-Lefevre, R. (1999). *Critical thinking in nursing: A practical approach* (2nd ed.). Philadelphia: W. B. Saunders.

Baird, A. (1998). Change theory and health promotion. *Nursing Standard, 12*(22), 34–36.

Barr, B. J. (2002). Managing change during an information systems transition. *AORN Online, 75*(6), 1085–088, 1090–1092.

Bennett, M. (2003). Implementing new clinical guidelines: The manager as agent of change. *Nursing Management, 10* (7), 20–23.

Bennis, W. G., Benne, K. D., & Chin, R. (Eds., 1985). *The planning of change* (4th ed.). New York: Holt, Rinehart & Winston.

Bozak, M. G. (2003). Using Lewin's force field analysis in implementing a nursing information system, *Computers, Informatics, Nursing, 21*(2), 80–85.

Ehrenfeld, M., Bergman, R., & Ziv, L. (1992, January/February). Academia: A stimulus for change. *International Nursing Review, 39,* 23–26.

Gruber, M. (2003). Cognitive dissonance theory and motivation for change. *Gastroenterology Nursing, 26*(6), 242–245.

Havelock, R. (1973). *The change agent's guide to innovations in education.* Englewood Cliffs. NJ: Educational Technology Publications.

Hein, E. C. 1998. *Contemporary leadership behavior: Selected readings* (5th ed.). Philadelphia: Lippincott.

Ingersoll, G. L., Fisher, M., Ross, B., Soja, M., & Kidd, N. (2001). Employee response to major organizational redesign. *Applied Nursing Research, 14*(1), 18–28.

Ingersoll, G. L., Kirsch, J. C., Merk, S. E., & Lightfoot, J. (2000). Relationship of organizational culture and readiness for change to employee commitment to the organization. *Journal of Nursing Administration, 30*(1), 11–20.

Lewin, K. (1948). *Resolving social conflicts.* New York: Harper and Brothers.

Lewin, K. (1951). *Field theory in social science.* New York: Harper and Row.

Lippitt, G. L. (1973). *Visualizing change: Model building and the change process.* La Jolla, Calif.: University Associates.

Lippitt, R., Watson, J., & Westley, B. (1958). *The dynamics of planned change.* New York: Harcourt Brace.

Manion, J. (1998). Understanding the seven stages of change. In E. C. Hein, *Contemporary leadership behavior: Selected readings* (5th ed., pp. 236–240). Philadelphia: Lippincott.

Mason, D., Leavitt, J., & Chaffee, M. (2002). *Policy and politics in nursing and health care* (4th ed.). St. Louis: W. B. Saunders.

Miller, C. E. (1999). Stages of change theory and the nicotine-dependent client: Direction for decision making in nursing practice. *Clinical Nurse Specialist, 13*(1), 18–22.

Rogers, E. M. (1995). *Diffusion of innovations* (4th ed.). New York: Free Press.

Rogers, E., & Shoemaker, F. (1971). *Communication of innovations: A crosscultural approach.* New York: The Free Press of Glencoe.

Sullivan, E. J., & Decker, P. (2001). *Effective leadership and management in nursing* (5th ed.). Upper Saddle River, NJ: Prentice Hall.

Tappen, R. M. (2001). *Nursing leadership and management: Concepts and practice* (4th ed.). Philadelphia: F. A. Davis.

Tiffany, C. R., & Lutjens, L. R. J. (1998). *Planned change theories for nursing: Review, analysis, and implications.* Thousand Oaks, CA: Sage Publications.

Tomey, A. M. (2000). *Guide to nursing management and leadership* (6th ed.). St. Louis: Mosby.

CHAPTER 15

Group Process

Outline

Objectives

- Differentiate between different types of groups.
- Discuss the stages of group development.
- Describe characteristics of effective groups.
- Describe the essential characteristics of group dynamics.
- Analyze group interactions to determine effective and ineffective group processes.
- Discuss the purposes of different types of health care groups.

M E D I A L I N K

Additional online resources for this chapter can be found on the companion Web site at http://www.prenhall.com/blais.

A group is defined by Adams and Galanes (2003, p. 11) as "three or more individuals who have a common purpose, interact with each other, influence each other, and are interdependent." Nurses belong to a variety of professional groups, ranging from the smallest group, consisting of two people, also called dyads, to large professional associations. In these groups the nurse may fill a variety of roles, including leader, advisor, elaborator, and encourager.

A group consists of people who share needs and goals and who take each other into account in their actions. People are usually born into a family group and interact with other groups at all stages of their lives through social, cultural, religious, and professional socialization. Groups are important in people's lives. The family provides for initial socialization, whereas other groups (e.g., peer, social, religious, work, political) are vehicles for continued learning and socialization. Group dynamics, or group process, is the way in which groups function. For group work to be accomplished and group goals to be achieved, group dynamics must be effective.

CHALLENGES AND OPPORTUNITIES

The changing health care system presents challenges for health care professionals if they are to be actively involved in decisions about health care policy and health care practice. Such decisions are rarely made by one person in isolation but rather by groups of people at all levels of society: think tanks, advocacy groups, professional groups, and politicians at local, regional, state, national, and international levels.

These challenges provide opportunities for nurses to participate as active members of the various decision-making groups. To be effective members of these groups, nurses must be knowledgeable about the dynamics of group work in addition to providing expert knowledge about nursing and health care.

GROUPS

Groups exist to help people achieve goals that might be unattainable by individual effort alone. By pooling the ideas and expertise of several individuals, groups can often solve problems more effectively than one person. Information can be disseminated to groups more quickly and with more consistency than to individuals. In addition, groups often take greater risks than do individuals as they support each other in decision making. Just as responsibilities for actions are shared by group members, so are the consequences of actions.

In the clinical setting, nurses work in groups as they collaborate with other nurses, other health care professionals, clients, and support persons when planning and providing care. Nurses also work in groups when joining professional and specialty organizations and civic and community groups to promote the goals of nursing on professional, civic, and political levels. Group skills are therefore important for nurses in all settings.

Types of Groups

Groups are classified as either primary or secondary, according to their structure and type of interaction. A **primary group** is a small, intimate group in which the relationships among members are personal, spontaneous, sentimental, cooperative, and inclusive. Examples are the family, a play group of children, informal work groups, and friendship groups. Members of a primary group communicate with each other largely in face-to-face interactions and develop a strong sense of unity, or "oneness." What belongs to one person is often seen as belonging to the group. For example, a success achieved by one member is shared by all and is seen as a success of the group.

Primary groups set standards of behavior for the members but also support and sustain each member in stressful situations he or she would otherwise not be able to withstand. Expectations are informally administered and involve primarily internal constraints imposed by the group itself. To its members, the primary group has a value in itself, not merely as a means to some other goal. The group has a sense of "we" and "our" to it, in contrast to "I" and "mine." Affective relationships are stressed.

The role of the primary group, particularly the family, in health care is increasingly recognized. It is to the primary group that people turn for help and support when they have health problems. Treatment and health care of individuals therefore are developing an expanded focus that includes the family.

A **secondary group** is generally larger, more impersonal, and less sentimental than a primary group. Examples are professional associations, task groups, ad hoc committees, political parties, and business groups. Members view these groups simply as a means of getting things done. Interactions do not necessarily occur in face-to-face contact and do not require that the members know each other in any inclusive sense.

Thus, there is little sentiment attached to such relationships. Expectations of members are formally administered through impersonal controls and external restraints imposed by designated enforcement officials. Once the goals of the group are achieved or change, the interaction is discontinued.

Functions of Groups

Sampson and Marthas (1990, pp. 3–21) describe eight functions of groups. See Table 15–1. Any one group generally has more than one function, and it may serve different functions for different group members. For example, for one member a group may provide support; for another, information.

Levels of Group Formality

There are three levels of group formality. Groups may be classified as formal, semiformal, or informal.

Formal Groups

The most common example of the formal group is the work organization. People become familiar with many different formal work groups during their lifetimes and spend a major part of their working hours in such groups. Formal groups usually exist to carry out a task or goal rather than to meet the needs of group members. An example of a formal group is the staff of a nursing unit where the nurse-manager provides the authority and structure for staff meetings. Traditional features of formal groups are shown in the box on page 270.

Semiformal Groups

Examples of semiformal groups include churches, lodges, social clubs, parent-teacher organizations, and some labor unions. Many of an individual's social and ego needs are often satisfied by membership in these

Table 15–1 Functions of Groups

Function	Description
Socialization	Primary socialization in growth and development. Professional socialization into nursing or to a change in position. Socialization into the culture of an organization (i.e., new customs and beliefs) when a hospital is taken over by a corporate organization.
Support	Provision of social support for the members, a source of collegiality, and a source of help when needed.
Task completion	Complete tasks that are beyond the scope of any one individual. Each person may bring specialized knowledge and skills. Cooperation is important in task completion.
Camaraderie	Provision of goodwill among the members, thereby providing moments of pleasure.
Information	Provide a context for defining social reality, for setting performance goals, for establishing priorities, and for sharing special knowledge.
Normative function	Develop definitions and standards and enforce those standards, thereby encouraging compliance and discouraging deviations.
Empowerment	Empowering people and thereby encouraging change. A group often has more power than any individual.
Governance	Groups are often active in making decisions and serving as a source of governance within an organization.

Source: Adapted from *Group Process for Health Professions,* by E. E. Sampson and M. Marthas (3rd ed.), 1990, Albany, NY: Delmar.

Characteristics of Formal Groups

- Authority is imposed from above.
- Leadership selection is assigned from above and made by an authoritative and often arbitrary order or decree.
- Managers are symbols of power and authority.
- The goals of the formal group are normally imposed at a much higher level than the direct leadership of the group.
- Fiscal goals have little meaning to the members of the group.
- Management is endangered by its aloofness from the members of the work group.

- Behavioral norms (expected standards of behavior), regulations, and rules are usually superimposed. The larger the turnover rate of members, the greater the structuring of rules.
- Membership in the group is only partly voluntary.
- Rigidity of purpose is often a necessity for protection of the formal group in the pursuit of its objectives.
- Interactions within the group as a whole are limited, but informal subgroups are generally formed.

groups. The groups are similar in form to formal groups, but exhibit slight differences. Features of semiformal groups are shown in the accompanying box.

Informal Groups

Most people, from childhood on, have membership in numerous informal groups. Informal groups are described by Crenshaw (2003) as groups "that provide much of a person's education and contribute greatly to his or her cultural values; members do not depend on one another." Five types of groups are representative of the numerous informal groups in existence:

- *Friendship groups.* The first groups formed in life are friendship groups. They are often formed on the basis of common interests. Many arise out of semiformal group interactions or are formed spontaneously from the work organization.
- *Hobby groups.* Hobby groups bring together people from all walks of life. Differences in members' personalities and backgrounds are largely ignored in the interests of the hobby itself.
- *Convenience groups.* Many examples of convenience groups are found both in and out of the work setting. Two examples are the carpool and the childcare group organized by mothers.
- *Work groups.* Informal work groups can make or break an organization. Managers need to be sensitive to such

Characteristics of Semiformal Groups

- The structure is formal.
- The hierarchy is carefully delineated.
- Membership is voluntary but selective and difficult to achieve.
- Prestige and status are often accrued from membership.
- Structured, deliberate activities absorb a large part of the group's meeting time.

- Objectives and goals are rigid; change is not recognized as desirable.
- In many cases, the leader has direct control over the choice of a successor.
- The day-to-day operating standards and methods (group norms) are negotiable. Because most people become bored at quibbling about norms, people can often "railroad" acceptance of a list of norms they desire.

groups and cultivate their cooperation and goodwill. Friendships often arise between a new member and the person who makes him or her feel a welcome addition to the group.

■ *Self-protective groups.* Self-protective groups can be found anywhere but are particularly common in work organizations. They arise spontaneously out of a real or perceived threat. For example, a supervisor may approach a worker too strongly and find a group of workers organizing a united front against the threat. Such groups dissipate as soon as the threat has subsided.

The main features of informal groups are shown in the accompanying box.

Group Development

The phases of group development have been variously described. Frisch and Frisch (2002) divide group development into three phases: orientation, working, and termination. In the *orientation phase*, group members seek to be accepted, and to find out how similar and different each one is from the other. Anxiety is often high during this period. The group is more likely viewed as a group of individuals than as a unified whole. Uncertainty and insecurity are often present in the group; safe topics are discussed.

In the *working phase*, group members feel more comfortable with one another, and group goals are established. Decisions are more likely to be made by consensus rather than by vote. Problem solving takes place, and frustration is often replaced by cautious optimism. Differences that are present are handled by adapting and problem solving rather than conflict. Disagreements are dealt with openly.

During the *termination phase*, the focus is on evaluating and summarizing the group experience. Feelings vary from frustration and anger to sadness or satisfaction, depending on whether the group has achieved its goals and attained group cohesion (group unity).

Crenshaw (2003) adds a fourth stage between the working and termination stages, the mature stage. In the *mature stage*, group members develop a group culture of acceptance and openness. There is a sense of "we" or cohesiveness as group members work to achieve the group goals. When conflict occurs, it is related to issues of significance rather than emotional issues.

Tuckman and Jensen (1977) identified six stages of group (team) development, which were further

Characteristics of Informal Groups

- The group is not bound by any set of written rules or regulations.

- Usually there is a set of unwritten laws and a strong code of ethics.

- The group is purely functional and has easily recognized basic objectives.

- Rotational leadership is common. The group recognizes that only rarely are all leadership characteristics found in one person.

- The group assigns duties to the members best qualified for certain functions. For example, the person who is recognized as outgoing and sociable will be assigned responsibilities for planning parties.

- Judgments about the group's leader are made quickly and surely. Leaders are replaced when they make one or more mistakes or do not get the job done.

- The group is an ideal testing ground for new leadership techniques, but there is no guarantee that such techniques can be transferred effectively to a large, formal organization.

- Behavioral norms are developed either by group effort or by the leader and adopted by the group.

- Deviance by one member from the group's behavioral norms is more threatening to the perpetuation of small, informal groups than to large, formal, heterogeneous groups. Conformity and group solidarity are important for the protection and preservation of small groups.

- Group norms are enforced by sanctions (punishments) imposed by the group on those who violate a norm. Different values are placed on norms in accordance with the values of the leader. One leader may regard the action as a gross violation, whereas another leader may find it quite acceptable.

- Interpersonal interactions are spontaneous.

Table 15–2 Stages of Team Development

Stage	Team Behaviors	Leadership Behaviors
Orientation	Uncertainty Unfamiliarity Mistrust Nonparticipation	Directive style Outline purpose Negotiate schedules Define the team's mission
Forming	Acceptance of each other Learning communication skills High energy, motivated	Plan/focus on the problem Positive role modeling Actively encourage participation
Storming	Team spirit developed Trust developed Conflict may arise Impatience, frustration	Evaluate group dynamics Focus on goals Conflict resolution Establish goals and objectives
Norming	Increased comfort Identify responsibilities Effective team interaction Resolution of conflicts	Focus on goals Attend to process and content Supportive style
Performing	Clear on purpose Unity/cohesion Problem solve and accept actions	Act as a team member Encourage increased responsibility Follow up on action plans Measure results
Terminating	Members separate Team gains closure on objectives	Reinforce successes Celebrate and reward

Source: From "Quality Work Improvement Groups: From Paper to Reality," by G. B. Smith and E. Hukill, July 1994, *Journal of Nursing Care Quality, 8,* 5. Used with permission.

described by Smith and Hukill (1994). Each group member should be aware of these stages and of the process of development in order to assess the developmental progress of the groups in which they participate. See Table 15–2.

Characteristics of Effective Groups

To be effective, a group must achieve three main functions: accomplish its goals, maintain its cohesion, and develop and modify its structure to improve its effectiveness.

See Table 15–3 for comparative features of effective and ineffective groups.

Reflect on...

■ your own involvements in groups. How many groups do you participate in? Which groups fulfill personal goals? Which groups fulfill professional goals? Which

groups are specific to fulfilling work goals? How does the organization of your different groups relate to the characteristics of the various types of groups described in this chapter?

Critical Thinking Exercise

List types of groups to which nurses belong. Identify primary and secondary groups and formal, semiformal, and informal groups in which nurses commonly participate. How does membership in these groups enhance the individual nurse, the goals of the organization, and the goals of professional nursing? How does nursing participation in these groups help to improve client/patient care?

Table 15–3 Comparative Features of Effective and Ineffective Groups

Factor	Effective Groups	Ineffective Groups
Atmosphere	Informal, comfortable, and relaxed. It is a working atmosphere in which people demonstrate their interest and involvement.	Obviously tense. Signs of boredom may appear.
Goal setting	Goals, tasks, and objectives are clarified, understood, and modified so that members of the group can commit themselves to cooperatively structured goals.	Unclear, misunderstood, or imposed goals may be accepted by members. The goals are competitively structured.
Leadership and member participation	Shift from time to time, depending on the circumstances. Different members assume leadership at various times, because of their knowledge or experience.	Delegated and based on authority. The chairperson may dominate the group, or the members may defer unduly. Members' participation is unequal, with high-authority members dominating.
Goal emphasis	All three functions of groups are emphasized—goal accomplishment, internal maintenance, and developmental change.	One or more functions may not be emphasized.
Communication	Open and two-way. Ideas and feelings are encouraged, both about the problem and about the group's operation.	Closed or one-way. Only the production of ideas is encouraged. Feelings are ignored or taboo. Members may be tentative or reluctant to be open and may have "hidden agendas" (personal goals at cross-purposes with group goals).
Decision making	By consensus, although various decision-making procedures appropriate to the situation may be instituted.	By the higher authority in the group, with minimal involvement by members; or an inflexible style is imposed.
Cohesion	Facilitated through high levels of inclusion, trust, liking, and support.	Either ignored or used as a means of controlling members, thus promoting rigid conformity.
Conflict tolerance	High. The reasons for disagreements or conflicts are carefully examined, and the group seeks to resolve them. The group accepts unresolvable basic disagreements and lives with them.	Low. Attempts may be made to ignore, deny, avoid, suppress, or override controversy by premature group action.
Power	Determined by the members' abilities and the information they possess. Power is shared. The issue is how to get the job done.	Determined by position in the group. Obedience to authority is strong. The issue is who controls.
Problem solving	High. Constructive criticism is frequent, frank, relatively comfortable, and oriented toward removing an obstacle to problem solving.	Low. Criticism may be destructive, taking the form of either overt or covert personal attacks. It prevents the group from getting the job done.
Self-evaluation of the group	Frequent. All members participate in evaluation and decisions about how to improve the group's functioning.	Minimal. What little evaluation there is may be done by the highest authority in the group rather than by the membership as a whole.
Creativity	Encouraged. There is room within the group for members to become self-actualized and interpersonally effective.	Discouraged. People are afraid of appearing foolish if they put forth a creative thought.

Source: From *Psychiatric Nursing* (5th ed., p. 736), by H. S. Wilson and C. R. Kneisl, 1996, Redwood City, CA: Addison-Wesley Nursing.

GROUP DYNAMICS

Group dynamics, or group processes, are related to how the group functions, communicates, sets goals, and achieves objectives (Marriner-Tomey, 2000). Every group has its own characteristics and ways of functioning. Seven aspects of group dynamics follow.

Commitment

The members of effective groups have a commitment (agreement, pledge, or obligation to do something) to the goals and output of the group. Because groups demand time and attention, members must give up some autonomy and self-interest. Inevitably, conflicts arise between the interests of individual group members and those of the group as a whole. However, members who are committed to the group feel close to each other and willingly work for the achievement of the group's goals and objectives. Some indications of group commitment are shown in the accompanying box.

Leadership Style

Leadership style refers to the different ways in which a leader combines task and relationship behaviors to influence others to accomplish goals (Huber, 2000). See Chapter 9 ⚭, The Nurse as Leader and Manager, for more information about leaders and leadership styles.

Decision-Making Methods

Making sound decisions is essential to effective group functioning. Effective decisions are made when the following things occur:

1. The group determines which decision method to adopt.
2. The group listens to all the ideas of members.
3. Members feel satisfied with their participation.

4. The expertise of group members is well used.
5. The problem-solving ability of the group is facilitated.
6. The group atmosphere is positive.
7. Time is used well; that is, the discussion focuses on the decision to be made.
8. Members feel committed to the decision and responsible for its implementation.

Three decision-making aids are described by Mc-Murray (1994, pp. 62–65): brainstorming, the nominal group technique, and the Delphi technique. According to McMurray, the idea behind **brainstorming** is that the interaction of several people in a group can generate more ideas about a subject than could the individuals by themselves. For brainstorming, (1) the individuals in the group must have a level of trust, (2) there must be a criticism-free atmosphere that allows ideas to flow freely, and (3) all ideas receive initial approval and are critically examined thereafter.

Nominal group technique (NGT) is also an aid to decision making. It is especially useful when numerous ideas from group members may result in conflict in reaching a decision. Adams and Galanes (2003, p. 246) describe nominal group technique as the process of alternating "between individual work and group work to help a group hear from every member when discussing a controversial issue." In this instance the individuals meet as a group, but they write their responses without discussion. The ideas are then collected and open discussion proceeds. The steps used for conducting nominal group technique are shown in Figure 15–1■.

The **Delphi technique** was originally used for technologic forecasting. It has been used for decisions that require more time or need responses from people in disparate locations. The participants maintain their anonymity, which eliminates peer pressure. Data are

Indications of Group Commitment

- Members feel a strong sense of belonging.
- Members enjoy each other.
- Members seek each other for counsel and support.
- Members support each other in difficulty.
- Members value the contributions of other members.

- Members are motivated by working in the group and want to do their tasks well.
- Members express good feelings openly and identify positive contributions.
- Members feel that the goals of the group are achievable and important.

Figure 15–1

Steps for Conducting Nominal Group Technique

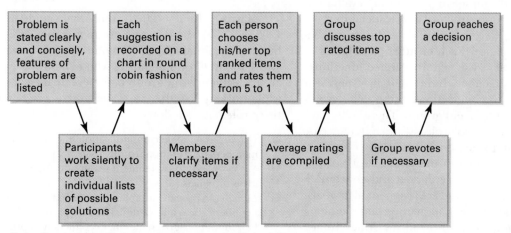

Source: From *Communicating in Groups: Applications and Skills* (p. 247), by K. Adams and G. J. Galanes 2003, Boston: McGraw-Hill. Reprinted with permission.

gathered through interviews or questionnaires in a series of rounds in which an initial question is posed. Once the responses are returned, they are compiled and redistributed. The participants do not know who said what: The comments or ratings are gathered for a compiled listing and are rated through averaging or statistical analysis. With the Delphi technique, agreement is reached as the process continues, either by consensus, voting, or mathematical average (McMurray, 1994, p. 64). See Table 15–4 for a comparison of brainstorming, nominal group technique, and the Delphi technique.

Table 15–4 Comparison of Brainstorming, Nominal Group Technique, and Delphi Technique

Brainstorming	Nominal Group Technique	Delphi Technique
Group activity, open discussion.	Group activity; initial silent interaction with later discussion.	No personal interaction; input is anonymous.
Can be conducted in one session.	Can be conducted in one session.	Takes place over three to four rounds of data collection and analysis.
Relaxed, noncritical atmosphere is essential.	Noncritical atmosphere desirable in discussion stage.	No interaction; responses are anonymous.
Largely unstructured format.	Structured format; sequential steps or stages to be followed.	Structured format; requires "rounds" of interaction.
Easy to conduct; requires little preparation or understanding.	Easy to conduct; requires little preparation or understanding.	Requires coordination of responses, can be time-consuming.
Promotes more ideas than do individuals acting alone.	Promotes more and better quality ideas than does brainstorming.	Promotes many high-quality ideas.
Possible influence of results by peer pressure.	Peer influence likely only in discussion phase.	Little peer pressure noted.

Source: From "Three Decision-Making Aids: Brainstorming, Nominal Group and Delphi Technique," by A. R. McMurray, March/April 1994, *Journal of Nursing Staff Development, 10,* 62–65. Used with permission.

Member Behaviors

The degree of input by members into goal setting, decision making, problem solving, and group evaluation is related to the group structure and leadership style, but members also have responsibilities for group behavior and participation. Each member participates in a wide range of roles (assigned or assumed functions) during group interactions. Individuals may perform different roles during interactions in the same group or may vary roles in different groups. These roles have been categorized as (1) task roles, (2) maintenance or building roles, and (3) dysfunctional roles.

Task roles are related to the task or work of the group. Their purpose is to enhance and coordinate the group's movement toward achievement of its goals. Some behaviors may be seen in many group members and some may not be seen at all. Marriner-Tomey (2000) and Adams and Galanes (2003, p. 176) describe the following task roles that facilitate group work:

- *Initiator-contributors* (orienters) propose goals, activities, or plans of action to achieve the goals. They usually act to identify the problem and clarify the goals. They may suggest items for discussion and set time limits.
- *Information givers* provide relevant facts, information, evidence, or experience useful in achieving the group task.
- *Information seekers* try to find factual data about the task. Information givers present facts and share experiences related to the task. The focus of information seekers and givers is facts rather than values and beliefs.
- *Opinion givers* state their own beliefs and thoughts about what they think the group values should be. The focus of opinion givers is on values and beliefs rather than facts.
- *Opinion seekers* clarify values associated with the problem or task and the possible solutions.
- *Clarifiers* interpret issues making vague or confusing statements clearer.
- *Elaborators* develop the ideas or suggestions. They take an idea and give substance to it. They may predict outcomes related to a particular approach.
- *Evaluators* assess the comparative worth of information or ideas. They may identify the advantages and disadvantages of various ideas.
- *Summarizers* review what has been discussed or decided throughout the decision-making process of the group.
- *Coordinators* organize the group's work.
- *Critics* evaluate the problem, its proposed solutions, and the group's work toward the solution. They may measure the group's work against a set of standards.
- *Consensus testers* determine if the group has reached agreement or a decision.
- *Energizers* stimulate the group to increase its productivity in both quantity and quality.

- *Recorders* take minutes of group meetings, keeping an account of the group's discussion, suggestions, and decisions.

Marriner-Tomey (2000) and Adams and Galanes (2003, p. 177) also describe group member roles that build and maintain the group continuity, cohesiveness, and stability. Group members who exhibit these roles are focusing on how group members treat each other while working together to achieve the goals. Some of these roles are as follows:

- *Gatekeepers* regulate communication to ensure that all members have an opportunity to be heard.
- *Supporters* express agreement or support for another's ideas or beliefs.
- *Encouragers* provide acceptance and support for group members' ideas and values. They are particularly helpful when a group member is reluctant to present or explore an idea that is controversial.
- *Harmonizers (tension-relievers)* try to maintain group cohesion. They may mediate group members' disagreements or use humor to relieve tension.
- *Compromisers* seek to achieve common ground within the group. They may modify their ideas to maintain group cohesiveness.

Group task roles and group maintenance roles are essential for the successful outcomes of group work. Group task roles provide the stimulus for achievement of the group goals; group maintenance roles serve the human needs for recognition and worth.

Other group member behaviors can interfere with the work of the group. Such interference may delay the work of the group or result in the group being unsuccessful in achieving its goals. These behaviors or roles are referred to as self-serving or dysfunctional roles. Often, these behaviors are more about the group member meeting his or her own needs rather than the group's needs. Marriner-Tomey (2000) identifies some of these behaviors as follows:

- *Aggressors* show disapproval of other group members by body language or verbal statements. They may disparage the ideas of another group member.
- *Dominators* assert their superiority by interrupting others or giving authoritative directions. They may make statements such as, "There is only one way to proceed . . . " (usually meaning their way).
- *Blockers* are negative, resistant to change, and disagreeable without apparent reason. They may make statements such as, "This is the way we have always done it," "Why do we need to do something different when what we are doing works just fine?" or "This is just not going to work."

- *Special-interest pleaders* focus on the needs of a specific interest group rather than the overall group task or goal.
- *Playboys* or *playgirls* demonstrate a lack of involvement in the group process. They may joke inappropriately or use the meeting time to gossip.

Interaction Patterns

Interaction patterns can be analyzed by using a sociogram, a diagram of the flow of verbal communication within a group during a specified period, for example, 5 to 15 minutes. This diagram indicates who speaks to whom and who initiates the remarks. Ideally the interaction patterns of a small group would indicate verbal interaction from all members of the group to all members of the group (Figure 15–2■). In reality, not all communication is a two-way process. In the sociogram shown in Figure 15–3■, the lines with arrowheads at each end indicate that the statement made by one person was responded to by the recipient; a short cross-line drawn near one of the arrowheads indicates who initiated the remark. One-way communication is indicated by lines with an arrowhead at only one end. Remarks made to the group as a whole are indicated by arrows drawn to the middle of the circle only. By using a sociogram, nurses can analyze strengths and weaknesses in a group's interaction patterns. Used in conjunction with member behavior tools, this can offer considerable data about the group's dynamics.

Cohesiveness

Groups that have the characteristic of **cohesiveness** possess a certain group spirit, a sense of being "we," and a common purpose. Adams and Galanes (2003, p. 187) define cohesiveness as the "attachment members feel toward each other, the group, and the task." When there is a high level of cohesiveness, group members feel greater satisfaction. Groups lacking cohesiveness are unstable and more prone to disintegration. See the box on page 278 for some of the attitudes and behaviors that reflect group cohesiveness.

Power

Patterns of behavior in groups are greatly influenced by the force of power. **Power** can be defined as the ability to influence another person in some way or the ability to do something, whether it is to decide the fate of a nation or to decide that a certain change in policy or practice is necessary.

Figure 15–2

An ideal interaction pattern of a small group. Each member interacts with all other members.

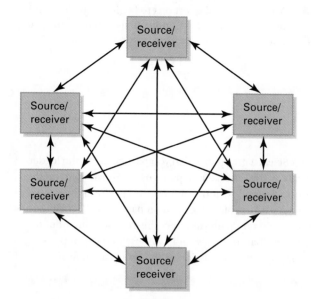

Figure 15–3

A sociogram indicating the flow of verbal communication within a group during a specific period. Note that five questions or comments calling for a response were directed at the leader.

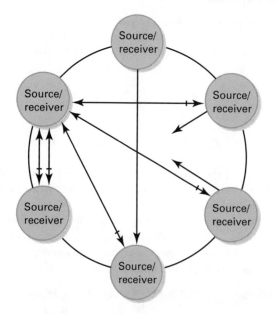

Attributes of Group Cohesiveness

MEMBERS' ATTITUDES AND BEHAVIORS

- Like each other, trust one another, and are friendly and willing to interact.
- Receive support from the group and praise one another for accomplishments.
- Have similar attitudes and beliefs.
- Are loyal to the group and defend it against outside criticism.
- Readily accept assigned roles and tasks.
- Influence each other and value being influenced by others.
- Feel satisfied and secure.
- Stay in the group and value group goals.

GROUP CHARACTERISTICS

- Goals are valued and are consistent with the goals of individuals.
- Activities are handled by group action.
- Actions are interdependent and cooperative.
- Goals that are difficult to achieve are met by persistent efforts.
- Participation is high.
- Commitment is high.
- Communication is high.
- "We" is frequently heard in discussions.
- Productivity is high.
- Norms are adhered to and protected.

Many people have a negative concept of power, likening it to control, domination, and even coercion of others by muscle and clout. However, power can be viewed as a vital, positive force that moves people toward the attainment of individual or group goals. The overall purpose of power is to encourage cooperation and collaboration in accomplishing a task. For more about power, see Chapter 11 ∞, The Nurse as Political Advocate.

Reflect on...

■ groups in which you are a participant. What level of commitment do the various group members exhibit? What is your own level of commitment to achieving the group goal(s)? How does the level of commitment exhibited by the individual group members affect the goal attainment of the group? What are the factors in the group process that increase/decrease your commitment to the group task?

FACILITATING GROUP DISCUSSION

A group leader can use certain techniques to facilitate group discussion. Smith and Hukill (1994, pp. 8–9) suggest the following:

■ Ask open-ended questions to begin discussions and to probe for details from individuals and from the group.
■ Encourage questions from group members.

Critical Thinking Exercise

Select a group in which you participate as a member. Analyze the interaction patterns demonstrated in the group. Identify group members who perform the various group tasks or roles described on pages 276–277. How do the interaction patterns affect the goal attainment of the group? What strategies could you use as a group member to improve the interaction of the group members?

Select a group in which you participate as the leader. Analyze the interaction patterns demonstrated in the group. Identify group members who perform the various group tasks or roles described on pages 276–277. How do the interaction patterns affect the goal attainment of the group? What strategies could you use as the group leader to improve the interaction of the group members?

Group Process Skills

- Active listening.
- Focusing discussions on the purpose.
- Checking perceptions of the group.
- Reflecting—the ability to convey the essence of what a group member has said so that others can understand it.
- Clarifying—focusing on key underlying issues and sorting out confusing and conflicting feelings and thinking.
- Summarizing—restating, reflecting, and summarizing major ideas and feelings by pulling important ideas together and establishing a basis for further discussion. Summarize points of agreement and disagreement among group members.

- Facilitating—assisting the members to express their feelings and thoughts openly and actively working to create a climate of openness and acceptance in which members trust one another and therefore engage in a productive exchange of ideas, opinions, and perceptions.
- Interpreting—offering possible explanations.
- Questioning—if overused, members can become frustrated and annoyed with continued questions.
- Confirming—restating a member's basic ideas by emphasizing the facts and encouraging further discussion.
- Encouraging—as a leader, don't agree or disagree with a member's ideas. Use noncommittal words with a positive tone of voice. Examples: "I see . . . "; "Uh-huh . . . "; "That's interesting . . . ."

■ Respond with positive statements or a summary each time a participant makes a contribution.

■ Reinforce participants' contributions by giving them your full attention.

■ Avoid making negative comments about group members' contributions. Instead, summarize or restate them and ask other team members for their thoughts about the idea.

■ Avoid taking sides on issues. Instead, summarize differences of opinion, stress that issues can be viewed from many different perspectives, and emphasize relative consensus.

■ When monitoring small break-out work groups, avoid becoming involved in any of the groups. Participants tend to expect the group leader to intervene, rather than focusing on the task themselves or seeking input from each other.

■ Seek equal contribution from all group members.

To conduct an effective group process, a leader needs to have certain skills. Some of these skills are listed in the accompanying box.

GROUP PROBLEMS

Problems that occur in groups include monopolizing, conflict, groupthink, scapegoating, silence and apathy, and transference and countertransference. These behaviors are described in the following sections.

Monopolizing

Because most group meetings have time restraints, domination of the discussion by one member seriously deprives others of their chances to participate. A sense of injustice develops, and ultimately members may direct their frustration and anger toward the group leader, who they think should do something to stop the monopolizer's behavior.

There may be several reasons for monopolizing behaviors, including anxiety, a need for attention, recognition, and approval. Whatever the reason, the goal of the leader is to assist the person to moderate his or her participation in the group. Often, compulsive talkers are unaware of their behavior and its effect on others and need help to recognize their behavior and its consequences.

Four strategies for dealing with monopolizing follow:

■ *Interrupt simply, directly, and supportively.* This strategy is an initial attempt to get the person to hear others.

■ *Reflect the person's behavior.* This strategy is an attempt to help the person become aware of the monopolizing behavior.

■ *Reflect the group's feelings.* This strategy is an attempt to help the person become aware of the effects of his or her behavior on others.

■ *Confront the person and/or the group.* This strategy can be directed toward the individual or toward the group to help members realize their own responsibility for the problem.

Conflict

Adams and Galanes (2003, p. 228) state "when group members think critically, disagreement almost always occurs. Conflict, expressed and managed appropriately, can help members sharpen their thinking and decide wisely." Conflict refers to disagreement, impatience, and argument among members. It can be either productive or nonproductive, and group leaders need to differentiate between destructive conflict and constructive conflict. Conflict is productive and beneficial when members feel involved, when the issue being discussed is important to them, and when they are working intensively on a problem. Productive conflict contributes to problem solving as long as the goal is clearly understood.

Nonproductive conflict leads the group astray and hinders the achievement of group goals. There are three common reasons for this type of conflict, as follows (Bradford, Stock, & Horwitz, 1974, p. 38):

1. The group has been given an impossible task, or the task is not clear. Members are frustrated because they feel unable to meet the demands on them.

2. The main concern of members is to find status in the group and to deal with their personal and individual tasks rather than the group problem.

3. Members are operating from unique, unshared points of view and may have competing loyalties to and conflicting interests in outside groups.

The nurse-leader should intervene early rather than later. In some instances, the nonproductive conflict is best avoided or played down rather than confronted. If the leader decides it is more beneficial for the group to face the issue directly, the leader can employ the following strategies (Sampson & Marthas, 1990, pp. 245–246):

- *Interpreting.* The leader explains her or his view of the problem. For example, the leader might say, "I think the group is having trouble making a decision because there are some distinct conflicts among several group members. Before we try to accomplish any other task I think we had better take some time and look at those conflicts."
- *Reflecting.* With this strategy, the leader points out certain behaviors of the members or points out his or her own feelings. To reflect behavior the leader may say, "I've noticed that several persons have been very quiet for some time, that others are talking a great deal but usually at cross-purposes, and that as a group we seem to be unable to focus our efforts on anything except disagreeing." To reflect feeling the leader may

say, "I'm not sure how anyone else feels, but I'm feeling frustrated and annoyed over the constant bickering. I know we have a job to do, and I'd like to get on with it."

- *Confronting.* With this strategy, the leader calls the group's attention to what she or he perceives is taking place with one or more of the members. For example, the leader may say, "Mrs. Purple, I think you are angry because . . . , and you seem to feel. . . . Is that why you are so distressed?" or "I think that Mr. Black and Ms. White are each trying to gain some points in this discussion, but this is not helping us deal with the task at hand. I wonder if you two could listen for a while and let us get back to our task?"
- *Voicing the unmentionable.* Here the leader states a belief or feeling which will be uncomfortable for the listener, for example, "I think you are afraid of losing power on your unit, and that is why you are disagreeing with everything that is being said without listening to the others."

Groupthink

Groupthink is defined by Adams and Galanes (2003, p. 232) as a "negative relational outcome of group decision making characterized by a group's failure to think critically about its decisions." Groupthink can occur in highly cohesive groups when group members do not want to disagree or criticize group thinking for fear of being considered disloyal. Symptoms of groupthink are shown in Table 15–5.

Scapegoating

Scapegoating is a process in which one or two members are singled out and agree, consciously or unconsciously, to be targets for group hostility or advice (Clark, 1994, p. 97). Scapegoating is a convenient method people use to negate any responsibility for what occurs in a group. By scapegoating, individuals can decrease their own anxiety. By also focusing on another's weakness, scapegoaters can minimize their own feelings of ineptitude.

For leaders to deal with scapegoating, they must be alert to its development and be prepared to accept anger when they confront the scapegoaters.

Silence and Apathy

Nonparticipation or **apathy** of one or more group members is sometimes best handled by nonintervention. Sometimes such silences are not a reflection of something in the immediate group setting but rather of some past experience. For example, after expressing an idea previously, this person may have been told,

Table 15–5   Symptoms of Groupthink

The Group Overestimates Its Power and Morality	The Group Becomes Closed-Minded	Group Members Experience Pressure to Conform
• Group believes its cause is right. • Members convince themselves they cannot fail.	• Group is selective in gathering information: chooses only information that supports its predisposition. • Group is biased in evaluating information. • Group excludes or ignores members and outsiders who seem to hold opposing views.	• Members censor their own remarks. • Members who voice contradictory opinions receive pressure from other members to conform. • Members have the illusion that the group opinion is unanimous.

Source: From *Communicating in Groups: Applications and Skills* (5th ed., p. 234), by K. A. Adams and G. J. Galanes, 2003, Boston: McGraw Hill. Reprinted with permission.

"That was a stupid thing to say." Having been hurt once in a group, such persons feel insecure about their views and are reluctant to express themselves again in groups.

Continued nonparticipation or apathy, however, needs to be dealt with by the leader, after a careful assessment of whether the apathy is a reflection of leadership style, task issues, or interpersonal conflicts.

For apathy reflecting the members' opinions that the task is unimportant, the leader may suggest, "I think there is general boredom with today's task. Do people feel that what we are doing is not really relevant or important?" After members have responded, the leader needs to ask, "What things would you prefer the group to do?"

For apathy related to members' feelings of inadequacy about handling the task or lack of the structure and organization needed for problem solving, the leader may ask, "Are people feeling generally that the group is not up to handling the task we are facing?" or "I think, because we're not really sure of what to do or how to go about dealing with the task facing us, that it may be helpful if we break up the task into smaller parts, decide what the important issues are, and develop a method for dealing with each part."

For apathy based on an interpersonal issue such as anger or fear and expressed by silence, the leader needs to decide whether to let the silence simply pass or intervene. If generally responsive group members suddenly become silent, it is important to note which issue or topic immediately preceded the silence. Some-

times a conflict among a few members has been uncovered or the group has been pushed into discussing a topic considered irrelevant or threatening. In this situation the leader may say, "I am wondering whether people are angry at what I've done," or "Are some of you anxious about bringing up that topic, since it may bring out bad feelings?" For apathy in response to an autocratic leadership style, the leader must implement measures to change the style and assist the group to work through and change their relationship with the leader.

Transference and Countertransference

Transference is the transfer of feelings that were originally evoked by parents or significant others to people in the present setting. An example is a group member who acts toward the leader as she or he would act toward a parent. In addition, members of a group can transfer to others in the group personal feelings of love, guilt, or hate.

When leaders respond to group members because of reactions from earlier relationships, they are engaging in countertransference. For example, if a group member reminds a leader of a teacher who was menacing and demanding, the leader is likely to react with anxiety and may become unreasonably fearful. It is therefore important that leaders recognize the possibility of overreaction because of countertransference and that it is not an unusual reaction among nurses who are highly involved in helping others.

Critical Thinking Exercise

Consider how problem behaviors, such as scapegoating, groupthink, apathy, transference, or countertransference, in an individual group effect achievement of the mission and goals of the organization as a whole. How might such problem behaviors in groups composed of nurses be viewed by nonnurses within an organization? How might this affect the role of nursing in the organization?

Reflect on...

- the personal goals that may be achieved by a group member who exhibits monopolizing, scapegoating, or apathetic behaviors. How might you, as the group leader, or other group members intervene to redirect such blocking behaviors?

TYPES OF HEALTH CARE GROUPS

Much of a nurse's professional life is spent in a wide variety of groups. As a participant in a group, the nurse may be required to fulfill different roles as member or leader, teacher or learner, adviser or advisee. Common types of health care groups include committees, teams, teaching groups, self-help groups, self-awareness/growth groups, therapy groups, work-related social support groups, and professional nursing organizations. There are similarities and differences among the characteristics of these various types of groups and the roles of nurses participating in them.

Committees or Teams

Committees are "relatively stable and formally composed" (Huber, 2000, p. 253). These are the most common types of work-related groups. They usually have a specific purpose that is part of the organizational structure and meet at defined intervals. Examples are policy committees, quality improvement committees, health care planning committees, nursing organization committees, and governmental affairs committees. Committees may also be referred to as teams, such as nursing care teams or wound-

care teams. Teams are defined as "a small number of consistent people committed to a relevant shared purpose, with common performance goals, complementary and overlapping skills, and a common approach to their work" (Manion, Lorimer, & Leander, 1996, p. 6).

The leader of a committee or team, usually called the chairperson, must be accepted by the members as an appropriate leader and, therefore, should be an expert in the area of the committee's focus. The chairperson's role is to identify the specific task, clarify communication, and assist in expressing opinions and offering solutions. Committee or team members are generally selected in terms of their individual functional roles and employment status rather than in terms of their personal characteristics. Committee members may reflect diverse expertise in order to assist the committee to achieve its purpose. Committee or team members are accountable for the group's results or outcomes.

Task Forces

Task forces or ad hoc committees are work groups that usually have a defined task that is limited in duration. In other words, the task force is brought together to perform a specific activity, such as preparation for a joint commission (JCAHO) visit or Nurse Week. When the activity is accomplished, the task force is dissolved. Task forces and ad hoc committees function in the same way as committees or work teams. The difference is in the duration of their work.

Teaching Groups

The major purpose of teaching groups is to impart information to the participants. Examples of teaching groups include group continuing education and client health care groups. Numerous subjects are often handled using a group teaching format: childbirth techniques, exercise for middle-aged and older adults, and instructions to family members about follow-up care for discharged clients. A nurse who leads a group in which the primary purpose is to teach or learn must be skilled in the teaching-learning process discussed in Chapter 8 ∞, The Nurse as Learner and Educator.

Self-Help Groups

A **self-help group** is comprised of individuals who come together to face a common problem or difficulty (Frisch & Frisch, 2002, p. 721). These groups

Evidence for Practice

Lin, M., Chang, Y., & Wang, C. (2000). The power of sharing groups: An exploration of nurse students' learning process in the clinical practice. *Journal of Nursing Research (China), 8*(5), 503–514.

The purpose of this qualitative study was to explore the learning process in a sharing group during nursing students' clinical practice and to determine its implications for interpersonal learning. The sample consisted of 14 senior baccalaureate nursing students in China. The students were invited to discuss their experiences in clinical practice during a focus interview process. All the interviews were recorded and transcribed. Narrative analysis was used to summarize the context of the learning process in the sharing group. Four categories were identified: (1) yielding to an open mind, (2) reflecting real self, (3) learning with regard for others, and (4) taking pleasure in learning. The interaction between the students in the sharing group provided a mechanism for self-understanding and change.

Using a sharing group process encourages more in-depth introspection and self-accommodation, which could help students better perform their professional roles. The findings may have implications for nurses working in stressful work areas, who may use the sharing group process to gain greater awareness and understanding about themselves and their co-workers.

Positive Aspects of Self-Help Groups

- Members can experience almost instant kinship, because the essence of the group is the idea that "you are not alone."

- Members can talk about their feelings and listen to the concerns of others, knowing they all share this experience.

- The group atmosphere is generally one of acceptance, support, encouragement, and caring.

- Many members act as role models for newer members and can inspire them to attempt tasks they might consider impossible.

- The group provides the opportunity for people to help as well as to be helped—a critical component in restoring self-esteem.

Source: From "Self-Help," by V. J. Gilbey, April 1987, *Canadian Nurse, 83,* 25.

are based on the helper-therapy principle: those who help are helped most. A central belief of the self-help movement is that persons who experience a particular social or health problem have an understanding of that condition which those without it do not. Alcoholics Anonymous (AA) is an example of a self-help group. Other support groups may consist of individuals who have specialized knowledge that enables them to assist individuals who have the problem in addition to individuals who have experienced the problem. Reach for Recovery (a support group to assist women with breast cancer) is an example of this type of group in which members may be victims of breast cancer or they may be other individuals who have the ability to help, such as oncology nurses. Positive aspects of these groups are outlined in the accompanying box.

Self-Awareness/Growth Groups

The purpose of self-awareness/growth groups is to develop or use interpersonal strengths. The overall aim is to improve the person's functioning in the group to which they return, whether job, family, or community. From the beginning, broad goals are usually apparent, for example, to study communication patterns, group process, or problem solving. Because the focus of these groups is interpersonal concerns around current situations, the work of the group is oriented to reality testing with a here-and-now emphasis. Members are responsible for correcting inefficient patterns of relating and communicating with each other. They learn group process through participation and involvement in guided exercises.

Evidence for Practice

Mok, E., & Martinson, I. (2000). Empowerment of Chinese patients with cancer through self-help groups in Hong Kong. *Cancer Nursing, 23*(3), 206–213.

The purpose of this study was to identify the process and outcomes of empowerment as experienced by Chinese Hong Kong patients with cancer through participation in cancer self-help groups. The sample consisted of 12 patients with cancer. Interviews of participants were conducted and observation of participants was done at self-help group meetings over a period of 6 months. Find-

ings indicated personal empowerment through interconnectedness, confidence and hope, support and affirmation, and a feeling of usefulness. At a social level, participants reported expanded social network and opportunities to participate in more activities.

Nurses should strongly consider referral of cancer patients to self-help groups. Although the study was done in Hong Kong, China, the findings should be considered for nurses working with cancer patients in other parts of the world.

Evidence for Practice

Adler, C. L. & Zarchin, Y. R. (2002). The "virtual focus group": Using the Internet to reach pregnant women on home bed rest. *JOGNN: Journal of Obstetric, Gynecologic, and Neonatal Nursing, 31*(4), 418–427.

The purposes of this qualitative study were to explore the lived experience of pregnant women confined to home bed rest following a diagnosis of preterm labor and to assess the value of a virtual focus group as an online peer support group for women on home bed rest. An additional purpose related to the study methodology: to examine the effectiveness of a "virtual focus group" as a mechanism to collect qualitative data. The investigators defined virtual focus groups as "an internet-based research method that utilizes electronic mail (email) to unite spatially and temporally separate participants in a text-based group discussion." Data were collected using the Internet. Participants included seven women who were on home bed rest for the treatment of preterm labor. Researchers presented over a 4-week period a series of questions to the participants using e-mail. Qualitative analysis identified three major categories or themes concerning the lived experience of home bed rest. They were (1) the effect of bed

rest on participants' lives, (2) the effect of bed rest on relationships with others, and (3) the effectiveness of the virtual focus group as an online peer support group. Seven subcategories were identified under the first two major categories. Subcategories identified under the effect of bed rest on the participants' lives included (1) transitioning onto bed rest, (2) loss of control and activities, (3) changes in identity and role, (4) coping and personal growth, and (5) transitioning off bed rest. Subcategories under the effect of bed rest on relationships with others included (1) relationships with the fetus and other children, (2) relationships with husbands, and (3) relationships with extended family members. All participants appreciated the use of the virtual focus group and indicated that participation was "valuable and beneficial in helping them to cope with the hardships of bed rest." A major implication of the study is that virtual focus groups are an effective tool for communicating and assisting preterm women who are confined to bed rest in their homes. The virtual focus group may also be useful for connecting other patient groups who are isolated or are homebound.

Therapy Groups

Therapy groups are comprised of people coming together to receive psychotherapy through which they work toward self-understanding, more satisfactory ways of relating or handling stress, and changing patterns of behavior toward health. Members are referred to as clients, participants, or, in some settings, as patients. They are selected by health professionals after extensive selection interviews that consider the pattern of personalities, behaviors, needs, and identification of group therapy as the treatment of choice. Duration of therapy groups is not usually set. A termination date is usually mutually determined by the therapist and members. Therapy groups are characterized by different approaches to psychotherapy, for example, interpersonal groups, existential groups, cognitive-behavioral groups, and psychodrama.

Work-Related Social Support Groups

Many nurses experience high levels of vocational stress, for example, hospice, emergency, and critical care nurses. Social support groups can help reduce stress for such nurses if various types of support are provided to buffer the stress. Group members who know about the work of others can encourage and challenge members to be more creative and enthusiastic about their work and to achieve more. For example, a nurse may help another group member consider alternative strategies for intervention. Members also can share the joys of success and the frustration of failure through active listening without giving advice or making judgments. This type of social support is best given outside the work-related support group.

Professional Nursing Organizations

Professional nursing organizations function as groups, and through smaller groups composed of organization members promote quality health care for all and support the needs of nurses. Professional nursing organizations can serve as task groups, teaching groups, self-help groups, and support groups. The effectiveness of professional nursing organizations is related to the commitment and effectiveness of their members.

Reflect on...

■ your own involvement in various work-related or professional groups. What are the purposes of the groups in which you participate? What are your reasons for participating in these groups? What are your roles in the groups? How does the work of these groups meet your own needs for professional fulfillment? How does your work in these groups help to fulfill organizational goals? Professional goals?

EXPLORE MEDIALINK

Questions, critical thinking exercises, essay activities, and other interactive resources for this chapter can be found on the Web site at http://www.prenhall.com/blais. Click on Chapter 15 to select activities for this chapter.

Critical Thinking Exercises

1. Identify teams, teaching groups, self-help groups, self-awareness groups, therapy groups, and work-related groups in your practice setting. What are the purposes of these various groups? In what way are nurses actively involved in these groups? If nurses are not involved in the various groups, how might the lack of their participation affect the perception of professional nursing? How might nurses become involved in these groups?

2. Identify the various health care groups in your community. Identify specific task groups, teaching groups, self-help groups, self-awareness groups, therapy groups, and work-related groups in your community. What are the purposes of these various groups? In what way are nurses actively involved in these groups? If nurses are not involved in the various groups, how might that affect the perception of professional nursing? How might nurses become involved in these groups?

3. Identify the various professional nursing organizations in your community, state, region. How effective are these organizations in promoting quality health care for the community, state, region, nation? What is your own involvement in these organizations?

Bookshelf

Adams, K. & Galanes, G. J. (2003). *Communicating in groups: Applications and skills* **(5th ed.). Boston: McGraw-Hill.**
This text provides a thorough discussion of the theory and practice of small group communication. Case studies and examples are used to demonstrate concepts related to group work. Unique to this text is a discussion of media and technology mediated group communication.

Donelson, R. F. (1998). *Group dynamics* **(3rd ed.). Stamford, CT: International Thomson Publishing.**
An introductory book to group processes integrating many areas of inquiry, including psychology, sociology, and other social sciences, this text features extended cases to illustrate applications.

Smith, K., & Berg, D. (1998). *Paradoxes of group life: Understanding conflict, paralysis, and movement in group dynamics.* **San Francisco: Jossey-Bass.**
This text approaches understanding groups by exploring the hidden dynamics that can prevent a group from functioning effectively and offers new ways of thinking about groups.

Stewart, G. L., Manz, C. C., & Sims, H. P. (1998). *Team work and group dynamics.* **New York: Wiley.**
The authors blend theory and practice with a realistic view of how teams function in actual work settings. The book is organized around input, process, and output.

SUMMARY

Groups can be classified as primary or secondary, according to their structure or their type of interaction. Groups can assume any one or more of eight functions: socialization, support, task completion, camaraderie, information, normative function, empowerment, and governance. They also can be described according to their formality, that is, as formal, semiformal, or informal.

According to Clark (1994) groups develop in three stages: orientation, working, and termination. Tuckman and Jensen (1977) describe six states: orientation, forming, storming, norming, performing, and terminating. Effective groups produce outstanding results, succeed in spite of difficulties, and have members who feel responsible for the output of the group.

Group dynamics (group process) are forces in the group situation that determine the behavior of the group and its members. Factors in group dynamics include commitment, leadership style, decision-making methods, member behavior, interaction patterns, cohesiveness, and power. Three decision-making aids are brainstorming, the nominal group technique, and the Delphi technique. Interaction patterns within a group can be assessed through the use of sociograms. Cohesive groups possess a common purpose and a group spirit. Groups lacking in cohesiveness are prone to disintegration.

Group discussion can be facilitated in eight ways, including asking open-ended questions and seeking equal contributions from all group members. Group leaders need certain skills to conduct an effective group process. A number of group problems can occur: monopolizing, conflict, groupthink, scapegoating, silence and apathy, and transference and countertransference.

Nurses often serve as members of committees, teams, teaching groups, self-help groups, self-awareness groups, work-related social support groups, and professional nursing organizations.

REFERENCES

Adams, K., & Galanes, G. J. (2003). *Communicating in groups: Applications and skills.* Boston: McGraw-Hill.

Adler, C. L., & Zarchin, Y. R. (2002). The "virtual focus group": Using the Internet to reach pregnant women on home bed rest. *JOGNN: Journal of Obstetric, Gynecologic, and Neonatal Nursing, 31*(4), 418–427.

Bradford, L. P., Stock, D., & Horwitz, M. (1974). How to diagnose group problems. In L. P. Bradford (Ed.), *Group development.* La Jolla, CA: University Associates.

Clark, C. C. (1994). *The nurse as group leader* (3rd ed.). New York: Springer.

Crenshaw, B. G. T. (2003). Working with groups. In W. K. Mohr (Ed.), *Johnson's psychiatric mental health nursing* (5th ed.). Philadelphia: Lippincott.

Frisch, N. C., & Frisch, L. E. (2002). *Psychiatric mental health nursing* (2nd ed.). Albany, NY: Delmar.

Gilby, V. J. (1987, April). Self-help. *Canadian Nurse, 83,* 23, 25.

Huber, D. (2000). *Leadership and nursing care management* (2nd ed.). Philadelphia: W. B. Saunders.

Kneisl, C. R., Wilson, H. S., & Trigoboff, E. (2004). *Contemporary psychiatric-mental health nursing.* Upper Saddle River, NJ: Prentice Hall.

Lin, M., Chang, Y., & Wang, C. (2000). The power of sharing groups: An exploration of nurse students' learning process in the clinical practice. *Journal of Nursing Research (China), 8*(5), 503–514.

Manion, J., Lorimer, W., & Leander, W. J. (1996). *Team-based health care organizations: Blueprint for success.* Gaithersburg, MD: Aspen.

Marriner-Tomey, A. (2000). *Guide to nursing management and leadership* (6th ed.). St. Louis: Mosby.

McMurray, A. R. (1994, March/April). Three decision-making aids: Brainstorming, nominal group and Delphi technique. *Journal of Nursing Staff Development, 10,* 62–65.

Mohr, W. K. (2003). *Johnson's psychiatric mental health nursing,* (5th ed.). Philadelphia: Lippincott.

Mok, E., & Martinson, I. (2000). Empowerment of Chinese patients with cancer through self-help groups in Hong Kong. *Cancer Nursing, 23*(3), 206–213.

Sampson, E. E., & Marthas, M. S. (1990). *Group process for the health professions* (3rd ed.). New York: Delmar.

Smith, G. B., & Hukill, E. (1994, July). Quality work improvement groups: From paper to reality. *Journal of Nursing Care Quality, 8,* 1–12.

Tuckman, B. W., & Jensen, M. A. (1977). Stages of small group development revisited. *Group and Organization Studies, 2,* 419–427.

Wilson, H. S., & Kneisl, C. R. (1996). *Psychiatric nursing* (5th ed.). Redwood City, CA: Addison-Wesley Nursing.

Technology and Informatics

Objectives

■ Define nursing informatics and technology assessment.

■ Describe current issues related to technology and informatics.

■ Identify applications of information technology in health care.

■ Discuss the role of nursing and health care informatics.

M E D I A L I N K

Additional online resources for this chapter can be found on the companion Web site at http://www.prenhall.com/blais.

Health care technologies and information management are two very important, closely related topics for professional nursing practice. For example, when a hospital installed point-of-care computers, nurses and other providers were given access to electronic patient records from any area in the facility. This was particularly important for error-free orders, capture and display of all current food and drug allergies, and documentation of medications to each electronic patient record. Acute care and outpatient services were subsequently linked, and departments such as physical therapy and respiratory therapy became paperless (Bishop, 2001).

With the availability of the World Wide Web, nurses can instantly draw upon current research, industry experiences, and publications for all aspects of health care and nursing. Health care consumers likewise have greater access to information. The use of computers in nursing and health care and the nurse's responsibility in using technological advances in the delivery of care is the focus of this chapter. Several nursing and health care technology frameworks guide the presentation of three current issues: ethics, confidentiality of patient records, and caring for clients in an increasingly technical environment.

CHALLENGES AND OPPORTUNITIES

Nurses are continuously challenged to provide effective, efficient, and accessible care in a range of environments. New technologies, particularly information systems, are changing and improving nursing practice, education, research, and administration. Computers in health care have dramatically changed nursing practice and outcomes over the past several years. Indeed, they hold promise as important tools for caring for individuals, families, and groups. There are, however, challenges to overcome before the adoption of new technologies and information systems. Nurses who design and use information technologies must be aware of confidentiality and security concerns. In addition, nurses are challenged to manage information technologies in a manner that supports quality nursing care.

The opportunities provided by information technology are vast. Applications can change the face of practice, education, research, and administration by providing powerful tools for educating student nurses, continuing education, informing nurses about outcome management, storing and accessing patient records, teaching patients about wellness, and public education. Health care information systems continue to evolve and are providing effective and efficient means to support nursing care.

Many new applications will be developed in the near future and nursing should be instrumental in the design and application of systems for every aspect of patient care. Examples of four important applications are considered in this chapter: physician order entries, clinical information systems, wireless and portable devices, and computer-based patient records.

NURSING INFORMATICS, HEALTH CARE INFORMATICS, AND TECHNOLOGY

The term **informatics** is used to describe all aspects of computers and information systems. **Health care informatics** is the application of information technology to

facilitate accountability, assist in cost containment, and enhance the quality of care (Ball & Douglas, 1997). According to Graves and Corcoran (1989), **nursing informatics** is the combination of computer and information science with nursing science. This combination assists in the management and processing of nursing data, information and knowledge in support of nursing practice, and the delivery of care. This definition is the historic one, and it remains relevant to the design, development, and implementation of health care information systems for nursing. Data, information, and knowledge are the core of informatics, and while computers are used to store, manipulate, and manage them, computers are not the focus of informatics science. The computer is simply a tool (Abbott, 2003).

Since the introduction of information systems to acute care in 1965, a blend of consumer informatics and patient-centered information systems has evolved through the current wide use of the Internet (Staggers, Thompson, & Snyder-Halpern, 2001). Nursing information systems are now modules within larger integrated health care information systems. For example, the nursing documentation features for perioperative care may be part of a larger surgical information system that includes patient registration, orders management, inventory control, scheduling, billing, and postoperative patient-discharge instruction.

Nursing Roles and Education

A discussion of the role and educational preparation for nursing informatics will help apply these definitions. The informatics nurse, a specialty that requires baccalaureate preparation, will generally find career opportunities in acute and ambulatory settings, academic institutions, application companies (vendors), and consulting firms. A recruiting advertisement for an informatics nurse might include the need for skills and experience to outline nursing functions to be automated, write technical manuals, manage projects, or train users. Informatics nurses design, develop, test, and evaluate new clinical applications and adapt existing systems to fit patient and provider requirements. Competencies vary and may include complex problem solving, database development, and application design and testing. In all cases, the prerequisite is clinical experience.

Nursing informatics is one of the newest specialties in professional nursing. It was recognized by the American Nurses Association (ANA) in 1992, and certification is available through the American Nurses Credentialing Center. The prerequisites for certification eligibility are shown in the box on page 291. A scope of practice and

Eligibility Requirements for Certification as a Nursing Informatics Specialist by the American Nurses Credentialing Center

1. Baccalaureate or higher degree in nursing or baccalaureate degree in relevant field
2. Active licensure as a registered nurse in the United States or territories
3. Minimum of 2 years practice as an RN
4. At least 2000 hours in informatics nursing within the past 3 years, *or*
   a. Completion of at least 12 semester hours of academic credits in a graduate program in informatics nursing with a minimum of 1000 hours in informatics nursing practice within the past 3 years; *or*
   b. Completion of a graduate program in nursing informatics that includes at least 200 hours of clinical practicum
5. Thirty continuing education contact hours applicable to the specialty area within the last 3 years unless 4b is met

Source: From American Nurses Credentialing Center, Certification Catalog, 2003, Washington, DC: ANCC.

standards documents were developed under the direction of the ANA in 1995 and revised in 2001.

A wide variety of educational preparation is available for the nursing informatics role. Educational opportunities for the nursing informatics specialization may be found at the Ph.D. level, in postmaster's certification, and in graduate nursing programs. The first two graduate programs in nursing informatics were established at the University of Maryland and University of Utah in 1988 and 1990, respectively. Undergraduate courses are often available as electives for nursing students. Conferences and weekend immersion programs are widely available to provide professional development and continuing education (Newbold, 2001).

Nursing roles in informatics are continually evolving. The work of an informatics nurse can involve any aspect of information systems, including design, development, marketing, testing, implementation, training, and evaluation. Informatics nurses are engaged in clinical practice, education, consultation, research, administration, and pure informatics (ANA, 2003). They may be entrepreneurs within start-up companies developing Web-based products or have their own business as health database designers.

All nurses need informatics competencies, whether or not they are specialists in that area. All nurses must be information- and computer-literate. These competencies may be categorized as computer skills, information literacy skills, or overall informatics competencies. Basic computer skills include such things as using a word processor, being able to communicate by e-mail, and using applications to document patient care. Information literacy skills include the ability to retrieve bibliographic information from the Internet and the ability to evaluate and use the information appropriately. Overall informatics competencies include implementing policies to protect privacy and confidentiality and security of information and recording data relevant to the nursing care of patients. These skills are basic to the entry-level nursing role. Experienced nurses should have even greater proficiency in a particular area, such as administration, education, or public health.

Reflect on...

■ how the informatics nurse might be implemented in your work setting. How might this assist the practicing nurse? The patient? Administration and management?

Technology and Informatics

The leap in the development and use of information technologies calls for close examination of all aspects as they relate to quality of care. The purpose is to improve patient care through a comprehensive evaluation of the safety, effectiveness, cost/benefit, and social impact of a specific technology. Technologies are drugs, devices, procedures, and systems. Evaluation is essential to protect patients and diffuse safe, cost-effective technologies. Part of the role of informatics nurses is to understand, apply, and disseminate the principles of health care technology assessment. The Health Care Technology Assessment (HCTA) framework was developed originally by the Office of Technology Assessment (Jacox, 1990; Office of Technology Assessment, 1982) and may be used to evaluate health care information systems.

Telehealth technologies, a part of communication and information system technologies, are beginning to play a major role in delivering quality health care to patients at a distance. These technologies assist nurses in delivering quality care to remote patients in underserved areas or in prisons. Telehealth is "the removal of time and distance barriers for the delivery of health care services or related health care activities" (Milholland, 1997, p. 4).

Informatics Frameworks

Several nursing and health care informatics models exist. Models or frameworks help clinicians understand how concepts are structured and operationalized. Four metastructures, or overarching concepts, are used in informatics theories and sciences:

>   Data, information, and knowledge
>
>   Sciences underpinning nursing informatics
>
>   Concepts and tools from information science and computer science
>
>   Phenomena of nursing

Data are discrete entities that are described objectively without interpretation. Information is data that have been interpreted, organized, or structured, and knowledge is synthesized information, whereby relationships are identified and formalized. Figure 16–1■, developed by Graves and Corcoran in 1989, depicts the relationship among the three entities. As data are transformed into information and information into knowledge, increasing complexity requires greater application of human intelligence. The circles overlap in these three concepts because the concepts are blurred, and there are multiple feedback loops. Nurses are processors of information. They use informatics to manage and communicate data, information, and knowledge to support patients, nurses, and other providers in making decisions. Informatics assists them in storing clinical data, translating clinical data into information, linking clinical data and knowledge, and aggregating clinical data.

The sciences underpinning nursing informatics are nursing science, information science, and computer science. They are used to manage and process nursing data, information, and knowledge to facilitate the delivery of health care. This combination of sciences creates a unique blend that can be used to solve information-management issues of concern to the discipline. Informatics nurse specialists often collaborate with other informaticists and may borrow concepts

Figure 16–1

Transformation of Data to Knowledge

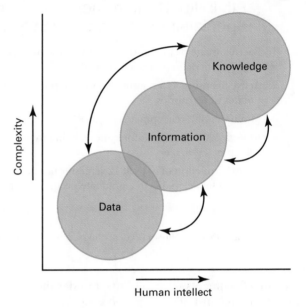

Source: From "The Study of Nursing Informatics," by J. R. Graves and S. Corcoran, 1989, *Image: Journal of Nursing Scholarship, 21*(4), 227–231. Used by permission.

from many sources, including linguistics, cognitive science, engineering, and a variety of others as needed.

The tools and methods derived from computer and information sciences include information technology, structures, management, and communication. Information technology includes computer hardware, software, communication, and network technologies. Human-computer interaction and ergonomics concepts are fundamental to the informatics nurse specialist. Ergonomics focuses on the design and implementation of the equipment related to human use. The goal is optimal task completion.

The metaconcepts of nursing are nurse, person, health, and environment. Decision making involves these four concepts, and nurses must make numerous decisions with important implications for quality of life and well-being of individuals, families, and communities. Nurses depend on data that have been transformed into information to determine interventions.

Turley (1997) proposed a model to describe nursing informatics. His major contribution was adding cognitive science to the model of Graves and Corcoran. He acknowledged the growing interdisciplinary nature of health care and focused on the unique contribution provided by nursing.

Goossen (1996) illustrated a nursing information reference model to structure nursing data and informa-

Figure 16–2

The Patient-Centered Informatics Model

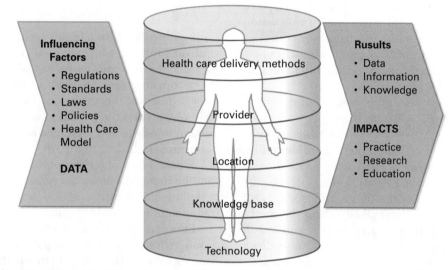

Patient-Centered Informatics Model

Influencing Factors
- Regulations
- Standards
- Laws
- Policies
- Health Care Model

DATA

Health care delivery methods

Provider

Location

Knowledge base

Technology

Rusults
- Data
- Information
- Knowledge

IMPACTS
- Practice
- Research
- Education

Source: From "An Operational Model for Patient Centered Informatics," by N. Staggers, C. B. Thompson, and B. A. Happ, 1999, *Computers in Nursing, 17*(6), 278–285. Used by permission.

tion. Staggers, Thompson, and Happ (1999) proposed a pragmatic, patient-centered informatics model (PCIM) that is an interdisciplinary framework to guide clinicians and systems developers. See Figure 16–2■. The model blends notions from prior conceptual models for a unique framework that enables users to evaluate the influencing factors in designing and implementing clinical systems. Influencing factors may be delivery methods, knowledge bases, and supporting technologies.

PCIM is important because it can be applied in the planning and integration of information systems. It also supports education and research by enabling technology assessment and critical thinking. PCIM is the only model that proposes a link to other disciplines. The Graves and Corcoran (1989) definition focuses on nursing phenomenon, but PCIM describes the relationship of nursing to other disciplines in planning and using information technologies. These models continue to evolve over time.

ISSUES RELATED TO INFORMATION TECHNOLOGY

As information technologies become basic tools for nurses, four issues need to be addressed: ethics, confidentiality, data integrity, and caring in a highly technical environment.

Ethical Concerns

The American Nurses Association code of ethics for nurses (2001) applies to the issues and dilemmas in informatics. Confidentiality, security, and privacy are of great concern. When medical data are stored electronically, special precautions are needed to be certain that unauthorized access is prevented.

Boykin (2000) elaborated on the basic principles that apply nursing ethics to the use of information technologies in health care. The concepts of autonomy, empowerment, accountability, and respect for the individual hold true for the practice of nursing informatics. Nurses have an ethical duty to protect patient confidentiality (ANA, 2001). All health care providers have a moral code that requires balancing the privacy of patients with the requirements for care, including access to patient records.

The expansion of guidelines for the ethical development of Internet sites has been ongoing since 1996, when Health on the Net Foundation (HON) became one of the very first Web sites to guide both patients and medical professionals to reliable sources of health care information on the Internet. HON's standards hold Web site developers to basic ethical standards in the presentation of information. The American Accreditation Healthcare Commission (2001) is also developing an accrediting process for health care Web sites.

Confidentiality of Medical Records and Data

An example of the blatant breach of the confidentiality of medical records and potential patient impact was reported in the February 12, 1999, *Detroit News* (Upton, 1999) issue. Records with identifying information (names, social security numbers, diagnostic codes) of thousands of University of Michigan health system patients were inadvertently placed on the Internet. This is one of the perils of automation.

There are many laws addressing confidentiality and patient privacy. The Health Insurance Portability and Accountability Act (HIPAA) has established policies and procedures that protect confidentiality. HIPAA requires improved efficiency of health care delivery by standardizing electronic data interchange and protection of confidentiality and security of health data through setting and enforcing standards. Unique health identifiers for all providers and health plans and security standards to protect the individual's identifiable health information, past, present, and future, for all health organizations—physicians' offices, health plans, employers, public health groups, life insurance companies, and information systems vendors—are required.

Another important law (Gramm-Leach-Bliley Act), required by most states as of July 1, 2001, calls for health plans and insurers to handle member and subscriber data in special electronic formats. The new legislation is expected to change the way nurses work, access data, and communicate health information (Judy, 2001). For health care organizations, the preparation to provide for patient confidentiality is much like the Y2K efforts in past years.

Data Integrity

Health care providers should have confidence in the accuracy and quality of the data that they access. Data integrity procedures instill trust with controls that avoid incomplete or inaccurate entry of data. Although the term *data integrity* is often linked to databases, it also refers to ensuring that data are entered correctly and that there are data quality-management procedures in place. The correctness of patient information is always essential. The quality of the data input into the computer is critical to ensuring quality output. Without processes and procedures in place, computers can replicate and speed up the communication of erroneous data. An example of a procedure to ensure the accuracy of data is when input fields are designed to check for correct data type. For example, if an alphabet character is entered and a numeric character should have been entered, an error message appears on the screen.

Caring in a High-Tech Environment

Caring for patients in a highly technical environment confronts nursing with potential conflict between using effective tools and methods and providing professional nursing care. Rinard (1996) and Brennan (2000) describe the impact of the increased use of technologies and the provision of nursing care. Introduction of new technologies leads to a transformation of nursing, according to Rinard. The author attributes the massive waves of technological change and related funding in health care delivery over time in part to the deskilling (substitution of less trained people) and fragmentation of nursing tasks.

Brennan (2000), on the other hand, described innovation (technological change) as a partnership or compensatory relationship between the care-delivery system, the patient, the environment, and the patient's health goals. When designing information technologies to improve health outcomes, the author advocates a partnership model in delivering nursing care.

The title of the book *Nursing Informatics: Where Caring and Technology Meet* (Ball, Hannah, Newbold, & Douglas, 2000) illustrates the related roles of nursing and informatics. Caring is an essential part of the provision of health. When technologies are introduced, informatics nurses may be the architects and bridges to improved patient outcomes.

The three issues, ethics, confidentiality, and caring, are important in a high-tech environment as the expansion of information technologies continues at a rapid pace. Informatics nurses are challenged to continue to research and apply the appropriate codes and laws to protect patients and to use information tools to improve the quality of patient care.

THE TECHNOLOGY EXPLOSION

Evolution of Technology

The growth of the Internet and information systems has been exponential. It was estimated that by the year 2002, 490 million people around the world had access to the Internet (Computer Industry Almanac, 2001). In April 2001, 57% of people using the Internet were searching for health-related information (Pew Foundation, 2001).

Nurses are often asked to verify information found on the Internet, and informatics nurses may be asked to explain and support research for more complex topics. Patients have come to expect health care information systems to provide services set by other industries.

Patient registration and billing should be as easy as the global ability to instantly authenticate accounts and access money online. Unfortunately, this may not always be the case. The evolution of new health care information technologies has not followed this pattern of revolutionary design and availability. Rather, traditional text-based health care records have been difficult to automate.

Managed-care funding for health care services has dwindled. New technologies have not only dramatically changed nursing and health care, but they have also added to the costs of patient care. Development of health care information systems generally is slower.

When the administration of a health care organization predicts physician and patient-care requirements, a study may be conducted and the system requirement may be added to the strategic plan. For example, when bedside computers were to be installed in a community hospital, a feasibility study was conducted and the system was tested on one unit. In addition, a cost-benefit study was undertaken. The board of trustees reviewed the new technology in light of the hospital strategic plan and recommended a phased approach, with careful analysis of patient outcomes and staff satisfaction.

The design of new patient-care systems has affected staff in regard to workflow, efficiency, and effectiveness. Development of information systems is not simply automating a paper system. It involves studying and improving the processes. From intensive care to hospice and assisted living, the venue for automation initiatives continues to expand and improve health care.

Reflect on...

- how the implementation of information technology has affected confidentiality in your work setting. Think of some ways that confidentiality could be enhanced.
- what ethical concerns you have about the inclusion of information systems in health care. How might nurses address these ethical concerns?
- whether increased uses of technology have affected the level of caring that nurses in your work setting have been able to deliver. What are some things nurses can do to increase caring in a highly technological care environment?

Evidence for Practice

Cader, R. C., Cambell, C., & Watson, D. (2003). **Criteria used by nurses to evaluate practice-related information on the World Wide Web.** *CIN: Computers, Informatics, Nursing, 21*(2), 97–102.

Health information of the World Wide Web (WWW) exists at varying levels of quality, validity, and reliability. This study was done to examine the process nurses in the United Kingdom use to evaluate nursing information on the WWW. This information is defined as that associated with the practice of nursing.

Nurses with more than 5 years of experience participated in semistructured face-to-face interviews about their frequency of Internet usage, purposes for using the Internet, favorite Web sites, quality of information of the WWW, and ways by which they assess practice-related information on the WWW. This qualitative study used a grounded theory approach to identify the process for assessing the information and the criteria for evaluating the information.

The process consisted of seven parts. They were identified as (1) evaluating publication source, (2) assessing author's background, (3) evaluating research evidence, (4) assessing application to practice, (5) making intuitive judgment, (6) assessing user-friendliness of the Web sites, and (7) assessing the nature of the WWW information.

Criteria for evaluating nursing information on the WWW were identified as:

Publication Source: Trustworthiness, Authority, and Cultural Identity

Author Background: Reputation, Clinical Credibility, and Cultural Identity

Research Evidence: Methodology and References

Practice Related: Nursing Care Oriented and Practice Enhancement

User-Friendliness: Clarity of Layout, Ease of Use, and Logical Presentation

Nature of Information: Purpose, Suitability, and Currency

The authors conclude that a reliable set of evaluative criteria is essential if the WWW is to become an effective information source of nurses.

Critical Thinking Exercise

Find a Web site with information on some aspect of nursing practice. Evaluate the information on that Web site using the process and criteria found in the Evidence for Practice box on p. 295.

Computer Technology in Practice, Education, Research, and Administration

New technologies have significantly changed the way nurses practice, conduct research, manage and administrate, and advance their education. Automation in health care has assisted in defining a standardized nomenclature for all disciplines. Standardization of terminologies for nursing is essential for delivering appropriate care and managing outcomes.

Nursing practice in an organization with an integrated clinical information system may include using an online Kardex, care protocols, bedside computers, or a personal digital assistant (PDA) for patient care. Orders, procedures, and appointments are automatically updated, and an online Kardex may be used as a primary communications tool. The automated Kardex shows allergies, interventions, specimens to be collected, current medications, diet, and patient weight. An automated rounds report allows providers to quickly view patient information, vital signs, intake and output, lab results, radiology reports, and patient-care notes. This increases accuracy and decreases redundancy and thus improves the efficiency and effectiveness of individual providers.

Orders-management systems streamline the entry, receipt, and monitoring of orders throughout the enterprise. Wireless bedside computers for patient documentation allow appropriate providers to enter and access patient records from anywhere at any time. Some institutions have been using wireless terminals successfully for several years.

Automated medication administration records that are integrated with orders-management, billing, and pharmacy systems proved effective and provided error-free access to drugs. When multiple medications are ordered, automated medication systems are programmed to scan for drug-drug interactions or other potential medication-related problems resulting in safer delivery of medications to the patient. Training for new applications and diverse equipment has become shorter and easier as nurses see the benefits and apply computer knowledge and skills from their everyday lives.

An informatics nurse's role in these new technologies is very important. It may involve examination and design of new workflow, development of an implementation plan, and training in and evaluation of the new technologies. Although patient access to the Internet may change the patient's level of knowledge about a health problem, patient education and counseling must be augmented and mediated by trained nurses for full understanding and compliance and subsequent improved patient outcomes. Overall, new information systems improve the efficiency, productivity, safety, and quality of care in an organization, but this is not always the case. Investment in information systems must be tied to an organization's strategic plan, sufficient resources must be in place, and a plan for managing the change must be implemented to see the full benefits.

The influence of new technologies on nursing education is changing the basic philosophies about the tools and methods for pedagogy. From online courses to virtual-reality intravenous training systems, students have benefited from improvements in educational information technologies. At this time, you may be at a computer accessing an Internet-based course with a virtual instructor or working hands-on with an intravenous simulator.

Automated research tools and the Internet facilitate nursing research. Research databases such as the *Cumulative Index for Nursing and Allied Health Literature* (CINAHL) or MEDLINE provide nurses with effective methods to quickly find current relevant literature and access appropriate psychometric tools from the computer desktop. Statistical tools like the Statistical Package for the Social Sciences (SPSS) help nurse researchers organize and analyze data when conducting research.

Nurse-administrators use information technologies to guide their management when they are uncertain about something, to satisfy multiple stakeholders, and to build and retain passionate workforces. Two elements moved nursing administration to embrace computers for decision making: the speed and accuracy needed and the financial constraints of managed care. Information systems enable nursing administration to manage budgets, collect and evaluate staff and patient data to track and forecast resource needs, and

Evidence for Practice

Larrabee, J. H., Boldreghini, S., Elder-Sorrells, K., Turner, A. M., Wender, R. G., Hart, J. M., & Lenzi, P. S. (2001). **Evaluation of documentation before and after implementation of a nursing information system in an acute care hospital.** *Computers in Nursing, 19*(2), 56–65.

The purpose of this quasi-experimental study was to evaluate the differences in documentation completeness, achievement of patient outcomes, and assessments before and after the implementation of a clinical computer system. The goal was to understand the relationship between quality of care and patient outcomes in order to improve both.

The study was conducted on two medical-surgical units and an intensive-care step-down unit in a 100-bed teaching facility in Tennessee. At least 90 records were examined retrospectively at each of three points in time over 18 months. The tool used was the Nursing Care Plan Data Collection Instrument developed by Larrabee in 1992. Interrater reliability before and during the data collection was acceptable (ANOVA, $P < .05$).

Mean scores for nurse assessment and nurse-perceived patient outcomes did not improve until 18 months after implementation, when the staff was retrained on the computer system. Although the clinical information system did not seem to improve care early in this study, continued training on the system helped to improve nursing care quality and patient outcomes.

- Standardized language/vocabularies
- Technology development to support practice and patient care
- Database issues
- Patient use of information technologies
- Use of telecommunications technology for nursing practice
- Putting technology into practice
- System-evaluation issues
- Information needs of nurses and other clinicians
- Nursing intervention innovations for professional practice
- Professional practice issues

Reflect on...

- how technology has changed nursing education since you were first introduced to nursing. What new skills do students need today compared to 5, 10, and 15 years ago?

CURRENT APPLICATIONS OF INFORMATION TECHNOLOGY IN PRACTICE

Four applications of information technology are of great importance to nursing: physician order entry, clinical information systems, wireless and portable devices, and the computer-based patient record.

Physician Order Entry

The Institute of Medicine (1999) report estimated that the number of deaths per year from medical errors is between 44,000 and 98,000. As part of the patient-safety strategy, strong consideration is being made for purchase and implementation of automated physician order entry systems. These systems enable appropriate providers (physicians and, in some states, nurse practitioners) to enter, edit, schedule, track, and discontinue treatment and diagnostic services electronically. In this way, orders can be checked against patient allergies, interactions with other medications or tests, dosage levels, and standards of practice for the institution. With computerized physician order entry, adverse events and costs may be reduced and length of patient stay may be shortened.

Automated physician order entry is generally part of an integrated enterprise system that allows direct entry by the physician and reduces the likelihood of transcription errors. It is a complex system interfaced with many other systems; in the past it has not been available because of the cost and complexity of development.

anticipate quality-management interventions. Data from clinical and financial information systems allow nurse-administrators to analyze data for trends in patient problems and reimbursement gaps. The availability of appropriate data minimizes risk taking. For instance, recruitment programs can be developed to improve staffing ratios when the seasonal influx of patients is higher than expected.

The introduction of information technologies continues to enhance nursing practice and to provide tools for research, administration, and nursing education. A survey of nursing informatics researchers identified ten priorities for research (Brennan et al., 1998):

There is a current sense of urgency to purchase this application for patient safety, and companies are now developing such products.

Clinical Information Systems

Another publication from the Institute of Medicine and National Academy Press (Committee on Quality of Health Care in America, 2001) highlighted the need for implementation of improved clinical information systems. The authors recommended a fundamental change and redesign of the health care system to promote evidence-based practice, strengthen clinical information systems, and lead to the elimination of most handwritten clinical data by the end of the decade.

Clinical information and financial and administrative systems are found in most health care entities and are generally integrated to serve patients and providers. Clinical systems may include patient registration, orders, and departmental systems such as nursing, dietary, radiology, pharmacy, cardiology, laboratory, and physical therapy. Although there are many independent systems, integration helps to ensure coordination of care across patient conditions, services, and settings over time.

Wireless and Portable Devices

Wireless and portable devices are bringing patient records and provider services to the point of care. When bedside computers emerged in the early 1990s, advances enabled access to patient information anywhere and at any time. The location of patient care at home, in an office, in a church, in a community center, or in a hospital makes wireless and portable devices an attractive vehicle for documentation and record access.

One type of device is the personal digital assistant (PDA). Two PDA functions allow nurses wireless access to patient records and reference databases such as MedCalc and ePocrates. RNpalm.com is a Web site dedicated to mobile computing for nurses. Wireless PDAs are being used to access medical records in some institutions.

Computer-Based Patient Record

Interest in a computer-based patient records (CPR) or electronically maintained information about an individual's lifetime health status and health began more than ten years ago when Dick and Steen (1991) conducted an important study on the value of a complete and accurate patient record. The text was updated in 1997 (Dick, Steen, & Detmer, 1997) and remains the seminal study for CPRs. These systems are not yet in use but are being developed with testing in some places.

The ideal CPR (also called electronic patient record or electronic medical record) will support users with reminders and alerts, clinical decision-support systems, and links to medical knowledge. The intent of a CPR is to capture quality measurements and clinical outcome data to support the analysis of patient problems. A CPR will affect quality improvements in patient care through effective documentation and monitoring.

An excellent example of a CPR is the system used by the Department of Veterans Affairs (VA). By leveraging the best parts of an older system and integrating commercial software applications, the VA has developed an advanced system that captures patient data in a provider-friendly way. Clinical documentation is standardized, accurate, always available, and very reliable throughout the inpatient areas and clinics in the VA system.

Beth Israel Deaconess Medical Center in Boston has an integrated online CPR-type information system with ready access to electronic patient records via a Web browser (Landro, 2000). This new system enables a clinician (with appropriate security clearance) in the emergency room to access patient records via the Web. This can cut the time for intervention and treatment, saving money and improving patient conditions.

These four applications of information technology in health care are but a few of the many important developments to support providers and patients. New applications are developed and become cost-effective as demand grows and system requirements are defined.

Reflect on...

■ the needs for changes in the technological environment of patient care in the future. What supports will nurses need to keep current with new technology applications? Are the current approaches to continuing education sufficient?

EXPLORE MEDIALINK

Questions, critical thinking exercises, essay activities, and other interactive resources for this chapter can be found on the Web site at http://www.prenhall.com/blais. Click on Chapter 16 to select activities for this chapter.

Bookshelf

Ellis, D., Campbell, M. L., Crandall, D. K., Peters, B. E., Ruff, C., & Seitz, K. (2000). *Technology and the future of health care: Preparing for the next 30 years.* **New York: Wiley.**
The author projects the rate of technological development into the next three decades of the health care industry. The idea is presented that the most visible technological advances such as MRI, CAT, and PET scanners are less important in the long run than the technological advances in streamlining administration of health care agencies and doctor's offices. Processing and storage of medical records and billing technology will have a greater impact.

Mascara, C., Czar, P., & Hebda, T. (2001). *Internet Resource Guide for Nurses and Healthcare Professionals* (2nd ed.). **Upper Saddle River, NJ: Prentice Hall.**

This book provides background information on Internet sources and can serve as a resource guide. It is written at an introductory level.

Fitzpatrick, J., Romano, C., & Chasek, R. (2001). *The nurses guide to consumer health web sites* (3rd ed.). **New York: Springer.**
Organized by topics, this is an annotated listing of Web sites.

Nicoll, L. (2001). *The nurses guide to the Internet* (3rd ed.). **Philadelphia: Lippincott.**
This is a guide to surfing the Web written with humor. It provides an overview and gives a directory of sites.

SUMMARY

Nursing informatics is the combination of computer and information science with nursing science. It is part of the larger health care informatics. Nurses are being prepared as specialists in this area, but every practicing nurse needs some level of expertise. Four current applications of information technology that are important for nursing are physician order entries, clinical information systems, wireless and portable devices, and computer-based patient records.

Several issues related to the increased use of technology in nursing include ethics, confidentiality, data integrity, and caring. Nurses are concerned with the ethical practices used in information access, storage, and retrieval. Ethical practices have a direct effect on confidentiality. The changes in technology of care also raise concerns about the caring practices that nurses implement. Advocacy is needed on the part of the nurse to see that patients, rather than equipment, remain the focus of care.

The application of computer technology has changed practice, education, and research. The skills required to interface with information systems at the point of care, to participate in educational programs that further one's career, and to manage research data have changed and will continue to change. This challenges continuing education both in its own application and in providing the means to learn new skills.

The ability of nurses to manage and use information systems is critical in improving outcomes, decreasing costs, and improving access to care. The 21st century will bring more and better technologies to challenge and enhance professional nursing. The role of the informatics nurse will expand, and confounding technology issues will multiply.

REFERENCES

Abbott, P. A. (2003). Nursing informatics: A foundation for nursing professionalism. *AACN Clinical Issues, 14*(3), 267–270.

American Accreditation Healthcare Commission. (2001). Healthcare website accreditation. http://www.urac.org/websiteaccreditation.htm.

American Nurses Association. (2001). *Code for nurses with interpretive statements.* Washington, DC: ANA.

American Nurses Association. (2003). *Informatics Nurse Certification.* http://www.nursingworld.org/ancc.

Ball, M. J., & Douglas, J. V. (1997 Winter). Health care informatics: Where caring and technology meet. *CommonHealth, 18.*

Ball, M. J., Hannah, K. J., Newbold, S. K., & Douglas, J. V. (2000). *Nursing informatics: where caring and technology meet* (3rd ed.). New York: Springer-Verlag.

Bishop, B. R. (2001, January). Informatics at the point of care: How one hospital integrated a new health information system with mobile documentation devices. *Advance for Nurses, 8.*

Boykin, P. (2000). *Confidentiality and security.* Presented at the 10th Annual Summer Institute in Nursing Informatics. Baltimore, MD. July 20.

Brennan, P. F. (2000). *Partnering with patients: Creating new pathways for innovation in health care.* Presented at the 10th Annual Summer Institute in Nursing Informatics. Baltimore, MD. July 19.

Brennan, P. F., Zielstorff, R. D., Ozbolt, J. G., & Strombom, I. (1998). Setting a national research agenda in nursing informatics. In B. Cesnik, A. T. McCray, & J.-R. Scherrer (Eds.), *Medinfo '98: Proceedings of the Ninth World Congress on Medical Informatics* (pp. 1188–1191). Amsterdam: IOS Press.

Cader, R., Campbell, S., & Watson, D. (2003). Criteria used by nurses to evaluate practice-related information on the World Wide Web. *CIN: Computers, Informatics, Nursing, 21*(2), 97–102.

Committee on Quality of Health Care in America. (2001). *Crossing the quality chasm: A new health system for the 21st century.* Washington DC: National Academy Press.

Computer Industry Almanac. (2001). http://www.ITAlmanac.com/italmanac/index.html.

Dick, R., & Steen, E. (1991). *The computer-based patient record: An essential technology for health care.* Washington, DC: National Academy Press.

Dick, R., Steen, E., & Detmer, D. (1997). *The computer-based patient record: An essential technology for health care.* Washington, DC: National Academy Press.

Goossen, W. (1996). Nursing information management and processing: A framework and definition for systems analysis, design and evaluation. *International Journal of Biomedical Computing, 40,* 187–195.

Graves, J. R., & Corcoran, S. (1989). The study of nursing informatics. *Journal of Nursing Scholarship, 21,* 227–231.

Health on the Net Foundation. (2001). http://www.hon.ch/.

Institute of Medicine. (1999). *To err is human: Building a safer health system.* Washington, DC: National Academy Press.

Jacox, A. (1990). Nursing and technology, technology assessment in reducing costs and improving care. *Nursing Economics, 8*(2), 116, 118.

Judy, K. (2001). Nursing informatics: What does HIPAA mean to you? *Advance for Nurses,* http://www.advancefornurses.com/feature4.html.

Landro, L. (2000). Deal with our doctors. *The Wall Street Journal,* November 13, R23.

Milholland, D. K. (1997). Telehealth: A tool for nursing practice. *Nursing Trends and Issues, 2,* 4.

Newbold, S. (2001). Nursing Informatics and Health Informatics Conferences. http://nursing.umaryland.edu/,snewbold/sknconf.htm.

Office of Technology Assessment. (1982). *Strategies for medical technology assessment.* Springfield, VA: NTIS.

Pew Foundation. (2001). Internet and American Life. http://www.pewinternet.org/reports/toc.asp?Report530.

Phoenix Health Systems. (2001). HIPA Advisory. http://www.hipaadvisory.com/.

Rinard, R. G. (1996). Technology, deskilling, and nurses: The impact of the technologically changing environment. *Advances in Nursing Science, 18*(4), 60–69.

Staggers, N., Thompson, C. B., & Happ, B. A. (1999). An operational model for patient-centered informatics. *Computers in Nursing, 17*(6), 278–285.

Staggers, N., Thompson, C. B., & Snyder-Halpern, R. (2001). History and trends in clinical information systems in the United States. *Journal of Nursing Scholarship,* First Quarter, 75–81.

Turley J. (1997). Toward a model for nursing informatics. *Image, 28,* 309–313.

Upton, J. (1999). U-M medical records end up on web. *The Detroit News,* Friday, February 12. http://detnews.com/1999/metro/9902/12/02120114.htm.

C H A P T E R   1 7

Nursing in an Evolving Health Care Delivery System

Outline

Objectives

- Examine the issues of cost containment and access to health care as they affect nursing.

- Differentiate health, wellness, and well-being.

- Compare selected models of health.

- Identify factors affecting health status, beliefs, and practices.

- Discuss the initiatives of the World Health Organization for the promotion of Health for All.

- Describe responses to the nursing shortage.

M E D I A L I N K

Additional online resources for this chapter can be found on the companion Web site at http://www.prenhall.com/blais.

Changes in the health care delivery system have had a dramatic impact on the practice of nursing. In the early 1900s nurses made home visits and focused on personal care of sick individuals. As hospitals became the workplace where physicians provided medical and surgical care, nurses were employed to provide nursing care, and nursing followed common organizational patterns by establishing specialty areas of practice such as psychiatric, pediatric, obstetrical, medical, and surgical nursing. As nursing education evolved and nurses

Comparison of Old Health Care Paradigm with New Paradigm

OLD PARADIGM	NEW HEALTH CARE PARADIGM
Hospital-based, acute care	Short-term hospital: same-day surgery, 23-hour stays; prehospital testing and precertification; telehealth/telemedicine; home health; mobile vans; school and mall clinics
Specialty units	Cross-training (multiskilled workers): LDRP, OR/PACU, CCU/telemetry
Hierarchical management	Decentralization (unit budget, scheduling, variance); shared governance; strategic plan
Physician "captain of ship"; others are followers	Inter/multidisciplinary team, collaboration; case management (registered nurse/broker)
Nurse as employee: job-focused, "refrigerator nurse"	Nurse as professional: career focused; clinical ladder; continuing credentials; tuition reimbursement, paid certification exam
Medical condition, focus on segment	Holistic person in family/community; pastoral care, parish nurse
"Sick care," focus on cure	Health care, health promotion, prevention programs; care and continuity of care; complementary health alternatives
Cost containment, focus on billing	Focus on patient and accountability of caregivers/agency; electronic patient record, continuous quality improvement, care maps
Written medical record	Integrated electronic records: smart card, bedside computers
Fee for service	Managed competition (HMO, PPO, IPA)
Physician as employer	Physician as employee; capitation system
One insurance plan	Variety of insurance options ("covered lives"): basic plan plus dental, eye, long-term care, cancer, disability
80–100% insurance	Greater deductible, lower percentage coverage, or copayment

Source: From *Health Policy and Politics: A Nurse's Guide* (2nd ed., p. 14) 2004, by J. A. Milstead, Jones and Bartlett, Sudbury, MA. Reprinted by permission.

began to understand more about what constituted the practice of nursing, the boundaries expanded. During the 1970s and 1980s nurses began to seek more autonomy in the practice of nursing, particularly with regard to physicians and hospital administration. Simultaneously, health care costs were rising at an alarming rate, so there was a congressional demand for cost containment related to the government-funded Medicare program. This began with a demand for prospective payment through diagnosis-related groups (DRGs). Private insurance companies followed suit, and hospital administrators were forced to cut costs to survive. Care became focused on costs and profit, with less concern about quality. Health care

providers were then forced to do more with fewer resources, resulting in stress, burn-out, and nurses leaving the profession. New models of care delivery emerged in response (Milstead, 2004). This resulted in major changes in the paradigm of health care, as shown in the accompanying box.

CHALLENGES AND OPPORTUNITIES

A commitment to high-quality care challenges nurses as never before to find ways of providing such care with fewer resources from the administrative levels of the health care organization. Creative ways of doing more with less while avoiding undue stress and burnout are needed. Traditional values, such as advocacy for the individual client, holistic care, and meeting the health care needs of individuals and populations, are at stake in the new health care arena.

The continued evolution of nursing and its place in health care delivery provides a wide range of opportunities for the future. Nursing is in a position to create new roles and redefine nursing in a way that can have a positive impact upon health care now and in the future.

Selected Issues

Two issues at the forefront of the nursing profession's response to health care changes are cost containment and access to health care. Third-party payers have shaped much of the change in an attempt to control rapidly increasing health care costs that many believe to be out of control. Many people are not covered by third-party payers and have few options. For the uninsured, there is little availability of health care, and they have been a concern in the shaping of care delivery in communities and in providing more primary and preventive care.

Cost-Containment Strategies

Many cost-containment strategies in health care have emerged in response to pressures from consumers and third party payers. The resulting changes in the economic structure will be discussed in Chapter 18 ∞, Health Care Economics. Some of the strategies used by nurses in an attempt to control costs and maintain quality include resource management, the development of critical pathways, and the utilization of assistive personnel.

Resource management is an important skill for successful, clinically competent nurses. It is of great importance that nurses be aware of limited resources and the consequences for health care delivery. Resource management uses cost-effective approaches to high-quality health care. The basic resources include financial, physical, and human, but others are organizational systems, information systems, and technical capabilities. Effective time management is an important resource-utilization skill consisting of the planned and organized assessment of when and how long it will take to complete an activity; consequently, control is exercised over what is responded to and the problems that are addressed. Responding to downsizing or the reduction in personnel has been a major challenge in resource allocation (Price, Koch, & Bassett, 1998).

The restructuring of care delivery has been a cost-containment response; one example of such an attempt has been the introduction of **critical pathways.** These are interdisciplinary plans for managing the care of clients that specify interdisciplinary assessments, interventions, treatments, and outcomes for specific health-related conditions across a timeline. Critical pathways are also called critical paths, interdisciplinary plans, anticipated recovery plans, interdisciplinary action plans, and action plans. Criticism has been that the plans are not individualized and that a patient's progress is dictated by a standardized timeline rather than by the professionals who are working with that patient. The argument is made that a nurse can better judge the progress made by individual patients and their readiness for the next step in the pathway. As a result, some hospitals are moving away from critical pathways to protocols that can more easily be adapted to the individual patient's needs.

The use of clinical nursing assistants (CNAs), also called certified nursing assistants or nurse aides, has been a controversial attempt at resource utilization. The intent of using these individuals in providing care has been to relieve the professional nurse of tasks that can safely and effectively be delegated to someone with less educational preparation who can provide that level of care more cost-effectively. Criticism of this approach has been that individuals in the role were placed in situations of care that went beyond their limited preparation and thereby jeopardized the quality of care provided. In many instances, the CNAs were thrust upon nursing without sufficient planning for the implementation of the role and without sufficient input from the nurses who would be working with them. Some have suggested that CNAs will be around for the foreseeable future because of the potential cost savings and because nursing needs to take charge of developing effective systems that maximize both the professional role of the nurse and the role of the CNA (Salmond, 1999).

Reflect on...

- what the wasted resources and wasted efforts found in health care are today.
- what nurses can do to increase cost-effective, quality health care.

Access to Health Care

The issue of access to health care has been a major factor in shaping the changes in nursing. Without universal health care coverage, about 40 million Americans are estimated to be uninsured at any one particular time, but nearly 60 million are without health insurance for a portion of the year (Congressional Budget Office, 2003). Many more are underinsured and economically limited from accessing health care. Barriers to accessing health care have been identified as cost of care, lack of insurance, problems with insurance, difficulty getting appointments, difficulty finding services, and lack of transportation (Glick, 1999).

The American Nurses Association (ANA) published *Nursing's Agenda for Health Care Reform* in 1991. This document represented the efforts of the ANA, the National League for Nursing (NLN), the American Association of Colleges of Nursing (AACN), and the American Organization of Nurse Executives (AONE). It provides for cost-effective, community-based delivery of care in a restructured health care system.

A central objective of this agenda was to provide a basic "core" of essential health care services for everyone. The statement called for a restructuring of the health care system to focus on consumers and their health needs. It also recommended that health care be delivered in such diverse settings as schools, workplaces, and homes and that the health care system shift its focus from illness and cure to wellness and care. See the box on page 305.

The 2003 ANA *House of Delegates Status Report* indicates that little improvement in the areas of quality, access, and cost have come about since the *Agenda for Health Care Reform* was released. In part this is due to the legislative failure of the Clinton administration's attempts at health care reform. Further, the report states that it is unlikely that broad reform will be accomplished in the near future because of overall fiscal restraints and the political climate. However, *Nursing's Agenda for Health Care Reform* is still used to guide ANA's responses to federal and state proposals addressing the health care system (ANA, 2003).

The AONE (1992, p. 42) writes that effective health care must do the following:

1. Encourage consumer partnerships so that consumers can take an active role in their health and their care and in decisions about their care.

2. Allow all U.S. citizens and residents access to basic health care services.

3. Increase health care access through the use of physician and nonphysician providers.

4. Create incentives that promote health, wellness, and prevention; individuals with chronic illnesses will not be penalized.

5. Promote affordable, safe, and effective health care.

6. Make provisions for skilled and long-term care.

7. Make provisions for catastrophic care, with some limitation on extraordinary procedures.

8. Finance health care through a combination of public- and private-sector funding.

Community nursing centers are innovative health care delivery models that represent a step in the paradigm shift from the centralized biomedical model of curing to the community-based and more holistic nursing model of caring (Glick, 1999). The purpose of these centers is to meet the needs of underserved populations by providing the public with direct access to a range of services that are not otherwise available in the community. Nursing centers provide a setting where patients' needs rather than medical diagnoses are the focus. They are located in places to which people have access, such as churches, mobile units, homeless shelters, and schools. Emphasis is on controlling costs by providing noninstitutional care through models that include community participation, care and case management, community health promotion, coordination of community resources, and referral.

This change in focus to prevention and community-based health care requires a shift in perspective from cure and treatment of illness to promotion of health, wellness, and well-being.

CONCEPTS OF HEALTH, WELLNESS, AND WELL-BEING

Nurses need to clarify their understanding of health and wellness because their definitions largely determine the scope and nature of nursing practice. Clients' health beliefs influence their health practices. Some people think of health and wellness (or well-being) as the same thing or, at the very least, as accompanying one another. However, health may not always accompany well-being: A person who has a terminal illness may have a sense of well-being; conversely, another person may lack a sense of well-being yet be in a state of good health.

For many years, the concept of disease was the yardstick by which health was measured. In the late nineteenth century, the "how" of disease (pathogenesis) was the major concern of health professionals. Currently, the emphasis on health and wellness (salutogenesis) is increasing.

Nursing's Agenda for Health Care Reform (Executive Summary)

The basic components of nursing's "core of care" include:

- A restructured health care system, which
  - Enhances consumer access to services by delivering primary health care in community-based settings.
  - Fosters consumer responsibility for personal health, self-care, and informed decision making in selecting health care services.
  - Facilitates utilization of the most cost-effective providers and therapeutic options in the most appropriate settings.
- A federally defined standard package of essential health care services available to all citizens and residents of the United States, provided and financed through an integration of public and private plans and sources.
  - A public plan, based on federal guidelines and eligibility requirements, will provide coverage for the poor and create the opportunity for small businesses and individuals, particularly those at risk because of preexisting conditions and those potentially medically indigent, to buy into the plan.
  - A private plan will offer, at a minimum, the nationally standardized package of essential services. This standard package could be enriched as a benefit of employment, or individuals could purchase additional services if they so choose. If employers do not offer private coverage, they must pay into the public plan for their employees.
- A phase-in of essential services, in order to be fiscally responsible.
  - Coverage of pregnant women and children is critical. This first step represents a cost-effective investment in the future health and prosperity of the nation.
  - One early step will be to design services specifically to assist vulnerable populations who have had limited access to our nation's health care system. A "Healthstart Plan" is proposed to improve the health status of these individuals.
  - Planned change to anticipate health service needs that correlate with changing national demographics.

- Steps to reduce health care costs include:
  - Required usage of managed care in the public plan and encouraged in private plans.
  - Incentives for consumers and providers to utilize managed care arrangements.
  - Controlled growth of the health care system by planning and prudent resource allocation.
  - Incentives for consumers and providers to be cost efficient in exercising health care options.
  - Development of health care policies based on effectiveness and outcomes research.
  - Assurance of direct access to a full range of qualified providers.
  - Elimination of unnecessary bureaucratic controls and administrative procedures.
  - Case management will be required for those with continuing health care needs. This will reduce the fragmentation of the present system, promote consumers' active participation in decisions about their health, and create an advocate on their behalf.
- Provisions for long-term care, which include:
  - Public and private funding for services of short duration to prevent personal impoverishment.
  - Public funding for extended care if consumer resources are exhausted.
  - Emphasis on the consumers' responsibility to financially plan for their long-term care needs, including new personal financial alternatives and strengthened private insurance arrangements.
  - Insurance reforms to improve access to coverage, including affordable premiums, reinsurance pools for catastrophic coverage, and steps to protect both insurers and individuals against excessive costs.
  - Access to services assured by no payment at the point of service and elimination of balance billing in both public and private plans.
  - Establishment of public/private sector review—operating under the federal guidelines and including payers, providers, and consumers—to determine resource allocation, cost reduction approaches, allowable insurance premiums, and fair and consistent reimbursement levels for providers. This review would progress in a climate sensitive to ethical issues.

Source: From *Nursing's Agenda for Health Care Reform* (PR-3 22M 6/91), by American Nurses Association, 1991, Washington, DC: ANA. Reprinted with permission.

Health

There is no consensus about any definition of health. There is knowledge of how to attain a certain level of health, but health itself cannot be measured.

Traditionally, **health** has been defined in terms of the presence or absence of disease. Nightingale defined health as a state of "being well and using every power the individual possesses to the fullest extent" (Nightingale, 1969 [1860], p. 334). At an international conference on global health issues in 1947, the World Health Organization (WHO) defined health as "a state of complete physical, mental, and social well-being, and not merely the absence of disease or infirmity" (WHO, 1947, p. 1). This definition does the following:

■ Reflects concern for the individual as a total person functioning physically, psychologically, and socially. Mental processes determine people's relationship with their physical and social surroundings, their attitudes about life, and their interaction with others.

■ Places health in the context of environment. People's lives, and therefore their health, are affected by everything they interact with—not only environmental influences such as climate and the availability of nutritious food, comfortable shelter, clean air to breathe, and pure water to drink but also other people, including family, significant others, employers, co-workers, friends, and associates of various kinds.

■ Equates health with productive and creative living. It focuses on the living state rather than on categories of disease that may cause illness or death.

In 1953 the (United States) President's Commission on Health Needs of the Nation made the following statement about health:

> *Health* is not a condition; it is an adjustment. It is not a state but a process. The process adapts the individual not only to our physical, but also our social environments. (President's Commission, 1953, p. 4)

This definition emphasizes health as an adaptive process rather than a state.

Health has also been defined in terms of role and performance. Parsons (1972, p. 107) wrote that health is "the state of optimum capacity of an individual for effective performance of his roles and tasks." Parsons further explained that when people feel well, they assume the health role; when they feel ill, in contrast, they assume the sick role. He describes the following four aspects of the sick role:

■ The person is not held responsible for the illness.
■ The person is exempt from the usual social tasks.
■ The person has an obligation to get well.
■ The person has an obligation to seek competent help to treat the illness.

Dubos (1968) viewed health as a creative process and described it as "a quality of life, involving social, emotional, mental, spiritual, and biological fitness on the part of the individual, which results from adaptations to the environment" (1968, p. 5). In Dubos's view, the individual must have sufficient knowledge to make informed choices about his or her health and also the income and resources to act on choices. Dubos (1978) believes that complete well-being is unobtainable, in contrast to the 1947 definition by the World Health Organization.

In 1980, the American Nurses Association (ANA) defined health in their social policy statement as "a dynamic state of being in which the developmental and behavioral potential of an individual is realized to the fullest extent possible" (ANA, 1980, p. 5). In this definition, health is more than a state or the absence of disease; it includes striving toward optimal functioning.

In recent years, the idea of health has come to include a more holistic approach and to encompass quality of life. Elements such as environmental, spiritual, emotional, and intellectual aspects have been included, and the term *wellness* has become more popular (Donatelle & Davis, 2000).

Wellness and Well-Being

Wellness is "a continual balancing of the different dimensions of human needs—spiritual, social, emotional, intellectual, physical, occupational, and environmental" (Anspaugh, Hamrick, & Rosata, 2000, p. v). It is a process of identifying needs for improvement and making choices that facilitate a higher level of health. Basic concepts of wellness include self-responsibility; an ultimate goal; a dynamic, growing process; daily decision making in the areas of nutrition, stress management, physical fitness, preventive health care, emotional health, and other aspects of health; and, most importantly, the whole being of the individual. See the box on page 307.

Well-being is a subjective perception of balance, harmony, and vitality. It is a state that can be described objectively, occurs at levels, and can be plotted on a continuum (Hood, 2003, p. 230).

Concepts of Wellness

- Wellness is a choice—a decision you make to move toward optimal health.

- Wellness is a way of life—a lifestyle you design to achieve your highest potential for well-being.

- Wellness is a process—a developing awareness that there is no end point, but that health and happiness are possible in each moment, here and now.

- Wellness is a balanced channeling of energy—energy received from the environment, transformed within you, and returned to affect the world around you.

- Wellness is the integration of body, mind, and spirit—the appreciation that everything you do, and think, and feel, and believe has an impact on your state of health and the health of the world.

- Wellness is the loving acceptance of yourself.

Source: From *Wellness Workbook* (3rd ed.), by W. Travis, and R. S. Ryan, Celestial Arts, Berkeley, CA. Reprinted with permission. © 1981, 1988, 2004 by John W. Travis. http://www.wellnessworkbook.com.

Illness and Disease

People may view illness and disease as the same entity; however, health professionals generally view them as completely separate. Emotions are not believed to cause disease, but they may create an environment in which disease can develop through their effect upon the immune system.

Illness is a highly personal state in which the person feels unhealthy or ill. Illness may or may not be related to disease. An individual could have a disease, for example, a growth in the stomach, and not feel ill. By the same token, a person can feel ill, that is, feel uncomfortable, yet have no discernible disease. Illness is highly subjective; only the individual person can say he or she is ill.

Disease is a term that can be described as an alteration in body functions resulting in a reduction of capacities or a shortening of the normal life span. Traditionally, intervention by physicians had the goal of eliminating or ameliorating disease processes. Primitive people thought disease was caused by "forces" or spirits. Later, this belief was replaced by the single-causation theory. Today, multiple factors are considered to interact in causing disease and determining an individual's response to treatment.

Another distinction needs to be made between disease and deviance. **Deviance** is behavior that goes against social norms. Some deviant behaviors may be considered diseases according to the earlier definition of disease. For example, alcoholism can result in an alteration of body functioning, a reduction in capacities, and a shortening of the life span. Other deviant behavior can be considered a disease, not because it alters the function of a body organ, but because it disrupts a family or a community. An example is drug addiction. However, differentiation between disease and deviance is not always clear and often depends on the perspective of the person observing the behavior.

Reflect on...

- what behaviors of others indicate to you that they are healthy or unhealthy.
- your own definition of health.
- whether you believe that your clients should agree with your definition of health.
- which factors you believe most affect your own sense of wellness.

Disease Prevention

Disease prevention is a part of health promotion. Health promotion is covered in greater detail in Chapter 7 ∞, The Nurse as Health Promoter and Care Provider. Prevention is taking action to avoid a later illness and is conceptualized in three levels: primary, secondary, and tertiary. **Primary prevention** is directed toward avoiding health problems before they begin and includes such activities as getting immunized and practicing safe sex. **Secondary prevention** occurs with the recognition of risk and taking action to reduce risk before disease gets a foothold. An example would be stopping smoking. **Tertiary prevention** refers to treatment or rehabilitation, such as physical therapy following an injury to restore function.

Evidence for Practice

Stuifbergen, A. K., Seraphine, A., & Roberts, G. (2000). An explanatory model of health promotion and quality of life in chronic disabling conditions. *Nursing Research, 49*(3), 122–129.

The objective of this study was to test an explanatory model of variables influencing health promotion and quality of life in persons living with multiple sclerosis. A sample of 786 completed a battery of instruments measuring severity of illness-related impairment, barriers to health-promoting behaviors, resources, self-efficacy, acceptance, health-promoting behaviors, and perceived quality of life. A causal model was created from the data using the software program LISREL8. The antecedent variables accounted for 58% of the variance in frequency of health-promoting behaviors and 66% of the variance in perceived quality of life. The effects of severity of illness on quality of life were mediated partially by health-promoting behaviors, resources, self-efficacy, and acceptance. The strength of the direct and indirect paths suggests the interventions to enhance social support, decrease barriers, and increase specific self-efficacy for health behaviors would result in improved health-promoting behaviors and quality of life.

MODELS OF HEALTH AND WELLNESS

Because health is such a complex concept, various researchers have developed models or paradigms to explain health and, in some instances, its relationship to illness or injury. Models can be helpful in assisting health professionals to meet the health and wellness needs of individuals. Nurses need to clarify their own understanding of health, wellness, and illness for the following reasons:

■ Nurses' definitions of health largely determine the scope and nature of nursing practice. For example, when health is defined narrowly as a physiologic phenomenon, nurses confine themselves to assisting clients regain normal physiologic functioning. When health is defined more broadly, the scope of nursing practice increases correspondingly.

■ People's health beliefs influence their health practices. Thus, a nurse's health values and practices may differ from those of a client. Nurses need to ensure that plans of care developed for individuals relate to the client's conception of health. Otherwise, clients may fail to respond to a health care regimen.

Leavell and Clark's Agent-Host-Environment Model

The *agent-host-environment model*, also called the *epidemiological triangle*, is a traditional approach to health and disease developed to address communicable disease and is one of the early models (Leavell & Clark, 1965). It has been expanded to other health conditions as a more general model, but it is still used primarily to predict illness. The three variables in the model are depicted as a triangle when they are in their normal state of equilibrium. A change in any of the three sides results in disequilibrium. In a healthy state, equilibrium exists (Anderson & McFarlane, 2000). The three dynamic interactive elements in this model are described as follows:

1. *Agent.* Any environmental factor or stressor (biologic, chemical, mechanical, physical, or psychosocial) that by its presence or absence (e.g., lack of essential nutrients) can lead to illness or disease.
2. *Host.* Person(s) who may or may not be at risk of acquiring a disease. Family history, age, and lifestyle habits influence the host's reaction.
3. *Environment.* All factors external to the host that may or may not predispose the person to the development of disease. Physical environment includes climate, living conditions, noise levels, and economic level. Social environment includes interactions with others and life events, such as the death of a spouse.

Because each of the agent-host-environment factors constantly interacts with the others, health is an ever-changing state. When the variables are in balance, health is maintained; when variables are not in balance, disease occurs.

Dunn's Levels of Wellness

Dunn described a health grid in which a health axis and an environmental axis intersect (1959a, p. 786). It demonstrates the interaction of the environment with the illness-wellness continuum (Figure 17–1■).

The health axis extends from peak wellness to death, and the environmental axis extends from very favorable to very unfavorable. The intersection of the two axes forms the following four health/wellness quadrants:

Figure 17–1

Dunn's Health Grid: Its Axes and Quadrants

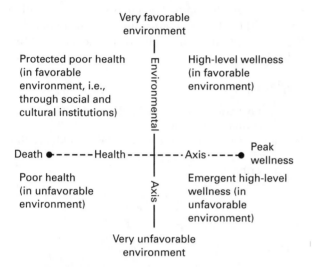

Source: From "High-Level Wellness for Man and Society," by H.L. Dunn, June 1959, *American Journal of Public Health, 49,* 788. Used with permission of the American Public Health Association.

1. *High-level wellness in a favorable environment.* An example of this is a person who implements healthy lifestyle behaviors and has the biopsychosocial, spiritual, and economic resources to support this lifestyle.
2. *Emergent high-level wellness in an unfavorable environment.* An example of this is a woman who has the knowledge to implement healthy lifestyle practices but does not implement adequate self-care practices because of family responsibilities, job demands, or other factors.
3. *Protected poor health in a favorable environment.* An example of this is an ill person (e.g., one with multiple fractures or severe hypertension) whose needs are met by the health care system and who has access to appropriate medications, diet, and health care instruction.
4. *Poor health in an unfavorable environment.* An example of this is a young child who is starving in a drought-stricken country.

In his book about high-level wellness in the individual, Dunn (1973) explored the concept of wellness as it relates to family, community, environment, and society. He believed that family wellness enhances wellness in individuals. In a well family that offers trust, love, and support, the individual does not have to expend energy to meet basic needs and can move forward on the wellness continuum. By providing effective sanitation and safe water, disposing of sewage safely, and preserving beauty and wildlife, the community enhances both family and individual wellness. Environmental wellness is related to the premise that humans must be at peace with and guard the environment. Societal wellness is significant because the status of the larger, social group, affects the status of smaller groups. Dunn believed that social wellness must be considered on a worldwide basis.

Health and Wellness Continuum

Health and illness or disease can be viewed as the opposite ends of a health continuum. The continuum ranges from optimum wellness to premature death and includes the six dimensions of health that affect movement along the continuum. These dimensions are described as follows:

- *Physical health*—Body size, sensory acuity, susceptibility to disease, body functioning, physical fitness, and recuperative abilities
- *Intellectual health*—Ability to think clearly and analyze critically to meet life's challenges
- *Social health*—Ability to have satisfying interpersonal relationships and interactions with others
- *Emotional health*—Appropriate expression of and control of emotions; self-esteem, trust, and love
- *Environmental health*—Appreciation of the external environment and the role one plays in preserving, protecting, and improving environmental conditions
- *Spiritual health*—Belief in a supreme being or a way of living prescribed by religion; a guiding sense of meaning or value in life

Many people believe optimum wellness is best achieved through a holistic approach by which there is a balance among the dimensions (Donatelle & Davis, 2000).

Reflect on...

- how the models of health and wellness fit your views.
- how the nurse might best care for a client with a belief in a model of health and wellness that differs from the nurse's.

HEALTH STATUS, BELIEFS, AND BEHAVIORS

The *health status* (state) of an individual is the health of that person at a given time. In its general meaning, the term may refer to anxiety, depression, or acute illness and thus describes the individual's problem in general.

Health status can also describe such specifics as pulse rate and body temperature. The *health belief* of an individual is a perception of the relationship between things such as actions or objects and health. Beliefs may or may not be founded on fact. Some of these are influenced by culture, such as the "hot-cold" system of some Hispanic Americans. In this system, health is viewed as a balance of hot and cold qualities within a person. Citrus fruits and some fowl are considered "cold" foods, and meats and bread are "hot" foods. In this context, "hot" and "cold" do not denote temperature or spiciness but innate qualities of the food. For example, a fever is said to be caused by an excess of "hot" foods.

Health behaviors are the actions people take to understand their health state, maintain an optimal state of health, prevent illness and injury, and reach their maximum physical and mental potential. Behaviors such as eating wisely, exercising, paying attention to signs of illness, following treatment advice, and avoiding known health hazards such as smoking are all examples. Many factors contribute to health behaviors. Figure 17–2■ shows a model of influences on these behaviors.

Reflect on...

■ what behaviors you consider to be the most likely to affect your own health.

■ how you would respond to a client who holds health beliefs that are contrary to the treatment that is prescribed.

Figure 17–2

Factors Influencing Health Behavior Change

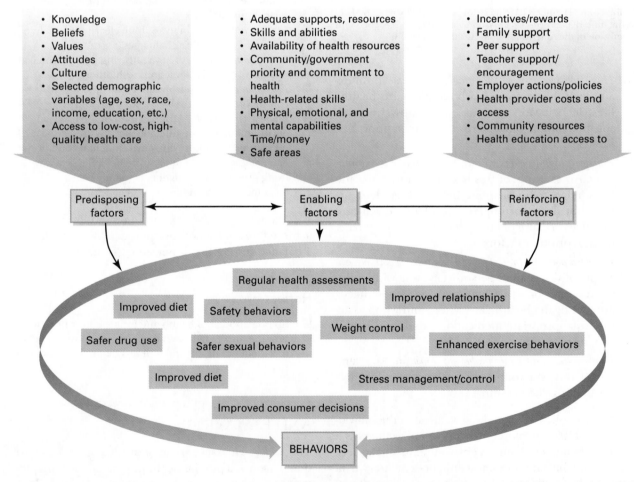

Source: From *Access to Health* (5th ed.), by R. J. Donatelle and L. G. Davis, Boston: Allyn and Bacon, Copyright © 1998. Reprinted with permission of Pearson Education, Inc.

HEALTH BELIEF MODELS

Several theories or health belief/behavior models have been developed to help determine whether an individual is likely to participate in disease prevention and health-promotion activities. These models can be useful tools in the development of programs for helping people change to healthier lifestyles and develop a more positive attitude to preventive health measures. See also Chapter 7 ⬚, The Nurse as Health Promoter and Care Provider.

Health Locus of Control Model

Locus of control is a concept from social learning theory that nurses may consider when determining who is most likely to take action regarding health, that is, whether clients believe that their health status is under their own or others' control. People who believe that they have a major influence on their own health status are internally controlled. They are more likely than others to take the initiative in their own health care, be more knowledgeable about their health, and adhere to prescribed health care regimens, such as taking medication, making and keeping appointments with physicians, and maintaining diets. By contrast, people who believe their health is largely controlled by outside forces (e.g., chance, luck, or powerful others) and is beyond their control are externally controlled and may need assistance to become more internally controlled if behavior changes are to be successful. Locus of control is a measurable concept that can be used to predict which people are most likely to change their behavior.

The results of a study by Lewis suggest that greater personal control over one's life is associated with higher levels of self-esteem, greater purpose in life, and decreased self-report of anxiety (Lewis, 1982, p. 113). Nurses can use this information about a client's locus of control to improve the client's self-care.

Rosenstock and Becker's Health Belief Model

In the 1950s, Rosenstock (1974) proposed a health belief model (HBM) in response to observations by public health providers that many people did not take advantage of low-cost preventive services, such as polio vaccines and tuberculosis screening. The model is based on subjective beliefs to predict which individuals would or would not use health care services. According to this model, behavior is influenced by multiple interacting beliefs, such as perceived susceptibility to and severity of

Evidence for Practice

Shaw, C., McColl, E., & Bond, S. (2003). The relationship of perceived control to outcomes in older women undergoing surgery for fractured neck of femur. *Journal of Clinical Nursing, 12,* 117–123.

The relationship between internal locus of control and recovery from surgery for fractured neck of the femur in women over the age of 65 years was investigated to inform strategies for nursing care. Structured interviews were carried out at 5 days and at 30 days post surgery with 112 women in five general hospitals in England. The average age of the subjects was 78.6 years. Locus of control was assessed related to outcomes of physical disability, measured as dependence in activities of daily living, and to psychologic distress, measured as anxiety and depression. Internal locus of control was significantly associated with less physical disability, but not with anxiety and depression at 30 days postsurgery. These findings suggest that nursing interventions to enhance perceived internal control during rehabilitation may result in more positive physical outcome and ability to perform self-care activities.

a condition, efficacy of alternative behaviors, barriers to action, and self-efficacy (Finfgeld et al., 2003).

The health belief model (Figure 17–3▪) is based on motivational theory. Rosenstock assumed that good health is an objective common to all people. Becker added "positive health motivation" as a consideration. Health behavior change happens because there is a readiness to take the action based upon the balance of multiple beliefs. Interventions based upon the health belief model are directed toward changing beliefs or activating those that already exist.

Becker (1974) modified the health belief model to include these components: individual perceptions, modifying factors, and variables likely to affect initiating action.

Individual perceptions include the following:

- *Perceived susceptibility.* A family history of a certain disorder, such as diabetes or heart disease, may make the individual feel at high risk.
- *Perceived seriousness.* The question here is: In the perception of the individual, does the illness cause death or have serious consequences? Concern about

Figure 17–3

The Health Belief Model

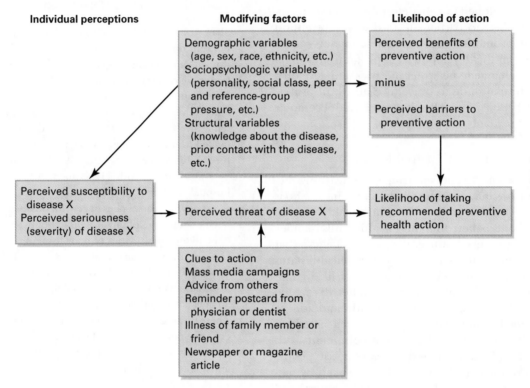

Source: From "Selected Psychosocial Models and Correlates of Individual Health-Related Behaviors," by M. H. Becker, D. P. Haefner, S. V. Dasi, 1977, *Medical Care, 15,* 27–46. Used with permission.

the spread of acquired immune deficiency syndrome (AIDS) reflects the general public's perception of the seriousness of this illness.

■ *Perceived threat.* According to Becker, perceived susceptibility and perceived seriousness combine to determine the total perceived threat of an illness to a specific individual. For example, a person who perceives that many individuals in the community have AIDS may not necessarily perceive a threat of the disease; if the person is a drug addict or a homosexual, however, the perceived threat of illness is likely to increase because of the combined susceptibility and seriousness.

Modifying factors are those that modify a person's perception, and they include:

■ *Demographic variables.* Demographic variables include age, sex, race, and ethnicity. An infant, for example, does not perceive the importance of a healthy diet; an adolescent may perceive peer approval as more important than family approval and participate as a consequence in hazardous activities or adopt unhealthy eating and sleeping patterns.

■ *Sociopsychological variables.* Social pressure or influence from peers or other reference groups (e.g., self-help or vocational groups) may encourage preventive health behaviors even when individual motivation is low. Expectations of others may motivate people, for example, not to drive an automobile after drinking alcohol.

■ *Structural variables.* Structural variables that are presumed to influence preventive behavior are knowledge about the target disease and prior contact with it. Becker found higher compliance rates with prescribed treatments among mothers whose children had frequent ear infections and occurrences of asthma.

■ *Cues to action.* Cues can be either internal or external. Internal cues include feelings of fatigue, uncomfortable symptoms, or thoughts about the condition of an ill person who is close.

Likelihood of action is the likelihood of a person taking the recommended preventive health action, which is based on the perceived benefits of the action minus the perceived barriers to the action.

Critical Thinking Exercise

Marcia Campbell is a 37-year-old woman who has recently immigrated to the United States from Jamaica. She tells you that she has never had a Pap smear and has only had pelvic exams when she had her two children. She says she has never known anyone who has had cervical cancer and doesn't think it is a very serious problem. She believes that she maintains her overall health by using herbal prepara-tions that she learned from her grandmother in Jamaica. This has kept her healthy so far and she hasn't had to have that "uncomfortable and embarrassing thing" done to her.

Based on the Health Belief Model, what is influenc-ing her decision to avoid preventive care? Based upon this information, devise a plan to help her change her readiness to take action.

- *Perceived benefits of the action.* Examples include refraining from smoking to prevent lung cancer, and eating nutritious foods and avoiding snacks to maintain weight.
- *Perceived barriers to action.* Examples include cost, inconvenience, unpleasantness, and lifestyle changes.

Nurses play a major role in helping clients imple-ment healthy behaviors. They help clients monitor health, supply anticipatory guidance, and impart knowledge about health. Nurses can also reduce barri-ers to action (e.g., by minimizing inconvenience or dis-comfort) and can support positive actions.

INTERNATIONAL INITIATIVE FOR HEALTH AND WELLNESS

Health for All has been proclaimed by the World Health Organization (WHO) as an international goal. The WHO constitution proclaims that the highest attain-able standard of health is "one of the fundamental rights of every human being without distinction for race, religion, political belief, economic or social con-dition" (WHO, 1998, 2000). *Health for All* was adopted in 1977 and launched at the Alma Ata Conference in 1978. A renewal was launched in 1995 to ensure that individuals, countries, and organizations are ready to meet the world's health care needs in the 21st century.

WHO (2000) published a document titled *Health for All in the Twenty-first Century.* It describes global pri-orities and targets for the first two decades of the cen-tury that will create conditions worldwide for people to reach and maintain the highest level of health. The goals are to achieve an increase in life expectancy and quality of life, to improve equity in health between and within countries, and to ensure access for all to sus-tainable health services and systems. Key values under-pining this effort are as follows:

- providing the highest attainable standard of health as a fundamental right
- strengthening application of ethics
- implementing equity-oriented policies and strategies
- incorporating a gender perspective to health policies and strategies

There are ten global targets that support *Health for All,* as shown in the box on page 314. Regional and na-tional targets will be developed within the framework of the global policy reflecting the diversity of needs and local priorities. The actions by all member states are to be guided by two policy objectives: making health central to human development and developing sustainable health systems to meet the needs of peo-ple. WHO will provide global leadership for attain-ment of *Health for All* and will promote international collective action. More information on healthy people can be found in Chapter 7 ∞, The Nurse as Health Promoter and Care Provider.

In the United States, goals for the health of indi-viduals, communities, and the nation are set forth by *Healthy People 2010,* a government document published by the Department of Health and Human Services (DHHS) in 2000, and *Healthy People* was originally a re-port of the Surgeon General in 1979. *Healthy People 2000* was published in 1989. Although only a few of the objectives of *Healthy People 2000* were met, the docu-ment raised consciousness and provided an impetus for health promotion. *Healthy People 2010* expands the objectives through two broad goals: increase in quality and years of healthy life and elimination of health dis-parities. The leading health indicators identified to re-flect major public health concerns and progress toward these goals are:

- Increased physical activity
- Weight management
- Reduction in tobacco use and substance abuse

Global Health Targets

1. Healthy equity: childhood stunting
2. Survival: MMR,[1] CMR,[2] life expectancy
3. Reverse global trends of five major pandemics
4. Eradicate and eliminate certain diseases
5. Improve access to water, sanitation, food, and shelter
6. Measures to promote health
7. Develop, implement, and monitor national HFA policies
8. Improve access to comprehensive, essential, quality health care
9. Implement global and national health information and surveillance systems
10. Support research for health

[1]MMR—maternal mortality rate.
[2]CMR—child mortality rate.
Source: From *Health for All in the Twenty-first Century* (executive summary, p. vi), by World Health Organization, 2000, Geneva: WHO.

■ Responsible sexual behavior
■ Promotion of mental health
■ Reduction of injury and violence
■ Improvement in environmental quality
■ Greater access to immunization and health care

Physical inactivity has been identified by WHO as a leading cause of disability (2002). At World Health Day in 2002, WHO issued a warning that a sedentary lifestyle could be among the 10 leading causes of death and disability in the world. It was estimated that 2 million deaths per year can be attributed to physical inactivity. Sedentary lifestyles can double the risk for cardiovascular disease, diabetes, and obesity. It increases the risk of colon cancer, hypertension, osteoporosis, and depression. WHO estimates that 60–85% of the world's population lead sedentary lives regardless of whether the country is developed or developing. It is estimated that about two thirds of children are inactive, thus increasing their risks for the future. Among the preventive measures promoted at World Health Day 2002 were exercise for 30 minutes per day, smoking cessation, and healthy nutrition. Among the measures recommended were implementing transportation policies that make it safer for people to walk or ride bicycles, building accessible parks and playgrounds and community centers, and promoting physical activity programs in schools, communities, and health services.

NURSING IN AN ERA OF SHORTAGE

The nursing profession has experienced cyclic periods of shortage throughout time. However, the current nursing shortage is predicted to last into 2020, with an estimated 400,000 job vacancies. Added to this is the finding that one out of three nurses in the United States younger than age 30 plans to leave their jobs within a year because of dissatisfaction and stress. This is attributable to several factors, including an increased average age of registered nurses and expanded opportunities for women in other careers. The nurses who are in the present workforce are faced with increased challenges and heavier workloads (Murray, 2002).

In the early 1980s, nursing was experiencing one of its cycles of shortage prompting a study by the American Academy of Nursing to investigate hospitals that were able to attract and retain nurses. Forty-one hospitals were identified as magnet hospitals and were found to have organizational traits that promoted and sustained professional nursing practice. These traits included flat organizational structure, unit-based decision making, an influential nurse executive, and an investment in the education and expertise of the nursing staff. In the early 1990s, the American Nurses Credentialing Center, an arm of the ANA, developed a formal procedure for recognition of magnet hospitals. It is called the Magnet Nursing Services Recognition Program (Bolton & Bennett, 2002).

To shape the future of nursing, nurses must be prepared to meet these challenges head on. Planning for anticipated changes requires becoming more proactive in the development of the future of the profession. The American Nurses Association along with other nursing organizations has developed an agenda for the future of nursing and a strategic plan to address the growing shortage and ensure that consumers have access to high-quality nursing care (ANA, 2002). The

Steering Committee for Nursing's Agenda for the Future

American Academy of Nursing	Emergency Nurses Association
American Association of Colleges of Nursing	Infusion Nurses Society
American Association of Critical-Care Nurses	National Black Nurses Association
American Association of Nurse Anesthetists	National Council of State Boards of Nursing
American Nurses Association	National League for Nursing
American Nurses Credentialing Center	National Student Nurses' Association, Inc.
American Organization of Nurse Executives	Nursing Organization Liason Forum
American Psychiatric Nurses Association	Obstetric and Neonatal Nurses
Association of Peri-Operative Registered Nurses	Oncology Nursing Society
Association of Women's Health	Sigma Theta Tau International Honor Society of Nursing

nineteen national nursing organizations that serve as the steering committee will guide and monitor the work on the initiative. These nursing organizations are listed in the accompanying box.

The Steering Committee identified the desired future for nursing as the following:

> Nursing is *the* pivotal health care profession, highly valued for its specialized knowledge, skill and caring in improving the health status of the public and ensuring safe, effective, quality care. The profession mirrors the diverse population it serves and provides leadership to create positive changes in health policy and delivery systems. Individuals choose nursing as a career, and remain in the profession, because of the opportunities for personal and professional growth, supportive work environments and compensation commensurate with roles and responsibilities. (ANA, 2002, p. 7)

Ten domains or areas of concern demanding action were identified. These included the following:

- *Leadership and planning*—calling for well-prepared nurse leaders to assume positions of power and influence on key decision making for nursing and health care
- *Economic value*—calling for recognition of nurses as providers of quality, cost-effective care and compensation of nurses for their value
- *Delivery systems/nursing models*—calling for the creation of integrated models of health care delivery through partnerships that improve the health of the nation

- *Work environment*—improvement of work environments so that quality patient care is optimized and professional nurses are retained
- *Legislation/regulation/policy*—calling for new collaborations that will increase nursing's role in shaping public policy
- *Public relations/communication*—demonstrating nursing's pivotal role in health care to various groups outside of nursing
- *Nursing/professional culture*—asserting nursing's high standards of professional practice, education, leadership and collaboration to enhance professionalism, image, and career satisfaction
- *Education*—reshaping nursing education to improve nursing practice, enhance image, and better meet patient care needs
- *Recruitment/retention*—attracting and sustaining excellent nurses for long, rewarding careers
- *Diversity*—aiming for diversity that reflects the patient population, to better meet population needs

From these 10 domains, the Steering Committee identified four as top priorities. These are Economic Value, Delivery Systems, Education, and Work Environment (ANA, 2002).

The aging population with its need for long-term care, advances in technology, the increases in the wellness movement, and economic trends will create changes in nursing. Whereas about 60% of nurses now work in acute-care settings, in the future more care will be delivered in the community and in the home. Computer technology and communications systems will reduce the need to see health care providers in person. Monitoring can be done from a distance.

Evidence for Practice

Ernst, M. E., France, M., Messmer, P. R., & Gonzalez, J. L. (2004). Nurses job satisfaction, stress, and recognition in a pediatric setting. *Pediatric Nursing, 30*(3), 219–227.

A survey design was used to identify a set of factors that describe nurses' satisfaction in a children's hospital. Nursing satisfaction, organizational work satisfaction, job stress, and nurse recognition were assessed by questionnaire for 534 nurses. Several factors were found to predict pediatric nurses' job satisfaction and organizational work satisfaction: pay, time to do the nursing care, confidence in one's ability, and task requirements. Nurses with more years of experience and longevity on the unit and at the hospital had more confidence, showed less concern about time demands, and were less concerned about pay and task requirements than younger nurses. Job stress correlated inversely with age, years as a nurse, and years in the organization. Older nurses were more satisfied with the recognition they received than were the younger nurses.

This study supports the need to focus on programs to increase the confidence of novice nurses, improve institutional nursing recognition for all levels of practice, enhance communication within the organization, and maintain competitive compensation.

Many procedures that have traditionally been invasive and required skilled care are being replaced by noninvasive procedures with a simplified recovery period. Hospitals and acute-care settings will likely be the site of intensive care units almost exclusively. The knowledge and skills that nurses use will be replaced more rapidly, requiring continuing education at a new level (Murray, 2002).

Nurses practice in virtually every health care setting and in all communities and are the largest health care profession, numbering about 2.7 million (ANA, 2002). The primary reason people are admitted to hospitals and acute-care settings is that they need nursing care. In addition to acute-care institutions, nurses provide long-term care, home care, primary and preventive care, health promotion, and public health. Nursing roles are evolving in new areas such as informatics and telehealth. One thing seems certain, that nurses will continue to acquire new skills, expanded roles, and new settings in the delivery of care.

EXPLORE MEDIALINK

Questions, critical thinking exercises, essay activities, and other interactive resources for this chapter can be found on the Web site at http://www.prenhall.com/blais. Click on Chapter 17 to select activities for this chapter.

Bookshelf

Anders, G. (1996). *Health against wealth.* **New York: Houghton Mifflin Company.**

This book discusses the background of the rise of HMOs and the breakdown of medical trust. It addresses ways to build a better system.

O'Brien, L. J. (1999). *Bad medicine: How the American medical establishment is ruining our healthcare system.* **Amherst, NY: Prometheus Books.**

This book analyzes the decline of health care services in the United States from the perspective of medicine and proposes approaches to change.

Weinberg, D. B. (2003). *Code green: Money-driven hospitals and the dismantling of nursing.* **Ithaca, NY: Cornell University Press.**

Discusses the reasons for the nursing shortage and the struggles of prestigious hospitals to fill vacancies. It shows the effects of hospital restructuring on nurses' ability to plan, evaluate, and deliver excellent care, and provides an indictment for the underestimation of the contribution nurses make to hospitals and to patient care.

SUMMARY

Changes in the delivery of health care have resulted in changes in the practice of nursing. Two influences on these changes are cost-containment measures mandated by third-party payers and the commitment to providing care that is accessible to people in their communities. Cost containment has resulted in more focus on resource management and created the need for nurses to become skillful in the utilization of scarce resources, the development of critical pathways that provide accountability for outcomes, and the use of unlicensed assistive personnel. Focus of care has expanded from acute inpatient care to include primary and preventive care that is community focused.

The changes in nursing require a new perspective on health as more than the absence of illness or disease, also involving a high level of wellness or the fulfillment of one's maximum potential for physical, psychosocial, and spiritual functioning. Wellness is an active, five-dimensional process of becoming aware of and making choices toward a higher level of well-being. The five dimensions of wellness are the physical, social, emotional, intellectual, and spiritual dimensions. Well-being is considered a subjective perception of balance, harmony, and vitality. It is a state rather than a process. Illness is usually associated with disease but may occur independently of it. Illness is a highly personal state in which the person feels unhealthy or ill. Disease alters body functions and results in a reduction of capacities or a shortened life span.

Because notions of health are highly individual, the nurse must determine each client's perception of health to provide meaningful assistance. This involves well-developed communication skills. Nurses also need to be aware of their own personal definitions of health. Many people describe health as freedom from symptoms of disease, the ability to be active, and a state of being in good spirits. Various models have been developed to explain health. They include the agent-host-environment model, the high-level wellness grid, and the health belief model.

A person's decision to implement health behaviors or to take action to improve health depends on a number of factors. Such factors include the importance of health to the person, perceived threat of a particular disease or severity of the health care problems, perceived benefits of preventive or therapeutic actions, inconvenience and unpleasantness involved, degree of lifestyle change necessary, cultural ramifications, and cost.

The movement toward health and wellness has an international impetus through the work of the World Health Organization. *Health for All* is promoted through international collaboration to meet global health targets set by the organization.

The nursing shortage in the United States has created a changed work environment for nurses and demands that action be taken to ensure high-quality health care for the nation. The Magnet Recognition Program for Excellence in Nursing Service provides recognition to hospitals. The goal of this recognition is to attract and retain nurses. It provides incentive for positive workplace change. *Nursing's Agenda for the Future* was developed by several professional organizations to provide a strategic plan to address the shortage.

REFERENCES

American Nurses Association. (1980). *Nursing: A social policy statement.* Kansas City: ANA.

American Nurses Association. (1991). *Nursing's agenda for health care reform.* Washington, DC: ANA.

American Nurses Association. (2002). *Nursing's agenda for the future.* Washington, DC: ANA.

American Nurses Association. (2003). *House of Delegates status report: Trends in the U.S. health care system.* Washington, DC: ANA.

American Organization of Nurse Executives. (1992). Eight premises for a reformed American health-care system. *Nursing Management, 23,* 42, 44.

Anderson, E. T., & McFarlane, J. (2000). Community as partner: Theory and practice in nursing. Philadelphia: J. B. Lippincott.

Anspaugh, D. J., Hamrick, M. H., & Rosata, F. D. (2000). *Wellness: Concepts and applications* (4th ed.). St. Louis: Mosby.

Becker, M. H. (Ed.). (1974). *The health belief model and personal health behavior.* Thorofare, NJ: Charles B. Slack.

Becker, M. H., Haefner, D. P., & Dasi, V. (1977). Selected psychosocial models and correlates of individual health-related behaviors. *Medical Care, 15,* 27–46.

Bolton, L. B., & Bennett, C. (2002). The ANCC Magnet Recognition Program and magnet hospitals. In D. Mason, J. Leavitt, & M. Chaffee, *Policy and Politics in Nursing and Health Care* (4th ed., pp. 324–327). St. Louis: W. B. Saunders.

Congressional Budget Office. (2003). *How many people lack health insurance and for how long?* http://www.cbo.gob/showdoc.cfm?index=4210&sequence=0.

Donatelle, R. J., & Davis, L. G. (2000). *Access to health* (6th ed.). Boston: Allyn and Bacon.

Dubos, R. (1968). *So human the animal.* New York: Scribners.

Dubos, R. (1978). Health and creative adaptation. *Human Nature, 74*(1).

Dunn, H. L. (1959a, June). High-level wellness in man and society. *American Journal of Public Health, 49,* 786.

Dunn, H. L. (1959b, November). What high-level wellness means. *Canadian Journal of Public Health, 50,* 447.

Dunn, H. L. (1973). *High-level wellness.* Arlington, VA: Beatty.

Finfgeld, D. L. (2003). Health belief model and reversal theory: a comparative analysis. *Journal of Advanced Nursing, 43*(3), 288–297.

Glick, D. F. (1999). Advanced practice community health nursing in community nursing centers: A holistic approach to the community as client. *Holistic Nursing Practice, 13*(4), 19–27.

Healthy People (2010). www.healthypeople.gov/Document/html/uih_bw/uih_2.htm.

Hood, L., (2003). *Pepper's conceptual bases of professional nursing* (5th ed.). Philadelphia: J. B. Lippincott.

Leavell, H. R., & Clark, E. G. (1965). *Preventive medicine for the doctor in his community* (3rd ed.). New York: McGraw-Hill.

Leddy, S., & Pepper, J. M. (1998). *Conceptual bases of professional nursing* (4th ed.). Philadelphia: J. B. Lippincott.

Lewis, F. M. (1982, March/April). Experienced personal control and quality of life in late-stage cancer patients. *Nursing Research, 31,* 113–118.

McAllister, G., & Farquhar, M. (1992, December). Health beliefs: A cultural division? *Journal of Advanced Nursing, 17,* 1447–1454.

Milstead, J. A. (2004). *Health policy and politics: A nurse's guide* (2nd ed.). Boston: Jones and Barlett.

Murray, M. K. (2002). The nursing shortage. Past present and future. *Journal of Nursing Administration, 32*(3), 79–84.

Nightingale, F. (1969). *Notes on nursing: What it is and what it is not.* New York: Dover Books. (Original work published 1860).

Parsons, T. (1972). Definitions of health and illness in the light of American values and social structure. In E. G. Jaco (Ed.). *Patients, physicians, and illness* (2nd ed.), New York: Free Press.

Pender, N. J. (1987). *Health promotion in nursing practice* (2nd ed.). Norwalk, CT: Appleton & Lange.

President's Commission on Health Needs of the Nation. (1953). *Building Americans' health* (Vol. 2) Washington, DC: U.S. Government Printing Office.

Price, S. A., Koch, M. W., & Bassett, S. (1998). *Health care resource management: Present and future challenges.* St. Louis: Mosby.

Rosenstock, I. M. (1974). Historical origins of the health belief model. In M. H. Becker (Ed.), *The health belief model and personal health behavior.* Thorofare, NJ: Charles B. Slack.

Salmond, S. W. (1999). Delivery-of-care systems using clinical nursing assistants: Making it work. In S. O. Turner, *Essential readings in nursing managed care.* (pp. 215–224) Gaithersburg, MD: Aspen Publications.

World Health Organization. (1947). *Constitution of the World Health Organization: Chronicle of the World Health Organization I.* Geneva: WHO.

World Health Organization. (1998). *The world health report 1998: Life in the 21st century—a vision for all.* Geneva: WHO.

World Health Organization. (2000). *Health for all in the twenty-first century.* Geneva: WHO.

World Health Organization. (2002). *World Health Day 2002. Move for Health.* http://www.who.int/archives/world-health-day.

U.S. Department of Health and Human Services. (2000). *Healthy People 2010: Understanding and Improving Health* (2nd ed.). Washington, DC: U.S. Government Printing Office.

Health Care Economics

Objectives

- Identify selected issues related to nursing and health care economics.
- Define common terms used in discussing health care financing.
- Discuss cost-containment strategies implemented in health care.
- Examine the economics of providing health care services.
- Apply economics to nursing.
- Describe approaches to financial management in health care.

M E D I A L I N K

Additional online resources for this chapter can be found on the companion Web site at http://www.prenhall.com/blais.

The decade of the 1990s focused on health care reform, accompanied by considerable debate regarding the resulting changes in health care financing. There was general recognition of the need for fundamental changes in health care delivery but no consensus about what these changes should be. There are several reform proposals; among them are (1) single-payer national health insurance with universal coverage, (2) expansion of public programs covering the poor, (3) requirement of employers to offer health insurance to all employees, and (4) use of credits for purchase of health insurance or using medical savings accounts.

Two central questions are raised by health care reform. Who should control the health care system? Who should pay for health care? Several issues must be addressed. People in the United States are paying more for health care and getting less in return for the amount paid. The cost of health care is implicated in the decline of the United States in the global economy. The cost of long-term care is a major concern, with a growing percentage of the population aging and a smaller workforce bearing the burden of providing services. Curbing the costs of prescription drugs and other medical technologies have been recent issues.

CHALLENGES AND OPPORTUNITIES

The economic changes in health care have made it necessary for nurses to find new ways of delivering needed services within new structures of payment. An era of cost cutting arising from changes in financing has resulted in reductions in nursing staff, higher nurse-patient ratios, and higher productivity expectations as values seemingly moved from quality of care to cost-effectiveness and profits.

The necessity of lowering the cost of health care has created many opportunities for nursing to expand practice and create new roles. Advanced practice nursing roles have increased as care moved from acute-care settings to outpatient and community settings. Nursing has an opportunity to exert its influence in new directions for policy and delivery of care.

ISSUES

Demand Versus Supply of Health Care

During the 1980s, the cost of medical care was increasing faster than the gross national product. Coupled with the increased expense of care was the consumer's expectation that any and all services should be available and paid for by third-party payers regardless of cost. The demand for expensive care was outstripping the ability of payers to pay and spiraling out of control, as consumers demanded a total continuum of care and unlimited access.

Further imbalance in supply and demand is created by the resulting increased cost of insurance coverage in the private sector. Many employers believe they cannot afford to provide coverage to employees at the levels previously provided. Individuals who must provide their own insurance because their employers do not offer that benefit can no longer afford premiums to maintain coverage. These increases in costs have resulted in a diminished ability of consumers to afford care, yet many continue to expect care on demand. Health care economics cannot supply health care at a level demanded by the public (Feldstein, 2003; Milstead, 2004).

When there is an imbalance of supply and demand, an outcome may be rationing of health care. No country can afford to provide unlimited amounts of medical services to everyone, and each must decide on a mechanism to ration, or limit access to, health care services. This can happen in two ways; the first is by having the government set limits. In this approach, the cost of services is kept low and people wait for availability. This type of rationing has been used in industrialized countries, such as Great Britain and Canada. Scarce services are kept at a reasonable cost, but they are allocated according to particular criteria, such as age or a waiting list. Even in these countries, those who can pay can access more services. In the United States, only Oregon has suggested such an approach. The Oregon legislature enacted a program to limit access to expensive procedures such as transplants and then increase Medicaid eligibility to a larger number of low-income people. The second rationing approach is to ration by ability to pay. This limits demand for more expensive procedures by offering them only to those who are willing and able to pay out of pocket or who have sufficient health insurance coverage (Feldstein, 2003).

There are important differences between these rationing methods. One is the freedom of the individual to choose the amount and type of health care used and to select who should deliver it. This has been a traditional value of health care consumers in the United States. Under a system of strict government rationing, a patient will not be able to purchase a service unless it has been made available to everyone by the government. Under a method using ability to pay, a consumer can spend as much as he or she can afford. For those who cannot afford it, that service is not an option. To decide on the rationing technique, decisions must be made regarding how much health care will be provided to whom and at what cost.

Paying for Health Care

The United States is the only industrialized nation without a national health policy. Although the specific details of coverage and the availability of certain services vary by country, those governments provide financing for health care (Powell & Wessen, 1999).

In the past, private insurers, for the most part, have paid for U.S. health care. In 1965 the federal government entered into health care financing with the passage of Medicare, followed by Medicaid. These programs have grown and expanded until nearly half of the cost of health care is covered by at least one of them. The dilemma in health care reform is whether the federal programs should continue to expand until there is a national health care payment structure or whether private insurance should continue. The debate about national health care versus private insurance has been vigorous, with significant support on each side of the issue (Feldstein, 2003).

Separate Billing for Nursing Services

Bills submitted to third-party payers and consumers from health care organizations such as hospitals continue to bundle nursing services with flat daily charges, such as the cost of the room and housekeeping. The specific cost of nursing has neither been separated out nor given a dollar value. This has hindered the ability of nurses to receive payment from third-party payers. Many nursing leaders think that for nursing to be a profession, nursing services must be accounted for separately from flat room fees to the health care institution.

Several developments within nursing have provided ways of quantifying nursing care (Abood & Franklin, 2002; Kerr, 2000; Peters, 2000). Some of the better-known projects have resulted in nursing diagnoses that can be used to categorize nursing interventions (NANDA), nursing intervention classification (NIC), and nursing outcome classification (NOC).

COST-CONTAINMENT STRATEGIES

Efforts have been made for many years to control health care costs, yet they continue to rise. Some of the main cost-containment strategies are competition, price controls, alternative insurance delivery systems, managed care, health promotion and illness prevention, alternative care providers, and vertically integrated health service organizations.

Competition

During the 1970s in the United States, regulations were changed to permit competition among the agencies that deliver health care and provide insurance. Currently, there appears to be little reduction in costs that can be attributed to competition. Competition has, however, led to the establishment of walk-in clinics, urgent-care clinics, and alternative health care providers, such as ad-

vanced registered nurse practitioners, which offer additional care choices for clients.

Price Controls

Price controls for health care services have been established in various ways. Freezes on physicians' fees have been imposed at various times for short periods, and many states limit reimbursement to physicians and hospitals for services provided to Medicaid clients. Group self-insurance plans are another means to reduce costs. These plans involve a designated group, such as employees in a large company, a group of companies, or a union, for example. The designated group assumes all or part of the costs of health care for its members. They can often provide coverage at a lower cost than insurance companies because they are exempt from certain taxes and fees.

The passage of the Tax Equity and Fiscal Responsibility Act (TEFRA) in 1982 brought about a dramatic restructuring of health care delivery in the United States. Through this act, the federal government changed the payment method for Medicare from a retrospective system to a **prospective payment system** (PPS). This legislation limits the amount paid to hospitals that are reimbursed by Medicare. Reimbursement is made according to a classification system known as **diagnosis-related groups** (DRGs). The system establishes pretreatment diagnosis billing categories and a payment schedule. Using DRGs, a hospital is paid a predetermined amount for clients with a specific diagnosis. For example, a hospital that admits a client with a diagnosis of myocardial infarction is reimbursed with a specific dollar amount, regardless of the cost of services, the length of stay, or the acuity or complexity of the client's illness. Before the DRG system, hospitals billed retrospectively, that is, after services were rendered. In contrast, prospective payment or billing is determined before the client is ever admitted to the hospital. DRG rates are set in advance of the year during which they apply and are considered fixed unless major, uncontrollable events occur.

This legislation has had a tremendous impact on health care delivery in the United States because hospitals and providers, rather than Medicare or other third-party payers, run the risk of monetary losses. If a hospital's costs exceed the fixed amount, the hospital loses money. Thus, this type of prospective payment system offers financial incentives for withholding unnecessary tests or procedures and avoiding prolonged hospital stays and excessive expenditures.

Notable effects of prospective payment systems include the earlier discharge of clients, a decline in admissions, a rise in the number and type of outpatient services, and an increased focus on the costs of care. One result of the decline in admissions is that most of those clients who are admitted to acute-care hospitals are seriously ill and have complex health care needs. The earlier discharge of clients has led to an expansion of home care services and an increased use of technology and specialists.

To protect clients from DRG abuses, Medicare introduced state **peer review organizations** (PROs). Made up of physicians, nurses, and other health care professionals, PROs are intended to monitor the hospitals and ensure high-quality care under DRGs. PROs have developed screening guidelines that determine whether admissions should occur or procedures should be performed. PROs also review health care records, render payment decisions, and handle related problems, such as admission criteria. Their goal is to improve the quality of services.

The cost-containment strategies have changed trends in health care delivery. These are shown in the accompanying box.

Trends in Health Care Delivery

FROM	TO
Illness emphasis	→ Preventive emphasis
Acute care	→ Preventive, home care
Hospital/institution-based	→ Noninstitution-based (clinic/home)
Fee-for-service (cost-based)	→ Prospective payment and managed care
Physician-directed	→ Diverse decision makers and managed care
If it helps (at all), use it (regardless of cost)	→ Outcomes measurement and cost-effectiveness
Independent decisions (practice variation)	→ Protocols/guidelines (best practice)
Local perspective (practice variation, standards/benchmarking)	→ Global perspective (protocols/guidelines/practice)
Introduce new technologies (regardless of cost)	→ Outcomes measurement and cost-effectiveness
Paper records, medical charts	→ Information systems, computer records

CHANGE IN
Orientation

Illness, crisis	→ Prevention
Specific, specialist	→ Holistic
Quantity of care	→ Quality of care

Location of Service

Inpatient	→ Outpatient, clinic, home

Payment Mode

Retrospective	→ Prospective
Fee-for-service	→ Managed care

Outlook

Just do it	→ Outcomes measurement
Just do it	→ Quality of care; quality of life

Source: From *Contemporary Nursing: Issues, Trends, and Management* (p. 162), by B. Cherry and S. R. Jacob, 1999, St. Louis, MO: Mosby. Used by permission.

Alternative Delivery Systems

With the advent of increased costs, alternative delivery systems were created. Private insurers created new programs, such as the health maintenance organization (HMO) and the preferred provider organization (PPO), as strategies to control costs. Insurers also encouraged outpatient diagnostic testing and surgery, required second opinions for surgery, and implemented a variety of other cost-cutting initiatives.

Health maintenance organizations are group health care agencies that provide basic and supplemental health maintenance and treatment services to voluntary enrollees. The enrollees or their employers prepay a fixed periodic fee that is set without regard to the amount or kind of services provided. To receive federal funds, an HMO must offer physician services, hospital and outpatient services, emergency services, short-term mental health services, treatment and referral for drug and alcohol problems, laboratory and radiological services, and preventive health services. By encouraging preventive and wellness services and by offering ambulatory services, HMOs have attempted to reduce the cost of health insurance to the consumer.

The **preferred provider organization** (PPO) emerged as another alternative health care delivery system. It consists of a group of physicians or a hospital that provides companies with health services at a discounted rate. Hospitals, physicians, and insurance companies are major sponsors of PPOs. Physicians can belong to one or more PPO, and the client chooses a primary care provider among the physicians who belong to a particular PPO.

Physician/hospital organizations (PHOs) are joint ventures between a group of private practice physicians and a hospital. PHOs combine both resources and personnel to provide managed care alternatives and medical services. PHOs work with a variety of insurers to provide services. A typical PHO will include primary care providers and specialists.

Managed Care

Managed care describes a health care system whose goals are to provide cost-effective, quality care that focuses on improved outcomes for groups of clients. In managed care, health care providers and agencies collaborate so as to render the most appropriate, fiscally responsible care possible. Managed care denotes an emphasis on cost controls, customer satisfaction, health promotion, and preventive services. Health maintenance organizations and preferred provider organizations are examples of provider systems committed to managed care.

Hospitals and other health care agencies have adopted many of the principles of managed care. Hospitals have developed strategies to reduce costs and ensure quality outcomes for groups of clients. These strategies have included case management, critical pathways, and patient-focused care. Collaboration among nurses, physicians, and ancillary providers is required to develop and implement health care.

Case management describes a model of integrating health care services for individuals or groups. Various case management models exist that strive to provide cost-effective care and ensure quality outcomes. Generally, case management reflects the shift from sickness to wellness as the health care system changed to funding that favored keeping people healthy. The case manager's intervention helps link people to appropriate resources and evaluates outcomes. The intervention is designed to prevent complications that are costly and may compromise future health status for the individual. Case managers suggest and assist with the initiation of services and link people to community resources. They assist with cost-efficiency by avoiding duplication of services, preventing gaps or delays in service, and facilitating movement through the health care system (Thurkettle & Noji, 2003). Key responsibilities for case managers are shown in the accompanying box.

Key Responsibilities of Case Managers

Assessing clients and their homes and communities

Coordinating and planning client care

Collaborating with other health professionals in the provision of care

Monitoring clients' progress

Evaluating client outcomes

Advocating for clients moving through the services needed

Seeking appropriate resources to fit a client's needs

Serving as a liaison with third-party payers in planning the client's care

Vertically Integrated Health Services Organizations

Before the 1970s, the typical delivery system for medical and surgical care was the single, not-for-profit hospital and its medical staff or small group practices. Very little care was provided in the home. In the current health care environment, new organizations have emerged, with new relationships between hospitals and physicians. The scope of responsibility has widened to wellness, ambulatory care, outpatient surgery, and home health services. Many physicians' practices are owned and managed by this new organization.

Two trends have contributed to this organizational change. The first—and probably the most important—is the change in payment structures, and the other is medical technology. Before the health care reform movement, hospitals and physicians were reimbursed separately on a fee-for-service basis regardless of how high the costs rose, as long as the patient had insurance coverage. Hospitals invested in services and facilities regardless of whether there was duplication in the community.

As insurers became more concerned about the rising costs of health care in the 1970s, hospitals began horizontal integration by forming multihospital systems. Thus, hospitals could band together to offer services within the community rather than duplicate them. The disadvantage was a loss of autonomy; as the system grew larger there was less control of operating budgets and decision making.

As a result of the changes in Medicare's payment under fixed-priced DRGs, the move to vertical integration began. Hospitals were then affected by physicians' hospital practices and began to monitor discharge practices and lengths of stay. It became more cost-effective to discharge some patients to another suitable setting such as a nursing home or the patient's home, and it became advantageous for hospitals to own or contract with agencies, such as home health, providing this type of care. This vertical integration allowed hospitals to reduce inpatient costs and receive additional Medicare revenues.

Advances in medical technology contributed to this move from a traditional hospital to an outpatient setting. Many surgeries, such as cholecystectomies, hernia repairs, and some orthopedic surgeries that had necessitated several days in the hospital at one time can now be done on an outpatient or ambulatory surgery basis. These outpatient services are less costly.

Another stimulus to vertical integration came with provider capitation payments. The move to paying for the full range of health care per person, rather than a per-diem amount for the stay, changed hospitals from profit centers to cost centers. In other words, it became more costly to the hospital to keep people in the hospital than treat them in other less costly settings.

Within the integrated system, there has been a goal to create a "seamless" system of patient care, in which movement from service to service is coordinated and well organized. Such a plan could improve quality of care and outcomes while increasing patient satisfaction. It provides better control of costs by more efficient use of resources. If it is efficient, it can decrease transaction costs and allow greater accountability.

A disadvantage of a vertically integrated organization is that the financial incentives need to be aligned among all the different providers within that organization. Medical groups must be well integrated both philosophically and in decision making regarding care.

HEALTH CARE ECONOMICS

Because health care is an exceedingly expensive entity in contemporary society, many approaches have been developed to finance it and, at the same time, maintain quality.

Billing Methods

There are three main types of billing for health care services: fee-for-service, capitation, and fee-for-diagnosis.

Fee-for-Service

In the fee-for-service method, clients pay the practitioner for each health service they receive. Physicians are not fiscally responsible for whatever they prescribe or for any resulting hospital costs. Ideally, clients choose the service they need and pay for this service. In reality, not all clients are willing or able to choose the service they require and not all health care providers are willing to relinquish their prescriptive power. Therefore, collaboration is required to select mutually acceptable health services in the fee-for-service billing.

Capitation

Under **capitation**, health care providers are paid a fixed dollar amount per person for providing an agreed-upon set of health services to a defined population for a specific period of time. If the costs of providing service are lower than the fixed amount, the provider organization makes a profit. If costs exceed payment, however, then the provider organization takes a financial loss.

HMOs, preferred provider organizations, and physician/hospital organizations discussed earlier are managed-care systems and thus subject to capitation. In other words, payers negotiate health care costs and the providers take both the potential financial risks and benefits.

Fee-for-Diagnosis

Fee-for-diagnosis is a type of prospective payment system (PPS). Agencies are provided with a fixed dollar amount for the care of a client based on the client's main and secondary diagnoses, demographic information (e.g., age and sex), and the usual treatment provided for the health problems. The DRG system is an example of a fee-for-diagnosis system. Because a diagnosis is needed to establish a fee for the health care provider, the fee-for-diagnosis system does not provide incentives for reducing costs by providing preventive care.

Payment Sources in the United States

In the United States, there are three main sources of payment: government health plans, private insurance, and personal payment.

Government Health Plans

The largest share of publicly funded health care expenditures are made by programs administered through the Center for Medicare and Medicaid Services (CMS). These include Medicare, Medicaid, and the State Children's Health Insurance Program (SCHIP).

Medicare was established in 1965 to provide medical care to the elderly, with coverage later added for certain disabled persons and for persons with renal disease. Medicaid was established to provide health care to the poor. In 2000 these programs accounted for about one third of the nation's total health care expenditures and nearly three-quarters of the public health care expenditures. Medicare covers 95% of the elderly, as well as many disabled people who are covered by Social Security.

MEDICARE   Medicare has traditionally consisted of two parts: Part A is known as Hospital Insurance (HI) and Part B is known as Supplemental Medical Insurance (SMI). In 1997 the Balanced Budget Act established Part C known as the Medicare+Choice program, which expanded the options for participation in private health care plans. The HI program is financed primarily through mandatory payroll taxation. The SMI program is financed through premium payments similar to traditional private insurance plans, but it also has contribution from the general fund of the U.S. Treasury. Capitation payment to the Medicare+Choice plans are financed from the HI and SMI trust funds. Fee-for-service is required for charges not covered by Medicare. There are three ways in which the fee-for-service charges can be covered: (1) by out of pocket payment by the beneficiary, (2) by Medi-gap coverage or private insurance for expenses not covered by Parts A and B, and (3) by Medicaid for those who are eligible.

The Medicare Modernization Act of 2003 strengthened the program by adding new prescriptive drug and preventive benefits. Medicare-approved Drug Discount Cards began in 2004 providing savings on prescription drugs through contractual agreements between Medicare and the drug manufacturers. Other new benefits were to be initiated over a three-year period (CMS, 2004).

MEDICAID   Medicaid pays for medical assistance for individuals and families with low income and few resources. It is jointly funded by federal and state governments and provides the largest source of funding for the poorest people in the United States. States have broad discretion in determining eligibility and which groups they will cover. However, states must provide certain required coverage as determined by the federal government. Medicaid operates as a vendor payment program. States pay providers directly on a fee-for-service basis or through prepaid arrangements such as an HMO.

Title XXI of the Social Security Act is known as the State Children's Health Insurance Program (SCHIP). It provides funds for states to expand Medicaid eligibility to include a greater number of children who are uninsured. It began in 1997 and included many children who would not have had coverage otherwise.

Long-term care is an important provision of Medicaid, and utilization of that provision will increase in the near future as the population ages. Medicaid paid for over 40% of cost of care for nursing facilities and home health services in 2000. Medicaid also provides supplemental services to people enrolled in Medicare. Medicaid provides some level of supplemental coverage for nearly 6.5 million Medicare beneficiaries (Hoffman, McFarland, & Curtis, 2002).

Private Insurance

In the United States, numerous commercial health insurance carriers offer a wide range of coverage plans.

Critical Thinking Exercise

Mrs. Helen Whitehead is a 70-year-old widow who recently retired from a job as a checkout clerk for a large supermarket chain. Before her retirement, she had group health insurance coverage through her employer. She no longer has her own coverage; she needs cataract surgery and has just been diagnosed with type II diabetes. She has no savings but she does collect Social Security benefits. Her two children live several hundred miles away from her, and she sees them only about twice a year. She owns her own house and drives her own car. She is an active member of her church which is also the source of her social group.

Discuss how Mrs. Whitehead might benefit from case management.

What options do you think she might have for health care?

There are two types of private health insurance: not-for-profit (e.g., Blue Cross–Blue Shield) and for-profit (e.g., commercial companies such as Metropolitan Life, Travelers, and Aetna). Private health insurance pays either the entire bill or, more often, there are co-payments required of the insured.

With these plans, insurance may be purchased either as an individual plan or as part of a group plan through a person's employer, union, student association, or similar organization. The individual usually pays a monthly premium to obtain this protection. Group plans offer premiums at lower costs. Some employers share the costs of the premiums, and this benefit is often a major item in labor contracts.

Personal Payment

Direct personal payment is money for services not covered by insurance paid by the recipient of care. The percentage of health care costs paid personally by an individual is higher in the United States than that paid by people in England, Germany, or Canada, for example.

The International Perspective

Values are important determinants of health care systems and policies. Most developed countries other than the United States have similar values with regard to health care. Table 18–1 contrasts those values. Two relatively new values are coming to the forefront in

Table 18–1 Comparison of Health Care Values Between the United States and Other Developed Countries

United States	Other Countries
Pluralism and choice	Universality
Individual accountability	Equity
Ambivalence toward government	Acceptance of the role of government
Progress, innovation, and new technology	Skepticism about markets and competition
Volunteerism and communitarianism	Global budgets
Paranoia about monopoly	Rationing
Competition	Technology assessment and innovation control

Source: From *Health Care in the New Millennium: Vision, Values, and Leadership,* (pp. 2–5), by I. Morrison, 2000, San Francisco: Jossey-Bass.

health care worldwide: consumerism and the Internet. The rise of consumerism reflects global education levels and communication; a corollary of this is a widening gap between the rich and the poor. The Internet has opened channels of communication without regard for national boundaries and this feeds consumerism (Morrison, 2000).

One thing that is fairly consistent around the world is that health care is in some level of crisis and countries are considering what would be appropriate health care reform and restructuring. Most countries, regardless of their level of funding for health care, have run out of ways to fund their expenditures through taxation or their existing channels. All are realizing they must contain costs in the future. Further, there is concern is Western European nations, Canada, and Australia about the increased sophistication and resulting expectations of their emerging middle classes.

Each country's health care system is unique, but four categories can be identified for the organization and financing of health care. The first is **socialized medicine**, in which the state owns and controls production. Examples are the United Kingdom, Sweden, and Denmark, where physicians derive virtually all their income from the government and have employment contracts with the state. **Socialized insurance** is a system in which all medically necessary services are covered, including physician care, hospital services, and to some extent prescription drugs. Canada, France, and Australia have this form of health care payment. **Mandatory health insurance** is found in Germany and Japan, where they have large, nonprofit health insurance organizations called "sickness funds." These sickness funds are usually organized around large employers or work-based associations. Government-sponsored programs cover citizens who are not part of a sickness fund. Everyone belongs to one of these two types of plans, thus ensuring universality. **Voluntary insurance** provides no guarantee of universality. The United States and South Africa both provide this kind of coverage. They are the only two developed countries where significant proportions of the population are uninsured (Morrison, 2000). An example of each of these is discussed.

Sweden, the United Kingdom, and Socialized Medicine

SWEDEN Good health and equal access to health care for all are the goals of the Swedish health care system. The fundamental principle is public sector re-

sponsibility for funding and provision of health services for the entire population. It represents the extreme of government financing and delivery of health care. County councils operate almost all the services and levy taxes to finance them. The central government establishes the basic principles for health services. Physicians are contracted and salaried by the county councils.

Patients may choose their health center, family physician, and hospital, but if that choice lies outside their county, a referral may be required. A care guarantee, in force since 1992, has reduced the wait for certain forms of treatment. Primary care services must offer help the same day that the patient contacts them, and there must be a medical consultation within eight days. The Swedish parliament has approved a plan for better coordination of health care implemented in 2001 to 2004. This is to improve access for certain groups such as the elderly and disabled (The Health Care System in Sweden, 2003).

GREAT BRITAIN Britain's National Health Service (NHS) provides remarkably comprehensive service to the entire population. It is tax-financed and free at the point of delivery. Although the quality of care is usually high, the environments are often dreary, and there are often long waits for service. Britain's system of primary health care contributes to the success of the system. A ten-year action plan was published in 2000 to increase funding by 6.3% over the five years to 2004. This plan prioritizes diseases that are the biggest killers and the changes needed to improve health and well-being and deliver modern, fair, and convenient services.

The NHS is funded by the taxpayer, accountable to parliament, and administered by the Department of Health. The overall health policy is set by the Department of Health. The United Kingdom stands out for the absence of income-related differences in access to health care, but waiting time is of great concern to the British public (Commonwealth Fund, 2001; National Health Service, 2004).

Canada, Australia, and Socialized Insurance

CANADA Canada's health care system is primarily publicly financed. Each province funds and administers its own health insurance plan that covers hospital and medical services. The federal government contributes financially on the condition that provinces meet national standards for eligibility and coverage. Most of the resources are in the private sector, and the system is often described as publicly funded and privately delivered. The aim of the Canada Health Act is to ensure that all eligible residents of Canada have reasonable access to medically necessary insured services on a prepaid basis without direct charges at the point of service.

There are five principles of the Canada Health Act: Public administration, Comprehensiveness, Universality, Portability, and Accessibility. The administration and operation of the insurance plan of a province or territory must be a carried out on a nonprofit basis by a public authority. The plans must insure all medically necessary services, and all insured persons are entitled to coverage on uniform terms. Residents moving to another province or territory must continue to be covered during a minimum waiting period imposed by the new province or territory. Reasonable access to medically necessary service must be unimpeded.

When Canadians need health care, they usually go to their family practitioner or local clinic and present their health insurance card. There is no direct payment, no forms filled out, and no deductibles or copayments for insured services. Health care in Canada is financed primarily through provincial and federal personal and corporate income taxes (Health Canada, 2002).

AUSTRALIA   The goal of national health care funding in Australia is to give universal access to health care while allowing choice through private sector involvement in delivery and funding. The major part of the national health care system is called Medicare, and it provides affordable and accessible care to all Australians that is often free of charge at the point of care. The system is financed from general taxation revenue based on a person's taxable income. The Medicare system also provides health care for New Zealand citizens, holders of permanent visas, or who are visitors from countries with which Australia has a health care agreement. The Medicare system consists of two parts: (1) free or subsidized treatment by a general practitioner, medical specialist, dentist or optometrist; and (2) free treatment as public patients in a public hospital. Clients may choose their own general practitioner; however, treatment by a specialist requires referral by a general practitioner.

If a client or client family spends in excess of the government-set amount on health care costs within a given year (A\$302.30 in 2001), the Medicare system will pay 100% of schedule fees for the remainder of that year through the Medicare Safety Net. This entitlement is designed to protect individuals and families from high medical expenses.

Australia's public hospital system is funded jointly by the commonwealth, state, and territory governments and is administered by the state/territory health departments. Medicare does not pay for private accommodation in either a public or private hospital, so individuals who choose to be treated as private patients must pay the difference between the amount Medicare subsidizes and the cost of service. Medicare pays 85% of the schedule fee for private physician services. Private patient services can also be paid for through private insurance (Australia Commonwealth Department of Health and Ageing, 2004).

Germany and Mandatory Health Insurance

Germany was the first country to institute national insurance-based social and health programs by adopting the Health Insurance Act in 1883, the Accident Insurance Law in 1884, and the Old Age and Invalidity Act in 1889 (Powell & Wessen, 1999, p. 49). Germany's health care system is based on private-practice physicians and on community, church, and municipality affiliated hospitals using a large number of nonprofit and for-profit insurers and autonomous sickness funds. An income-adjusted fee pays the cost of the sickness fund; the worker pays half of this fee and the employer pays half. Individuals and their families are obligated to become members of a sickness fund if they fall below certain income levels or are in certain occupations. It is a pluralistic, private system that ensures universal coverage and contains costs. It is based on a principle of *solidarity* that treats all persons as equals who received treatment according to their needs rather than ability to pay. In 1977, the need for more effective cost-containment efforts led to the creation of an advisory group called Concerted Action in Health Care, with the very specific duty of maintaining stability in the contribution rates to the sickness funds by placing expenditure controls on the funds. This required changes in provider-payment methods.

There are concerns today about the loss or compromise of the solidarity principle as German faces the same demographic problems encountered in the United States; that is the aging population with fewer in the workforce to support the program and it's increasing demand for services.

Voluntary Insurance and the United States

The voluntary nature of insurance means that the population has a choice about carrying health insurance. It is provided by private insurance companies most of which are for-profit and individuals pay their own premiums. The voluntary nature means that some segments of the population are not covered. This was the predominant means of insurance prior to the establishment of Medicare and Medicaid, which have increasingly become health care payers since the 1960s.

NURSING ECONOMICS

Few efforts have been made to determine the actual costs of nursing care. Traditionally, the cost of nursing services has been included in the average hospital bill within the general category of "room rate." Often, the number of patients determined the number of nurses needed. However, when the PPS was introduced, it became necessary for hospitals to determine their staffing needs more efficiently. In the early 1960s, a patient classification system (PCS) was developed at Johns Hopkins Hospital that identified the needs for nursing care in quantitative terms. Since that time, various PCSs have been developed that assess the acuity of illness and the corresponding complexity and amount of nursing care required.

Quality care and cost trade-offs in hospitals dominate the literature of the past decade. Both consumers and health care professionals are expressing concerns about diminished quality of care resulting from cost constraints, early discharge, nursing shortages, and the increased use of unlicensed assistive personnel (UAPs). Determining the precise cost of nursing services is a major challenge for nursing. What are the exact costs of high-quality nursing care? How many nursing care hours are required for each DRG? What is the best skill mix—that is, ratio of registered nurses to licensed practical nurses and nursing assistants—on each hospital unit? Since 1983, many studies have been undertaken to determine the actual costs of nursing care and the cost-effectiveness of nursing care. Researchers have investigated such topics as the impact of nurse-physician collaboration; new cost-effective interventions; cost benefits of primary nursing, nurse practitioners, and nurse midwives; cost-effectiveness of home care; and so on. The quality of the nursing care of the future will rely on ongoing research.

Reflect on...

- whether cost-containment programs implemented in your agency have influenced nursing care.
- measures that have been implemented in your agency to relieve nurses of nonnursing tasks.

- the role nurses play in maintaining quality nursing care in your agency.
- what cost-effective care nurses could provide that may substitute for physicians' services in your community.
- who should reimburse the nurse for services.

The Nursing Shortages

Since the 1940s, there have been periods of concern over a national shortage of nurses. The shortages have been cyclic in their occurrence; there have been periods in which the shortage has seemed to be acute, followed by a period of time in which the problem seems to have been resolved, only to have it emerge again. The measure commonly used to indicate a shortage of nurses is the nursing vacancy rate, or the percent of unfilled positions for which an organization is recruiting. When the national nursing vacancy rate is high, commissions and committees study the problem and make recommendations. The federal government has spent billions of dollars in nursing education through the Nurse Training Act that was passed in 1964 (Feldstein, 2003).

In theory, the reason for a nursing shortage is that organizations cannot hire enough nurses at the wage offered. If the demand for nurses exceeds the supply, then organizations will compete to employ them and wages will increase. As the wages increase, nurses who are not employed in nursing or who are working part time either seek employment or increase their work time. As the organizations are able to fill the positions, they no longer need to compete with higher wages until employment falls off and another shortage begins.

In part, this theory explains the cycles, but trends of the past 15 years in health care have added to the complexity of the problem. When length of stay decreased, patients were sent home "sicker and quicker." The acuity level within inpatient settings increased, and care shifted to the home, outpatient settings, and skilled-nursing facilities. Cost-containment companies began hiring nurses to do utilization review and case management. For a period of time, hospitals were downsizing nursing departments as a cost-cutting measure and adding unlicensed assistive personnel. Some nurses experienced disillusionment with health care and left the profession, feeling that they could no longer provide quality care.

Ending the cycle of nursing shortages will require some adjustment to the approaches used by employers and nurses. New opportunities and new roles for nurses may attract more people into the profession. To the extent that RNs are able to perform more highly valued functions, their presence will be more valuable to administrators in health care organizations.

FINANCIAL MANAGEMENT

Profit Versus Not-for-Profit Organizations

Hospitals in the United States have three forms of ownership: public, private for-profit, and private nonprofit (Baker et al., 2000). Federal, state, or local government agencies govern public nonprofit hospitals, which provide care regardless of the client's ability to pay. Private for-profit hospitals are owned by private investors to make profits, and they primarily serve paying clients. They provide limited charitable care. Private not-for-profit hospitals are owned by a voluntary board of trustees to provide care for both paying clients and those who require charitable care.

Health care in the United States has been and continues to be mostly a nonprofit enterprise. The for-profit sector has accounted for about 15% of hospital beds over the past 20 years (Morrison, 2000). For-profit organizations have shareholders who invest money and expect a return on the investment. Not-for-profit organizations operate according to mission statements that usually refer to community service. The not-for-profit organizations are often referred to as the public sector; they receive tax exemptions based on their benefits to the community. The for-profit organizations are often referred to as the private sector and are taxed by the government.

During the health care reform movement of the 1980s, the shift of hospitals and physician groups to the private sector was referred to as the corporatization of health care. The emphasis placed upon profits for shareholders led to the criticism that quality of care was no longer important; rather, the focus was on cost cutting and revenue production.

Increased attention has been paid to the for-profit sector because of its visibility in acquiring struggling hospitals and HMOs and creating corporate chains. The pattern has been for these chains to undergo turmoil as a result of low profits or even losses, with the divesting of struggling organizations and the buyout of other institutions. According to Morrison (2000, p. 64), "It is likely that when the accounting is all done, the net amount of capital brought into health care from shareholders exceeds the amount of capital that has gone out of the system in the form of profits." In other words, the for-profit organizations have not been profitable.

Evidence for Practice

Baker, C. M., Messmer, P. L., Gyurko, C. C., Domagala, S. E., Conly, F. M., Eads, T. S., Harshman, K. S., & Layne, M. K. (2000). Hospital ownership, performance, and outcomes: Assessing the state-of-the-science. *Journal of Nursing Administration*, *30*(5), 227–244.

An analysis of the research literature from 1985 to 1999 was done to achieve three objectives related to hospital ownership, performance, and outcomes: (1) identify research evidence, (2) assess the state of the science in acute-care hospitals, and (3) identify measurable components of performance and outcomes. Examination and synthesis of the published research indicated that hospital ownership has an impact on hospital performance in relation to costs, prices, financial management issues, and personnel issues. For-profit hospitals offer fewer unprofitable services, but regardless of ownership, market share influences the availability of services and pricing. The for-profit hospitals also employ fewer employees and fewer full-time-equivalent employees, and they offer lower salaries, except in competitive markets. Hospital ownership has an impact on type and degree of community benefits. The association with patient outcomes varies with the dimension measured; the evidence is mixed or inconclusive regarding access to care, morbidity, and mortality.

Assessment of the state of the science was determined to be in its infancy. The evidence is described as fragmented. There is a need for better-defined and more consistent outcome measurements for performance and outcomes.

The not-for-profit organizations operate in much the same way as the private sector in that their leaders use the language of business and they pay attention to financial margins. They are also under pressure to show evidence of community benefit, as required by their tax-exempt status. Because much of the cost cutting was generated by changes in health care financing by third-party payers rather than by a profit motive, public institutions have suffered the same impact of tightened financial resources.

Evidence for Practice

Tu, H. T., & Reschovsky, J. D. (2002). Assessments of medical care by enrollees in for-profit and nonprofit health maintenance organizations. *The New England Journal of Medicine, 346*(17), 1288–1293.

This study analyzed the relationship between the profit status of HMOs and the enrollees' assessments of their care. Data from two national surveys were combined to provide information on 13,271 people under the age of 65 years; this included 10,654 adults and 2,617 children. All had employer-sponsored insurance for health care provided by an HMO, but some HMOs were for-profit and some were nonprofit. Health status was self-reported by the enrollees to be excellent, very good, good, fair, or poor. Satisfaction with the primary health care provider was indicated by ratings on a five-point Likert scale using items related to the thoroughness of the examination, how well the doctor listened, how well the doctor explained things, and trust in physicians. Enrollees in the nonprofit plans were more likely to be very satisfied with their overall care than were enrollees in the for-profit plans. Sick enrollees (those who rated their health as fair or poor) were more likely to report unmet needs or delayed care, organizational or administrative barriers to care such as difficulty getting referrals and delays in appointments, and higher out-of-pocket spending for health care. Among the nonprofit HMO enrollees, sick enrollees expressed more trust in doctors to refer when needed and had more trust in their physician to put their medical needs first. Comparison of the assessments of all enrollees in for-profit and nonprofit HMOs showed significant differences among both sick and healthy; nonprofit HMOs were given higher ratings in satisfaction.

Costs and Budgeting

It is extremely important for nurses to understand the business of health care. Financial considerations and accounting drive many management decisions, and familiarity with the basic concepts can empower nurses.

Cost accounting is used by hospitals and other organizations; it is a method of accounting for total costs of the business and tracking and allocating those costs to the specific service. For instance, the cost of providing a service is calculated and then used to determine the charge for the service. In the mid-1980s this was applied to DRGs. This method is used when the organization negotiates capitated rates.

Total costs of care are a sum of fixed costs and variable costs. Fixed costs are those that do not fluctuate with census or volume. Examples are salaries of managers and salaries of the minimum number of nurses needed to staff a unit. Variable costs are a function of census or volume and are over and above the fixed costs. An example is medical supplies for a particular patient. The total costs are used to calculate the cost per unit of service, which in many hospitals is the cost per patient day.

Full costing includes direct and indirect costs. Direct costing compares a department's actual outflow with its inflow from the services it delivers. Indirect costs are necessary but not directly related to delivery of service; examples are administrative salaries or bed linens. Productivity measures also figure in determining costs. These measure how efficiently resources are utilized in providing the service. For nursing, productivity is often measured in hours per patient day and compares actual staffing with projected hours under some patient acuity classification system.

Costing and productivity measures are used to develop a budget for the unit of service. The budget is an educated guess or estimate of the expenses to be encountered in the next year. It operationalizes management functions of planning, ongoing activities, and spending control. There are different budgeting methods that may be used. The simplest method is the flat percentage increase that develops a budget based on year-to-date expenses and multiplies it by the inflation rate. Management by objective supports programs and services that assist the organization to reach its predetermined goals and usually requires cost-benefit analysis. Zero-based budgeting requires analysis of services on three levels: minimum, current, and improvement levels. It requires ranking by priorities.

Marketing concepts are applied to health care to maximize the potential utilization and satisfaction with a service. Four variables are involved in marketing:

1. *Product*—the service to be provided
2. *Place*—the agency where the service is to be provided
3. *Promotion*—advertising and publicity
4. *Price*—the charge for the service

The goals of marketing are to maximize marketplace consumption of a service and to maximize customer satisfaction to create more demand. Marketing of nursing's product or services may emphasize the quality of nursing provided in the organization compared to others. Many public relations campaigns emphasize care that is more family-centered, for example, so that the potential customer will want to receive care at that agency. Some marketing strategies may focus more on one variable than others, but health care marketing tends to focus more on the product or quality of a particular service (Turner, 1999).

Reflect on...

- how your organization values nursing.
- how your organization fits into the vertical integration of health care.
- how nursing can work toward achieving a seamless health care delivery system.
- marketing strategies that could be used to promote nursing.

 EXPLORE MEDIALINK

Questions, critical thinking exercises, essay activities, and other interactive resources for this chapter can be found on the Web site at http://www.prenhall.com/blais. Click on Chapter 18 to select activities for this chapter.

Bookshelf

Armstrong, H., Armstrong, P., & Fegan, C. (1998). *Universal healthcare: What the United States can learn from the Canadian experience.* New York: New Press: Distributed by W. W. Norton.
This book compares the U.S. and Canadian systems and examines the mechanisms of care that are universal, accessible, comprehensive, portable, and publicly administered.

Andrews, C. (1995). *Profit fever: The drive to corporatize health care and how to stop it.* Monroe, ME: Common Courage Press.
The author is an advocate of single-payer health care coverage. From this perspective, the history of health insurance in the United States is provided.

Berwick, D. M. (2003). *Escape fire: Designs for the future of health care.* San Francisco: Jossey-Bass, Inc.
This book comprises 11 speeches delivered by the author at the Institute for Healthcare Improvement's annual forum. He offers hope to health care professionals and explores the need to ensure care based on the best scientific knowledge.

SUMMARY

The demand for controlling the spiraling costs of health care resulted in changes in health care financing. Cost containment became the goal of many changes in the way health care is delivered and paid for. Billing, which was once retrospective payment for services rendered, is now done through capitation or costs allowed for particular diagnoses on a prospective basis. Alternative health care delivery systems have arisen such as Health Maintenance Organizations (HMOs) and Preferred Provider Organizations (PPOs). Managed care has emerged to provide cost-effective care and improved outcomes. Case managers work to integrate health services and guide people through appropriate services in a timely manner and evaluate the outcomes. Vertical integration has occurred as hospitals attempt to make the most of capitation funding by providing a full range of services rather than refer patients out for service.

Billing methods include fee-for-service, capitation, and fee-for-diagnosis. Payment sources can be public or private. As health care reform progresses, controversy regarding universal health care arises. There is little agreement in the United States about who should pay. Third-party payers in the form of insurance companies and the federal government (Medicare and Medicaid) provide the vast majority of financing, with self-pay by consumers accounting for a very small percentage.

Internationally, health care systems provide one of four systems: socialized medicine, socialized insurance, mandatory insurance, and voluntary insurance. The United States is the only developed country without a national health plan and has the largest uninsured segment of population.

Nursing is attempting to meet the challenge of payment for nursing care by developing its business savvy. One of these attempts is the development of ways of documenting the costs of nursing by using outcomes and measurements that allow nursing to be separated from the indirect and direct costs of the health care institution. Hospitals and health care organizations, whether they are for-profit or not-for-profit, are being managed in a business-oriented manner, and nurses need to be familiar with costing, budgeting, and marketing. Changes in health care delivery and financing are challenging the traditional practice of nursing.

The challenges produced by changes in health care economics have provided opportunities for the nursing profession to take a leadership role in shaping the future of health care.

The cycle of nursing shortages over the years has not resulted in the wage gains that could be explained by supply and demand. Trends of cost containment over the past few decades have added complexity to the problem.

REFERENCES

Abood, S., & Franklin, P. (2002). Billing for nursing services. *Nevada Reformation, 11*(2), 12.

About Medicare (Australia). (2001). http://www.hic@gov.au/yourhealth/our_services/am.htm.

Aiken, L. H., Clarke, S. P., & Sloane, D. M. (2000). Hospital restructuring: Does it adversely affect care and outcomes? *Journal of Nursing Administration, 30*(10), 457–465.

American Nurses Association. (1985). *Code for nurses with interpretive statements.* Kansas City, MO: ANA.

American Nurses Association. (1991). *Nursing's agenda for health care reform.* Washington, DC: ANA.

American Nurses Association. (2000). *Achieving access for all Americans: A proposal from the American Nurses Association for Health Coverage 2000.* http://www.nursingworld.org/ readroom/rwjpaper.htm.

American Nurses Association. (2000). *Nursing's values challenged by managed care: Executive summary.* http://www.nursingworld.org/products/nti0198.htm.

Australia Commonwealth Department of Health and Ageing. (June, 2004). *The Australian Health Care System: An Outline.* http://www.health.gov.au/statistics.

Baker, C. M., Messmer, P. L., Gyurko, C. C., Domagala, S. E., Conly, F. M., Eads, T. S., Harshman, K. S., & Layne, M. K. (2000). Hospital ownership, performance, and outcomes: Assessing the state of the science. *Journal of Nursing Administration, 30*(5), 227–245.

Center for Medicare and Medicaid Services. *The facts about upcoming new benefits in Medicare.* Publication # CMS-11054, February 17, 2004.

Cherry, B., & Jacob, S. R. (1999). *Contemporary nursing: Issues, trends, and management.* St. Louis, MO: Mosby.

Commonwealth Fund. (2001). *United Kingdom adults' health care system views and experiences.* Publication No. 554. New York: The Commonwealth Fund.

Day, P., & Klein, R. (1991). The British health care experiment. *Health Affairs, 10*(3), 39–59.

Feldstein, P. J. (2003). *Health policy issues: An economic perspective on health reform* (3rd ed.). Chicago: Health Administration Press.

Haugh, R. (2000). *New directions in managed care: Hospitals and health networks.* http://www.hhnmag.com.

Health Canada. (2002). *Canada's health care system at a glance.* http://www.hc-sc.gc.ca.

Hoffman, E. O., McFarland, C. M., & Curtis, C. A. (2002). *Briefd summaries of Medicare and Medicaid.* Office of the Actuary, Centers for Medicare and Medicaid Services, Department of Health and Human Services. Washington DC.

Immergut, E. (1992). *Health politics: Interests and institutions in Western Europe.* Cambridge, UK: Cambridge University Press.

Kerr, P. (2000). Comparing two nursing outcome reporting initiatives. *Outcomes Management for Nursing Practice, 4*(3), 144.

Mark, B. A., Salyer, J., & Wan, T. T. H. (2000). Market, hospital, and nursing unit characteristics as predictors of nursing unit skill mix: A contextual analysis. *Journal of Nursing Administration, 30*(11), 552–560.

Milstead, J. A. (2004). *Health policy and politics: A nurse's guide* (2nd ed.). Boston, MA: Jones and Bartlett Publishers.

Morrison, I. (2000). *Health care in the new millennium: Vision, values, and leadership.* San Francisco: Jossey-Bass.

National Health Service United Kingdom. (2004). *The National Health Service explained.* http://www.nhs.uk

Peters, R. M. (2000). Using NOC outcome of risk control in prevention, early detection, and control of hypertension. *Outcomes Management for Nursing Practice, 4*(1), 39–45.

Powell, F. D., & Wessen, A. F. (Eds). (1999). *Health care systems in transition: An international perspective.* Thousand Oaks, CA: Sage.

Rambur, B. (1998). Ethics, economics, and the erosion of physician authority: A leadership role for nurses. *Advances in Nursing Science, 20*(4), 62–71.

Sweden, S. E. (2003). *The health care system in Sweden.* http://www.sweden.se/templates/FactSheet__6856.asp.

Thurkettle, M. A., & Noji, A. (2003). Shifting the healthcare paradigm: The case manager's opportunity and responsibility. *Lippincott's Case Management, 8*(4),160–165.

Turner, S. O. (1999). *The nurse's guide to managed care.* Gaithersburg, MD: Aspen.

Providing Care in the Home and Community

Objectives

- Describe the roles of the home health and community health nurse.
- Compare differences in applying the nursing process in the home setting versus the hospital setting.
- Describe characteristics of a healthy community.
- Differentiate between community health nursing and community-based nursing.
- Discuss various settings for community-based nursing practice.
- Apply the nursing process to the community as client.
- Discuss the interrelationship between the home health and community health nurse.

M E D I A L I N K

Additional online resources for this chapter can be found on the companion Web site at http://www.prenhall.com/blais.

In the past decade there has been an increase in the delivery of nursing services in home and community settings. Several factors have contributed to this trend, among them rising health care costs, an aging population, and a growing emphasis on managing chronic illness and stress, preventing illness, and enhancing quality of life. Important concepts related to providing nursing care in the home and community include the following:

- The goals of home and community nursing practice are health promotion, disease prevention, health maintenance, and health restoration.
- Increasing access to preventive health services is a goal of *Healthy People 2010*. This goal can best be achieved by delivering services where people live, work, play, or attend school, in their homes and communities.
- For the home- and community-based nurse, nursing care generally focuses on the individual client and the persons who provide support for that client.
- Community health nursing focuses on local, state, federal, and international health initiatives. For the community health nurse, there are three general types of clients: individuals, families, and groups. Groups may be communities, at-risk aggregates, or persons with similar problems and needs.
- Home health nursing practice and community-based nursing practice differ from nursing in acute-care settings in many ways. For example, home- and community-based nurses assume a higher degree of autonomy and independence as they work with patients/clients who have greater control of their health care decision making.

CHALLENGES AND OPPORTUNITIES

One of the greatest challenges of the 21st century will be for nurses to continue to work within the health care system to provide safe and effective nursing and health care for all, regardless of race, religion, age, gender, sexual orientation, political belief, or other characteristic that serves to marginalize segments of the population. For those with limited access to health care, nurses in the community provide a most important link to health care knowledge and services. As rising health care costs result in decreased hospital lengths of stay, patients are being sent home "quicker and sicker." Nurses will be required to apply the nursing knowledge and skills previously applied primarily in acute-care settings to the care of patients in their homes and other residential settings. Nurses will need to join community leaders in advocating for those who need quality health care. Gottschalk and Baker (2004) describe the challenges as follows:

> If current trends are any indication, the peoples and nations of the 21st century will continue to face many of the same health-related problems that we struggle with today: poverty, hunger, unemployment, homelessness, illiteracy, racism, sexism, ageism, environmental deterioration, militarism, and human rights violations. (p. 6)
>
> Together with others in their communities, [nurses] commit themselves to the attainment of health for all. Their goal is only achieved when the human rights of all, especially women, children, and those most marginalized and vulnerable, are promoted and protected. In other words, community health nurses direct their efforts to the achievement of social justice and equity for all. (p. 3)

The opportunities for addressing these problems will increase. Technology will provide opportunities for instant communication in the most remote areas of the world. New and effective partnerships with communities will be developed. Nurses will have the responsibility to be on the forefront of planning for the nation's health care future.

HOME HEALTH NURSING

Historically, nurses who provided direct services in the home were strong generalists who focused on long-term preventive, educational, remedial, and rehabilitative outcomes. Today, **home health** services center on individualized, episodic care with curative, short-term outcomes. Many home health care nurses are generalists or specialists possessing high-technology skills that were formerly used only in acute-care settings. For example, nurses provide a variety of intravenous therapies in the home setting and monitor clients who are dependent on technologically complex medical equipment, such as ventilators and central lines. These nurses collaborate with physicians and other health care professionals in providing care; usually, third-party payers pay for their services.

Home nursing care reached a peak in 1997 and then slowly declined in the years up to 2000 (National Center for Health Statistics, 2004). The declines occurred in both the number of patients cared for and the number of home health agencies to provide care. In 2000, approximately 1.4 million patients were cared for by care providers from 7200 agencies in the United States. The largest percentage, approximately 70.5% in 2000, of these patients was 65 years of age or older, and, of these, 75.3% were over 75 years of age. The majority of home health care patients are older women (44.2%) rather than men, and white (61.6%) rather than minority.

Several factors contributed to the growth of home health care in the 1980s and early 1990s. These factors include (1) the increase in the older population, who are frequent recipients of home care; (2) third-party payers who favor home care to control costs; (3) the ability of agencies and institutions to successfully deliver high-technology services in the home; and (4) consumers who prefer to receive care in the home rather than an institution (Stulginsky, 1993a, p. 402). In an effort to decrease governmental health care costs related to Medicare and Medicaid reimbursement, clients were encouraged to assume more responsibility for care more quickly as the average length of service decreased to an average of 69 days.

Definitions of Home Health Nursing

The delivery of nursing services in the home has been called by a variety of terms, including home health nursing, home care nursing, and visiting nursing. In 1980 (Warhola, 1980), The Department of Health and Human Services defined home health care as

> ... that component of a continuum of comprehensive health care whereby health services are provided to individuals and families in their place of residence for the purposes of promoting, maintaining or restoring health, or of maximizing the level of independence while minimizing the effects of disability and illness, including terminal illness.

The National Center for Health Statistics (2004) defines home health care as "care provided to individuals and families in their place of residence for promoting, maintaining or restoring health or for minimizing the effects of disability and illness including terminal illness." Allender and Spradley (2005, p. 909) define home health care as "all of the services and products provided to clients in their homes to maintain, restore, or promote their physical, mental, and emotional health." Stanhope and Lancaster (2004, p. 963) add that "home health care cannot simply be defined as 'care at home' but includes an arrangement of disease prevention, health promotion, and episodic illness-related services provided to people in their places of residence." This suggests that home health nursing services are not only provided in private homes, but also in long-term care facilities, residential hospices, residential shel-

ters for abused women and children and the homeless, and adult congregate living facilities (ACLFs). Allender and Spradley (2005, p. 886) further define home health nursing as

> the provision of nursing to acute, chronic, and terminally ill clients of all ages in their homes, while integrating community health nursing principles that focus on the environmental, psychosocial, economic, cultural, and personal health factors affecting the client's and family's health status and well-being.

Today, home health nurses work primarily with ill clients. In 2000, the most frequent diagnosis of clients being cared for in their place of residence was heart disease, followed by diabetes, cerebral vascular disease, COPD, cancer, congestive heart failure, osteoarthritis, fractures, and hypertension (National Center for Health Statistics, 2004). Although home health nurses provide physical care, they must also incorporate their knowledge of social, economic, and environmental influences on health when planning care. The primary focus is on the individual, but the family also must be considered.

Perspectives of Home Health Nursing

Stulginsky (1993a, p. 404) interviewed home health care nurses who identified their practice as "meeting the acute and chronic care needs of patients and their families in the home environment." These nurses maintained that care focuses on the client and that the nurse's role is to advocate for the client despite possible conflict in the opinions and needs of various care providers. Because the home is the family's territory, power and control issues in delivering nursing care differ from those in the institution. For example, entry into a home is granted, not assumed; the nurse must therefore establish trust and rapport with the client and family. Families also may feel more free to question advice, to ignore directions, to do things differently, and to set their own priorities and schedules.

Clark (2003, pp. 498–499) describes six advantages of home health care: convenience, access, information, relationship, cost, and outcomes. Because care is provided in the home, it is convenient and accessible for clients who are immobile or have difficulty with transportation to a clinic, doctor's office, or hospital. The home setting is intimate, enabling nurses to develop a better relationship with the client and the client's family or caregivers. This intimacy fosters familiarity, information sharing, connections, and caring among clients, families, and their nurse. Behaviors are more natural, cultural and spiritual beliefs and practices are more visible, and multigenerational interactions tend to be displayed. Home health care nurses become realistic about what they can remedy and learn how to provide various supports and use creative interventions for what they cannot remedy.

Home health care nurses have also identified issues that negatively affect care in the home. More than any other care providers, these nurses have firsthand knowledge and experience about the burden of caregiving. In the interest of cutting health care costs; policy makers, third-party payers, and medical providers are placing increasingly complex responsibilities on clients' families and significant other(s). Caregiving demands may go on for months or years, placing the caregivers themselves (many of whom are older adults) at risk for physiologic and psychosocial problems. This is especially so for parents who have the responsibility of care for a disabled child or the spouse who has the responsibility of care for a spouse with Alzheimer's disease. This may also be true for adult children, sometimes referred to as the "sandwich generation," who have responsibility for their own children while also providing care for elderly parents. Additionally, nurses enter homes where the living conditions and support systems may be inadequate. When additional support or improved caregiving cannot be obtained for the client, home health care nurses face difficult decisions (Stulginsky, 1993a, p. 406).

Because home health care nurses must function independently in a variety of home settings and situations, employers generally prefer that the nurse be prepared at the baccalaureate level or above. In 1995 ("ANCC approves," 1995), the American Nurses Credentialing Center (ANCC) approved a certification for clinical specialist in home health nursing. This certification requires a baccalaureate degree in nursing, 2000 hours of clinical practice in the previous three years, 30 contact hours of continuing education within the last three years, in addition to licensure as a registered nurse in the United States (ANCC, 2004). Many nurses are choosing to leave the stresses of acute-care nursing to provide more holistic care in the home health setting.

Hospice nursing is often considered a subspecialty of home health nursing because hospice services are frequently delivered to terminally ill clients in their residence. See the box on page 339 for an interview of a hospice nurse.

Evidence for Practice

Flynn, L., & Deatrick, J. A. (2003). Home care nurses' description of important agency attributes. *Journal of Nursing Scholarship, 35*(4), 385–390.
The purpose of this study was to identify attributes of home care agencies that nurses described as important to their professional practice and job satisfaction. Seven focus groups composed of 58 home health care staff nurses were conducted at six home care agencies located in three states in the Mid-Atlantic region of the United States.

Six major categories and eight subcategories of organizational attributes were described by the home care nurses as important to the support of their practice and job satisfaction. The six major categories identified were (1) extensive preceptor-based orientation, (2) an organized and supportive office environment, (3) reasonable working conditions, (4) accessible field security, (5) competent and supportive management, and (6) a patient-centered vision. An organized and supportive office environment included (a) real-time phone support, (b) interdisciplinary coordination, and (c) scheduled time off. Reasonable working conditions included (a) realistic workload, (b) adequate staffing, and (c) scheduled time off. Competent and supportive management included (a) competent nursing supervisors and (b) supportive administrative practices.

The authors stated that the attributes identified in this study of home care nurses were similar to those described by hospital-based nurses in the literature about magnet hospitals. The implications of this study are important for home care agency administrators in planning for an effective work environment for their home health nurses. Additionally, nurses considering working in the home health setting may use these attributes to identify a supportive work environment when interviewing for a position with a home health agency.

Interview – *Hospice Nurse*

Jace Martinson, RN, BSN, MSN

Why did you choose this practice setting? I worked in an intensive care unit in Alaska and found that I was very comfortable and effective in dealing with families before and after their loved one died. I also liked the flexible schedule and autonomy that hospice nursing offers.

What qualities do you think are necessary to be a nurse in this setting? The most important quality is compassion. Additionally, it is important to be truly empathetic and sympathetic but also therapeutic during interactions with families.

What has been your most gratifying moment as a nurse in this setting? Hospice nursing is the only job I ever had in which I entered the client's home as a stranger and two hours later emerged as part of the family. I watched families come together, become prepared, and know what to expect before and after their family member's death.

What encouragement would you give a nurse considering practice in your setting? I would encourage nurses to be well aware of their feelings about death and their own mortality. I would tell them that the job is very satisfying, and that the client and family really do benefit from the service.

The majority of reimbursement payments for home health services are from Medicare. This federally funded insurance covers services for those over age 65 and the disabled. Medicare eligibility criteria for home care services require the need for skilled nursing or physical, occupational, or speech therapy. The client must be homebound and receive restorative care on an intermittent basis. In the past, agencies were reimbursed for each visit. Currently, reimbursement is based on a prospective payment system, similar to acute-care reimbursement. This type of reimbursement has resulted in a decreased number of home visits a client may receive for each diagnosis. Medicare also provides reimbursement for hospice care.

Evidence for Practice

Cramer, L. D., McCorkle, R., Cherlin, E., Johnson-Hurzeler, R., & Bradley, E. H. (2003). Nurses' attitudes and practice related to hospice care. *Journal of Nursing Scholarship, 35*(3), 249–255.

The purpose of this study was to describe characteristics, attitudes, and communications of nurses regarding hospice and caring for terminally ill patients. A questionnaire related to hospice-related training, knowledge and attitudes, demographic and practice characteristics, and personal experience with hospice was administered to 180 randomly selected nurses (174 responded) from six randomly selected community hospitals in Connecticut.

Participants self-rated their knowledge about hospice care as low, with only about 30% of nurses agreeing that they felt well trained to care for terminally ill patients or knowledgeable enough to discuss hospice. A large majority (81.4%) of the nurses thought "it is essential for a dying patient to be told his/her prognosis," 72.2% indicated "that many patients would benefit if hospice care were initiated earlier in the course of their illness," and 81.4% indicated that "hospice care generally meets the needs of the family better than conventional care."

Characteristics of the nurses related to discussion of hospice with terminally ill patients and their families were greater religiousness, having a close family member or friend who had used hospice, and reporting personal satisfaction with hospice caregivers. Results of the study suggest the importance of interventions focused on increasing nurses' knowledge and positive attitudes about hospice might improve nurses' tendency to discuss hospice with terminally ill patients and their families.

Medicaid is the largest source of reimbursement for home care services. This state-funded insurance is provided for medically indigent clients of all ages. Medicaid also provides for clients with chronic conditions needing custodial care. Through Medicaid, many frail, elderly clients can remain in their own homes with the services of a home health aide.

Private insurance, managed-care plans, worker's compensation insurance, and private pay are other methods of home care reimbursement. Free or sliding-scale fees are often provided by home care agencies such as the Visiting Nurse Association (Stackhouse, 1998).

Applying the Nursing Process in the Home

The application of the nursing process is focused on the needs of individual clients and their caregivers. According to the ANCC (2004),

> the framework of home health practice is care management, which includes: the use of the nursing process to assess, diagnose, plan, and evaluate care; performing nursing interventions, including teaching; coordinating and using referrals and resources; providing and monitoring all levels of technical care; collaborating with other disciplines and providers; identifying clinical problems and using research knowledge; supervising ancillary personnel; and advocating for the client's right to self-determination.

ASSESSING   Nurses must assess the health care needs of the client and family in the context of the home and community environment. The home health nurse obtains a health history from the client, reviews documents from the referral agency, examines the client, observes the client and caregiver relationship, and assesses the home and community environment. Parameters of assessment of the home environment include client and caregiver mobility, client ability to perform self-care, the cleanliness of the environment, the availability of caregiver support, safety, food preparation, financial supports, and emotional status of the client and caregiver.

DIAGNOSING   In addition to nursing diagnoses specific to the client's health needs, nursing diagnoses related to the home environment may be identified.

Nursing diagnoses that might be used for clients in the home environment include Deficient Knowledge (specify), Impaired Home Maintenance, Ineffective Coping, and Caregiver Role Strain. In forming nursing diagnoses related to clients in their places of residence, the nurse must consider not only the needs of the client but also the needs of the client's family members or caregivers. The nurse must also consider the characteristics of the home environment, for example, poor lighting or increased clutter in the home environment might yield the nursing diagnosis Risk for Falls.

PLANNING AND INTERVENTION   Planning and intervention, done in collaboration with the client and caregivers, focuses on establishing a realistic plan for home health management, teaching the client and family the techniques of home care, and identifying appropriate resources to assist the client and family in maintaining self-sufficiency.

EVALUATING   Evaluation can be done by the nurse on subsequent home visits by observing the same parameters assessed on the initial home visit. The nurse can also teach caregivers parameters of evaluation so that they can obtain professional intervention if needed.

Differences Between Home Health Nursing and Hospital Nursing

The role of the home care nurse is different from the role of the nurse in acute care. Stackhouse (1998) identified the following major considerations that differentiate home health nursing from hospital nursing:

- The nurse works within the client's environment. The nurse is a guest in the client's home. In the hospital, there is often the feeling that the nurses and doctors own the hospital and the client is a guest.
- The need for clear and complete communication is essential because other health team members are usually not present with the nurse.
- Knowledge of reimbursement systems is essential. Clients must know what services are available, because most people do not pay directly for services.
- The home health nurse works alone. The hospital nurse is surrounded by other colleagues, whereas the home health nurse has only a telephone.
- The nurse in the hospital setting has a large variety of supplies and equipment. The home health nurse often must create or adapt equipment to fit the home.

■ Knowledge of community resources is important. Community resources can often bring a great deal of improvement to the client's quality of life. Home health nurses should have a resource file to share with the client and the client's family.

Reflect on...

■ the differences in professional autonomy between the home health care nurse and the hospital nurse. What are the legal and ethical implications of the independence experienced by the home health care nurse?

■ how the availability of computer technology assists the home health care nurse in providing and documenting better nursing care.

COMMUNITY NURSING

The goal of many public and private efforts is to develop and maintain healthy communities. Characteristics of a healthy community are described in the accompanying box. Nursing, as a caring profession, exists because individuals, families, and groups (and, therefore, communities) are not always healthy or self-sufficient. The focus in community nursing is the community: it is a practice that is comprehensive and continuous, takes place in a wide variety of settings, is directed toward all age-groups, and commands the utilization of all professional nursing roles. Although definitions of community health nursing by the American Nurses Association, the American Public Health Association Public Health Nursing

Section, and the 1990 Task Force on Community Health Nursing Education, Association of Community Health Nursing Educators vary, they all agree that community health nurses focus on nursing service to the population as a whole. Providing care for individuals, families, and groups in the community enhances the health of the community as a whole.

Allender and Spradley (2005, pp. 18–22) describe eight characteristics of community health nursing practice as an area of specialization. Community health nursing:

1. is a field of nursing that has specialized knowledge and skills and focuses on a particular group of people receiving its services
2. combines public health science with nursing science
3. is population focused
4. emphasizes prevention, health promotion, and wellness
5. promotes client responsibility and self-care
6. uses aggregate measurement and analysis
7. uses principles of organizational theory
8. involves interprofessional collaboration

The **community health nurse specialist** is prepared in graduate nursing programs. These programs usually prepare the nurse for leadership and coordinating functions in the community. The many roles of the community health nurse can include care provider, client advocate, consultant, coordinator, manager, educator,

---

Ten Characteristics of a Healthy Community

A healthy community:

• Is one in which members have a high degree of awareness that "we are a community."

• Uses its natural resources wisely while taking steps to conserve them for future generations.

• Openly recognizes the existence of subgroups and welcomes their participation in community affairs.

• Is prepared to meet crises.

• Is a problem-solving community; it identifies, analyzes, and organizes to meet its own needs.

• Possesses open channels of communication that allow information to flow among all subgroups of citizens in all directions.

• Seeks to make each of its systems' resources available to all members of the community.

• Has legitimate and effective ways to settle disputes that arise within the community.

• Encourages maximum citizen participation in decision making.

• Promotes a high level of wellness among all its members.

Source: Adapted from *Community Health Nursing: Concepts and Practice* (6th ed., p. 425), by J. A. Allender and B. W. Spradley, 2005, Philadelphia: Lippincott Williams & Wilkins.

Interview – *Community Health Nurse*

Mary Jorda, ARNP, BSN, MPH

Why did you choose this practice setting? After a year of working in a poor public hospital in Honduras (when I was in the Peace Corps), I noticed that the same patients were returning frequently with the same problems. I began to think that a more effective solution would be to provide education and health promotion in the community.

What qualities do you think are necessary to be a nurse in this setting? Working in the community requires patience, persistence, understanding, and flexibility. The clients set the agenda and priorities; we as health care workers are "guests" in assisting communities to realize their goals in improving health.

What has been your most gratifying moment as a nurse in this setting? While I was working in a refugee camp in Honduras, we transported a young girl who was very ill to a makeshift hospital. She was diagnosed with typhoid fever and started on IV antibiotics. The next morning I found her back in her hut. Her brother reported that "spirits" had entered her body through the IV. I realized that she had been delirious, but her family would not return her to the hospital. I conferred with the family and neighbors and we developed a plan to care for the girl in the camp. I administered antibiotics and bathed her, and her family gave her fluids. Some neighbors prayed; others boiled water. I also provided continuing education in the camp on the transmission of the disease. She survived. It was gratifying to see her well again and to realize the important role the family and community played in recovery.

What encouragement would you give a nurse considering practice in your setting? If you believe in preventing health problems before they arise, then community health nursing is the place to be.

---

collaborator, and researcher. These nursing roles are explored in more detail in Chapters 7 though 12 ∞. See the accompanying interview box for a community health nurse specialist's description of her practice.

Definitions of Community and Community Nursing

To understand community nursing one must first define the word *community* and other terms associated with community nursing. The World Health Organization (1974, p. 7) defined community as "a social group determined by geographic boundaries and/or common values and interests. Its members know and interact with one another. It functions within a particular social structure and exhibits and creates norms, values and social institutions." Allender and Spradley (2005, p. 392) define **community** as "a group of people who have some characteristics in common, are bounded by time, interact with one another, and feel a connection to one another." Groups that constitute a community because of common member interests are often referred to as a *community of interest* (e.g., religious and ethnic groups). A community also can be defined as a *social system* in which the members interact formally or informally and form networks that operate for the benefit of all people in the community. Five functions of the community are described in the box on page 343.

In community health, a community may be viewed as having a common health problem, for example, community populations in which there is a high incidence of infant mortality or communicable disease, such as tuberculosis or HIV infection. These communities may be geographic communities, such as nations, states, or provinces, or cities, or clusters of population within or crossing a geopolitical boundary.

Critical Thinking Exercise

Consider the different roles of the professional nurse as described in Chapters 7 through 12 ∞. Identify how these roles might be operationalized differently in the practice of the home health care nurse and the hospital nurse. What new knowledge does the nurse need to transition from hospital-based nursing to home health nursing?

Five Functions of a Community

1. *Production, distribution, and consumption of goods and services.* These are the means by which the community provides for the economic needs of its members. This function includes not only the supplying of food and clothing but also the provision of water, electricity, police and fire protection, and the disposal of refuse.

2. *Socialization.* Socialization refers to the process of transmitting values, knowledge, culture, and skills to others. Communities usually contain a number of established institutions for socialization: families, places of religious worship, schools, media, voluntary and social organizations, and so on.

3. *Social control.* Social control refers to the way in which order is maintained in a community. Laws are enforced by the police; public health regula-

tions are implemented to protect people from certain diseases. Social control is also exerted through the family, religious organizations, and schools.

4. *Social interparticipation.* Social interparticipation refers to community activities that are designed to meet people's needs for companionship. Families and places of worship have traditionally met this need; however, many public and private organizations also serve this function.

5. *Mutual support.* Mutual support refers to the ability to provide resources at a time of illness or disaster. Although the family is usually relied on to fulfill this function, health and social services may be necessary to augment the family's assistance if help is required over an extended period.

One must also differentiate between community-based nursing and community health nursing. Community-based nursing is defined by Stanhope and Lancaster (2004, p. 14) as the "provision or assurance of personal illness care to individuals and families in the community." In contrast, community health nursing is the provision of strategies or interventions to prevent disease and promote health for populations and communities as a whole." Clark (2003, p. 172) defines community health nursing as "a synthesis of nursing knowledge and practice and the science and practice of public health, implemented via systematic use of the nursing process and other processes, designed to promote health and prevent illness in population groups." The major goal of the community health nurse is to promote health and prevent illness in populations. Zotti, Brown, and Stotts (1996, p. 212) describe the four major assumptions of this philosophy as follows:

- Health is a political and social right. Equity is fundamental and universal coverage is the norm, with care provided according to need.
- The community as a whole, rather than the individual, is the client, and the community determines its greatest priority and resources allocation in health care. Thus the overall public good is promoted, but needs of individuals may go unmet.
- Because conditions in many sectors of communities affect health, multisectoral cooperation is necessary

to promote, maintain, or improve the health of the community.
- The philosophy of primary health care can be applied to any country or community.

The U.S. Department of Health and Human Services has identified *Healthy People 2010* as the prevention agenda for the nation, its citizens, and its communities. This statement of national health objectives is designed to identify significant preventable threats to health and the establishment of goals to reduce these threats. Nurses in the home and community will have increasing responsibilities in assisting individuals, families, and groups in meeting these goals. Discussion of *Healthy People 2010* can be found in Chapter 7 ∞, The Nurse as Health Promoter and Care Provider.

Keller et al. (1998) identified 17 interventions taken by public health nurses on behalf of communities, systems, individuals, or families in an effort to improve or protect their health status. See the box on page 344.

Settings for Community-Based Nursing Practice

Community-based nursing is practiced in diverse settings, including community centers, schools, and the workplace, among others.

Public Health Interventions

- *Surveillance* is the ongoing and systematic collection, analysis, and interpretation of health data for the purpose of planning, implementation, and evaluation.
- *Disease investigation* is the process of gathering and analyzing data regarding threats to the health of populations.
- *Outreach* is the process of locating populations of interest or at risk in order to provide information.
- *Screening* is the process of identifying individuals with unrecognized or asymptomatic health conditions.
- *Case-finding* locates individuals and families with identified risk factors.
- *Referral and follow-up* assist individuals, families, and groups to obtain resources.
- *Case management* is the process of coordinating services for optimal use.
- *Delegated functions* are those direct-care tasks that the RN carries out or delegates under the nurse practice act.

- *Health teaching* is the communication of facts, ideas, and skills in order to change knowledge, behavior, attitudes, values, and practices of others.
- *Counseling* is the engaging of the family, individual, or group at an emotional level in order to establish an interpersonal relationship.
- *Consultation* is interactive problem solving through the community system, family, or individual.
- *Collaboration* is two or more persons working together to achieve a goal.
- *Coalition building* is the process of promoting and developing alliances and linkages with organizations and constituencies to solve problems or provide for a common goal.
- *Community organizing* is the working together of groups to identify and solve common problems.
- *Advocacy* is acting on behalf of oneself or another to plead a cause.
- *Social marketing* uses marketing principles and technology to influence the behaviors, attitudes, knowledge, values, and practices of a population.
- *Policy development* is the placement of issues on a decision maker's agenda.

Source: From "Population-Based Public Health Nursing Interventions: A Model from Practice," by L. O. Keller, S. Stohschein, B. Kia-Hoagberg, and M. Schaffer, 1998, *Public Health Nursing, 115*(3), 207–215.

Community Centers

Community nurses and advanced nurse practitioners practice in a variety of community sites. In community centers, the client is usually a group of individuals with common needs or interests. In recent years, nurse-managed community nursing centers have emerged, where care is provided by center nurses and advanced nurse practitioners. Community nursing centers may be outreach clinics provided by large hospital organizations. They may be based in colleges/universities or schools to provide family health services or health services for students or employees, or they may be freestanding. Advanced nurse practitioners may diagnose and treat common health problems in community nursing centers or refer clients for more complex care by physicians or in acute-care facilities such as hospitals.

Community nurses may provide services through organized community health care programs in various settings in the community. Nursing services may include activities such as health-related education and influenza immunizations for older adults in an adult day-care center, blood pressure screenings and nutritional counseling at a community health fair, stress management group discussion at a local church, or a cardiopulmonary resuscitation (CPR) class in a school. Nurses and advanced nurse practitioners also staff stationary or mobile clinics that provide primary care and health screening services for the medically indigent or disadvantaged. Providing care through community health centers or clinics increases nurse efficiency and decreases nurse travel time. Nurses and advanced nurse practitioners in the community also collaborate with other health and

Interview – *School Nurse*

Nancy Humbert, ARNP, MSN

Why did you choose this practice setting? I chose school health in order to participate in holistic, family-centered, and multidisciplinary nursing practice.

What qualities do you think are necessary to be a nurse in this setting? To function effectively in a school health setting, a nurse must have clinical expertise in public health and pediatrics. The school health nurse must be flexible, patient, creative, and culturally competent.

What has been your most gratifying moment as a nurse in this setting? My most gratifying moment as a school

health nurse was when I helped empower an adolescent to overcome a severe case of bulimia.

What encouragement would you give a nurse considering practice in your setting? I would encourage any nurse to consider the school health practice setting after first developing strong basic nursing skills. School health is by far the most rewarding and challenging setting I've ever encountered. One must love change, challenge, and children.

---

community professionals, such as social workers, nutritionists, or environmental engineers.

Schools

Community schools reflect the greater community of which they are a part. Today, schools are encountering increasingly complex health-related problems in students, including substance abuse and teen pregnancies; dealing with major environmental risks, such as violence and poverty; and accommodating children with significant physical and psychosocial impairments. School nurses are responsible for providing nursing care to the students and staff of the school. They help children who have disabilities or complex medical regimens to stay in school. In their role as health educator, school nurses provide individual health counseling for students and teach health education classes. They consult with teachers regarding student learning and behavioral problems to assess health-related factors.

Allender and Spradley (2005, p. 662)) identify the primary responsibilities of the school nurse as preventing illness and promoting and maintaining the health of the school community, including individuals, families, and groups. The core components of a **school health** program are health services, health education, and a healthy environment. Nursing services are an integral part of the school health program. School nurses provide direct care in school clinics, manage immunization programs, provide health education in classrooms, offer health-related expertise during student conferences, coordinate student health services, pro-

mote safety, and advocate for student health programs at the local and state levels. Many school systems recognize that providing health services is an investment in children's future, and they directly or indirectly support health services at school sites by, for example, maintaining primary care clinics. Nurses who wish to pursue a specialty in school nursing will find a variety of graduate programs that provide advanced degrees leading to certification in this field. See the accompanying interview box, in which a school nurse describes her role.

Faith Communities

Parish nursing is practiced in faith communities, such as churches, synagogues, temples, and other places of worship. Parish nursing has its historical foundations in the religious foundations of nursing starting with the early Roman deaconesses who provided care based on early Christian values and continuing through the Middle Ages, when men and women of faith provided care to those who were in need. Although parish nursing is associated with the Christian faith, the concept of parish nursing is also practiced in Jewish and Muslim faith communities. In contemporary society, parish nursing began in the United States in the late 1960s, when churches used nurses to provide health care to their congregations. Parish nurses are defined by the American Nurses Association (1998, p. 7) as registered nurses "who serve as members of the ministry staff of a faith community to promote health as wholeness of the faith community, its family and individual members, and the community it serves." The International

Evidence for Practice

Kelly, C. S., Morrow, A. L., Shults, J., Nakas, N., Strope, G. L., & Adelman, R. D. (2000). **Outcomes evaluation of a comprehensive intervention program for asthmatic children enrolled in Medicaid.** *Pediatrics, 105*(5), 1029–1035.

The purpose of this study was to evaluate health care and financial outcomes in a population of Medicaid-insured asthmatic children after a comprehensive asthma intervention program. The subjects were eight children 2 to 16 years old with a history of frequent use of emergent health care services for asthma in a pediatric allergy clinic. Children in the intervention group received asthma education and medical treatment in the setting of a tertiary care pediatric allergy clinic. An asthma outreach nurse maintained monthly contact with the families enrolled in the intervention group. Baseline demographics did not differ significantly between the two groups. In the year before the study there were no significant differences between intervention and control children in emergency department visits (mean = 3.5 per patient), hospitalizations (mean = 0.6 per patient), or health care charges (mean = $2969 per patient). During the study year, emergency department visits decreased to a mean of 1.7 per patient in the intervention group and 2.4 in the control group, whereas hospitalizations decreased to a mean of 0.2 per patient in the intervention group and 0.5 in the control group. Asthma health care charges decreased by a mean of $721 per child per year in the intervention group and by a mean of $178 per child per year in the control group.

The conclusion is that a comprehensive asthma intervention program for Medicaid-insured asthmatic children can significantly improve health outcomes while reducing health care costs, decreasing emergency department visits, and decreasing hospitalizations.

Parish Nurse Resource Center (2001) describes the role of the parish nurse as one that balances "knowledge and skill, the sciences, theology, and humanities; service and worship; and nursing care with pastoral care functions." Ryan (1997, p. 4) states the following:

> intent of parish nursing is to create the environment within which the parish nurse, patient, family, and congregation can interact, understand, and care for one another in light of their relationships to God, themselves, each other, the congregation, and the community around them.

Parish nursing is nondenominational and includes nurses of all religious faiths. Parish nurses are found in nations around the world, including Canada, Australia, New Zealand, Russia, and Jamaica. See the interview box on page 347 in which a parish nurse describes her role. More information about the role of the nurse in meeting the spiritual needs of patients and clients can be found in Chapter 22 ⚭, Nursing in a Spiritually Diverse World.

Occupational Health

Occupational health nurses focus on the promotion, prevention, and restoration of health within a safe and healthy work environment. They work in private industry and governmental agencies and have responsibilities not only for providing health care services directly to employees but also for ensuring a safe work environment. The primary functions of the occupational nurse are to provide emergency treatment and promote worker health and safety; however, rapid changes in technology, the health care system, and societal expectations have expanded the nurse's role and made it increasingly complex. Occupational health nurses may now develop and carry out health promotion, health maintenance, and risk-management programs and consult with their employers in reducing health-related costs. They may offer direct care to employees, manage program evaluation, and analyze work-related injuries and illnesses. In companies in which management positions have been reduced, the occupational health nurse may assume expanded responsibilities in job analysis, safety, and benefits management. Specialization in the field is often a requirement for additional responsibilities. Nurses who wish to pursue specialization and certification in occupational health will find a number of graduate programs that offer advanced education in this field. See the interview box on page 347, in which an occupational health nurse describes her practice.

Interview – *Parish Nurse*

Dorothy Guida, RN, PhD

What attracted you to parish nursing? I've always believed the spiritual aspect of nursing is important, and that it is not being adequately addressed in care. By including the spiritual dimension, the nurse provides more complete health care. Believing this promotes the idea that we humans have to be seen in the delicate web and fiber of our context which includes God, nature, others, and self.

What qualities should a parish nurse have? A parish nurse needs experience in all areas of nursing. It is not a job for the new graduate. The parish nurse has to understand the complexities of the needs of the individual and the community. Sometimes the person has no insurance, no family nearby, and is fearful of making an office visit for health care. The parish nurse must have an advanced level of assessment skill to appropriately intervene. I believe that a graduate degree is necessary to provide the breadth and depth of knowledge needed for the job.

What is your most positive experience as a parish nurse? It is helping those who do not know whom to go to for help. For example, a man came to me with some symptoms that he was concerned about. He had no insurance and a low income. He had been to the emergency department of a local hospital, but refused hospitalization for further testing. He described his symptoms to me, and I was concerned for him. I called the Family Life Center for a referral and he was seen fairly quickly. As it turned out, he had five-way cardiac bypass surgery. Now he is on Medicaid, lives in subsidized housing, and works part-time. He obtained charity for payment of his surgery from the Sisters of Mercy of Holy Cross Hospital after appropriate forms were filed.

What advice would you give someone who is interested in being a parish nurse? Practice in medical-surgical nursing or home health to get experience then shadow a parish nurse in her practice to see the day-to-day concerns. There are a variety of things that are addressed. The parish nurse might run support groups or plan educational programs on health-related topics. Sometimes the focus is on the individual and sometimes on the entire congregation. The attitudes and expectations held by the nurse, the pastor, and the parish staff, regarding the parish nurse role, are important. The four functional or service areas of the parish nurse are counseling, teaching, advocacy, and coordinating congregational activities.

Interview – *Occupational Health Nurse*

Ethel Oatman, RN, BSN, MS

Why did you choose this practice setting? I found that I enjoyed working with adults in an ambulatory setting. There is so much to offer in the field of occupational health. The workplace is a natural environment for building a rapport with employees. Even though there is treatment of injuries and illnesses, much more can be done through employee health education, especially in the areas of health promotion and disease and injury prevention.

What qualities do you think are necessary to be a nurse in this setting? It is helpful to have medical-surgical and emergency nursing skills and be able to work independently. To be credible and effective, occupational health nurses must possess skills and knowledge in the areas of workers' compensation, health education, counseling, and human relations. Good verbal and written skills are also required.

What has been your most gratifying moment as a nurse in this setting? The focus of many of our clinics is on prevention and early detection of disease. I was coordinating a skin cancer clinic, and three malignant melanomas were found. All of the melanomas were in the early, treatable stage, so I feel I saved three lives that day.

What encouragement would you give a nurse considering practice in your setting? To stay in business, companies must address health cost containment, usually through managed care. Occupational health nurses have opportunities to assume leadership roles in ensuring high-quality, appropriate health care while remaining a client advocate.

Reflect on...

■ organizations within your community where health care is currently delivered or where health and nursing services could be delivered. What are the advantages to delivering health care in these various settings?

■ whether nursing and health services are better provided to the traditionally underserved (e.g., the poor, older adults, minorities) by providing that care in the community and in the home.

■ which nursing services can be effectively delivered in the home and community. Are there any nursing services that can be delivered only in the hospital? If yes, which services and why? Are there nursing services that are more effectively delivered in the home or community? If yes, which services and why?

APPLYING THE NURSING PROCESS IN THE COMMUNITY

Assessing

In developing an understanding of a community, the nurse uses a systematic approach in identifying community needs, defining problems, and determining community resources. Nurses assess community health by using epidemiologic studies and by using an established community assessment framework or tool.

Epidemiologic Studies

Epidemiology is "the study of the determinants and distribution of health, disease, and injuries in human populations" (Allender & Spradley, 2005, p. 154). Epidemiologic studies provide health professionals with information about the health and illness patterns of a specified population, the people involved, and any causal factors. Most health problems are currently thought to be the result of multiple causes. For example, multiple factors interact to result in illnesses such as coronary heart disease, injuries such as those experienced in motor vehicle accidents, or other health problems, including teenage pregnancy.

Epidemiologists use three types of studies: analytic, descriptive, and experimental. In analytic studies, the epidemiologist uses prospective (forward-looking) and retrospective (backward-looking) and/or experimental studies to test hypotheses about health and illness. A *prospective study* starts with an event and then goes forward in time to look at outcomes such as follow-up studies. For example, a nurse researcher may implement an educational intervention with ninth-grade stu-

dents to prevent teenage pregnancy in a specific high school. The researcher then gathers data about the incidence of pregnancy among those students through their graduation. The researcher can then make judgments about the effectiveness of the educational intervention. In a *retrospective study* the investigator starts with an event, such as an outbreak of food poisoning, and then looks at past records to determine the possible causes.

A *descriptive study* relies primarily on existing data. The epidemiologist describes the people most likely to be affected by a disease, the geographic region in which it will occur, when it will occur, and its overall effect.

An *experimental study* is often conducted to determine the effectiveness of a particular therapeutic modality. Subjects are assigned to one or more groups: a control group and one or more experimental groups. People in the experimental group(s) are, for example, exposed to one or more conditions thought to improve health, to prevent disease, or to influence a person's health status in some manner, such as implementing a specific exercise program. The members of the control group are not exposed to the experimental condition(s). Any subsequent differences in the health patterns between the groups are then attributed to the manipulated factor(s). More information about the research process can be found in Chapter 10 ∞, The Nurse as Research Consumer.

Two types of rates are commonly used when describing health patterns in a population: the incidence rate and the prevalence rate. The **incidence rate** reflects the number of people with a particular health problem or characteristic over a given unit of time, such as a year. The **prevalence rate** describes a situation at a given point in time. For example, if 63 students in a school of 1000 students have chickenpox, the number of students who have the disease is divided by the number of students in the school, resulting in a prevalence rate of 0.063 or 6.3%.

Community Assessment Framework

There are many sources for obtaining data for community assessment (see the box on page 349). Anderson and McFarlane (2004) developed a systems framework for assessing communities. Their community assessment framework is conceptualized by a wheel consisting of an inner core called the community core and a surrounding circle consisting of eight

Sources of Community Assessment Data

- City maps to locate community boundaries, roads, churches, schools, parks, hospitals, and so on.
- State or provincial census data for population composition and characteristics.
- Chamber of commerce for employment statistics, major industries, and primary occupations.
- Municipal, state, or provincial health departments for location of health facilities, occupational health programs, numbers of health professionals, numbers of welfare recipients, and so on.
- City or regional health planning boards for health needs and practices.
- Telephone book for location of social, recreational, and health organizations, committees, and facilities, and individual health care providers.
- Public and university libraries for district social and cultural research reports.
- Health facility administrators for information about employee caseloads, prevalent types of problems, and dominant needs.
- Recreational directors for programs provided and participation levels.
- Police department for incidence of crime, vandalism, domestic violence, and drug addiction.
- Teachers and school nurses for incidence of children's health problems and information on facilities and services to maintain and promote health.
- Local newspapers for community activities related to health and wellness, such as health lectures or health fairs.
- Online computer services that may provide access to public documents related to community health and census data.

community subsystems: Recreation, Physical Environment, Education, Safety and Transportation, Politics and Government, Health and Social Services, Communication, and Economics (see Figure 19–1■).

Assessment of the community core includes an examination of the history of the community, its demographics, and its values and beliefs. In examining the history of the community the nurse might seek to find out if this is an older established community with little population shift or a new community. Is it a community where a large percentage of the population moves in and out in a more transient way? What are the members of the community proud of—its programs for children, for the elderly, for other specific populations?

In assessing the demographics of the community, the observer would collect data about population size, rate of growth, density, and composition; life expectancy; overall health status of individuals the types of people and families living in the community and their age, ethnicity, languages spoken, marital status, and other demographic characteristics that might indicate the health needs of the community. Consider that a specific community might

provide comfort and a home to population groups that are sometimes marginalized by general society, such as homeless communities, gay and lesbian communities, and so on.

The values and beliefs of the community are assessed by noting the numbers and types of houses of faith, including churches, temples, synagogues, mosques, and so on and signs of culture and community heritage, cleanliness, and green spaces. Faith communities are an important component of the community because members of faith communities often draw upon support from spiritual leaders and family and friends of faith during times of crisis. In assessing faith communities, the observer also notes the number and types of programs provided by religious communities to assist members, such as youth recreation programs, meal programs for older adults, health ministry (parish nursing), and other community service programs.

Assessing the community subsystems of physical environment, health and social services, economy, transportation and safety, politics and government, communication, education and recreation, the observer can use the Learning About the Community on

Figure 19–1

The Community Assessment Wheel

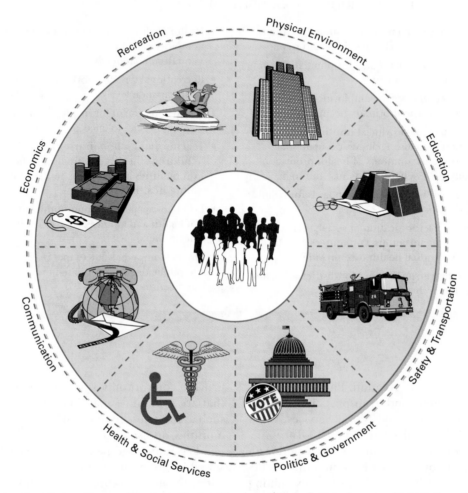

Source: From *Community as Partner: Theory and Practice in Nursing* (4th ed., p. 170), by E. T. Anderson and J. McFarlane, 2004, Philadelphia: Lippincott Williams & Wilkins.

Foot instrument developed by Anderson and McFarlane (2004). See Table 19–1.

Diagnosing

After gathering and analyzing the community assessment data, the nurse identifies community diagnoses that describe the health situation in the community and the etiology, or reason, for health problems that exist. Nursing diagnoses are those actual or potential health problems that the nurse is qualified to treat based on scope of practice and licensure. Community nursing diagnoses focus on a community or an aggregate of people rather than individuals, for example, high infant mortal-

Critical Thinking Exercise

Select a community of interest in your area. Using Anderson and McFarlane's assessment model, Learning About the Community on Foot, assess your community. What are your findings? What are the strengths of the community? What are the weaknesses?

Table 19–1   Learning About the Community on Foot

Subsystem	Observations	Data
Physical Environment	• How does the community look? • What do you note about air quality, flora, housing, zoning, space, green areas, animals, people, human-made structures, natural beauty, water, climate? • Can you find or develop a map of the area? • What is the size of the community (e.g., square miles)?	
Health and Social Services	• Is there evidence of acute or chronic health conditions? • Are there shelters (e.g., homeless shelters for victims of domestic violence, etc.)? • Is there evidence of "traditional" healers (curandero[a]s, botanicas, etc.)? • Are there clinics, hospitals, health care providers' offices, public health services, home health agencies, emergency centers, nursing homes, social service facilities, mental health services, hospices? • If not available within the community, are there resources outside the community accessible to the community's residents?	
Economy	• Does the community appear to be "thriving" or does it appear to have "fallen on hard times"? • Are there stores, places for employment, industries? • Where do people shop? Are there signs that food stamps are used/accepted? • What is the unemployment rate?	
Transportation and Safety	• How do people get around? • What type of private and public transportation is available? • Do you see buses, bicycles, taxis? • Are there sidewalks, bike trails? • Is getting around in the community possible for people with disabilities? • What types of protective services are there (e.g., police, fire, sanitation)? • Are air and water quality monitored? • What are the number and types of crimes committed? Do people feel safe?	
Politics and Government	• Are there signs of political activity (e.g., posters, meetings)? • What party affiliation predominates? • What is the governmental jurisdiction of the community (e.g., elected mayor, city council with single member districts)? • Are people involved in decision making in their local government?	

Table 19–1   Learning About the Community on Foot (Cont.)

Subsystem	Observations	Data
Communication	• Are there "common areas" where people gather?	
	• What newspapers do you see in the stands?	
	• Do people have televisions and radios? What do they watch/listen to?	
	• What are the formal and informal methods of communication?	
Education	• Are there schools in the area?	
	• How do they look?	
	• What is the reputation of the schools?	
	• What are the dropout/graduation rates?	
	• Are extracurricular activities available? Are they used?	
	• Is there a school health service? A school nurse?	
	• Is there a local board of education? How does it function?	
	• Are there libraries in the community?	
	• What are the major educational issues?	
Recreation	• Where do children play? Where do families or adults play?	
	• What are the major forms of recreation? Who participates?	
	• What facilities for recreation do you see?	

Source: Adapted from *Community as Partner: Theory and Practice in Nursing,* (4th ed., pp. 172–173), by E. T. Anderson and J. McFarlane, 2004, Philadelphia: Lippincott Williams & Wilkins.

ity rate, high rate of sexually transmitted diseases (STDs) or HIV/AIDS among teenagers and young adults, or high rate of morbidity/mortality related to motor vehicle accidents (MVAs) among the elderly.

A community nursing diagnosis not only states the problem, it also includes the etiology of the problem and the signs and symptoms or characteristics of the problem. For the examples given above, the etiology statements could be:

- High infant mortality rate related to lack of prenatal care as manifested by
  - insufficient public prenatal clinics
  - inaccessibility of available prenatal clinics
- High rate of STDs and HIV/AIDS related to lack of school-based health education programs, as manifested by
  - insufficient or inaccurate sexual health knowledge of teenagers and young adults in the community

- unavailability of sexual health education programs in community schools
- unavailability of sexual health education programs in community faith communities
- High rate of morbidity/mortality related to motor vehicle accidents among the elderly as manifested by
  - insufficient public transportation resources
  - lack of safe driving education programs for older adults

It is important to note that although the community nursing diagnoses are related to health problems in the community, the data supporting the diagnosis may come from any of the subsystems of the community. In the examples given above, the subsystems of education, transportation and safety, and health and social services are all involved in the problems cited. Therefore, the solutions need to focus on the appropriate subsystems of the community if they are to be successful.

Planning and Implementing

Planning community health may be oriented toward improved crisis management, disease prevention, health maintenance, or health promotion. The responsibility for planning at the community level is usually broadly based. The exact resources and skills of members of the community will often depend on the size of the community. A broadly based planning group is most likely to create a plan that is acceptable to members of the community. Also, people who are involved in planning become educated about the problems, the resources, and the interrelationships within the subsystem relative to health and problems.

When setting priorities, health planners must work with consumers, interest groups, or other involved persons to prioritize health problems. The priority areas established in *Healthy People 2010* can be used as a guide in this stage (USDHHS, 2004). It is important to take into consideration the values and interests of community members, the severity of the problems, and the resources available in order to identify and act on the problems. Because any plan will probably result in change, members of the planning group should be cognizant of and employ planned change theory. (See Chapter 14 ∞, Change Process.)

Establishing goals also requires consumer participation. The goals should reflect a desirable state, for example, to reduce infant mortality by 15%. National statistics and/or *Healthy People 2010* goals may be helpful in keeping goals realistic. Among the many other factors that must be considered are the traditions of people in the community, vested interests, current organizations, and resources, all of which may be barriers to change. An example of a goal for a community would be to reduce the incidence of motor vehicle accidents among older adult drivers.

Outcome criteria or objectives are specific, measurable targets. An example of such an objective is an increase in immunization levels by 20%, to be achieved by September 2006.

Implementing nursing strategies in community health is generally a collaborative action. Nurses are also frequently catalysts and facilitators in implementation of plans.

Evaluating

In community health, evaluation determines whether the planned interventions have led to the achievement of the established goals and objectives; for example, whether the rate of STDs and HIV/AIDS in teenagers and young adults was decreased. Because community health is usually a collaborative process between health providers, including nurses, community leaders, politicians, and consumers, all may be involved in the evaluation process. Often the community health nurse is the agent of evaluation in collecting evaluation data that determines the effectiveness of implemented programs. Evaluation data may include community statistics related to changes in disease incidence rates, mortality and morbidity rates, the costs to provide programs and the availability of required financial and other resources, and citizen program utilization and satisfaction rates. Leaders must decide whether the benefits of a program merit the costs in money, time, and other resources. Based on such evaluation, effective programs may be continued, ineffective programs may be discontinued, existing programs may be modified, or new programs might be implemented.

Reflect on...

■ the responsibility and role of the hospital-based nurse in promoting community health. What activities can you pursue to promote community health in your various communities?

■ the value of collaboration among various health professionals in promoting community health. How can you, as a nurse, influence legislators and policy makers, who have little or no knowledge and experience related to health care, to make wise and effective decisions regarding community health? (See Chapter 12 ∞ for more information about the nurse as a collaborator.)

INTEGRATION OF HOME AND COMMUNITY NURSING

"Home care has been an organized system of care in the United States for more than 100 years. Home care was developed in response to (1) the needs and preferences of families to care for ill and infirm members at home and (2) limitations and costs of institutional care" (Barkauskas, 1990, p. 394). The focus of home nursing has always been on the individual client and his or her family. Community nursing has an equally prestigious history as nurses focused on the health needs of the community as a whole. In many ways the roles and practice settings of the home health care nurse and the community health nurse are separate and distinct. For example, the home health care nurse works exclusively in the client's residence. Community nurses may work in the home but are more frequently found in clinics, immigrant and refugee centers, public health centers, community nursing centers, and other community-based settings for care outside the home or hospital. The home health care nurse is usually providing care to a client who is recovering from illness or injury; the community health nurse is usually working in areas of health promotion and illness prevention.

The home health care nurse is the care provider, teacher, and advocate for the client and the client's family. The nurse may intervene to mobilize the resources of the community or the hospital to meet the client's identified needs, but the focus remains the client and family. The community nurse may work with the individual client and the client's family but often must subjugate the needs of the individual to the needs of the community. For example, a client with a highly communicable disease may have his or her freedom of movement restricted in order to protect the community, or a client diagnosed with an STD may have to defer his or her right of confidentiality for the identification and treatment of the client's contacts.

Some consider home health nursing an aspect of community nursing because the client's residence is within his or her community and the strengths and weaknesses of the community affect the client's ability to stay well or recover from illness in the home. Although the issue of whether home health nursing is community nursing may be debated, it is more important that nurses recognize the wide range of professional opportunities for nurses to influence the health of individuals, and families, in their homes and communities.

Reflect on...

- your thoughts about autonomy in decision making and practice between the hospital nurse, the home care nurse, and the community nurse. Do you believe that one type of nurse has greater autonomy than another, or are there simply differences in the types of independent decision making and practice? What is your level of autonomy in your current area of practice? How does it compare to the autonomy experienced by home health nurses or community nurses?

EXPLORE MEDIALINK

Questions, critical thinking exercises, essay activities, and other interactive resources for this chapter can be found on the Web site at http://www.prenhall.com/blais. Click on Chapter 19 to select activities for this chapter.

Critical Thinking Exercise

Using the American Credentialing Center for Nurses (AACN) guidelines, what academic and experiential qualifications should a nurse have to practice in the home or community setting? What are the differences in knowledge and skill required to become certified as a home care nurse or a community health nurse? How do your nursing experiences prepare you to function in the community as either a home health nurse or a community health nurse?

Bookshelf

Anderson, E. T., & McFarlane, J. (2004). *Community as partner: Theory and practice in nursing* **(4th ed.). Philadelphia: Lippincott Williams & Wilkins.**
This text is an excellent resource for nurses in assessing the health of communities. Using Anderson and McFarlane's guide for assessing communities and the nursing process, the reader is taken through the model using case studies as examples of various types of communities.

Friedman, M., Bowden, V. R., & Jones, E. G. (2003). *Family nursing: Research, theory and practice* **(5th ed.). Upper Saddle River, NJ: Prentice Hall.**
This text focuses on the practice of family nursing using a holistic approach. It describes the theoretical foundations of family nursing in addition to nursing theories in family nursing practice. Various models of family assessment are discussed in detail.

Friedemann, M. (1995). *The framework of systemic organization: A conceptual approach to families and nursing.* **Thousand Oaks, CA: Sage Publications.**
The author provides a theoretical framework for assisting families within the context of their various communities—social, environmental, cultural, and economic. The author guides the reader through the application of family theory to practice and research as the practitioner seeks to advocate and support health and well-being in individuals and families.

SUMMARY

Because of changing demographics and a need for health care cost containment, the focus of health care has shifted from hospital-based illness treatment to community-based health promotion and disease prevention in home and community settings. Although not new nursing practice settings, this shift in focus has created new opportunities for nurses to influence the health of individuals, families, and communities.

Home health care nursing is a rapidly growing industry providing a wide range of nursing services to clients in their places of residence. It may include the administration of physician prescribed treatments, independent nursing interventions, and high-technology therapies, including chemotherapy and dialysis. The home health care nurse assesses the care needs of clients in their home; plans, implements, and supervises that care; teaches clients and their families self-care; and mobilizes the resources of hospitals, physicians, and community agencies in meeting the needs of the clients and their families.

Community health nurses may provide nursing services in the home, but are more frequently found in clinics, schools, and other community-based settings. Community health nurses focus on the health needs of the community as a whole, providing health education, illness prevention through immunization programs, and communicable disease follow-up.

Both home health care nurses and community health nurses are essential components of a health care delivery system that ensures access to quality health care at an affordable cost.

REFERENCES

Allender, J. A., & Spradley, B. W. (2005). *Community health nursing: Promoting and protecting the public health* (6th ed.). Philadelphia: Lippincott Williams & Wilkins.

American Nurses Association. (1992). *A statement on the scope of home health nursing practice.* Washington, DC: ANA.

American Nurses Association. (1998). *Scope and standards of parish nursing practice.* Washington, DC: ANA.

American Nurses Credentialing Center. (2004). *Specialty nursing practice certifications.* Washington, DC: ANA. http://www.nursingwolrd.org/ancc/certifcations/cert/certs/specialty.html. Retrieved July 9, 2004.

ANCC approves new certification program for clinical specialist in home health nursing. (1995, July 4). *Vital signs: The pulse of Florida's health care opportunities* (p. 11).

Anderson, E., & McFarlane, J. (2004). *Community as partner* (4th ed.). Philadelphia: Lippincott Williams & Wilkins.

Barkaukas, V. H. (1990). Home health care: Responding to need, growth, and cost containment. In N. L. Chaska (Ed.), *The nursing profession: Turning points* St. Louis: Mosby.

Clark, M. J. (2003). *Nursing in the community* (4th ed.). Norwalk, CT: Appleton & Lange.

Clemen-Stone, S., McGuire, S. L., & Eigsti, D. G. (1998). *Comprehensive community health nursing: Family, aggregate, and community practice* (5th ed.). St. Louis: Mosby.

Cramer, L. D., McCorkle, R., Cherlin, E., Johnson-Hurzeler, R., & Bradley, E. H. (2003). Nurses' attitudes and practice related to hospice care. *Journal of Nursing Scholarship, 335*(3), 249–255.

Flynn, L., & Deatrick, J. A. (2003). Home care nurses' descriptions of important agency attributes. *Journal of Nursing Scholarship, 35*(4), 385–390.

Giese, D. J. (2004). Community-oriented nurse in home health and hospice. In M. Stanhope & J. Lancaster, *Community & public health nursing* (6th ed.). St. Louis: Mosby.

Gottschalk, J., & Baker, S. S. (2004). Primary health care. In E. Anderson & J. McFarlane, *Community as partner? Theory and practice in nursing* (4th ed.). Philadelphia: Lippincott Williams & Wilkins.

International Parish Nurse Resource Center. (2001). *What is parish nursing?* http://www.advocatehealth.com/about/faith/parishn/index.

Keller, L. O., Stohschein, S., Kia-Hoagberg, B., & Schaffer, M. (1998). Population-based public health nursing interventions: A model from practice. *Public Health Nursing, 115*(3), 207–215.

Kelly, C. S., Morrow, A. L., Shults, J., Nakas, N., Strope, G. L., & Adelman, R. D. (2000). Outcomes evaluation of a comprehensive intervention program for asthmatic children enrolled in Medicaid. *Pediatrics, 105*(5), 1029–1035.

National Association of Home Care. (2001). *Basic statistics about home care.* http://www.nahc.org/consumer/hcstats.html. Retrieved July 8, 2004.

National Center for Health Statistics. (2004). *Home health care.* Washington, DC: USDHHS. http://www.cdc.gov/nchs/fastats/homehealthcare.htm. Retrieved July 5, 2004.

National Center for Health Statistics. (2004). *Hospice care.* Washington, DC: USDHHS. http://www.cdc.gov/nchs/fastats/hospicecare.htm. Retrieved July 5, 2004.

National Hospice and Palliative Care Organization. (2004). *Hospice and palliative care.* http://www.nhpco.org. Retrieved July 8, 2004.

Ryan, J. (1997). Assuring the future quality of parish nursing practice. *Perspectives in Parish Nursing Practice, 5*(3), 4.

Stackhouse, J. (1998). *Into the community.* Philadelphia: Lippincott.

Stanhope, M., & Lancaster, J. (2004). *Community & public health nursing* (6th ed.). St. Louis: Mosby.

Stulginsky, M. M. (1993a, October). Nurses' home health experience. Part 1: The practice setting. *Nursing & Health Care, 14*(8), 402–407.

Stulginsky, M. M. (1993b, November). Nurses' home health experience. Part 2: The unique demands of home visits. *Nursing & Health Care, 14*(9), 476–485.

U.S. Department of Health and Human Services. (2004). *Healthy people 2010 national health promotion and disease prevention objectives.* http://www.helth.gov/healthypeople. Retrieved July 5, 2004.

Warhola, C. (1980, August). *Planning for home health services: A resource handbook.* (Pub No. HRA 80–14017). Washington, DC: USDHHS, Public Health Service.

World Health Organization. (1974). *Community health nursing: Report of a WHO expert committee.* Tech Rep Series No. 558. Geneva: WHO.

Zotti, M., Brown, P., & Stotts, C. (1996). Community-based nursing versus community health nursing. What does it all mean? *Nursing Outlook, 44*(5), 211–217.

Nursing in a Culture of Violence

Objectives

- Define domestic violence and abuse.

- Recognize the incidence of violence within the family, in the community, and in the workplace.

- Discuss theoretical perspectives of violence.

- Identify essential aspects of assessing the effects of violence and abuse.

- Explain the nurse's role in assisting victims of abuse and violence.

- Discuss methods of violence prevention.

- Identify risks to the public health from violent events such as terrorism.

M E D I A L I N K

Additional resources for this chapter can be found on the companion Web site at http://www.prenhall.com/blais.

Violence and abusive behavior have become major health problems in the United States, and they are the source of injury and both physical and mental morbidity in people of all ages. The context of the violence and abuse may be the family, the community, or the workplace.

- In 2001, 1300 children died from maltreatment; 35% was from neglect and 26% was from physical abuse (National Center for Injury Prevention and Control, 2004a).
- In 2002, more than 877,700 young people ages 10 to 24 years were injured from violent acts. Approximately

1 in 13 required hospitalization (National Center for Injury Prevention and Control, 2004b).

■ The costs of intimate partner rape, assault, and stalking exceed $5.8 billion each year, and nearly $4.1 billion is for direct medical and mental health services (National Center for Injury Prevention and Control, 2003).

■ Seventy-one percent of public elementary and secondary schools experience at least one violent incident during the school year (National Center for Educational Statistics, 2004).

■ Violence in the workplace is a serious safety and health issue. There were 639 homicides in the workplace in 2001 (FBI, 2004)

■ Elder abuse in domestic settings affects hundreds of thousands of elderly across the United States; the problem is likely underreported, and the reported incidents may be only the tip of the iceberg (National Center on Elder Abuse, 2004).

CHALLENGES AND OPPORTUNITIES

The high incidence of violence in society affects large segments of the population, with direct impact on health care. Nurses are challenged in their practice to identify and intervene when providing care for a victim of violence. Because the victims often attempt to hide the fact that they have been attacked, detection requires high levels of skill in communication and assessment on the part of the nurse. Terrorist events and weapons of mass destruction have created new challenges to the public health system. New ways of treating and preventing large-scale injury and disease are needed.

In meeting the challenge of providing care for victims of violence, the nurse has an opportunity to have a positive impact on client outcomes. Nurses are strategically placed to have a role in primary and secondary prevention programs. The focus on the community that is embraced by professional organizations, such as the American Nurses Association (ANA) Agenda for Health Care Reform, places nurses in roles and settings that enable them to have influence on reducing the effects of violence within the community and within families. New systems are being created to meet public health challenges for large-scale injury and disease, and nurses will be involved in these new programs.

FAMILY VIOLENCE AND ABUSE

Traditionally the term *domestic abuse* has been thought of as violence against a woman by a spouse or boyfriend. More recently, the term has expanded to include other forms of violence, such as child abuse, elder abuse, abuse of male partners, and violence between same-sex partners. The Centers for Disease Con-

trol now uses the term **intimate partner violence**, which is defined as "the intentional emotional and/or physical abuse by a spouse, ex-spouse, boyfriend/girlfriend, ex-boyfriend/ex-girlfriend, or date" (CDC, 2000).

Domestic Violence

Family violence includes intimate partner abuse, child abuse, and elder abuse, ranging from verbal abuse to light slaps to severe beatings to homicide. It occurs in all strata of society; it crosses all racial, religious, ethnic, socioeconomic, and educational boundaries, and it is not confined to any particular age-group or occupation. It is a myth that domestic violence occurs only in poor minority families.

Emotional abuse is equally damaging. Words can hit as hard as a fist, and the damage to self-esteem can last a lifetime. Emotional abuse involves one person shaming, embarrassing, ridiculing, or insulting a loved one. It may include the destruction of personal property or the killing of pets in an effort to frighten or control the victim. Emotional abuse may also include statements that are devastating to the victim's self-esteem, such as, "You can't do anything right," "You're ugly and stupid—no one else would want you," "I wish you had never been born" (Fontaine, 1996, p. 565).

Abusive individuals come from all walks of life but have the following traits or characteristics in common:

■ Overpossessiveness: viewing family members in terms of ownership and property
■ Excessive jealousy
■ Desire to control and dominate
■ Poor control of impulses
■ Low tolerance for frustration
■ Belief that physical measures are necessary to control children
■ Dependence on an elder for financial support and accommodation
■ Drug or alcohol abuse
■ History of poor mental health or a personality disorder
■ History of abuse as a child by own parents

Intimate Partner Abuse

Most intimate partner abuse is perpetrated by men against women; however, abuse is also perpetrated by women against men and between partners of the same gender. Women are more vulnerable, generally speaking, to this violence because of their disadvantage in size and strength and their social and economic dependence on men. However, men who are victimized in this way have fewer resources available, such as 24-hour toll-free-assistance numbers or shelters. Abused men may be less likely to seek help because of the stigma.

Societal acceptance regarding violence against women by husbands has existed historically; it was considered a private domestic matter. Before 1700, laws allowed a husband to chastise his wife with any reasonable instrument, such as a rod not thicker than the husband's thumb (the origin of the phrase "rule of thumb") (Henderson, 1992, p. 27). Today, there are cultures that have a greater acceptance of abuse than other cultures and may view women and children as possessions. This may exist within a larger culture that does not condone such action.

Abuse can be categorized as physical abuse, sexual abuse, psychosocial abuse, and property violence. *Physical abuse* involves any physical harm or nonconsensual touching. It may involve pushing and shoving, dragging or pulling; kicking, hitting, or beating with fists or objects; locking a person out of the home or in a room or closet or abandoning him or her in a dangerous place; or biting, choking, or physically restraining; or threatening with a weapon. *Sexual abuse* involves any forced or nonconsensual sex. It includes sexually criticizing the person, hurting during sex, and/or treating that person as property or a sex object. *Psychosocial abuse* can involve threats of harm, abuse of pets, constant criticism and downgrading in front of others, insulting family or friends, keeping the person from talking to or seeing friends and family, and threats to kidnap the children. It may involve keeping the person from working or going to school, censoring mail, taking away car keys or money, accusations of having affairs, or forbidding use of the telephone. *Property violence* is threatened or actual destruction of material possessions.

It is especially difficult for many victims to leave an abusive relationship. Women who do leave an abusive relationship attempt an average of three to five separations before finally ending the relationship. Some women are threatened with loss of children or with death if they do not return home. Social and cultural beliefs also play a role. Women have been socialized to be self-sacrificing for the good of others and feel responsible for keeping the family together at almost any cost. Cultural beliefs about loyalty and duty may reinforce the role of victim. In addition, many women are financially dependent on their abusive partners; if they have outside employment, they are unlikely to earn as much as their male counterparts. If there are children, the woman may desperately need child support, and many fathers do not honor this obligation and default on the payments. The burdens of child care have traditionally fallen entirely on the mother. Thus, lack of affordable and adequate child care facilities has become a major problem for the single mother seeking employment.

Many people believe that abused spouses can end the violence by divorcing their abuser or that the victim can learn to stop doing those things that provoke violence. These beliefs are myths and not supported by facts. In many cases, the separation process brings on an increased level of harassment and violence, including homicide. In a battering relationship, moreover, the abuser needs no provocation to become violent. Violence is the abuser's pattern of behavior, and the victim cannot learn how to control it. Even so, many victims blame themselves for the abuse, feeling guilty—even responsible—for doing or saying something that triggers the abuser's behavior. They then suffer a loss of self-esteem. Friends, family, and service providers reinforce this attitude by laying the blame and the need to change on the shoulders of the victim. Many people who do try to disclose their situation are met with disbelief or denial; this discourages them from persevering.

Evidence for Practice

Yarn, M. (2000). Seen but not heard: Battered women's perceptions of the ED experience. *Journal of Emergency Nursing, 26*(5), 464–470.

This qualitative study described battered women's perceptions of their experience in the emergency department. A phenomenological approach was used to interview women recruited from shelters for battered women. Participants in the study had been treated at a hospital emergency department for abuse-related injuries within the past 12 months. In-depth interviews and a demographic data sheet were used to collect the data. Data analysis used Colaizzi's procedural steps.

Several categories emerged from the data. Feelings experienced during the ED visit were fear of their partner, concern for the children, and loneliness. The women's perceptions were that nurses in the ED do not understand abuse. They were satisfied with the treatment of the injuries but dissatisfied with how the issue of abuse was managed. They indicated that they had difficulty disclosing the abuse due to fear, embarrassment, and a lack of resources. They wanted health care professionals to be compassionate, provide referrals, and offer options.

Effects of Domestic Violence on Children

Children experience domestic violence as victims and as witnesses, affecting not only their physical health and safety but also their psychological adjustment, social relations, and academic achievement. The experience affects their perception of the world, self-concept, ideas about the purpose of life, future expectations, and moral development (Margolin & Gordis, 2000). Domestic violence violates a child's safe haven, and the immediate reaction is likely to be helplessness, fear, anger, and high arousal, which can disrupt the child's efforts in age-appropriate academic and social pursuits.

Children of any age, race, religion, or socioeconomic status can be victims of abuse and neglect. Perpetrators may be parents, siblings, a boyfriend or girlfriend, or a baby-sitter, and the form of the abuse may be physical battering, physical neglect, sexual abuse, or emotional abuse and neglect. Laws mandate the reporting of suspected child abuse to child-protection authorities, and these laws also protect health care professionals from any liability that might result from their reporting, in good faith, suspected cases of child maltreatment.

Physical abuse is nonaccidental injury of a child and is relatively easy to recognize and treat. The most common types of physical abuse are burns, bruises, fractures, abdominal injuries, and head or spinal injuries. The location and pattern of injuries help determine the likelihood of abuse. For example, accidental scalds usually occur on the front of the body; scald burns on the back and feet are suspicious. Bruises over bony surfaces such as the shin, forehead, knees, forearms, and chin are common occurrences among active children; bruises on the cheek, abdomen, back, buttocks, and thighs raise suspicion of abuse.

Whiplash-shaking can lead to severe injury in infants. Cerebral damage, neurological defects, blindness, and mental retardation can result. These findings are often seen without external evidence of head injury. Nurses should suspect **shaken baby syndrome** (SBS) in infants less than one year of age who present with apnea, seizures, lethargy or drowsiness, bradycardia, respiratory difficulty, coma, or death. Subdural and retinal hemorrhages accompanied by the absence of external signs of trauma are hallmarks of the syndrome.

Another common, but often unrecognized, form of family violence occurs between siblings (Fontaine, 1996, p. 522). Many people assume that it is natural, and even appropriate, for children to use physical force with one another: "It is a good chance for him to learn how to defend himself," "She had a right to hit him; he was teasing her," or "Kids will be kids." These attitudes teach children that physical force is an appropriate method of resolving conflicts. Sibling violence is highest in the early years and decreases with age. In all age-groups, girls are less violent toward their siblings than are boys.

Physical neglect is failure to meet the basic needs of children by those persons responsible for doing so. Basic needs include adequate nourishment, clothing, housing, supervision, and medical care. Nurses must exercise caution, however, "not to define as willful neglect a case in which an impoverished or uneducated family is providing . . . the best care possible within their means" (Srnec, 1991, p. 476).

Child sexual abuse is the occurrence of any sexual activity between an adult and child. It includes either *assaultive abuse*, which produces physical injury and severe emotional trauma, or *nonassaultive abuse*, which produces minimal or no physical trauma. Nonassaultive abuse may not involve physical contact but may involve visual acts and is often chronic and severely disruptive of the child's sexual development. Children who have been sexually abused may demonstrate the following clinical signs: perineal rashes, genital-rectal irritation or tissue trauma, frequent urinary tract infections, evidence of vaginal or anal penetration by a foreign body, presence of sexually transmitted disease, and an unusually mature knowledge of sexual terminology and slang. Some children may become involved in promiscuous sexual activities and juvenile prostitution or pornography. Because child sexual abuse often involves the parent of the child, this form of abuse is the least reported.

Emotional abuse and neglect is failure to provide an environment in which the child can thrive, learn, and develop. Obviously, this type of abuse is more difficult to identify and manage than physical abuse.

Abused children manifest various characteristics (see the box on page 361). Childhood abuse may have far-reaching consequences for the victim's health. Empirical data link child maltreatment and exposure to domestic violence with numerous outcomes, including aggression and violent behavior problems with peers, delinquency, depression, delayed cognitive functioning, poor academic performance, and symptoms of post–traumatic stress disorder (Margolin & Gordis, 2000).

Behavioral Characteristics of Abused Children

The child may

- Be unusually aggressive, withdrawn, overly compliant, or attention seeking.
- Appear afraid of a parent or wary of physical contact with an adult.
- Be inappropriately clothed during winter.
- Manifest developmental delay and failure to thrive.
- Express violence toward pets.

- Run away from home.
- Demonstrate changes in school performance.
- Be habitually late for school or avoid spending time at home by arriving early and staying late.
- Verbalize fault for injuries: "I deserved it."
- Attempt suicide or abuse alcohol or drugs.

Elder Abuse

Older adults who can no longer live independently may be vulnerable to mistreatment in the forms of physical abuse, psychologic or emotional abuse, sexual abuse, financial manipulation, or neglect. The most likely perpetrators are persons in continual contact with the dependent elder and could be family or nonfamily caregivers such as spouses, children, or professional caregivers (Marshall, Benton, & Brazier, 2000). Federal definitions of elder abuse, neglect, and exploitation first appeared in the Amendments to the Older Americans Act in 1987 and appeared as guidelines for identifying problems, not for law-enforcement purposes (National Center on Elder Abuse, 2000). Currently, elder abuse is defined by state laws, and definitions vary somewhat by state.

According to the National Center on Elder Abuse (2000), there are three categories of elder abuse: (1) domestic elder abuse, (2) institutional elder abuse, and (3) self-neglect. *Domestic abuse* refers to any of several forms of maltreatment of an older person by someone who has a special relationship with the elder. *Institutional abuse* refers to abuse occurring in residential facilities such as nursing homes. *Self-neglect* is characterized as the behavior of the elderly person that threatens health and safety; it is usually a failure to provide sufficiently for himself or herself.

The types of abuse that can occur are physical abuse, which includes not only striking, but also inappropriate use of drugs, physical restraints, and force-feeding. Sexual abuse is nonconsensual sexual contact of any kind, even if the elder is not capable of giving consent. Emotional or psychological abuse is defined as the infliction of anguish, pain, or distress through verbal or nonverbal acts. Neglect is the refusal or failure to fulfill any part of a person's obligations or duties to an elder, such as providing medication or food. Abandonment is the desertion by an individual who has assumed responsibility for providing care for the elder. Financial exploitation is the illegal or improper use of an elder's funds, property, or assets, such as cashing checks or forging the signature, or improper use of a power of attorney.

Elder abuse is complex, but some of the reasons researchers have found to be associated with it are caregiver stress, impairment of the dependent elder, continuation of a cycle of violence (because the tendency for violent responses is perpetuated in some families), and personal problems of the abusers. Typically, the abusers are adult children. The incidence is probably underreported because of the dependent status of the abused and their embarrassment at disclosing abuse or fear of retribution (Beers & Berkow, 2000). The box on page 362 describes clinical situations suggestive of elder abuse. Although the incidence is difficult to determine, it is estimated that there are about 1 million known cases annually in the United States and that reported numbers in Canada and Western Europe are comparable (Beers & Berkow 2000; Marshall et al., 2000).

Reflect on...

- how a nurse's previous abusive relationships might affect his or her practice with victims of domestic violence.
- the available resources for victims of abuse in your area of practice. What additional resources might be needed?

Clinical Situations Suggestive of Elder Abuse

- When there is a delay between the injury or illness and the seeking of medical attention
- When the accounts of the patient and caregiver do not agree
- When the severity of the injury does not fit the explanation given by the caregiver
- When the explanation of the patient or caregiver is implausible or vague
- When visits to the emergency department for chronic disease exacerbations are frequent despite an appropriate care plan and adequate resources
- When a functionally impaired patient presents to the physician without a designated caregiver in attendance
- When laboratory findings are inconsistent with the history
- When the caregiver is reluctant to accept home health care (e.g., a visiting nurse) or to leave the elderly person alone with a health care practitioner

Source: From *The Merck Manual of Geriatrics* (3rd ed., p.152), by M. H. Beers and R. Berkow (Eds.), 2000, Whitehouse Station, NJ: Merck Research Laboratories. Used by permission.

Evidence for Practice

Early, M. R., & Williams, R. A. (2002). Emergency nurses' experience with violence: Does it affect nursing care with battered women? *Journal of Emergency Nursing, 28*(3), 199–204.

One hundred and ninety-five emergency nurses were surveyed on the personal experiences with violence involving patients or intimate partners. They then responded to two vignettes of women-battering scenarios using a Nursing Care Checklist consisting of 27 nursing actions that might be indicated for partner battering. Seventy percent of the nurses surveyed had been hit by a patient and 40% had been hit by a partner. Further, 19% reported having used force against their intimate partner. Only about 20% reported no experience with patient or partner assault. The experience of being a victim of violence did not make a difference in the nursing care actions selected by the nurses in response to the vignettes. What was most startling was the high incidence of being a victim of violence in this sample of nurses. Findings point to the need to increase safety for nurses in the workplace and provide employee assistance to help nurses confront violence at home.

Violence in the Community

Violence in the community has ripple effects. People who are not directly victimized may observe violent acts or at the least may hear about them repeatedly from the news media. Data suggest that in inner-city neighborhoods, one third or more of children have been directly victimized, and almost all children have been exposed to community violence (Margolin & Gordis, 2000). Children are particularly vulnerable because violence can result in a disruption of the normal developmental trajectory. Anxiety, depression, and post–traumatic stress syndrome symptoms are results that can disrupt the child's developing socialization, social interactions, and concentration in school. In Western culture, the home and the neighborhood are considered safe havens for children, but they lose those protective and comforting qualities in the aftermath of violence in the community. Exposure to community violence has been linked to the development of aggressive and antisocial behavior on the part of the child (Miller et al., 1999).

Although exposure to violence clearly puts children at risk for developing psychological problems, these negative outcomes are not inevitable. It is important for nurses to identify those factors that mediate or moderate the effects and use them to help children who experience violence in the community. Mediating factors identified in research fall into three categories: (1) child characteristics; (2) factors related to the frequency, severity, and chronicity of the violence; and (3) quality of family and social relations, along with the level of disruption and chaos in the child's life (Hughes, 1997).

The elderly are particularly vulnerable to violence in the community. They are often easy victims of crimes such as mugging, theft, and robbery. In addition, the threat of violence in the community may keep them from leaving the perceived safety of their homes to go out alone. This contributes to isolation, loneliness, fear, and depression.

The causes of violence have been investigated extensively by many disciplines in the social sciences. According to a review by Gilligan (2000), the experience of shame and humiliation is at the root of violent behavior, along with a lack of guilt or remorse. When individuals experience shame and humiliation without the ability to feel guilt or remorse, they may be prone to violence as a way of striking out without self-control. Worldwide, the most powerful predictor of the murder rate is the size of the gap between the income of the rich and the poor. The primary prevention suggested is to ensure that people have access to the means by which they can achieve feelings of self-worth, such as education and employment and equitable levels of income, wealth, and power.

Nurses need to be involved in creating safer communities through social policies. This may be approached with political advocacy, as discussed in Chapter 11 ⚭, The Nurse as Advocate.

School Violence

School shootings have raised concern about the risk of violence by children and youths. Risk factors have been investigated so that violence potential can be identified and preventive measures can be implemented. The Seattle Social Development Project conducted a prospective study of a panel of youths and studied potential risk factors for violence at age 18. They sampled the risk factors at ages 10, 14, and 16 years. The parent rating of hyperactivity, low academic performance, peer delinquency, and availability of drugs in the neighborhood predicted violence at all three ages. Multiple risk factors increased the likelihood of later violence. The recommendation from the project was that prevention efforts must be comprehensive and developmentally sensitive, responding to populations exposed to multiple risks (Herrenkohl et al., 2000).

Other research has identified the victimization by peers as a risk factor. Violent acts committed at school are often associated with bullying and ostracizing of the perpetrators (Hanish & Guerra, 2000). The National School Safety Center has made recommenda-

tions for school personnel to help create a safe school environment (Miller et al., 2000). School nurses may be directly involved in prevention measures.

Violence in the Workplace

Workplace violence may consist of a violent act or the threat of violence against workers and can consist of physical assault and homicide, as well as threats and verbal abuse. The costs of workplace violence include loss of productivity, work disruptions, employee turnover, litigation and legal costs, and other incident-related costs. About 2 million American workers are victims of workplace violence, and some workers are at greater risk than others. The workers at greatest risk are those who exchange money with the public, make deliveries, carry passengers in vehicles, work alone or in small groups during late night or early morning hours, or work in community settings in high crime areas. Workplace homicides are the second leading cause of job-related deaths. Robbery is the primary motive of job-related homicide, and along with disputes among co-workers and with customers or clients accounted for most fatalities (OSHA, 2002).

In the United States, health care workers are at greater risk for violence than other service workers, and nurses are the health care workers at greatest risk. The problem is international in scope. National Health Service staff in the United Kingdom report a 40% incidence of bullying in the workplace. In Australia, 67% reported they experienced physical or psychological violence in 2001; and in that same year health care personnel in Bulgaria, South Africa, Thailand, and Brazil reported the incidence of physical or psychological violence ranged from 76% to 47% (United Nations International Labor Organization, 2002).

The U.S. Occupational Safety and Health Administration (OSHA) has published Guidelines for Preventing Workplace Violence for Health Care and Social Service Workers (2002). These guidelines consist of four main components: (1) management commitment and employee involvement, (2) worksite analysis, (3) hazard prevention and control, and (4) safety and health training. The training for employees should include recognizing potential violence, defusing violence, and dealing with the aftermath of violence. Topics suggested for the training programs are:

- The institution's workplace violence prevention policy
- Early recognition of escalating behavior
- Ways of defusing volatile situations, managing anger, and appropriately using medications

Evidence for Practice

Nabb, D. (2000). Visitor's violence: The serious effects of aggression on nurses and others. *Nursing Standard, 14*(3), 36–38.

One hundred British nurses in acute medical, rehabilitation, and long-term care units caring for older people completed a questionnaire and a personal interview. A majority (59%) reported they had experienced verbal abuse from patient's visitors within the past 12 months and 72% of those incidents had been repeated from two to five times. Twenty percent of the nurses reported experiencing some sort of physical violence within that same period of time; for these nurses, it occurred from one to five times. The type of physical violence included being pushed, grabbed, and being struck. Eighty-four percent of the nurses believed that violence from visitors is increasing.

Analysis of the interview data identified effects of the violence on the nurses. They reported (1) increased incidence of illness, (2) not wanting to come to work, (3) thinking about leaving, and (4) feeling vulnerable.

■ The location and operation of safety devices such as alarms
■ Policies and procedures for obtaining medical care, counseling, workers' compensation, and legal assistance in the aftermath of a violent event.

ASSESSING THE EFFECTS OF VIOLENCE AND ABUSE

Often the nurse is the first one outside a person's family to discover that the person is being abused. Some victims may not disclose the abuse, or they may minimize its impact. However, it is the nurse's responsibility to assess all clients at each visit for and be alert to signs of abuse and not deny the violence.

During the assessment interview, the nurse must ensure privacy. The victim must feel safe from the perpetrator. It may be difficult for the client to admit to the reality of family violence until a trusting nurse-client relationship evolves. The nurse should assure the client of a genuine desire to help the entire family system. The nurse should also approach this topic as if it were any other health risk. In addition, the nurse can offer the option of answering questions about incidents of abuse with "sometimes" instead of "yes" or "no"; this may encourage the client to make a first step to acknowledge the abuse.

Victims of violence enter the health care system for a variety of conditions associated with abuse. For example, common physical complaints include chronic pelvic pain, headache, irritable bowel syndrome, arthritis, pelvic inflammatory disease, and neurological damage. Psychiatric illness (e.g., alcoholism) may also be the result of a history of sexual or physical abuse. Depression is also common.

Victims of physical abuse may suffer a variety of injuries. During a head-to-toe assessment, the nurse may observe for indications of abuse, such as the following:

■ *Head:* Bald patches on the scalp where hair has been pulled out; evidence of trauma from blows to the head, such as hematoma, facial bruises, facial fractures, bruised or swollen eyes, hemorrhages into the eyes; petechiae around the eyes from attempted strangulation.
■ *Skin:* Swelling or tenderness, bruises, burns, or scars of past injuries on the skin, genitals, and rectal areas.
■ *Musculoskeletal system:* Fractures or evidence of previous fractures, particularly of the face, arms/legs, and ribs; dislocated joints, especially in the shoulder when the victim is grabbed or pulled by the arm.
■ *Abdomen:* Bruises, wounds, or intra-abdominal injuries, especially if the person is pregnant.
■ *Neurological system:* Hyperactive reflexes due to neurological damage; paresthesias, numbness, or pain from old injuries.

If the nursing assessment reveals possible domestic violence, a team assessment needs to take place. The victim's medical condition and emotional state must be assessed. The severity and potential fatality of the situation must be considered, as well as the needs of dependent children and the legal ramifications.

The American Academy of Pediatrics (AAP, 1999) has published guidelines for the evaluation of sexual abuse of children. These were developed by the committee on child abuse and neglect and are available from the AAP.

Reflect on...

■ nursing and medical assessment instruments used in your practice setting. Are there areas or questions that specifically assess for abuse or violence? Do self-report instruments ask questions that would elicit a history of abuse?
■ the possibility that abuse is underreported in practice settings whose staff are not attuned to the signs and symptoms of violence. How might the

ignorance of health care providers exacerbate the problem of abuse?

■ the responsibility of the nurse if evidence of abuse is detected during assessment.

PLANNING/IMPLEMENTING INTERVENTIONS FOR THE ABUSED

The goals of treating abuse are (1) to empower the client to take control, (2) to support the client, and (3) to maximize the client's safety (CNA, 1992, p. 10).

Most people involved in intrafamily violence are disturbed by this behavior and would like it to end. Even though they want help to stop the abuse, they may not know how to seek the assistance they need. It is extremely important for nurses to be nonjudgmental in their interactions with all family members. The abusers may be distrustful of the motives of the nurse. Initially, the victims may be unwilling to trust because of family shame and fear of being blamed for remaining in the violent situation. The nurse should convey a nonjudgmental manner; in other words, the nurse should avoid blaming the victim or the abuser or looking for pathological elements in anyone's behavior. It is vital not to impose personal values on the family by offering quick and easy solutions to intrafamily violence (Fontaine, 1996).

Short-Term Interventions

Because the nurse may have the only contact with the client, it is essential that the nurse (1) determine the immediacy of danger, (2) convey that the person is not to blame and has the right to be safe, (3) explore options for help, and (4) provide information regarding available services.

It is important that the nurse avoid a judgmental attitude and support the person's choice about whether to leave the unsafe situation or return to the abusive relationship. Because severely battered women are at risk for homicide, the nurse needs to inform the client about associated risk factors and determine the immediacy of danger.

A collaborative team of nurse administrators and clinical nurses at Harris County Health Department in Houston, Texas, developed a screening and intervention triage tool for abuse. The triage structure facilitates appropriate intervention according to screening data. Each of the triage levels includes related interventions and essential documentation. See Table 20–1.

It should be noted that research on the effectiveness of screening for family violence as a routine part of health care has resulted in reduction of abuse (Nelson et al., 2004). Therefore, nurses must detect signs of abuse

Table 20–1 Screening and Intervention Triage for Abuse

Steps	TRIAGE		
	Level I	Level II	Level III
SCREEN	No history or present threat of abuse.	Recent or present abuse.	Client presents with injuries.
INTERVENE	Group or individual education about domestic violence; give handouts and pamphlets of community resources to client.	Crisis intervention; individual counseling; assist client with escape plan; identify shelter and other emergency resources; assist client in contacting shelter.	Crisis intervention; notify police; refer client to hospital for treatment (call ambulance); notify shelter; transport patient to shelter.
DOCUMENT	Statement of no abuse or threat of abuse; give handouts/education materials to client.	Statement of present or recent abuse; counsel client; give numbers to shelter and police; plan escape route; note if client declines shelter assistance at this time, or if shelter should be contacted per client's request.	Give statement of medical care given; notify emergency services; note where client was transported and in what condition.

Source: From "Establishing a Screening Program for Abused Women," by M. V. Lazzaro and J. McFarlane, October 1991, *Journal of Nursing Administration, 21,* 10. Reprinted with permission.

when patients come to a health care facility and know what to do when family violence is detected. The abuse should be carefully documented, and the patient should receive appropriate treatment for injuries both physical and psychological. Information should be given about protective services. Follow-up during future visits is important (United States Preventive Services Task Force, 2004). Several guidelines for the screening and management of intimate partner violence have been published. A critical pathway, developed with funding from the Agency for Healthcare Research and Quality, is organized into the categories of physical assessment and treatment, psychiatric/mental health assessment and treatment, and social assessment and treatment (Dienemann & Wiederhorn, 2003). This can provide guidance across all health care settings. There is evidence from numerous studies that women who use a shelter for protection experience a reduced rate of reabuse and an increased quality of life when they also receive advocacy and counseling services. Without those services, there is little data to support the effectiveness of shelter stays to reduce violence (Wathen & MacMillan, 2003).

Abused children need to be encouraged to talk, but they must also be protected from having to provide multiple reports. Nurses need to tell an abused child that they believe the story, and they must reassure the child that he or she has done nothing wrong. The nurse should also avoid making negative comments about the abuser and to follow established protocols for mandatory reporting, documentation, and use of available support services (e.g., the police department, social service agencies, and child welfare agency).

Interventions for abused older adults include developing a positive relationship with both the victim and the abuser, exploring ways for the older person to maximize independence, and exploring the need for additional home care services or alternative living arrangements.

Nurses must familiarize themselves with agency protocols and resources available for victims of domestic violence. Most municipalities have crisis helplines and hotlines to provide assistance to victims of abuse. The nurse should also keep a record of telephone numbers for transition houses and rape crisis centers, alcohol and drug abuse information, support groups, religious organizations, and legal services. There are also several national organizations that offer toll-free contacts, such as the National Organization for Victim Assistance, the National Coalition Against Domestic Violence (in the United States), and the National Clearinghouse on Family Violence (in Canada).

Long-Term Interventions

Goals for ongoing counseling and care may include (1) helping the client continue to choose to be safe from violence, (2) helping the client explore options for self-development, and (3) helping the client improve quality of life through increasing self-esteem (CNA, 1992, p. 14).

Usually, the best way to treat violent families is a multidisciplinary approach involving nurses, physicians, social workers, police, protective services personnel, and, often, lawyers. Most families are more open to accepting help during a time of crisis than at other times.

Ciritical Thinking Exercise

Lucy Barnes, a 30-year-old woman who is 25 weeks pregnant, comes to the emergency department of Parkfield Community Hospital. She says she fell and hit her head at home and is having headaches. During the assessment the nurse notices multiple bruises in various stages of healing over her body and asks Lucy how she got them. Lucy says that she is just clumsy and falls a lot. While the nurse is assessing Lucy, another nurse enters the room to tell Lucy that her boyfriend is there to take her back home. At that point, Lucy becomes frightened and tells the nurse that her boyfriend has hit her many times before and had knocked her down today. She says he has threatened to kill her if she tells anyone and she does not want to leave with him.

Make a list of questions that the nurse could use in continuing her assessment and in documenting the discussion with Lucy.

What other people should be involved in Lucy's care in the Emergency Department?

Who should make the decision about where Lucy should go?

What should be done with the boyfriend?

They most likely will be willing to develop new behavior patterns for a short time following a crisis. If they are not helped during that time, they will most likely return to previous behavior patterns, including violence.

Nurses should know the laws associated with reporting abuse. In the United States and Canada, nurses are required to report any suspected child abuse. The courts and child protective agencies make decisions in the child's interest. They may allow a child to remain in the home but under court supervision; they may remove the child from the home; and, in some instances, they may terminate parental rights if the abuse was severe.

State and provincial laws about reporting adult and elder abuse vary. Domestic violence is considered a violent crime; the victim has a right to be protected, and the perpetrator of the violence can be prosecuted.

PREVENTION OF VIOLENCE AND ABUSE

Nurses in all areas of practice (e.g., maternal/child health; school; community and occupational health; mental health; primary and acute care; and academic settings) need to take a proactive role to prevent family violence. Early screening of vulnerable people and efforts to promote a change in attitudes and beliefs about family violence are essential.

If they are to assist victims effectively, nurses must be aware of their own feelings about family violence. Nurses who are unclear about their own feelings about family violence may deny its existence, blame the victim in crisis, or minimize the effects of the violence (CNA, 1992, p. 8).

Nurses also can be instrumental as advocates in developing policies and programs, and providing in-service training and education to health care professionals and the public. Comprehensive violence prevention programs require a variety of disciplines and organizations working together, such as state or provincial and local health care agencies, criminal justice agencies, and social service agencies.

Many of these programs are generated by *Healthy People 2010*, a national health-promotion and disease-prevention initiative to increase health for all. The objectives for violence and abuse prevention are shown in Table 20–2 (USDHHS, 2000, pp. 45–60).

Table 20–2 *Healthy People 2010* Objectives for Violence and Abuse Prevention

Objective	Target	Baseline
Reduce homicides	3.0 per 100,000 population	6.5 per 100,000 population in 1998
Reduce maltreatment of children	10.3 per 1000 children under 18 years	12.9 per 1000 in 1998
Reduce child maltreatment fatalities	1.4 per 100,000 children under 18 years	1.6 per 100,000 in 1998
Reduce the rate of physical assault by current or former intimate partners	3.3 per 1000 persons aged 12 years and older	4.4 per 1000 persons aged 12 years and older in 1998
Reduce the annual rate of rape or attempted rape	0.7 per 1000 persons	0.8 per 1000 persons aged 12 years and older in 1998
Reduce sexual assault other than rape	0.4 per 1000 persons aged 12 years and older	0.6 per 1000 persons aged 12 years and older in 1998
Reduce physical assaults	13.6 per 1000 persons aged 12 years and older	31.1 per 1000 persons aged 12 years and older in 1998
Reduce physical fighting among adolescents	32%	35% in grade 9 through 12 within a year in 1999
Reduce weapon carrying by adolescents on school property	4.9%	6.9% of students in grades 9 through 12 during a 30-day period in 1999

VIOLENCE AND PUBLIC HEALTH

Terrorism and Weapons of Mass Destruction

Terrorism has become a major challenge to public health worldwide. It affects health in many ways. It causes injury, illness, and death, but it also creates fear and anxiety. *Terrorism* is defined as "politically motivated violence or the threat of violence, especially against civilians, with the intent to instill fear" (Levy & Sidel, 2003). It is intended to have effects beyond the immediate victims and intimidate a wider population.

The U.S. Department of Justice (DOJ) Office for Domestic Preparedness (ODP) was established in 1998 to help provide training to first responders on a national level as part of an integrated effort (ODP, 2002). Emergency Responders Guidelines were developed to guide training at three levels: Awareness, Performance, and Planning and Management. This training has intensified in the aftermath of September 11, 2001, and plans are developed to implement the training in communities nationwide in coordination with state and regional plans.

While the role of first responders is of utmost importance following a terrorist event, mental health and social needs are created and preparation is necessary for meeting those needs. A wide range of public health professionals have become involved in plans for responding to terrorist events and the threats of future terrorist events. The interdisciplinary approach includes epidemiologists, health educators, nurses, mental health specialists, social workers, and vaccine developers, for example. These groups must plan responses to terrorist acts and work to prevent future terrorism, as well as to reduce or prevent inappropriate responses.

The role of public health in any emergency is to promote physical and mental health and prevent disease, injury, and disability. The Centers for Disease Control and Prevention (CDC) has published basic competencies in emergency preparedness and bioterrorism readiness for all public health workers. These basic competencies are shown in the accompanying box.

Acts of terrorism often involve weapons of mass destruction and are usually motivated by political differences. Weapons of mass destruction are grouped into three categories: nuclear, biological, and chemical. Nuclear weapons involve the spread of radioactive material. Biological agents can cause diseases such as anthrax and smallpox through the dissemination of materials such as bacteria, viruses, fungi, and toxins. Chemical agents can cause injury by skin contact and inhalation, for example, and may require decontamination of the victim. Chemical agents may also cause explosions that result in injury. The recognition of signs and symptoms as well as the appropriate management for each are important training and education needs for those health care workers who will be providing that care should an act of terrorism happen.

Emergency Preparedness: Core Competencies for All Public Health Workers

1. Describe the public health role in emergency response in a range of emergencies that might arise.

2. Describe the chain of command in emergency response.

3. Identify and locate the agency emergency response plan (or the pertinent portion of the plan).

4. Describe his or her functional role(s) in emergency response and demonstrate his or her roles in regular drills.

5. Demonstrate correct use of all communication equipment used for emergency communication.

6. Describe communication roles in emergency response within the agency, with media, with the general public, and in personal situations.

7. Identify limits to own knowledge/skill/authority and identify key system resources for referring matters that exceed these limits.

8. Recognize unusual events that might indicate an emergency and describe appropriate action.

9. Apply creative problem solving and flexible thinking to unusual challenges within his or her functional responsibilities and evaluate effectiveness of all actions taken.

Source: From *Bioterrorism and Emergency Readiness: Competencies for All Public Health Workers,* Centers for Disease Control and Prevention (p. 4), 2002. Used by permission.

Hospitals and health care groups have had mass casualty plans and drills for decades, but the breadth of those plans and drills have expanded greatly. Early mass casualty plans were developed for incidents of natural disasters such as hurricanes and mass injuries such as airline crashes. The planning for terrorist events includes broader collaboration among communities and adds procedures such as decontamination.

Strengthening the Public Health System

The Metropolitan Medical Response System (MMRS) program of the Department of Health and Human Services (DHHS) has provided funds to major U.S. cities "to help them develop plans for coping with the health and medical consequences of a terrorist attack with chemical, biological, or radiological (CBR) agents" (Institute of Medicine, 2002, p. 1). By the spring of 2002, 122 cities had signed contracts to develop these programs under the auspices of the Office of Emergency Preparedness. The development of these plans must be a continual process involving formative evaluation. Twenty-three essential capabilities have been set forth for evaluation of a community's program; they are shown in the accompanying box.

An essential part of the evaluation is the demonstration of competency through field exercises and drills, particularly in the absence of real events.

Current improvements in public health are concerned with disease surveillance and epidemiology. Improvements in laboratory capabilities and in reporting among local, state, and federal agencies are underway. Research on improving vaccines, antitoxins, and antimicrobials is being funded at higher levels than previously. The potential threats to food, water, and air have created new challenges for the public health system. This has stepped up surveillance. Arising from the concerns about protecting the public from attack have come concerns about protecting civil liberties and the balance between freedom and regulation (Levy & Sidel, 2003).

EXPLORE MEDIALINK

Questions, critical thinking exercises, essay activities, and other interactive resources for this chapter can be found on the Web site at http://www.prenhall.com/blais. Click on Chapter 20 to select activities for this chapter.

Essential Response Capabilities to Incidents of Chemical, Biological, and Radiological Weapons

1. Relationship development (partnering)
2. Communication system development
3. Hazard assessment
4. Training
5. Equipment and supplies
6. Mass immunization and prophylaxis
7. Addressing the information needs of the public and the news media
8. First responder protection
9. Rescue and stabilization of victims
10. Diagnosis and agent identification
11. Decontamination of victims (at site of exposure or at hospital or treatment site)
12. Transportation of victims
13. Distribution of supplies, equipment, and pharmaceuticals
14. Shelter and feeding of evacuated and displaced persons
15. Definitive medical care
16. Mental health services
17. Volunteer utilization and control
18. Crowd and traffic control
19. Evacuation and quarantine decisions and operations
20. Fatality management
21. Environmental cleanup, physical restoration of facilities, and certification of safety
22. Follow-up study of responder, caregiver, and victim health
23. Process for continuous evaluation of needs and resources

Source: From *Preparing for Terrorism: Tools for Evaluating the Metropolitan Medical Response System Program: Executive Summary* (p. 9), by F. J. Manning, and L. Goldfrank (Eds.), 2002, Washington, DC: National Academy Press. Used by permission.

Bookshelf

Coloroso, B. (2003). *The bully, the bullied, and the bystander.* **New York: Harper Collins.**
This book is directed at parents and teachers to help them understand the triad of bully, bullied, and bystander. It provides guidance in helping to break the cycle.

Levy, B. (1998). *In love and in danger: A teen's guide to breaking free of abusive relationships.* **Seattle: Seal Press.**
The book examines abusive relationships among teenagers. It is appropriate for grades 9 and up.

Plain, B. (1994). *Whispers.* **New York: Dell Publishing.**
This novel is the story of a contemporary family and the story beneath the surface of their perfect lives. A woman struggles to free herself from the cycle of violence–contrition–more violence and finally emerges in triumph.

Rodriguez, S. (1999). *Time to stop pretending: A mother's story of domestic violence, homelessness, poverty, and escape.* **Middlebury, VT: P. S. Eriksson.**
This book is one woman's story of her life of domestic violence, poverty, and homelessness with her eight children in New York City.

Victor, B. (1996). *Getting away with murder: Weapons for the war against domestic violence.* **New York: Simon and Schuster.**
This text gives interviews with victims and abusers, as well as police, social workers, district attorneys, and judges about the violent crimes committed against women by intimate partners. Suggestions are given from each of these sources regarding how to stop the attacks.

SUMMARY

The prevalence of violence and abusive behavior in the United States is alarming. National health care organizations now view violence as a major health problem and are directing attention to its recognition, prevention, and treatment. Nurses need to know how to identify victims of violence, to appreciate potential risk factors for future injury, to understand some of the unique considerations regarding care of victims of abuse, and to intervene effectively. Acts of violence often escalate in frequency and severity and may ultimately result in homicide.

Family violence includes intimate partner abuse, child abuse and neglect, and elder abuse, neglect, or mistreatment. It occurs in all strata of society. Abusive individuals have certain traits in common, such as overpossessiveness, desire to dominate, poor control of impulses, and a history of drug or alcohol use. Victims of domestic violence most often are women, many of whom have difficulty leaving the abusive relationship largely because of fear, shame, guilt, and economic dependence. Laws mandate the reporting of suspected child abuse. Elder abuse can involve not only physical, sexual, or emotional abuse but also active or passive neglect, violation of human or civil rights, and financial abuse. Those most vulnerable to elder abuse are females over 75 years of age, physically or mentally impaired individuals, and those dependent for care on the abuser.

Often the nurse is the first one outside the family to discover that a person is being abused. Appropriate assessment, intervention, and documentation are essential to prevent the abuse from continuing. The nurse needs to empower the client to take control, provide support, and maximize the client's safety. Treatment of violent families requires a multidisciplinary approach among nurses, social workers, physicians, family therapists, vocational trainers, police, protective services personnel, and lawyers.

If they are to assist victims effectively, nurses need to be aware of their own feelings about family violence. They also need to take a proactive role in preventing family violence. Nurses can advocate in developing programs and policies and provide inservice training and education to other health care professionals and the public.

Terrorism is a form of violence that affects the community. Terrorism often involves weapons of mass destruction that affect large numbers of the population. Nurses are involved in interdisciplinary efforts toward preparedness and prevention so these events may be avoided or the effects minimized.

REFERENCES

American Academy of Pediatrics. (1999). Guidelines for the evaluation of sexual abuse in children: Subject review. *Pediatrics, 103*(1), 186.

Beers, M. H., & Berkow, R. (2000). *The Merck manual of geriatrics* (3rd ed.). White House Station, NJ: Merck Research Laboratories.

Bureau of Labor Statistics. (1998). *National census of fatal occupational injuries, 1997.* http://www.bls.gov/opub.

Canadian Nurses Association. (1992). *Family violence: Clinical guidelines for nurses.* Ottawa: CNA.

Centers for Disease Control. (2000). What is domestic violence? http://www.cdc.gov/ncipc/dvp/fivpt/spotlite/home. htm.

Centers for Disease Control and Prevention. (2002). *Bioterrorism and emergency readiness. Competencies for all public health workers.* http://www.trainingfinder.org/competencies.

Chiocca, E. M. (1995, January/February). Shaken baby syndrome: A nursing perspective. *Pediatric Nursing, 21,* 33–38.

Devlin, B. K., & Reynolds, E. (1994, March). Child abuse: How to recognize it, how to intervene. *American Journal of Nursing, 94,* 26–32.

Dienemann, J. C., & Wiederhorn, N. (2003). A critical pathway for intimate partner violence across the continuum of care, *Journal of Obstetric, Gynecologic, and Neonatal Nursing, 32*(5), 594–603.

Federal Bureau of Investigation. (2004). *Work place violence: Issues in response.* Washington, DC: FBI.

Fontaine, K. L. (1996). Rape and intrafamily abuse and violence. In H. S. Wilson & C. R. Kneisl, *Psychiatric nursing* (5th ed., pp. 555–584). Menlo Park, CA: Addison-Wesley Nursing.

Frost, M. H., & Willette, K. (1994, August). Risk for abuse/neglect: Documentation of assessment data and diagnoses. *Journal of Gerontological Nursing, 20,* 37–45.

Gilligan, J. (2000). Violence in public health and preventive medicine. *Lancet, 355,* 1802–1804.

Hall, L. A., Sachs, B., Rayens, M. K., & Lutenbacher, M. (1993, Winter). Childhood physical and sexual abuse: Their relationship with depressive symptoms in adulthood. *Image: Journal of Nursing Scholarship, 25*(4), 317–323.

Hanish, L. D., & Guerra, N. G. (2000). The roles of ethnicity and school context in predicting children's victimization by peers. *American Journal of Community Psychology, 28*(2), 201–223.

Henderson, A. (1992, February). Critical care nurses need to know about abused women. *Critical Care Nurses, 12*(2), 27–30.

Herrenkohl, T. I., Maguin, E., Hill, K. G., Hawkins, J. D., Abbott, R. D., & Catalano, R. F. (2000). Developmental risk factors for youth violence. *Journal of Adolescent Health, 26*(3), 176–186.

Hoag-Apel, C. (1994, September). Protocol for domestic violence intervention. *Nursing Management, 25,* 81–83.

Hughes, H. M. (1997). Research concerning children of battered women: Clinical implications. In R. Geffner, S. B. Sorenson, & P. K. Lundberg-Love (Eds.), *Violence and sexual abuse at home: Current issues in spousal battering and child maltreatment* (pp. 225–244). New York: Haworth.

Institute of Medicine. (2002). *Preparing for terrorism: Tools to evaluate the Metropolitan Medical Response System Program.* http://www.iom.edu/report.asp?id=4449.

Lenius, P. (1999, October). Workplace violence is a growing concern. *Contractor.*

Levy, B. S., & Sidel, V. W. (2003). *Terrorism and public health.* New York: Oxford University Press.

Manning, F. J., & Goldfrank, L. (Eds.). (2002). *Preparing for terrorism: Tools for evaluating the Metropolitan Medical Response System Program.* Washington, DC: National Academy Press.

Margolin, G., & Gordis, E. B. (2000). The effects of family and community violence on children. *Annual Review of Psychology, 51,* 445–479.

Marshall, C. E., Benton, D., & Brazier, J. M. (2000). Elder abuse: Using clinical tools to identify clues of mistreatment. *Geriatrics, 55,* 42–53.

Miller, L. S., Wasserman, G. A., Neugebauer, R., Gorman Smith, D., & Kamboukos, D. (1999). Witnessed community violence and antisocial behavior in high-risk urban boys. *Journal of Clinical Child Psychology, 28,* 2–11.

Miller, T. W., Clayton, R., Miller, J. M., Bilyeu, J., Hunter, J., & Kraus, R. F. (2000). Violence in the schools: Clinical issues and case analysis for high-risk children. *Child Psychiatry and Human Development, 30*(4), 255–272.

National Center for Educational Statistics. (2004). *Crime and safety in America's public school.* Washington, DC: Department of Education.

National Center for Injury Prevention and Control. (2003). *Costs of intimate partner violence against women in the United States.* Atlanta: Centers for Disease Control and Prevention. http://www.cdc.gov/ncipc.

National Center for Injury Prevention and Control. (2004a). *Child maltreatment: Fact sheet.* Atlanta, GA: Centers for Disease Control and Prevention.

National Center for Injury Prevention and Control. (2004b). *Youth violence: Fact sheet.* Atlanta, GA: Centers for Disease Control and Prevention.

National Center on Elder Abuse. (2000). *What is elder abuse?* http://www.elderabusecenter.org/basic/indes.html.

National Center on Elder Abuse. *Trends in elder abuse in domestic settings. Elder abuse information series No. 2.* Washington, DC: National Center on Elder Abuse. Retrieved August 20, 2004, http://www. elderabusecenter.org.

National Institute for Occupational Safety and Health. (1996). Violence in the workplace: Risk factors and prevention strategies. *NIOSH Current Intelligence Bulletin, 57.*

Nelson, H. D., Nygren, P., McInerney, Y., & Klein, J. (2004). Screening women and elderly adults for family and intimate partner violence: A review of the evidence for the U.S. Protective Services Task Force. *Annals of Internal Medicine, 140*(5), 487–396.

Occupational Safety and Health Administration. (2002). *Workplace violence.* http://www.osha.gov/oshinfo/priorities/ violence.html.

Office for Domestic Preparedness. (2002). *Emergency responder guidelines.* http://www.ojp.usdoj.gov/odp.

Srnec, P. (1991, September). Children, violence, and intentional injuries. *Critical Care Nursing Clinics of North America, 3,* 471–478.

Tjaden, P., & Thoennes, N. (1998, November). *Prevalence, incidence, and consequences of violence against women: Findings from the National Violence Against Survey.* Institute of Justice, Research in Brief.

United Nations International Labor Organization Joint Task Force. (2002). *Framework guidelines for addressing workplace violence in the health sector.* Geneva, Switzerland: ILO.

United States Department of Health and Human Services. (1990, September). *Healthy people 2000: National health promotion and disease prevention objectives.* DHHS Publ. No. (PHS) 91–50212. Washington, DC: Government Printing Office.

United States Department of Health and Human Services. (2000). *Healthy people 2010 injury and violence prevention objectives* (pp. 15.3–15.60). Washington, DC: U.S. Government Printing Office.

United States Department of Justice, Federal Bureau of Investigation. (1986). *U.S. Department of Justice crime reports: Crime in the U.S. 1985.* Washington, DC: U.S. Department of Justice.

United States Preventative Services Task Force. (2004). Screening for family and intimate partner violence: Recommendation statement. *Annals of Internal Medicine, 140*(5), 382–386.

Wang, C. T., & Daro, D. (1998). *Current trends in child abuse reporting and fatalities: The results of the 1997 annual fifty-state survey.* Chicago: National Committee on the Prevention of Child Abuse.

Warchol, G. (1998). *Workplace violence, 1992–1996. National Crime Victimization Survey.* Report No. NCJ-168634.

Wathen, C. N., & MacMillan, H. L. (2003). Interventions for violence against women: Scientific review. *Journal of the American Medical Association, 289*(5), 589–600.

Yarn, M. (2000). Seen but not heard: Battered women's perceptions of the ED experience. *Journal of Emergency Nursing, 26*(5), 464–470.

Nursing in a Culturally Diverse World

Objectives

■ Analyze concepts related to cultural diversity in nursing.

■ Discuss components of culture pertinent to nursing care.

■ Describe the components of Leininger's Sunrise Model.

■ Describe barriers to cultural competence.

■ Assess clients from a cultural perspective.

■ Plan and implement culturally competent care.

M E D I A L I N K

Additional online resources for this chapter can be found on the companion Web site at http://www.prenhall.com/blais.

Nurses need to become informed about and sensitive to culturally diverse subjective meanings of health, illness, caring, and healing practices. A transcultural care perspective is now considered essential for nurses and other health care professionals to deliver quality health care to all clients.

The United States and Canada are home to many cultural groups. Table 21–1 provides statistical data

Table 21–1 Population Diversity of the United States 1990–2000

Race	1990 (%)	2000 (%)
One race*		
White	80.3	75.1
African American/Black	12.1	12.3
American Indian and Alaska Native	00.8	00.9
Asian	02.8	03.6
Native Hawaiian/Other Pacific Islander	00.1	00.1
Other race	03.9	05.5
Two or more races*		02.4
Hispanic or Latino†	09.0	12.5

* In the 2000 census, participants could select multiple races for the first time if they were of mixed race heritage, therefore, the total can exceed 100%.
† Persons of Hispanic origin may be of any race.
Source: by *Census 2000 Redistricting Data (P.L. 94–171) Summary File for States,* U.S. Census Bureau. Retrieved June 23, 2004, from http://www.census.gov/stab.www/poprace.html.

reflecting the diversity of the United States. In addition to the indigenous peoples (Native Americans and Aboriginals), there is much diversity in immigrant groups in North America. The term *cultural mosaic* is used to describe the way in which many people of different cultures maintain the cultural values, beliefs, traditions, and practices of their homelands for many generations. These diverse cultural beliefs and practices influence health care decision making.

Nurses must understand how their own cultural beliefs and biases relate to people whose beliefs are different. Health care professionals are not expected to know and understand all cultures of the world; it is possible, however, for health care professionals to develop an awareness of those cultural belief systems that are prevalent in the community or region where they practice. Awareness of and sensitivity to potential differences is important to provide culturally competent care.

Nurses must be aware that although people from a given ethnic group share certain beliefs, values, and experiences, often there is also widespread intra-ethnic

diversity. Major differences within ethnic groups may be related to such factors as age, sex, level of education, socioeconomic status, religious affiliation, area of origin in the home country (rural or urban), and the length of time living in the new country. These factors influence the client's beliefs about health and illness, health and illness practices, health-seeking behaviors, and expectations of health professionals.

In 1991 the American Nurses Association stated, "culture is one of the organizing concepts upon which nursing is based and defined" (ANA, 1991, p. 1). This position was reaffirmed in the document *Nursing: Scope and Standards of Practice* (ANA, 2004, p. 2), which states "the cultural, racial, and ethnic diversity of the patient must always be taken into account in providing nursing services." Nurses need to understand how cultural groups understand life processes, how cultural groups define health and illness, what cultural groups do to maintain wellness, what cultural groups believe to be the causes of illness, how healers cure and care for members of cultural groups, and how the cultural background of a nurse influences the way in which the nurse provides care. Because a nurse is expected to provide individualized care based on an assessment of the client's physiologic, psychologic, and developmental status, the nurse must understand how the client's cultural beliefs and practices can affect the client's health and illness.

CHALLENGES AND OPPORTUNITIES

The challenges of working in a culturally diverse environment require nurses to be open to differences in beliefs about health and illness, different types of cultural healers and healing behaviors, and the use of traditional healing practices that may be considered untested to modern health practitioners. Establishing trust with people whose beliefs are different depends on a nurse's willingness to accept difference and to work with the client's different beliefs to effect a healing relationship.

Working with clients of different cultural beliefs provides nurses with the opportunity to enrich their own lives through an understanding of the differences of others. Traditional remedies such as acupuncture, massage, meditation, and some herbs increasingly are being shown to have healing properties. Researchers are examining the effects of complementary, also referred to as alternative, healing methods, often derived from cultural healing practices, on health and healing. New knowledge derived from traditional beliefs and practices can provide new ways of healing and helping.

CONCEPTS RELATED TO CULTURE

All groups of people face similar issues in adapting to their environment: providing nutrition and shelter, caring for and educating children, division of labor, social organization, controlling disease, and maintaining health. Humans adapt to varying environments by developing cultural solutions to meet these needs. An understanding of the cultural dimension of people is the focus of the field of anthropology. Cultural anthropologists attempt to understand culture by studying both similarities and differences among human groups. Nurses use the cultural information gained by cultural anthropologists to understand and help clients (individuals, their families, or groups) to achieve optimum health.

Culture is a universal experience, but no two cultures are exactly alike. Two important terms identify the differences and similarities among peoples of different cultures. Culture-universals are the commonalities of values, norms of behavior, and life patterns that are similar among different cultures. Culture-specifics are those values, beliefs, and patterns of behavior that tend to be unique to a designated culture and do not tend to be shared with members of other cultures. For example, most cultures have ceremonies to celebrate the passage from childhood to adulthood; this practice is a culture-universal. However, different cultural groups celebrate this important life event in very different ways. In Latin or Hispanic cultures, the "quince" or "quinceañero" party, which celebrates a girl's fifteenth birthday, signifies that the young girl has now become a woman. In the Jewish tradition, the bar mitzvah (for boys) and the bat mitzvah (for girls) are celebrations of the passage to adulthood.

Anthropologists have also traditionally divided culture into material and nonmaterial culture. **Material culture** refers to objects (such as dress, art, religious artifacts, or eating utensils) and ways these are used. **Nonmaterial culture** refers to beliefs, customs, languages, and social institutions.

The terms *culture, diversity, ethnicity,* and *race* are often used interchangeably, but they are not synonymous. **Culture** is defined as "the learned, shared, and transmitted values, beliefs, norms, and lifeway practices of a particular group that guide thinking, decisions, and actions in patterned ways" (Leininger, 1988, p. 158). The Office of Minority Health further defines culture as "the thoughts, communications, actions, customs, beliefs, values, and institutions of racial, ethnic, religious, or social groups" (Office of Minority Health, 2002, p. 131).

Because cultural patterns are learned, it is important for nurses to note that members of a particular group may not share identical cultural experiences. Thus, each member of a cultural group will be somewhat different from his or her own cultural counterparts. For example, third-generation Japanese Americans, or *Sansei,* will differ in cultural understandings from first-generation Japanese Americans, or *Issei.*

Large cultural groups often have cultural subgroups or subsystems. A subculture is usually composed of people who have a distinct identity and yet are also related to a larger cultural group. A subcultural group generally shares ethnic origin, occupation, or physical characteristics with the larger cultural group. Examples of cultural subgroups include occupational groups (e.g., nurses), societal groups (e.g., homeless people), and ethnic groups (e.g., Cajuns, who are descendants of French Acadians).

Bicultural refers to the integration of two cultures within the individual. In the 2000 U.S. census, individuals could identify themselves as multiracial for the first time. For an immigrant, biculturalism is the integration of the culture of the native country, or homeland, with the culture of the new country. Children whose parents are from two different cultures may grow up in an environment that practices and respects both cultures. The values, beliefs, rituals, and traditions of both cultures may be practiced. For example, a young man whose father is Native American and whose mother is European American may maintain his traditional Native American heritage while also being influenced by his mother's cultural values.

Diversity refers "to differences in race, ethnicity, national origin, religion, age, gender, sexual orientation, ability/disability, social and economic status or class, education, and related attributes of groups of people in society" (Andrews & Boyle, 2003, p. 5). Diversity therefore occurs not only between cultural groups but also within cultural groups.

The term *ethnic* has been used to describe a group of people who share a common and distinctive culture and who are members of a specific group. An ethnic group is a subgroup of a larger social system whose members "have common ancestral, racial, physical or national characteristics and who share cultural symbols such as language, lifestyle, religion, and other characteristics that are not fully understood or shared by outsiders" (Andrews & Boyle, 1999, p. 10). The characteristics of the group give an individual a sense of cultural identity. Ethnicity has been defined by Sprott (1993, p. 190) as "a consciousness of belonging to a group that is differentiated from others by symbolic markers (culture, biology, territory). It is rooted in bonds of a shared past and perceived ethnic interest." Giger and Davidhizar (2004, p. 67) state that "the most important characteristic of ethnicity is that members of an ethnic group feel a sense of identity." Other factors that help to define ethnicity are religion and geographic background of the family. Discussion of religion as an influence on health care will be presented in Chapter 22 ⊙, Nursing in a Spiritually Diverse World.

Race is the classification of people according to shared biologic characteristics, genetic markers, or features. They have common characteristics such as skin color, bone structure, facial features, hair texture, and blood type. Different ethnic groups can belong to the same race, and different cultures can be found within the same ethnic group. For example, the terms *Caucasian* and *European American* describe the race of people whose origins are in Europe. Whereas British Americans are a subgroup of European Americans, Scottish Americans (an ethnic subgroup of British Americans) may share different cultural practices than other British Americans. It is important to understand that not all people of the same race have the same culture. Culture should not be confused with either race or ethnic group.

Acculturation is the process of "becoming a competent participant in the dominant culture" (Spector, 2004, p. 17). Acculturation, also referred to as assimilation, is the integration of the cultural patterns of the dominant or host culture into the person's way of life. Spector suggests that it takes three generations for a family to become fully assimilated into the American culture.

The cultural beliefs and practices regarding the health and illness of North America's many different ethnic and cultural groups are important considerations for nurses when planning nursing care. Nursing ethnoscientists study the health beliefs of cultures so that nurses can provide culturally competent care to clients of different cultures. Madeleine Leininger, a nurse theorist and anthropologist, described **transcultural nursing** as the study of different cultures and subcultures with respect to nursing and health illness caring practices, beliefs, and values (1978, p. 493). The goal of transcultural nursing is to provide culture-specific and culture-universal nursing care. Cultural awareness and cultural sensitivity are prerequisite to the provision of culturally competent nursing care. **Cultural awareness** is the conscious and informed recognition of the differences and similarities between varied cultural or ethnic groups. Cultural awareness is not knowledge derived solely from myths and stereotypes. **Cultural sensitivity** is the respect and appreciation for cultural behaviors based on an understanding of the other person's perspective. Cultural competence is "having an awareness of one's own existence, sensations, thoughts, and environment without letting them have an udue influence on those from other backgrounds" (Purnell & Paulanka, 2003, p. 352). Spector (2004, p. 5) describes cultural and linguistic competence as the "ability by health care providers and health care organizations to understand and respond effectively to the cultural and linguistic needs brought to the health care experience." The culturally competent nurse, therefore, works within the cultural belief system of the client to resolve health problems. To provide culturally competent care, nurses need data about the client's personal and cultural views regarding health and illness. To make valid assessments, nurses need to try to see and hear the world as their clients do. When developing care plans, nurses need to consider the client's world and daily experiences. Although a client's needs and behaviors can be better understood when particular cultural health norms are identified, nurses must take care to avoid stereotyping clients by unfounded culture norms. This allows for individualized care.

Culture shock can occur when members of one culture are abruptly moved to another culture or setting. **Culture shock** is the state of being disoriented or unable to respond to a different cultural environment because of its sudden strangeness, unfamiliarity, and incompatibility to the stranger's perceptions and expectations (Leininger, 1978, p. 490). For example, when immigrants first enter the United States or Canada, language and behavior differences may initially cause them difficulty in carrying out normal activities. People can also experience culture shock when they are abruptly thrust into the health care subculture. Nursing students, for example, may experience culture shock when they enter nursing school and must learn medical terminology (a new language) and provide care for clients in clinical environments with which they are unfamiliar. Expressions of culture shock can range from silence and immobility to agitation.

Reflect on...

■ your own cultural values, beliefs, and practices. How do you describe yourself culturally? What meaning does your cultural identification have for you? How do you celebrate your cultural identification?

Characteristics of Culture

Culture exhibits several characteristics.

- *Culture is learned.* It is neither instinctive nor innate. It is learned through life experiences from birth.
- *Culture is taught.* It is transmitted from parents and primary caregivers to children over successive generations. All animals can learn, but only humans can pass along culture. Verbal and nonverbal communication patterns are the transmitters of culture.
- *Culture is social.* It originates and develops through the interactions of people: families, groups, and communities.
- *Culture is adaptive.* Customs, beliefs, and practices change as people adapt to the social environment and as biologic and psychologic needs of people change. Some traditional norms in a culture may cease to provide satisfaction and are eliminated. For example, in many cultures it is customary for family members of different generations to live together (extended family); however, education and employment considerations may require children to leave their parents and move to other parts of the country. In such cases, the extended family norm may change.
- *Culture is satisfying.* Cultural habits persist only as long as they satisfy people's needs. Gratification strengthens habits and beliefs. Once they no longer bring gratification, they may disappear.
- *Culture is difficult to articulate.* Members of a specific cultural group often find it difficult to articulate their own culture. Many of the values and behaviors are habitual and are carried out subconsciously.
- *Culture exists at many levels.* Culture is most easily identified at the material level. For example, art, tools, and clothes usually reveal aspects of a culture relatively readily. More abstract concepts, such as values, beliefs, and traditions, are often more difficult to discover. Nurses may need to ask culturally sensitive questions of the client or support persons to obtain this information.

Components of Culture

Cultures are very complex. They consist of facets that relate to all aspects of life: language, art, music, values systems (beliefs, morals, rules), religion, philosophy, family interaction, patterns of behavior, childrearing practices, rituals or ceremonies, recreation and leisure activities, festivals and holidays, nutrition, food preferences, and health practices. Many facets of culture such as social structures and gender relationships; health and illness practices; attitudes about touch, territory and privacy; childbirth and childrearing practices; and death and dying practices have an impact on nursing practice.

Critical Thinking Exercise

Compare the various cultural and ethnic groups in your community. Consider the values, beliefs, and practices of the cultural and ethnic groups in your community. Is cultural difference valued? If cultural and ethnic difference is valued, in what ways is this value manifested in your community, the nation, and the world? In what ways are negative responses to cultural difference manifested in your community, the nation, and the world?

Reflect on...

- your own cultural or ethnic background. What are your values, beliefs, and practices about health and health care? How might they affect your nurse-client interactions? How do they influence your practice as a nurse?

CULTURE AND HEALTH CARE

Two transcultural health care systems generally exist side by side with limited awareness by practitioners of both systems: an indigenous health care system and a professional health care system (Leininger, 1993, p. 36). The *indigenous health care system* refers to traditional folk health care methods, such as folk medicines and other home treatments. The modern *professional health care system* refers to a structured system maintained by individuals who have engaged in a formal program of study. The indigenous system is the older system and has often provided health care long before a professional system enters the culture. According to Leininger, few professional health care workers are knowledgeable about the indigenous health care system or its practitioners. Some professionals regard the indigenous system as unscientific, "primitive," or even "quackery." Leininger emphasizes that the goal of health care should be to use the best of both systems and that health professionals need to consider ways to interface with the two systems for the benefit of the people served. "Every culture has health, caring, and curing processes, techniques, and practices viewed as important to the people" (p. 38).

Currently there is much interest in and inquiry into the efficacy of folk healing methods and herbal remedies. These healing practices are considered complementary or alternative to Western or scientific medicine. In 1998 the National Center for Complementary and Alternative Medicine (NCCAM) was established at the National Institutes of Health to stimulate, develop, and support research on the benefits of complementary and alternative medicines (CAM) to the public (NCCAM, 2001).

Leininger's Sunrise Model

Leininger produced the Sunrise Model to depict her theory of cultural care diversity and universality (Figure 21–1■). This model emphasizes that health and care are influenced by elements of the social structure, such as technology, religious and philosophical factors, kinship and social systems, cultural values, political and legal factors, economic factors, and educational factors. These social factors are addressed within environmental contexts, language expressions, and ethnohistory. Each of these systems is part of the social structure of any society; health care expressions, patterns, and practices are also integral parts of these aspects of social structure (Leininger, 1993).

Technological factors, such as the availability of technical and electrical equipment, greatly determine what health equipment will be used. For example, many European Americans regard resuscitative equipment as essential. The *economic* system determines the quality of health care within a culture, for example, the availability of funds for health care services materially affects the health of the culture's infants and older adults. The *political* system is a major determinant of what health programs will be available and which health practitioners may provide health services. *Legal* aspects govern the roles, functions, and standards of health professionals within cultures. *Kinship* and the *social system* often influence who will or will not receive health care and how promptly it will be provided. For example, in some cultures a person of high status (e.g., tribal leader, CEO, or king) may receive prompt care; a person of lower status (e.g., a peasant, housewife, or child) may experience a considerable waiting period for care. Because of male dominance in many cultures, men may receive care before a wife or female child. *Cultural, educational, religious,* and *philosophical* factors are closely related. They influence the type, quality, and quantity of health care considered desirable, appropriate, or acceptable to the culture. *Environmental* and *demographic* factors relate to the health needs of the culture and which strategies of care can be used in the setting.

Since the development of Leininger's Sunrise Model, several other transcultural nursing models have been developed. These include Murdock's Outline of Cultural Material, appropriate for community cultural assessment (Murdock, 1971); Bloch's Assessment Guide for Ethnic/Cultural Variation (Orque, Bloch, & Monrroy, 1983); Giger and Davidhizar's Model of Cultural Assessment (1995); The Felder Cultural Diversity Practice Model (Felder, 1995); Purnell's Conceptual Model for Cultural Competence (Purnell & Paulanka, 1998); and the Model for Developing Cultural Sensitivity (Baldwin et al., 1996). All models are useful for assessing the belief systems and health practices of individuals and groups of different cultures.

CULTURALLY SENSITIVE CARE

Kittler and Sucher (1990) suggest a four-step process to improve cultural sensitivity:

1. *Become aware of one's own cultural heritage.* Nurses should identify their own cultural values and beliefs. For example, does the nurse value stoic behavior in relation to pain? Are the rights of the individual valued over and above the rights of the family? Only by knowing one's own culture (values, practices, and beliefs) can a person be ready to learn about another's.

2. *Become aware of the client's culture as described by the client.* It is important to avoid assuming that all people of the same ethnic background have the same culture. When the nurse has knowledge of the client's culture, mutual respect between client and nurse is more likely to develop.

3. *Become aware from the client of adaptations made to live in a North American culture.* During this interview, a nurse should also identify the client's preferences in health practices, diet, hygiene, and so on.

4. *Form a nursing care plan with the client that incorporates his or her culture.* In this way, cultural values, practices, and beliefs can be incorporated with care and judgment.

Barriers to Cultural Sensitivity

Many factors can be barriers to providing culturally sensitive or culturally competent care to clients and their support persons. These factors can also affect communication and working relationships with other health care personnel. Ethnocentrism, stereotyping, prejudice, and discrimination are some of these factors.

Ethnocentrism refers to an individual's belief that his or her culture's beliefs and values are superior to those of other cultures. In the health care area, ethnocentrism means that the only valid health care beliefs

Figure 21-1

Leininger's Sunrise Model

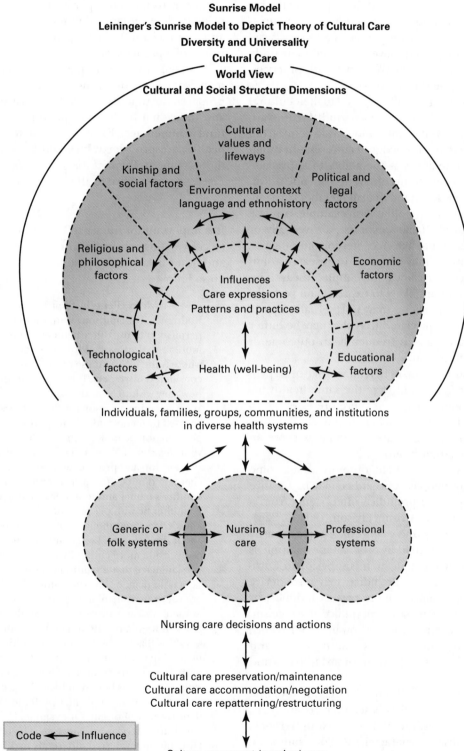

Source: From *Culture Care Diversity and Universality: A Theory of Nursing* (p. 43), by M. Leininger, 1991, New York: National League for Nursing Pub. No. 15-2402. Reprinted with permission.

and practices are those held by the health care culture. Nurses who take a transcultural view, however, value their own beliefs and practices while respecting the beliefs and practices of others. It is important for nurses to realize that although many people of differing racial and religious backgrounds have combined their traditional health practices with Western health practices, other people may be unable to do so.

Most people are gradually exposed to their cultural beliefs, values, and practices over a period of years starting at birth. Ethnocentricism is thought to result from lack of exposure to or knowledge of cultures other than one's own. **Ethnorelativity** is the ability to appreciate and respect other viewpoints different from one's own.

Stereotyping is assuming that all members of a culture or ethnic group are alike. For example, a nurse may assume that all Italians express pain verbally or that all Chinese people like rice. Stereotyping may be based on generalizations founded in research, or it may be unrelated to reality. For example, research indicates that Italians are likely to express pain verbally; however, an Italian client may not verbalize pain. Stereotyping that is unrelated to reality may be either positive or negative and is frequently an outcome of racism or discrimination.

It is important for nurses to realize that not all people of a specific group will have the same health beliefs, practices, and values. It is therefore essential to identify a specific client's beliefs, needs, and values rather than assuming they are the same as those attributable to the larger group.

Prejudice is strongly held opinion about some topic or group of people. A prejudice may be positive or negative. A positive prejudice often stems from a strong sense of ethnocentrism (Eliason, 1993, p. 226), that is, beliefs held by one's cultural group are vastly superior to the beliefs held by others. One example is that American nursing education is superior to European nursing education. Prejudice may also derive from ignorance, misinformation, past experience, or fear. Other types of negative prejudice are ageism, which includes negative attitudes toward older adults; sexism, such as negative attitudes toward women; and homophobia, which is negativism toward lesbians and gay men.

Discrimination is the differential treatment of one person or group over another based on race, ethnicity, gender, age, social class, disability, sexual preference, or other distinguishing characteristic. For example, a nurse takes a child who is waiting in an emergency department ahead of another child. The child taken first appears clean, is neatly dressed, and is smiling; the other child appears dirty, is wearing worn clothes, and is angry. **Racism** is a form of discrimination related to ethnocentrism where a person believes that race is the primary determinant of human traits and capacities and that racial differences produce an inherent superiority of a particular race.

In 2002, the U.S. Department of Health and Human Services through the Office of Minority Health prepared documents to help health care organizations and individual health care providers assess their cultural competence. Examples of statements assessing health care provider values and beliefs contained in the document *Potential Measures/Indicators of Cultural Competence* are shown in the box on page 381.

Conveying Cultural Sensitivity

It is important for nurses to be culturally sensitive and to convey this sensitivity to clients, support persons, and other health care personnel. Some of the ways to do so follow.

■ Always address clients by their last names (e.g., Mrs. Rodriguez, Dr. Simpson) until they give you permission to use other names. In some cultures, the more formal style of address is a sign of respect, whereas the informal use of first names may be considered disrespect. It is important to ask clients how they wish to be addressed.

■ When meeting a person for the first time, introduce yourself by name, and, when appropriate, explain your position, for example, "I'm Mary Johnson and I will be your Registered Nurse today." This helps establish a relationship and provides an opportunity for both clients and nurses to clarify pronunciation of one another's names and to understand the expected roles.

■ Be authentic with people, and share your lack of knowledge about their culture. When possible, ask about their cultural beliefs and practices so that you can provide more culturally appropriate care.

■ Use language that is culturally sensitive; for example, say gay, lesbian, or bisexual rather than homosexual; do not use man or mankind when referring to a woman or women. African American is currently preferred over Black, however, recent immigrants to the United States as well as Black people whose family history includes many generations in the United States, may view the term African American as referring to individuals whose ancestry is bound in the culture of slavery. Therefore, some people may prefer to be referred to by their country of origin, for example, Haitian American, Jamaican American, or Nigerian. The terms Latino and Hispanic are preferred differently in different regions of the country, for example, Latino is currently preferred in California and Texas, whereas Hispanic is preferred in Florida. Asian may be more acceptable

Measures/Indicators of Cultural Competence Values and Attitudes

- I recognize and accept that folk and religious beliefs may influence a family's reaction and approach to a child born with a disability or later diagnosed with a disability or special health care needs.

- I understand that traditional approaches to disciplining children are influenced by culture.

- I understand that families from different cultures will have different expectations of their children for acquiring toileting, dressing, feeding, and other self-help skills.

- I accept and respect that customs and beliefs about food and its value, preparation, and use are different from culture to culture.

- Before visiting or providing services in the home setting, I seek information on acceptable behaviors, courtesies, customs, and expectations that are unique to families of specific cultures and ethnic groups served by my program or agency.

- I seek information from family members or other key community informants, which will assist in service adaptation to respond to the needs and preferences of culturally and ethnically diverse children and families served by my program or agency.

- I advocate for the review of my program's or agency's mission statement, goals, policies, and procedures to ensure that they incorporate principles and practices that promote cultural diversity and cultural competence.

- I avoid imposing values that may conflict or be inconsistent with those of cultures or ethnic groups other than my own.

- In group therapy or treatment situations, I discourage children from using racial and ethnic slurs by helping them understand that certain words can hurt others.

- I intervene in an appropriate manner when I observe other staff within my program or agency engaging in behaviors that show cultural insensitivity or prejudice.

- I understand and accept that family is defined differently by different cultures.

- I recognize and accept that individuals from culturally diverse backgrounds may desire varying degrees of acculturation into the dominant culture.

- I accept and respect that male-female roles in families may vary significantly among different cultures.

- I understand that age and life cycle factors must be considered in interactions with individuals and families (e.g., high value placed on the decisions of elders or the role of the eldest male in families).

- Even though my professional or moral viewpoints may differ, I accept the family/parents as the ultimate decision makers for services and supports for their children.

- I recognize that the meaning or value of medical treatment and health education may vary greatly among cultures.

- I accept that religion and other beliefs may influence how families respond to illnesses, disease, and death.

Indicate A = things I do frequently, B = things I do occasionally, C = things I do rarely or never.

Source: From *Attachment 3: Potential Measures/Indicators of Cultural Competence* by Office of Minority Health, 2002, Washington, DC: U.S. Department of Health and Human Services. Retrieved May 26, 2004, from http://www.hrsa.gov/OMH/cultural/attachment3.htm.

than Oriental. It is important for nurses to keep up with language changes or specific language preferences appropriate to their region of practice.

■ Find out what the client knows about his or her health problems, illness, and treatments. Assess whether this information is congruent with the dominant health care culture. If the beliefs and practices are incongruent, establish whether this will have a negative effect on the client's health.

■ Do not make any assumptions about the client, and always ask about anything you do not understand.

■ Respect the client's values, beliefs, and practices, even if they differ from your own or from those of the dominant culture. If you don't agree with them, it is important to respect the client's right to hold these beliefs.

■ Show respect for the client's support people. In some cultures males in the family make decisions affecting the client, whereas in other cultures females make the decisions.

■ Make an effort to obtain the client's trust, but do not be surprised if it develops slowly or not at all.

SELECTED CULTURAL PARAMETERS INFLUENCING NURSING CARE

This section outlines selected cultural and ethnic phenomena of significance to nursing.

Health Beliefs and Practices

Andrews and Boyle (2003, p. 75–77) describe three health belief views: magico-religious, scientific, and holistic. In the **magico-religious health belief view**, health and illness are controlled by supernatural forces. The client may believe that illness is the result of "being bad" or opposing God's will. Getting well is also viewed as dependent on God's will. The client may make statements such as, "If it is God's will, I will recover," or "What did I do wrong to be punished with cancer?" Some cultures believe that magic can cause illness. A sorcerer or witch may put a spell or hex on the client. Some people view illness as possession by an evil spirit. Although these beliefs are not supported by empirical evidence, clients who believe that such things can cause illness may, in fact, become ill as a result. Such illnesses may require magical treatments in addition to scientific treatments. For example, a man who experiences gastric distress, headaches, and hypertension after being told that a spell has been placed on him may recover only if the spell is removed by the culture's healer.

The scientific, or **biomedical health belief view** is based on the belief that life and life processes are controlled by physical and biochemical processes that can be manipulated by humans (Andrews & Boyle, 2003, p. 76). The client with this view will believe that illness is caused by germs, viruses, bacteria, or a breakdown of the human machine, the body. This client will expect a pill, or treatment, or a surgery to cure health problems.

The **holistic health belief view** holds that the forces of nature must be maintained in balance or harmony. Human life is one aspect of nature that must be in harmony with the rest of nature. When the natural balance or harmony is disturbed, illness results. The Medicine Wheel is an ancient symbol used by Native Americans of North and South America to express many concepts. Related to health and wellness, the Medicine Wheel teaches the four aspects of the individual's nature: the physical, the mental, the emotional, and the spiritual. Each of the dimensions must be in balance to be healthy. The Medicine Wheel also can be used to express the individual's relationship with the environment as a dimension of wellness. The concept of yin and yang in the Chinese culture and the hot/cold theory of illness in many Spanish cultures are examples of holistic health beliefs. When the client has a yin illness, or a "cold" illness, the treatment will need to include a yang, or "hot" food. For example, a Chinese client who has been diagnosed with cancer, a yin disease, will want to eat cultural foods that have yang properties. What is considered as hot or cold varies considerably across cultures. In many cultures, the mother who has just delivered a baby should be offered warm or hot foods and kept warm with blankets, because childbirth is seen as a cold condition. Conventional scientific thought recommends cooling the body to reduce a fever. The physician may order liquids for the client and cool compresses to be applied to the forehead, the axillae, or the groin. Many cultures believe that the best way to treat a fever is to "sweat it out." Clients from these cultures may want to cover up with several blankets, take hot baths, and drink hot beverages. Giger and Davidhizar (2004) state that the nurse must keep in mind that a treatment strategy that is consistent with the client's beliefs may have a better chance of being successful. For example, the Mexican-American client who avoids "hot" foods when he has a stomach disturbance such as an ulcer may be eating foods consistent with the bland diet that is normally prescribed by physicians for clients with ulcers.

Sociocultural forces, such as politics, economics, geography, religion, and the predominant health care system, can influence the client's health status and health care behavior. For example, people who have limited access to scientific health care may turn to folk medicine or folk healing. **Folk medicine** is defined as those beliefs and practices relating to illness prevention and healing that derive from cultural traditions rather than from Western medicine's scientific base. The nurse may recall special teas or "cures" that were used by older family members to prevent or treat colds, fevers, indigestion, and other common health problems. For example, many people continue to use chicken soup as a treatment for flu.

There are many reasons why individuals use their traditional folk healing methods. Folk medicine, in contrast to biomedical health care, is thought to be more humanistic. The consultation and treatment takes place in the community of the recipient, frequently in the home of the healer. It is less expensive than scientific or biomedical care because the health problem is identified primarily through conversation with the client and the family. The healer often prepares the treatments, for example, teas to be ingested, poultices to be applied, or charms or amulets to be worn. A frequent component of treatment is some ritual practice on the part of the healer or the client to cause healing to occur. Be-

---

Critical Thinking Exercise

Consider nursing situations in your experience that reflect each of the health belief views as described by Andrews and Boyle: the magico-religious health belief view, the biomedical health belief view, and the holistic health belief view. Describe culturally competent nursing interventions that would be appropriate for each of your nursing situations.

---

cause folk healing is more culturally based, it is often more comfortable and less frightening for the client.

It is important for the nurse to obtain information about folk or family healing practices that may have been used prior to the client's seeking Western medical treatment. Often clients are reluctant to share home remedies with health care professionals for fear of being laughed at or rebuked. Nurses must remember that clients may continue to use these practices in lieu of or in addition to prescribed "Western" or scientific treatments. The nurse should remember that treatments once considered to be folk treatments, including acupuncture, therapeutic touch, and massage are now being investigated for their therapeutic effect.

Family Patterns

The family is the basic unit of society. Cultural and religious values can determine communication within the family group, the norm for family size, and the roles of specific family members. In some families the man is usually the provider and decision maker. The woman may need to consult her husband before making decisions about her medical treatment or the treatment of her children (Galanti, 1991). Some families are matriarchal; that is, the mother or grandmother is viewed as the leader of the family and is the decision maker. The nurse needs to identify who has the "authority" to make decisions in the client's family. If the decision maker is someone other than the client, the nurse needs to include that person in health care discussions.

The value placed on children and elderly within a society is culturally derived. In some cultures, children are not disciplined by spanking or other forms of physical punishment. Rather, children are allowed to interact with their environment and to learn from their environment while caregivers provide subtle direction to prevent harm or injury. In other cultures, the eld-

erly are considered the holders of the culture's wisdom and are therefore highly respected. Responsibility for caring for older relatives is determined by cultural practices. In many cultures, older relatives who cannot live independently often live with a married daughter and her family.

Culture and religious norms about sex-role behavior may also affect nurse-client interaction. In some countries, the male dominates and women have little status. The male client from these countries may not accept instruction from a female nurse or physician but be receptive to the same instruction given by a male physician or nurse (Galanti, 1991). In some cultures, there is a prevailing concept of machismo, or male superiority. The positive aspects of machismo require that the adult male provide for and protect his family, including extended family members. The woman is expected to maintain the home and raise the children.

Cultural family values may also dictate the extent of the family's involvement in the hospitalized client's care. In some cultures, the nuclear and the extended family will want to visit for long periods of time and participate in care. In other cultures, the entire clan may want to visit and participate in the client's care (Galanti, 1991). This can cause concern on nursing units with strict visiting policies. The nurse should evaluate the positive benefits of family participation in the client's care and modify visiting policies as appropriate.

Cultures that value the needs of the extended family as much as those of the individual may hold the belief that personal and family information must stay within the family. Some cultural groups are very reluctant to disclose family information to outsiders, including health care professionals. This attitude can present difficulties for health care professionals who require knowledge of family interaction patterns to help clients with emotional problems.

In many cultures naming systems differ from those in North America. In some cultures (e.g., Japanese and Vietnamese) the family name comes first and the given name, second. One or two names may or may not be added between the family and given names. Other nomenclature may be used to delineate gender, child, or adult status. For example, in traditional Japanese culture, adults address other adults by their surname followed by *san*, meaning *Mr., Mrs.,* or *Miss.* An example is Murakami-san. The children are referred to by their first names followed by *kun* for boys and *chan* for girls. Sikhs and Hindus traditionally have three names. Hindus have a personal name, a complimentary name, and then a family name. Sikhs have a personal name, then the title Singh for men and Kaur for women, and lastly the family name. Names by marriage also vary. In Central America, a woman who marries retains her father's name and takes her husband's. For example, if Louisa Viccario marries Carlos Gonzales she becomes Louisa Viccario de Gonzales. The connecting de means "belonging to." A male child will be Pedro Gonzales Viccario. Nurses need to become familiar with appropriate ways to address clients. In many cultures, using a client's first name is considered offensive or patronizing.

Communication Style

Communication style and culture are closely interconnected. Through communication, the culture is transmitted from one generation to the next, and knowledge about the culture is transmitted within the group and to those outside the group. Communicating with clients of various ethnic and cultural backgrounds is critical to providing culturally competent nursing care. Luckmann (2000, p. 15) identifies the following influencing factors for implementing transcultural communication:

1. The increase in ethnic, racial, and cultural diversity in the United States
2. The increase in cultural, ethnic, and disenfranchised populations who seek health care
3. Multicultural and multinational settings for health care delivery
4. The commitment of health care professions to provide high-quality, culturally appropriate care

Verbal Communication

The most obvious cultural difference is in verbal communication: vocabulary, grammatical structure, voice qualities, intonation, rhythm, speed, pronunciation, and silence (Giger & Davidhizar, 2004, p. 25). In North America, the dominant language is English; however, immigrant groups who speak English still encounter language differences, because English words can have different meanings in different English-speaking cultures. For example, in the United States a boot is a type of footwear that comes to the ankle or higher; in England, a boot also can be the trunk of a car. Spanish is spoken by people in several regions of the world: Spain, South America, Central America, Mexico, the Caribbean, and the Philippines. It is the second most commonly spoken language in the United States. Nevertheless, each cultural group that speaks Spanish may use different vocabulary, apply rules of grammar differently, and use different pronunciation, so that often two people of different Latino cultures, speaking Spanish together, may not completely understand each other.

Initiating verbal communication may be influenced by cultural values. The busy nurse may want to complete nursing admission assessments quickly. The client, however, may be offended when the nurse immediately asks personal questions. In some cultures, it is believed that social courtesies should be established before business or personal topics are discussed. Discussing general topics can convey that the nurse is interested in the client and has time for the client. This enables the nurse to develop a rapport with the client before progressing to more personal discussion.

Verbal communication becomes even more difficult when an interaction involves people who speak different languages. Both clients and health professionals experience frustration when they are unable to communicate verbally with each other. For clients who have limited knowledge of English, the nurse should avoid slang words, medical terminology, and abbreviations. Augmenting spoken conversation with gestures or pictures can increase the client's understanding. The nurse should speak slowly, in a respectful manner and at a normal volume. Speaking loudly does not help the client understand and may be offensive. The nurse must also frequently validate the client's understanding of what is being communicated. The nurse must be wary of interpreting a client's smiling and head nodding to mean that the client understands; the client may only be trying to please the nurse and not understand what is being said.

For the client who speaks a different language, a translator may be necessary. Andrews and Boyle (2003) suggest that it is best to use a professional medical interpreter who can facilitate communication between people speaking different languages in a health care setting. Guidelines for using an interpreter are shown in the box on page 385.

Translators should be objective individuals who can provide accurate translation of the client's information and of the health professional's questions, information, and instruction. Many institutions that are located in culturally diverse communities have translators available on staff or maintain a list of employees who are fluent in other languages. Embassies, consulates, ethnic churches (e.g., Russian Orthodox, Greek Orthodox), ethnic clubs (e.g., Polish American Club, Italian American Club) or telephone communication companies may also be able to provide translating services. Nursing and other health personnel can use pictures and gestures to augment verbal communication. Some schools of nursing and health care institutions do not permit nursing students to translate for a procedure consent because a lack of knowledge about the procedure may lead the student to give inaccurate information. The student should check the

Using an Interpreter

- Avoid asking a member of the client's family, especially a child or spouse, to act as interpreter. The client, not wishing family members to know about his or her problem, may not provide complete or accurate information.

- Be aware of gender and age differences; it is preferable to use an interpreter of the same sex as the client to avoid embarrassment and faulty translation of sexual matters.

- Avoid an interpreter who is politically or socially incompatible with the client. For example, a Bosnian Serb may not be the best interpreter for a Muslim, even if he speaks the language.

- Address the questions to the client, not to the interpreter.

- Ask the interpreter to translate as closely as possible to the words used by the nurse.

- Speak slowly and distinctly. Do not use metaphors, for example, "Does it swell like a grapefruit?" or "Is the pain stabbing like a knife?"

- Observe the facial expressions and body language that the client assumes when listening and talking to the interpreter.

institution's policy before agreeing to translate for institutional staff and physicians.

Nurses and other health care providers must remember that clients for whom English is a second language may lose command of their English when they are in stressful situations. It is not uncommon for clients who have used English comfortably for years in social and business communication to forget and revert back to their primary language when they are ill or distressed. It is important for the nurse to assure the client that this is normal and to promote behaviors that facilitate verbal communication.

Nonverbal Communication

To communicate effectively with culturally diverse clients, the nurse needs to be aware of two aspects of nonverbal communication behaviors: what nonverbal behaviors mean to the client and what specific nonverbal behaviors mean in the client's culture. It is not required that the nurse be knowledgeable about the nonverbal behavior patterns of all cultures; however, before the nurse assigns meaning to nonverbal behavior, the nurse must consider the possibility that the behavior may have a different meaning for the client and the family. Furthermore, to provide safe and effective care, nurses who work with specific cultural groups should learn more about cultural behavior and communication patterns within those cultures.

Nonverbal communication can include the use of silence, touch, eye movement, facial expressions, and body posture. It also includes cultural perceptions of

space orientation and distance. Some cultures are quite comfortable with long periods of silence, whereas others consider it appropriate to speak before the other person has finished talking. Many persons value silence and view it as essential to understanding a person's needs or use silence to preserve privacy. Some cultures view silence as a sign of respect, whereas to other persons silence may indicate agreement (Andrews & Boyle, 2003, p. 27).

Touch and touching is a learned behavior that can have both positive and negative meanings. In the American culture, a firm handshake is a recognized form of greeting that conveys character and strength (Giger & Davidhizar, 2004, p. 31). In some European cultures, greetings may include a kiss on one or both cheeks along with the handshake. In some societies, touch is considered magical and because of the belief that the soul can leave the body on physical contact, casual touching is forbidden. In the Hmong culture, only certain elders are permitted to touch the head of others, and children are never patted on the head. Nurses should therefore touch a client's head only with permission (Rairdan and Higgs, 1992, p. 55). The sex of the person touching and being touched often has cultural significance. Purnell and Paulanka (2003, p. 16) describe how among Egyptian-Americans, touch between men and women is accepted "in private and only between husband and wife, parents and children, and adult brothers and sisters."

Cultures also dictate what forms of touch are appropriate for individuals of the same sex and opposite sex. In many cultures, for example, a kiss is not appropriate for a public greeting between persons of the opposite sex, even those who are family members; however, a kiss on the cheek is acceptable as a greeting among individuals of the same sex. The nurse should watch interaction among clients and families for cues to the appropriate degree of touch in that culture. The nurse can also assess the client's response to touch when providing nursing care, for example, by noting the client's reaction to the physical examination or the bath.

Facial expression can also vary between cultures. Giger and Davidhizar (2004, p. 32) state that Italian, Jewish, African-American, and Spanish-speaking persons are more likely to smile readily and use facial expression to communicate feelings, whereas Irish, English, northern European, and Asian persons tend to have less facial expression and are less open in their response, especially to strangers. Facial expression can also convey the opposite meaning of what is felt or understood. For example, clients who have difficulty understanding English may smile and nod their heads as though they understood what is being said, when, in fact, they do not understand at all, but do not want to displease the caregiver.

Eye movement during communication has cultural foundations. In Western cultures, direct eye contact is regarded as important and generally shows that the other is attentive and listening. It conveys self-confidence, openness, interest, and honesty. Lack of eye contact may be interpreted as secretiveness, shyness, guilt, lack of interest, or even a sign of mental illness. Other cultures may view eye contact as impolite or an invasion of privacy. In the Hmong culture, continuous direct eye contact is considered rude, but intermittent eye contact is acceptable (Rairdan & Higgs, 1992, p. 53). The nurse should not misinterpret the character of the client who avoids eye contact.

Body posture and gestures are also culturally learned. Finger pointing, the "V" sign with the index and middle fingers, and the "thumbs up" sign may have different meanings. For example, the "V" sign means victory in some cultures, whereas it may be an offensive gesture in other cultures (Galanti, 1991, p. 22). In the Hmong culture, bowing the head slightly when entering the room where an elder is present or using both hands to give something to someone are considered signs of respect (Rairdan & Higgs, 1993, p. 52).

Communication is an essential part of establishing a relationship with a client and his or her family. It is also important for developing effective working relationships with health care colleagues. To enhance their practice, nurses can observe the communication patterns of clients and colleagues and be aware of their own communication behaviors. The accompanying box provides strategies for communicating with clients from different cultures. The same strategies can be used in communication with professional colleagues.

Strategies for Communicating with Clients from Different Cultures

- Consider the cultural component of communication, and integrate it into the relationship.

- Encourage the client to communicate cultural interpretations of health, illness, treatments, and planned care. Incorporate this into the plan of care so that it is congruent with the client's lifestyle and needs as the client views them.

- Understand that respect for clients and their communicated needs is crucial to the effective helping relationship.

- Use an open and attentive approach so that the client knows you are really listening.

- Relate to the client in an unhurried manner that considers the social and cultural amenities. Give the client time to answer. Engage in appropriate social conversation before discussing more intimate or personal details.

- Use validation techniques while communicating to check that the client understands. Note that big smiles and frequent head nodding may indicate merely that the client is trying to please you, not necessarily that the client understands you.

- Sexual concerns may be difficult for clients to discuss. Try to have a nurse of the same sex as the client discuss sexual matters.

- Use alternative methods of communication for clients who do not speak English: foreign language dictionaries or phrase books, interpreter, gestures, pictures, facial expressions, tone of voice.

- Learn key phrases in languages that are commonly spoken in the community. For example, medical phrase books are available in Spanish and French.

Reflect on...

■ your own values, beliefs, and practices related to verbal and nonverbal communication. How might your values, beliefs, and practices related to communication conflict with those of people from the different cultural groups in your community? What strategies will you implement to improve your communication with people of other cultures?

Space Orientation

Space is a relative concept that includes the individual, the body, the surrounding environment, and objects within that environment. The relationship between the individual's own body and objects and persons within space is learned and is influenced by culture. For example, in nomadic societies space is not owned; it is occupied temporarily until the tribe moves on. In Western societies people tend to be more territorial, as reflected in phrases such as "This is my space" or "Get out of my space." In Western cultures, spatial distances are defined as the intimate zone, the personal zone, the social zone, and the public zones. The intimate zone is the smallest area of space around the individual, the public zone the largest area. The size of these areas may vary within different cultures. Nurses move through all four zones as they provide care for clients: the intimate zone when they listen to heart and breath sounds, the personal zone when adjusting an intravenous flow rate, and the social zone when greeting the client on entering the room. Nurses who are teaching community education classes are working in the public zone. The nurse needs to be aware of the client's response to movement toward the client. The client may physically withdraw or back away if the nurse is perceived as being too close. The nurse will need to explain to the client why there is a need to be close to the client. To assess the lungs with a stethoscope, for example, the nurse needs to move into the client's intimate space. The nurse should first explain the procedure and await permission to continue.

Clients who reside in long-term care facilities, or are hospitalized for an extended time, may want to personalize their space. They may want to arrange their space differently and control the placement of objects on their bedside cabinet or over-bed table. The nurse should be responsive to clients' needs to have some control over their space. When there are no medical contraindications, clients should be permitted and encouraged to wear their own clothing and have objects of personal significance. Wearing cultural dress or having personal, cultural, and spiritual items in one's environment can increase self-esteem by promoting not only one's individuality but also one's cultural identity. Of course, the nurse should caution the client about responsibility for loss of personal items.

Time Orientation

Time orientation refers to an individual's focus on the past, the present, or the future. Most cultures combine all three time orientations, but one orientation is more likely to dominate. The European American focus on time tends to be directed to the future, emphasizing time and schedules (Purnell & Paulanka, 2003). Nursing students know what times they "must" be in class or clinical. They know what courses they will take in future semesters. European Americans often plan for next week, their vacation, or their retirement. Other cultures may have a different concept of time. Leininger (1978, pp. 256, 262) describes the Navajo emphasis as "on the flow of life within the natural environment without specific time boundaries." For example, a Navajo mother may not be concerned about when her child achieves developmental milestones, such as walking or toileting.

The culture of nursing and health care values time. Appointments are scheduled and treatments are prescribed with time parameters (e.g., changing a dressing once a day). Medication orders include how often the medicine is to be taken and when (e.g., digoxin 0.25 mg, once a day, in the morning). Nurses need to be aware of the meaning of time for clients. Giger and Davidhizar (2004, p. 112) state that when caring for clients who are "present-oriented," it is important to avoid fixed schedules. The nurse can offer a time range for activities and treatments. For example, instead of telling the client to take digoxin every day at 10:00 A.M., the nurse might tell the client to take it every day in the morning, or every day after getting out of bed.

Nutritional Patterns

Most cultures have staple foods, that is, foods that are plentiful or readily accessible in the environment. For example, the staple food of Asians is rice; of Italians, pasta; and of Eastern Europeans, wheat. Even clients who have been in the United States or Canada for several generations often continue to eat the foods of their cultural homeland.

The way food is prepared and served is also related to cultural practices. For example, in the United States, a traditional food served for the Thanksgiving holiday is stuffed turkey; however, in different regions of the country the contents of the stuffing may vary. In Southern states, the stuffing may be made of cornbread; in New England, of seasoned bread and chestnuts.

The ways in which staple foods are prepared also varies. For example, some Asian cultures prefer steamed rice; others prefer boiled rice. Southern Asians from India prepare unleavened bread from wheat flour rather than the leavened bread of Anglo-Americans.

Food-related cultural behaviors can include whether to breast-feed or bottle-feed infants, and when to introduce solid foods to them. Food can also be considered part of the remedy for illness. Foods classified as "hot" foods or foods that are hot in temperature may be used to treat illnesses that are classified as "cold" illnesses. For example, corn meal (a "hot" food) may be used to treat arthritis (a "cold" illness). Each cultural group defines what it considers to be hot and cold entities.

Reflect on...

- the nutritional content of the foods of various cultures. Identify the food preferences of cultural groups in your community. How do these diets fulfill nutritional requirements? What nutritional deficiencies exist in these diets?

Pain Responses

Research has demonstrated that beliefs about and responses to pain vary among ethnic/racial groups. Cultural response to pain must be viewed in relation both to the actual perception of pain and to the meaning or significance of pain to the client and family. In some cultures, pain may be considered a punishment for bad deeds; the individual is, therefore, to tolerate pain without complaint in order to atone for sins. In other cultures, self-infliction of pain is a sign of mourning or grief. In other groups, pain may be anticipated as a part of the ritualistic practices of passage ceremonies, and therefore tolerance of pain signifies strength and endurance. In yet other cultures, the expression of pain elicits attention and sympathy, while in other cultures, boys especially are taught "to take pain like a man" and "big boys don't cry."

Cavillo and Flaskerud (1991, p. 16) found that nurses and clients assess pain differently. In a study of Mexican American clients with pain, they found that nurses and physicians tend to underestimate and undertreat their client's pain in relation to the client's expression of pain. Client responses to pain should be assessed within the context of their culture. If the client does not complain of pain, it should not be assumed that the client is not experiencing pain. The nurse must be aware of what conditions are likely to cause pain and offer clients pain relief as appropriate.

Evidence for Practice

McCarthy, P., Chammas, G., Wilimas, J., Alaoui, F. M., & Harif, M. (2004). Managing chilren's cancer pain in Morocco. *Journal of Nursing Scholarship*, *1*(36), 11–15.

The purpose of this study was to identify issues related to the management of pain in children with cancer in two pediatric oncology centers in Morocco. Focus groups were conducted with pediatric oncology nurses and physicians to determine their concerns in the management of pediatric cancer pain. Four themes were identified: (1) Moroccan nurses and physicians who participated in the study had an overwhelming concern about children's cancer pain; (2) training and resources for children's cancer pain management are lacking in Morocco; (3) some barriers to pain relief were verbalized, such as a stoic approach to suffering and limited use of some drugs; and (4) there is a critical need for a comprehensive pain management approach for children with cancer in Morocco. The study helped the participating nurses increase their knowledge of pediatric pain assessment and management, and cultural issues related to pain management in children with cancer in Morocco.

Treatment for pain may also vary with culture. In European American cultures, medication is typically used for pain relief. In other cultures, heat, cold, relaxation, meditation, or other techniques and treatments may be used.

Childbirth and Perinatal Care
Prenatal Care

In North America, emphasis is placed on regular prenatal medical visits, dental care, prenatal classes for both parents, and avoidance of communicable disease. These practices are accepted in varying degrees by people of other cultures. To some, for example, regular medical checkups are often avoided because they are equated with problems or abnormalities. Traditionally, these women will see a physician only if there is a problem.

Many immigrants may also prefer not to attend prenatal classes for a variety of reasons. Some of these relate to language problems or discomfort and embarrassment about doing exercises in front of others, discussing sexual matters, or seeing movies about childbirth.

Because in many cultures pregnancy and childbirth are considered the exclusive realm of women, some women prefer to have a female friend or relative attend prenatal classes and the birth rather than the husband. Nurses need to respect this choice. However, some new immigrant husbands, in the absence of a mother, mother-in-law or other female, may indicate interest in attending prenatal classes and the birth, if only to act as interpreters for their wives.

Prenatal practices vary in regard to safeguarding the health of the fetus and mother. People in several cultures (e.g., Mexican Americans, Asians, Chinese) emphasize the equilibrium model of health—that is, balancing yin and yang or "hot" and "cold"—during pregnancy. Pregnant women therefore avoid too much "hot" or "cold" food as determined by their culture. Some women believe that "hot" foods during the first trimester of pregnancy can cause miscarriage or a premature delivery; as a result, they emphasize the ingestion of "cool" foods, such as some fruit, coconut, buttermilk, and yogurt, and the avoidance of "hot" foods, such as meat, nuts, and eggs, during this period. It is important to note that "hot" and "cold" do not necessarily relate to the temperature of the food, but rather to the balancing or holistic characteristic of the food.

Labor and Delivery

In some cultures, pregnant women traditionally return to their parents' home for the delivery of the first child and, sometimes, subsequent births. Births in the home are usually managed by a midwife with the assistance of the woman's mother, mother-in-law, or married sister. Traditionally, the husband is not present. In other cultures, childbirth takes place in homes, hospitals, and clinics and is attended by physicians and certified midwives.

Positions used for delivery vary from the standard lithotomy position of North Americans. For example, squatting, kneeling, sitting, or standing may be preferred.

Responses to labor pain vary. Some women of certain cultures tolerate considerable pain and stoically accept pain for many reasons. They may, for example, want to avoid showing weakness or calling undue attention to themselves for fear of shaming themselves and their families, or they may act accordingly simply because it is expected behavior within their culture. In other cultures, women express pain and anguish more freely. For example, screaming and sobbing are acceptable and expected responses. It is important for the nurse to know that the absence of crying and moaning does not necessarily mean that pain is absent, nor does the presence of crying and moaning necessarily mean that pain relief is desired at that moment. With clients from some cultures, nurses may use touching and the support of others (husband, female relative, or friend) to decrease pain during labor. Various other cultures may or may not value the same comfort measures. Pain-relief medications may also be used, but some clients are hesitant to request them.

Postpartum Care

Most cultures emphasize certain postpartal routines or rituals for mother and baby. These are frequently designed to restore harmony or the "hot"-"cold" balance of the body. In many cultures, the mother's health status is classified as "cold" due to stress and the loss of blood. Thus, people take care to warm the body and to avoid cold after birth. This prohibition includes cold air and wind, as well as designated foods and fluids. Showers, tub baths, and shampoos are restricted, often until the lochia stops or longer, to avoid chilling. Sponge baths may be taken using warm water and/or special products that have medicinal properties. Foods considered "hot" by the specific culture are provided, whereas foods considered "cold" are avoided. Some women may wear binders around the abdomen and perineum not only to protect the body from cold but also to aid the uterus to return to its normal size. Mexican Americans may also cover the head, body, and feet to avoid cold air, infection, and other problems, such as sterility.

Confinement periods also vary and in many cultures are considerably longer than that of the health care system of North America. For example, traditional Chinese practice a "sitting in" period for one month to avoid cold winds. This confinement also applies to the newborn. New Mexican American mothers may remain in bed for three days following delivery, begin to walk inside the home after one week, and may go outside after two weeks.

For most cultures, the extended family frequently plays an essential role during the postnatal period. A grandmother, mother, mother-in-law, aunt, or married sister may be the primary helper for the mother and newborn. This gives the new mother time to rest as well as access to someone who can help with problems and concerns as they arise.

THE NEWBORN   Breast-feeding is the traditional feeding method in most cultures. However, bottle-feeding is becoming more common among women who are employed. The current emphasis in North America on breast-feeding is confusing to some new immigrants because effective advertising campaigns have convinced women of the superiority of bottle-feeding; they believe babies grow faster on the formulas. Nurses need to provide additional encouragement and clear explanations for these women. In some cultures, newborn babies may have a coin placed on the umbilicus or their waist tied with a belly-band to prevent a protruding umbilicus or hernia.

It is important to remember that younger members of a specific cultural group may have been acculturated to the dominant culture and no longer follow traditional practices. In other instances, they follow some practices but not others. Sensitive nurses can work toward a blending of old and new behaviors to meet the goals of all concerned.

Death and Dying

Death is a universal experience, and people want to die with dignity. Various cultural traditions and practices associated with death, dying, and the grieving process help people cope with these experiences. Nurses are often present through the dying process and at the moment of death, especially when it occurs in a health care facility. Knowledge of the client's cultural heritage helps nurses provide individualized care to clients and their families, even though they may not participate in the rituals associated with death.

Dying in solitude is generally unacceptable in most cultures. In many cultures, people prefer a peaceful death at home rather than in the hospital. Some ethnic groups may request that health professionals not reveal the prognosis to dying clients. They believe the person's last days should be free of worry and pain. People in other cultures prefer that a family member (preferably a male in some cultures) be told the diagnosis so that the client can be tactfully informed by a family member in gradual stages or not be told at all. Nurses also need to determine whom to call, and when, as the impending death draws near.

Beliefs and attitudes about death, its cause, and the soul also vary among cultures. Unnatural deaths, or "bad deaths," are sometimes distinguished from

Evidence for Practice

Carolan, M. (2000). Menopause: Irish women's voices. *Journal of Obstetric, Gynecologic, and Neonatal Nursing, 29*(4), 397–404.

This phenomenological study focused on understanding the cultural meanings of menopause for Irish women. Colaizzi's method of qualitative analysis was used to analyze the stories of Irish women. Six Irish women were interviewed 1 to 6 years after menopause; they were each the mother of five or more surviving children. Women who wished for more children were excluded from the study. They lived in small villages in rural southern Ireland and were interviewed in their homes.

Three themes were predominant in the stories of the women. One was a sense of relief, principally relief from continued childbearing. The second theme was acceptance as a natural event; they expressed that life was as full as ever, and menopause had not significantly affected their lives. The third theme was a sense of satisfaction at having successfully raised their families; they looked forward to a quieter life invested in grandparenting.

These results were interpreted in the sociocultural context of a predominantly Catholic religion with high values on family. Family sizes tend to be large and spacing options for births are limited. The women have very busy lives with homemaking, child care, and farmwork. Rural Irish women experience menopause as a normal process of aging and do not associate it with illness. This supports the view that menopause is a complex phenomenon experienced within a sociocultural context.

"good deaths." The death of a person who has behaved well in life is considered less threatening because that person will be reincarnated into a good life.

Reflect on...

- personal cultural beliefs and practices related to death and dying.
- cultural beliefs and practices related to death and dying among people of the different cultural groups in your community. How can the nurse support the client and family in the performance of death and dying practices?

PROVIDING CULTURALLY COMPETENT CARE

All phases of the nursing process are affected by the client's and the nurse's cultural values, beliefs, and behaviors. As the client and the nurse come together in the nurse-client relationship, a unique cultural environment is created that can improve or impair the client's outcome. Self-awareness of personal biases can enable nurses to modify behaviors or (if they are unable to modify behaviors) to remove themselves from situations where care might be compromised. Nurses can become more aware of their own cultural values through values-clarification activities. Nurses must also consider the cultural values of the health care setting because they, too, may influence a client's outcome.

To obtain cultural assessment data, nurses use broad statements and open-ended questions that encourage clients to express themselves fully. The important principle to remember when conducting an assessment is that "the client is the teacher and expert regarding his or her culture, and the nurse is the learner" (Rosenbaum, 1995, p. 188). At this stage nurses make no conclusions but obtain information from clients.

There are several cultural assessment tools available. Nurses need to use tools that are appropriate to the situation and adapt them as required. For example, a nurse in an emergency department of an urban hospital may need a different format than a nurse working in a home care setting. It is unnecessary to complete a total cultural assessment for every client. Instead, nurses need to collect enough basic data to identify patterns of behavior that may either facilitate or interfere with a nursing strategy or treatment plan.

Anderson et al. (1990, pp. 256–262) emphasize the following points relevant to cultural assessment.

- A cultural assessment takes time and usually needs to extend over several time periods.
- Recognition of one's own ethnicity and social background is essential. Even when the nurse and client share the same ethnic background, the nurse should expect differences in beliefs and values.
- The process of assessment is important. How and when questions are asked requires sensitivity and clinical judgment.
- The timing and phrasing of questions need to be adapted to the individual. Timing is important in introducing questions. Sensitivity is needed in phrasing questions.
- Trust needs to be established before clients can be expected to volunteer and share sensitive information.

The nurse, therefore, needs to spend time with the clients, introduce some social conversation, and convey a genuine desire to understand their values and beliefs.

Before a cultural assessment begins, the nurse determines what language the client speaks and the client's degree of fluency in the English language. The nurse can also learn about the client's communication patterns and space orientation by observing both verbal and nonverbal communication. For example, does the client speak for himself or herself or defer to another? What nonverbal communication behaviors does the client exhibit (e.g., touching, eye contact)? What significance do these behaviors have for the nurse-client interaction? What is the client's proximity to other people and objects within the environment? How does the client react to the nurse's movement toward the client? What cultural objects within the environment have importance for health promotion/health maintenance?

For the initial cultural assessment, regardless of the approach used, nurses should ask themselves the following questions (Grant, 1994, pp. 180–181):

- What does the client think about the nature of the illness? What does the client believe to be its cause? How does the client usually deal with the problem? How can others help?
- What support systems are available to the client? Is support from family, religious, community, or ethnic groups available to the client during and after treatment? Does the client need assistance contacting these individuals?
- What treatments is the client using to maintain health and fight illness? Are nontraditional healers involved? What remedies or treatments are ongoing or under consideration? What assistance will be needed from the health care institution or staff to accommodate a combined approach to the problem?
- What biologic and social factors should the nurse consider when planning client care? What health care risks and individual needs characterize the client's culture? What communication problems might occur?
- What does the client want from traditional medicine? What problems are foreseeable? What decisions can be anticipated? How might any legal or ethical problems be addressed?

As the client answers these questions, the sensitive nurse will identify other concerns and issues that can be queried. Examples of open-ended questions to elicit cultural data are shown in the box on page 392.

To provide culturally congruent care that benefits, satisfies, and is meaningful to the people nurses serve,

Examples of Open-Ended Questions for a Cultural Assessment

CULTURAL AFFILIATION

I am interested in learning about your cultural heritage. Can you tell me about your cultural group, where you were born, and how long you have lived in this country?

BELIEFS ABOUT CURRENT ILLNESS

What do you call your problem? What name do you give it? What do you think has caused it? Why did it start when it did? What does your sickness do to your body? How severe is it? What do you fear most about your sickness? What are the chief problems your sickness has caused for you personally, for your family, and at work?

HEALTH CARE PRACTICES

What kinds of things do you do to maintain health? For example, what types of food do you eat to maintain health? What foods do you eat during illness, and how is food prepared? What other activities do you or your family do to keep people healthy (e.g., wearing amulets, religious or spiritual practices)? How do you know when you are healthy?

ILLNESS BELIEFS AND CARE PRACTICES

What kinds of things do you do to treat illnesses? Do you use traditional healers (shaman, curandero, priest, spiritualist, minister, monk)? Who determines when a person is sick? How would you describe your past experiences with cultural healers and Western health professionals? What special remedies are generally used for the illness you have? What remedies are you currently using (e.g., herbal remedies, potions, massage, wearing of talismans, copper bracelets, or charms)? What remedies have you used in the past, and which did you find helpful? What remedies or treatments are you considering now, and how can we help?

FAMILY LIFE AND SUPPORT SYSTEM

I would like to learn about your family. Who are the members of your family? What family duties do women and men usually perform in your culture? Whom do you consult when making health care decisions (e.g., other family member, cultural or religious leader)? Who will be able to help you during and after treatment? Do you need help to contact these people?

Sources: From *Transcultural Concepts in Nursing Care* (4th ed.), by M. M. Andrews and J. S. Boyle, 2003, Philadelphia: Lippincott. *Cross Cultural Caring: A Handbook for Health Professionals in Western Canada* (pp. 245–267) by N. Waxler-Morrison, J. Anderson, and E. Richardson (Eds.), 1990, Vancouver, BC: UBC Press, "A Cultural Assessment Guide: Learning Cultural Sensitivity," by J. N. Rosenbaum, April 1991, *Canadian Nurse, 88,* 32–33; and "Culture, Illness and Care," by A. Kleinman, L. Eisenberg, and B. Good, 1978, *Annals of Internal Medicine, 88,* 251–258.

Leininger (1991, pp. 41–42) conceptualizes three major modes to guide nursing judgments, decisions, and actions:

1. *Cultural care preservation and/or maintenance.* The nurse accepts and complies with the client's cultural beliefs. For example, the nurse provides herbal tea to ease a "nervous stomach," a practice the client says has worked well in the past.

2. *Cultural care accommodation and/or negotiation.* The nurse plans, negotiates, and accommodates the client's culturally specific food preferences, religious practices, kinship needs, child-care practices, and treatment practices.

3. *Cultural care repatterning or restructuring.* The nurse is knowledgeable about cultural care and develops ways to repattern or restructure nursing care.

Cultural care preservation may involve, for example, encouraging the use of cultural health care prac-

tices, such as ingesting herbal tea, chicken soup, or "hot" or "cold" foods to the ill client. Accommodating the client's viewpoint and negotiating appropriate care require expert communication skills, such as responding empathetically, validating information, and effectively summarizing content. Negotiation is a collaborative process. It acknowledges that the nurse-client relationship is reciprocal and that differences exist between the nurse and client about notions of health, illness, and treatment. The nurse attempts to bridge the gap between the nurse's (scientific) and the client's (cultural) perspectives. During the negotiation process, the nurse first elicits the client's views and acknowledges these views and then, if appropriate, provides relevant scientific information. If the client's views reveal that certain behaviors would not affect the client's condition adversely, then the nurse incorporates these views in planning care. If the client's views can lead to harmful behaviors, then the

Critical Thinking Exercise

Interview a client using the open-ended questions in the box on page 392. Observe their verbal and non-verbal communication. What nursing interventions will be required to provide culturally competent care to this client? How will you identify and evaluate the client's response to your interventions? What other family members or significant others will be important in the delivery of culturally competent nursing care to this client?

nurse attempts to shift the client's perspectives to the scientific view. Negotiation therefore occurs when cultural treatment practices conflict with those of the health care system and when the cultural practices are considered harmful to the client's well-being. The nurse must determine precisely how the client is managing the illness, what practices could be harmful, and which practices can be safely combined with Western medicine. For example, reducing dosages of an antihypertensive medication or replacing insulin therapy with herbal measures may be detrimental. In situations where harm may occur, the nurse needs to inform the client about possible outcomes. When a client chooses to follow only cultural practices and refuses all prescribed medical or nursing interventions, the

Critical Thinking Exercise

Interview a colleague of a different culture than yourself about his or her beliefs and practices related to communication, health and illness care, family and kinship patterns, space orientation, time orientation, nutritional patterns and preferences, pain responses, childbirth practices, childrearing practices, and death and dying. How do your colleague's beliefs and practices differ from your own? What did you learn from this interview that would help you provide more culturally competent care to clients of different cultures?

nurse needs to adjust the client's goals. Anderson et al. (1990, p. 264) point out that monitoring the client's condition to identify changes in health state and to recognize impending crises before they become irreversible may be all that is realistically achievable. At a time of crisis, the nurse may then have the opportunity to renegotiate the original care approach.

Transcultural nursing care is challenging. It requires discovery of the meaning of the client's behavior, flexibility, creativity, and knowledge to adapt nursing interventions. For example, a culturally sensitive nurse knows that a Chinese woman who has just given birth and refuses to eat fruit and vegetables, refuses to drink the cold water at her bedside, stays in bed, and refuses to take sitz baths, baths, or showers needs to increase the return of yang forces. The nurse will make plans to adapt nursing interventions accordingly.

Nurses also need to identify community resources that are available to assist clients of different cultures. Nurses should try to learn from each transcultural nursing situation they encounter to improve the delivery of culture-specific care to future clients. The accompanying box offers suggestions for providing culturally competent nursing care.

Providing Culturally Competent Care

- Learn the rituals, customs, and practices of the major cultural groups with whom you come into contact. Learn to appreciate the richness of diversity as an asset rather than a hindrance in your practice.

- Identify personal biases, attitudes, prejudices, and stereotypes.

- Incorporate culture practices into care. Recognize that cultural symbols and practices can often bring a client comfort.

- Include cultural assessment of the client and family as part of overall assessment.

- Recognize that it is the client's (or family's) right to make their own health care choices.

- Provide the services of an interpreter if one is needed.

- Convey respect and cooperate with traditional healers and caregivers.

Reflect on...

■ resources (e.g., churches, synagogues, or mosques; civic groups; embassies or consulates; and so on) available in your community that will assist health care providers in delivering culturally competent care.

■ the value of learning the language of culturally different clients in your community. What resources are available in your community for nurses to learn different languages or phrases related to health care?

EXPLORE MEDIALINK

Questions, critical thinking exercises, essay activities, and other interactive resources for this chapter can be found on the Web site at http://www.prenhall.com/blais. Click on Chapter 21 to select activities for this chapter.

Bookshelf

Books that describe the African American experience:
Angelou, M. (1997). *I know why the caged bird sings.* **New York: Bantam Books.**
Ellison, R. (1947). *Invisible man.* **New York: Vintage.**
Walker, A. (1982). *The color purple.* **New York: Washington Square Press.**
Books that describe the Asian experience:
Tan, A. (1989). *The joy luck club.* **New York: Vintage.**
Books that describe the Hispanic experience:
Marquez, G. G. (1985). *Love in the time of cholera.* **New York: Penguin Books.**

Santiago, E., & M. Asher. (1994). *When I was Puerto Rican.* **Cambridge, MA: Perseus Publishing.**
Book that describes the Irish American experience:
McCourt, F. (1999). *Angela's ashes.* **New York: Simon & Schuster.**
Book that describes the Indian American experience:
Lahiri, J. (2003). *The namesake.* **New York: Houghton Mifflin Company.**

SUMMARY

North Americans come from a variety of ethnic and cultural backgrounds, and many North Americans retain at least some of their traditional values, beliefs, and practices. Many groups in North America are bicultural; that is, they embrace two cultures: their original ethnic culture and a North American culture. An individual's ethnic and cultural background can influence values, beliefs, and practices. Through acculturation, most ethnic and cultural groups in North America modify some of their traditional cultural characteristics.

Health beliefs and practices, family patterns, communication style, space and time orientation, nutritional patterns, pain response, childbirth and perinatal care, death and dying practices, and ethnic-related problems influence the relationship between a nurse and a client who have different cultural and spiritual backgrounds.

Nurses must be aware of their own cultural beliefs because they may affect the care they give. When assessing a client, a nurse considers the client's cultural values, beliefs, and practices related to health and health care. It is the responsibility of nurses not only to be aware of cultural difference, but also to be culturally sensitive and to provide culturally competent nursing care.

REFERENCES

American Nurses Association. (1991). *Position statement on cultural diversity in nursing practice.* Washington, DC: ANA.

American Nurses Association. (2004). *Nursing: Scope and standards of practice.* Washington, DC: ANA.

Anderson, J. M., Waxler-Morrison, N., Richardson, E., Herbert, C., & Murphy, M. (1990). Delivering culturally-sensitive health care. In N. Waxler-Morrison, J. Anderson, & E. Richardson, *Cross cultural caring: A handbook for health professionals in Western Canada* (pp. 245–267). Vancouver, BC: UBC Press.

Andrews, M. M., & Boyle, J. S. (1999). *Transcultural concepts in nursing care,* (3rd ed.). Philadelphia: Lippincott.

Andrews, M. M., & Boyle, J. S. (2003). *Transcultural concepts in nursing,* (4th ed.). Philadelphia: Lippincott.

Baldwin, D., Cotanch, P., Johnson, P., & Williams, J. (1996). *An Afrocentric approach to breast and cervical cancer early detection and screening.* Washington, DC: ANA.

Calvillo, E. R., & Flaskerud, J. H. (1991, Winter). Review of literature on culture and pain of adults with focus on Mexican Americans. *Journal of Transcultural Nursing, 2,* 16–23.

Carolan, M. (2000). Menopause: Irish women's voices. *Journal of Obstetric, Gynecologic, and Neonatal Nursing, 29*(4), 397–404.

Eliason, M. J. (1993, September/October). Ethics and transcultural nursing care. *Nursing Outlook, 41,* 225–228.

Felder, E. (1995). Integrating culturally diverse theoretical concepts into the education preparation of the advanced practice nurse: The cultural diversity practice model. *Journal of Cultural Diversity, 2,* 88–92.

Galanti, G. (1991). *Caring for patients from different cultures.* Philadelphia: University of Pennsylvania Press.

Giger, J. N., & Davidhizar, R. (1995). *Transcultural nursing: Assessment and interventions* (2nd ed.). St. Louis: Mosby.

Giger, J. N., & Davidhizar, R. (2004). *Transcultural nursing: Assessment and interventions* (4th ed.). St. Louis: Mosby

Grant, A. B. (1994). *The professional nurse: Issues and actions.* Springhouse, PA.: Springhouse.

Kavanaugh, K. H., & Kennedy, P. H. (1992). *Promoting cultural diversity.* Newbury Park, CA: Sage Publications.

Kittler, P. G., & Sucher, K. P. (1990). Diet counseling in a multicultural society. *Diabetes Educator, 16,* 127–134.

Kleinman, A., Eisenberg, L., & Good, B. (1978). Culture, illness and care. *Annals of Internal Medicine, 88,* 251–258.

Lea, A. (1994, August). Nursing in today's multicultural society: A transcultural perspective. *Journal of Advanced Nursing, 20,* 307–313.

Leininger, M. M. (1978). *Transcultural nursing: Concepts, theories, and practices.* New York: Wiley.

Leininger, M. M. (1988, November). Leininger's theory of nursing: Cultural care diversity and universality. *Nursing Science Quarterly, 14,* 152–160.

Leininger, M. M. (Ed.). (1991). *Culture care diversity and universality: A theory of nursing.* New York: National League for Nursing Press. Pub. No. 15–2402.

Leininger, M. M. (1993, Winter). Towards conceptualization of transcultural health care systems: Concepts and a model. *Journal of Transcultural Nursing, 4,* 32–40.

Luckmann, J. (2000). Transcultural communication in health care. Albany, NY: Delmar.

McCarthy, P., Chammas, G., Wilimas, J., Alaoui, F. M., & Harif, M. (2004). Managing chilren's cancer pain in Morocco. *Journal of Nursing Scholarship, 36*(1), 11–15.

Murdock, G. (1971). *Outline of cultural materials,* (4th ed.). New Haven, CT: Human Relations Area Files.

Murray, R. B., & Zentner, J. P. (2001). *Health promotion strategies through the life span.* Upper Saddle River, NJ: Prentice Hall.

National Center for Complementary and Alternative Medicine. (2001). http://nccam.nih.gov.

Office of Minority Health. (2002). *Attachment 3: Potential Measures/Indicators of Cultural Competence.* Washington, DC: US Department of Health and Human Services. Retrieved on May 26, 2004, http://www.hrsa.gov/OMH/cultural/attachment3.htm.

Orque, M. S., Bloch, B., & Monrroy, L. S. A. (1983). *Ethnic nursing care: A multicultural approach.* St. Louis: Mosby.

Purnell, P. D., & Paulanka, B. J. (1998). *Transcultural health care: A culturally competent approach.* Philadelphia: F. A. Davis.

Purnell, P. D., & Paulanka, B. J. (2003). *Transcultural health care: A culturally competent approach* (2nd ed.). Philadelphia: F. A. Davis.

Rairdan, B., & Higgs, Z. R. (1992, March). When your patient is a Hmong refugee. *American Journal of Nursing, 92,* 52–55.

Rosenbaum, J. N. (1991). A cultural assessment guide: Learning cultural sensitivity. *Canadian Nurse, 88,* 32–33.

Rosenbaum, J. N. (1995, April). Teaching cultural sensitivity. *Journal of Nursing Education, 34,* 188–189.

Spector, R. E. (2004). *Cultural diversity in health and illness* (6th ed.). Upper Saddle River, NJ: Prentice Hall Health.

Sprott, J. (1993). The black box in family assessments: Cultural diversity. In S. Feetham, S. Meister, J. Bell, & C. Gilliss (Eds.), *The nursing of families: Theory, research, education, practice* (pp. 189–199). Beverly Hills, CA: Sage Publications.

United States Census Bureau. (2001). *USA statistics in brief: Population and vital statistics.* http://www.census.gov/statab/www/part1.

Nursing in a Spiritually Diverse World

Objectives

■ Analyze concepts related to spirituality and religion in nursing and health care.

■ Differentiate between spirituality, religion, and faith.

■ Describe the spiritual development of the individual across the life span.

■ Discuss the influence of spiritual beliefs about diet, dress, prayer and meditation, and birth and death on health and healing.

■ Assess clients from a spiritual perspective.

■ Plan and implement spiritually competent care.

MEDIALINK

Additional online resources for this chapter can be found on the companion Web site at http://www.prenhall.com/blais.

In viewing people holistically, nurses must consider the spiritual and religious beliefs of clients when providing care. The United States and Canada have a diversity of spiritual and religious beliefs; therefore, nurses must be informed about and sensitive to the spiritual and religious influences on the beliefs and practices related to health and illness (Table 22–1). Nurses should understand how individuals' spiritual beliefs influence their health decision making, providing strength during illness and times of adversity, and how spiritual and faith communities can provide support for health, healing, and dying.

Table 22–1 United States Religious Diversity 1995/2002

Religion	1995 (%)	2002 (%)
Protestant	56	53
Catholic	27	25
Jewish	2	2
Orthodox	1	1
Mormon	1	2
Other*	5	8
None	8	9

* Other includes Muslim, Buddhist, Unitarian, Hindu, Bahai, Taoist, Rastafarian, Sikh, Santeria, and others, each with less than 1%.
Source: Statistical Abstracts of the United States, 2002. http://www.census.gov/prod/2004pubs/03statab/pop.pdf.

Nurses must also understand how their own spiritual beliefs affect their ability to relate to people whose beliefs are different from their own. Health care professionals are not expected to know and understand all spiritual and religious belief systems of the world. It is possible, however, for health care professionals to develop an awareness of those spiritual and religious belief systems that are prevalent in the community where they practice.

CHALLENGES AND OPPORTUNITIES

The challenges of working in a spiritually diverse environment require nurses to be open to differences in beliefs about health and illness, and the importance of faith and spiritual beliefs and practices in healing. Establishing trust with people whose spiritual beliefs are different depends on the nurse's willingness to accept difference and to work with the client's different beliefs in achieving a healing relationship. Spiritual beliefs influence clients' beliefs about cause of illness, acceptance of treatment recommendations, and response to treatments. Questions about illness and health that are founded in spiritual and religious beliefs include: Is illness the result of God's will? Is it punishment for doing evil? Can prayer heal? Can faith prevent illness? It is im-

portant for nurses to respect clients' spiritual beliefs and integrate them into care.

Working with clients of different spiritual beliefs provides nurses with the opportunity to enrich their own lives through an understanding of the differences of others. Faith-based remedies such as prayer and meditation are increasingly being shown to have an effect on healing. Researchers are examining the effects of prayer and faith on health and healing. New knowledge derived from traditional beliefs and practices can provide new ways of healing and helping.

CONCEPTS RELATED TO SPIRITUALITY

Spiritual beliefs and religious traditions are an integral part of a person's belief and value system and can influence a client's beliefs about the cause of illness, healing practices, and the choice of healer or health care provider. Spiritual and religious beliefs can be a source of strength and comfort for clients experiencing illness, a crisis, or approaching death.

Spirituality, Religion, and Faith

Spirituality, religion, and faith, although often used interchangeably, are different. The nurse must be aware of the differences to understand the depth of feeling that clients have about their beliefs.

Spirituality

The word *spiritual* derives from the Latin word *spiritus,* which means "to blow" or "to breathe" (the same word origin for *inspire* and *respiration*), and has come to mean that which gives life or essence to the soul. Mauk and Schmidt (2004, p. 15) define spirituality as "the core of a person's being, involving one's relationship with God or a higher power." According to O'Brien (1999, p. 6), spirituality includes "love, compassion, caring, transcendence, relationship with God, and the connection of body, mind, and spirit." **Spirituality** is the belief in or relationship with a higher power, creative force, divine being, or infinite source of energy. For example, a person may believe in God, Jehovah, Allah, the Creator, or a Higher Power.

Burkhardt and Nagai-Jacobson (2002) state that there are different ways in which people express or experience their spirituality. Some express their spirituality through the practice of a particular religion, whereas others express their spirituality outside specific organized religious systems. An example of spirituality outside an organized religious system is the Native American traditional belief system. According to Lowe and Struthers (2001, p. 282), the Native American concept of spirituality includes the five characteristics of relationship, unity, honor, balance, and healing. The spiritual components of relationship include touching, learning, and using cultural traditions in all relationships. A second cultural concept related to spirituality is connectedness and includes the connectedness with all others, with the environment, and with the Creator (Lowe & Struthers, 2001, p. 281). (See accompanying Evidence for Practice Box.) Still others express their spirituality through the blending of different religious and philosophical traditions. Burkhardt (1993, p. 12) describes the following aspects of spirituality:

- Dealing with the unknown or uncertainties in life
- Finding meaning and purpose in life
- Being aware of and able to draw upon inner resources and strength
- Having a feeling of connectedness with oneself and with God or a Higher Being

"The spiritual dimension tries to be in harmony with the universe, strives for answers about the infinite, and especially comes into focus or sustaining power when the person faces emotional stress, physical illness, or death. It goes outside a person's own power" (Murray & Zentner, 2001, p. 116). Characteristics of spirituality are listed in the box on page 400.

Religion

Religion is defined by Dossey, Keegan, and Guzzetta (2000, p. 92) as "an organized system of beliefs shared by a group of people and the practices, including worship, related to that system." It provides a way of spiritual expression that guides people in responding to life's questions and crises. According to Vardey (1995, p. xv), the organized religions offer (1) a sense of community bound by common beliefs; (2) the collective study of scripture (the Bible, Torah, Koran, or others); (3) the performance of ritual; (4) the use of disciplines and practices, commandments, and sacraments; and (5) ways of taking care of the person's soul (such as fasting, prayer, and meditation). Many traditional religious practices and rituals are related to life events such as birth, transition from childhood to adulthood, marriage, illness, and death. Religious rules of conduct, like cultural beliefs, may also apply to matters of daily life such as dress, food,

Evidence for Practice

Lowe, J., & Struthers, R. (2001). A conceptual framework of nursing in Native American culture. *Journal of Nursing Scholarship, 33*(3), 279–283.

The purpose of this study was to describe the phenomenon of nursing in the Native American culture. Focus groups consisting of 203 Native American nurses, nursing students, and others who provide health care to Native American people were conducted on the Flathead Reservation in Montana. The participants represented many Native American tribes across the United States. Native American nurses were facilitators for the focus groups. Seven dimensions of Native American culture were identified: caring, traditions, respect, connection, holism, trust, and spirituality. Each dimension is considered essential to the practice of nursing in Native American culture.

The dimension of spirituality consisted of five characteristics: relationship, unity, honor, balance, and healing. Relationship included touching, learning, and utilizing traditions. "The art of touching someone has spiritual power." Unity is described as transcending boundaries and pursuing oneness. The characteristic of honor includes appreciation and respect: "It is an honor to be present at birth and at death." The characteristic of balance involves destiny and "centering oneself with Mother Earth." It also includes caring for oneself. The characteristic of healing includes gifting, praying, and resonating with the "Great Mystery."

Nursing implications: Using the spirituality dimension of the Native American Cultural Framework can help nurses, both Native American and non–Native American, support Native American clients in the practice of their spiritual traditions during times of illness and healing. Examination of these beliefs and practices may also have implications for non–Native American patients.

Characteristics of Spirituality

PERSONAL CONNECTEDNESS

- Awareness and acceptance of self (self-esteem, self-knowledge)
- Ability for self-reflection
- Inner strength
- Attitude of trust, optimism

CONNECTEDNESS TO OTHERS

- Sharing self with others in a caring relationship
  - Caring for family (children, parents, siblings, extended family)
  - Caring for friends
  - Caring for others
- Sharing knowledge and resources

CONNECTEDNESS TO THE ENVIRONMENT

- Feeling of harmony with the environment
- Respect for nature
- Protection of the environment

CONNECTEDNESS TO A SUPREME BEING

- Feelings of belief and faith
- Religious or nonreligious belief
- Prayer and/or meditation
- Use of religious articles (symbols, sacred writings)
- Participation in religious/spiritual rituals

Evidence for Practice

Meisenhelder, J. B. (2003). Gender differences in religiosity and functional health in the elderly. *Geriatric Nursing, 24*(6), 343–347.

The purpose of this study was to examine community-dwelling residents over 65 years of age regarding the relationship between importance of faith, frequency of prayer, and religious coping and eight categories of functional health. Because the sample was evenly divided by gender, gender differences were examined. Half the sample was Protestant, a third was Catholic, 4% were Jewish, and 6% were atheist. A survey was conducted using the Medical Outcomes Study Health Survey Short-Form 36. Eight health outcomes were measured: physical functioning, physical limitations to role functioning, extent of bodily pain, general health, vitality or energy level, health limitations to social functioning, emotional limitations to role functioning, and mental health. Gender differences occurred on all three religious variables. Women rated importance of their faith and frequency of prayer higher than the men. The difference in religious coping showed the same gender trend but was not statistically significant.

A correlation matrix using Pearson product-moment correlations was used to examine the relationship of religious dimensions and demographic variables with the eight health subscales separately for men and women. Mental health was the only outcome related to the spiritual indicators for both genders, although it was used differently. Men who prayed more often had higher mental health scores. Reliance on religious coping and a high importance of one's faith were positively related to mental health for women. Physical functioning was related to religious coping for men only, men with poorer physical functioning tended to rely more on religious coping.

The implication of this study is the importance for nurses to promote and support older clients' religious and spiritual beliefs and practices as part of promoting health and wellness.

social interaction, and sexual relationships. Religious development of an individual refers to the acceptance of specific beliefs, values, rules of conduct, and rituals. Religious development may or may not parallel spiritual development. For example, a person may follow certain religious practices yet not internalize the symbolic meaning behind the practices.

Faith

Faith is "deeper and more personal than organized religion. . . . [It relates] to one's transcendent values and relationship with a higher power, or God"

Table 22–2 Westerhoff's Four Stages of Faith

Stage	Age	Behavior
Experienced faith	Infancy and early adolescence	Experiences faith through interaction with others who are living a particular faith tradition
Affiliative faith	Late adolescence	Participates in activities that characterize a particular faith tradition; experiences awe and wonderment; feels a sense of belonging
Searching faith	Young adulthood	Through a process of questioning and doubting own faith, acquires a cognitive as well as an affective faith
Owned faith	Middle adulthood and old age	Puts faith into personal and social action and is willing to stand up for beliefs even against the nurturing community

Source: Adapted from *Will Our Children Have Faith?* (pp. 79–103), by J. Westerhoff, 1976, New York: Seabury Press.

(O'Brien, 1999, p. 58). Faith is belief in something that cannot be directly observed (Mauk & Schmidt, 2004). Faith is about expectation. A person who has faith in God has certain expectations of God; for example, a person may have faith in God that He will heal them or provide the strength to cope with pain or illness.

Reflect on...

■   your own spiritual and/or religious beliefs. What is the source of your spirituality? How does your spirituality sustain you when you have to deal with difficult personal situations? Professional situations?

Spiritual Development

Spiritual development is also referred to as faith development and spiritual formation. As with other types of growth and development, spiritual or faith development occurs in a linear fashion, and a person can be in more than one stage at a time. The work of Westerhoff (1976) and Fowler (1981) serve as the foundation of our understanding of spiritual development. Westerhoff describes four stages of faith: experienced faith, affiliative faith, searching faith, and owned faith. Fowler describes seven stages of faith development that parallel the developmental stages described by Piaget (cognitive development), Kohlberg (moral development), and Erikson (socioemotional development). Tables 22–2 and 22–3 present Westerhoff's and Fowler's stages of faith development.

Prayer and Meditation

Prayer is a communication or petition to God in word or thought. Meditation is an internal reflection or contemplation. Prayer and meditation are part of most religions. Depending on the specific religion, prayer is a communication with God, Jehovah, Allah, or some Higher Power. In some religions, prayers may be channeled through another; for example, Catholics may pray to God through a saint or the Virgin Mary. Prayers may be a petition or request (e.g., cure from illness or relief from pain), a thanksgiving (e.g., for healing), or a spiritual communion (e.g., to find peace or acceptance). Dossey (1993) identifies seven forms of prayer that may be used when someone is ill (see the box on page 403). Some religions have formal prayers that are printed in a prayer book, such as the Anglican or Episcopal Book of Common Prayer or the Catholic Missal. Some religious prayers are attributed to the source of faith; for example, the Lord's Prayer is attributed to Jesus, and the first sutra for Muslims is attributed to Mohammed.

Daily prayers are prescribed by some religions. For example, Muslims perform the five daily prayers, or Salat, while facing toward Mecca, at dawn, noon, midafternoon, sunset, and evening. Jews may say the Kaddish daily for the first year after the death of a loved one. People who are ill may want to continue their prayer practices. Moschella et al. (1997) report that patients may even increase their prayer practices in response to illness. People may memorize prayers during childhood, and their repetition becomes a source of

Table 22–3 Fowler's Stages of Faith Development

Stage	Description	Developmental Tasks
Infancy	Primal Faith—original or primitive faith	• Separation without anxiety, developing trusting relationships • Consistent, loving, respectful responses from parents/caregivers/nurturers
Early Childhood	Intuitive Faith—without conscious reasoning Projective Faith—impulsive	• Listening and reacting to spiritual stories, songs, and religious celebrations
Childhood and Beyond	Mythic Faith—imaged Literal Faith—realistic, factual	• Development of concrete images of God, heaven, and hell • Adherence to scripture-based codes of behavior • Acceptance that scriptures are truth
Adolescence and Beyond	Synthetic Faith—composed Conventional Faith—ordinary and commonplace, generally accepted	• Talking with others about the meaning of faith or spirituality • Believing that God is the only one who really knows them • Questioning the existence of God
Young Adulthood and Beyond	Individuative Faith—unique, independent, distinct Reflective Faith—thoughtful, considered	• Struggling with faith • Developing an intimacy with or a withdrawal from faith
Early Midlife and Beyond	Conjunctive Faith—connected	• Discussions of early midlife in relation to faith • Discussions of ecumenism and religious diversity/pluralism • Prayers of contemplation and meditation
Midlife and Beyond	Universalizing Faith—holistic	• Serving in social ministries, such as soup kitchens, food pantries, hospices, or prison ministries • Living a lifestyle that places faith as the basis and framework for living

Sources: From *Spiritual Care in Nursing Practice,* by K. L. Mauk, and N. K. Schmidt, 2004, Philadelphia: Lippincott Williams & Wilkins; *Stages of Faith,* by J. Fowler, 1981, New York: Harper & Row.

comfort during illness or adversity. Clients may need uninterrupted quiet time or want to have their sacred writings, books of daily meditations, prayer books, rosaries, prayer beads, or other sacred symbols available to them. Some clients may want their minister, priest, rabbi, imam, or other spiritual advisor with them when they pray. There may be times when the patient asks the nurse or physician to pray with them.

Reflect on...

■ your own spiritual and religious beliefs. How do they affect your beliefs about health and illness? How

important would it be for you to be able to practice your spiritual and religious traditions if you were ill?

■ your comfort with patients/clients who ask you to pray with them or for them. How would you respond to patients or clients who ask you to pray with them? Do you think that nurses should pray with patients and/or their families when requested to do so?

■ the various spiritual and religious groups in your community. Is religious difference valued? Where could you go to learn more about the religious groups in your community? In what ways could you as a professional nurse support the spiritual and religious practices of your clients?

Types of Prayer

Petition	Asking something for oneself
Intercession	Asking something for another
Confession	Repentance of wrongdoing and asking forgiveness
Thanksgiving	Offering gratitude
Adoration	Giving honor and praise
Invocation	Summoning the presence of the Almighty
Lamentation	Crying in distress and asking for vindication

Source: Adapted from *Healing Words: The Power of Prayer and the Practice of Medicine* (p. 5), by L. Dossey, 1993, New York: Harper San Francisco.

SELECTED SPIRITUAL AND RELIGIOUS BELIEFS INFLUENCING NURSING CARE

This section discusses some selected spiritual phenomena of significance to nursing. Nurses should be aware of holy days, sacred writings and symbols, beliefs about dress, and spiritual beliefs and practices as they relate to health and nursing care of people of the predominant religious groups in their community.

Holy Days

A holy day is a day set aside for special religious observance (Blais, 2000, p. 223). In addition to special holy days observed throughout the year, most religions have a weekly day set aside for rest, prayer, reading of sacred writings, and worship. Most Christians observe the Sabbath Day on Sunday as a day of rest and worship in remembrance of Christ's resurrection. Other Christian religious groups observe Saturday as the Sabbath. Jews observe the time from sundown on Friday until sundown on Saturday as a holy day of rest and worship in commemoration of the final day of Creation and observance of the biblical injunction to "remember the Sabbath day and keep it holy." Muslims observe Friday as a day of meditation and worship.

Holy days also can be special days of celebration and feasting that occur once a year, such as the Christ-ian celebrations of Christmas that celebrates the birth of Christ and Easter, an observance of the death and resurrection of Christ. The Jewish celebration of Sukkoth, the Feast of Tabernacles, celebrates the end of the harvest. The Eid al Fitr celebrates the end of the month of Ramadan in the Muslim religion. Solemn religious observances throughout the year may be referred to as high holy days and may include fasting, reflection, and prayer. Examples of such holy days are Good Friday, the day of Christ's crucifixion, in the Christian religion. In the Jewish religion, Rosh Hashanah, also called the Day of Judgment or Day of Remembrance, is the start of the Jewish New Year. Rosh Hashanah begins a ten-day period that culminates in Yom Kippur or Day of Atonement, a day of fasting and purification. In the Muslim religion, Ramadan is the month-long observance of daylight fasting and meditation that ends with Lailat Al-Qadr, a commemoration of the revelation of the Qur'an (Koran) to the Prophet Mohammed, and the Eid al Fitr, or the breaking of the month-long fast.

Many religions require fasting, extended prayer, and reflection or ritual observances on sacred days; however, believers who are seriously ill are often exempted from such requirements. Many hospitals and health organizations facilitate ritual observances for patients, clients, and staff on religious holy days. For example, a hospital may provide fish or other nonmeat entrée on Good Friday for Catholic patients. Because many religions, such as the Jewish, Muslim, and Hindu faiths, follow a calendar of religious observances different from the Gregorian calendar, a calendar that lists the holy days of the major religions is useful in anticipating patients' spiritual needs.

Sacred Writings and Symbols

Sacred writing or scriptures are believed to be the thought or word of God or the Supreme Being and are held to have been written by that deity's appointed disciples or prophets. Each religion has its sacred writings that tell the stories of the religions' leaders, kings, and heroes, such as the stories of Abraham and Solomon in both Jewish and Christian scriptures. Sacred writings also contain rules or commandments or other guidelines for living. For example, dietary laws of the Jewish religion are contained in the Torah, and literal interpretations of the Bible provide guidelines for relationships, health and hygiene, and dress. Religious laws or commandments are often used as the basis for secular law, such as those derived from the Ten Commandments, contained in the Old Testament of the Bible, that forbid killing, stealing, adultery, and so on. Religious interpretations of these laws provide the foundations for ethical debates about abortion and euthanasia.

Religious law may affect a client's willingness to accept treatment suggestions. For example, blood transfusions are in conflict with the religious teachings of Jehovah's Witnesses. People who are ill or in distress often gain comfort and hope from reading religious writings. Examples of sacred stories that may give comfort to patients are Job's suffering in both the Jewish and Christian scriptures and Jesus healing people who were physically or mentally ill in the New Testament of the Bible. See Table 22–4 for a listing of selected sacred writings of selected religious or spiritual belief systems.

Symbols of religious belief include jewelry, medals, amulets, icons, totems, or body ornamentation (e.g., tattoos) that carry religious or spiritual significance. They may be worn as an assertion of one's faith, to provide protection, or as a source of comfort or strength. People may wear religious medals at all times, and they may wish to wear them when undergoing diagnostic studies, medical treatment, or surgery. People who are

Catholic may carry a rosary for prayer and a Muslim may carry prayer beads.

Other religious symbols include pictures or statues of saints or religious prophets. They may be found in the believer's home, car, or workplace as a reminder of their faith. Some people may have personal alters in their homes that include icons, candles, incense, or other articles of faith. Patients in hospitals or residents of long-term care facilities may want to have their spiritual symbols at their bedside as an expression of faith and a source of comfort.

Dress

Many religions have laws or traditions that dictate dress. For example, Orthodox and Conservative Jewish men believe that it is important to have their head covered at all times and therefore wear a yarmulke. Orthodox Jewish women may wear a wig or scarf to cover their hair as a sign of respect to God. Muslim men wear a head covering during prayer and may wear head coverings at all times. Muslim women may wear a hijab or headscarf that fully covers the hair. In strict Muslim countries, women may wear the chador, a body-enveloping robe. While people in Western coun-

Table 22–4 Supreme Being, Major Earthly Incarnation or Prophet, and Sacred Writings of the Major Religions and Spiritual Beliefs Systems

Religion	Supreme Being/Earthly Incarnation or Prophet	Sacred Writings
Christianity	God/Jesus Christ	Bible
Judaism	Jehovah/Abraham	Torah Talmud
Islam/Muslim	Allah/Muhammad	Koran (Qur'an) Hadith
Hindu	Vishnu and Lakshmi; the Supreme Being has the ability to take on many forms	Vedas
Sikh	God/Guru Nanak	Adi Granth Guru Granth Sahib
Buddhism	A spiritual philosophy/Buddha	Vedas
Baha'i	Baha'u'llah	Writings of Baha'u'llah
Confucianism	A spiritual philosophy but not a religion/Confucius	The *Four Books* and the *Five Classics* of Confucius
Taoism	Multiple deities/Lao-tzu	Tao-Te Ching

tries often view the chador as a sign of women's oppression, many Muslim women feel that the chador protects them.

Some religions (e.g., Seventh Day Adventist, Mormon, and so on) require that women dress in a conservative manner. These religions may have restrictions against wearing sleeveless or low-cut tops and skirts that are above the knees. Clients who are trying to comply with religious rules about dress may feel uncomfortable about wearing or refuse to wear hospital gowns.

Health Beliefs and Practices

Andrews and Boyle (2003, pp. 75–76) describe the magico-religious and holistic health belief systems. Both health belief systems have spiritual and religious connotations to consider. In the magico-religious health belief view, health and illness are controlled by supernatural forces. The client may believe that illness is the result of "being bad" or opposing God's will. For example, the diagnosis of cancer may be considered a punishment from God, as expressed by the statement, "What did I do wrong that God gave this to me?" Getting well also may be viewed as dependent on God's will. The client may make statements such as, "Only through God's will can I recover." Some cultures believe that magic can cause illness. A sorcerer or witch may put a spell or hex on the client. Some people view illness as possession by an evil spirit. Although these beliefs are not supported by empirical evidence, clients who believe that such things can cause illness may, in fact, become ill as a result. Such illnesses may require magical treatments in addition to scientific treatments for healing to occur. For example, a man who experiences gastric distress, headaches, and hypertension after being told that a spell has been placed on him may recover only if the spell is removed by a spiritual healer.

The holistic health belief view is based on the spiritual belief systems of many cultures and holds that the forces of nature must be maintained in balance or harmony. Human life is one aspect of nature that must be in harmony with the rest of nature. When the natural balance or harmony is disturbed, illness results. The Medicine Wheel is an ancient symbol used by Native Americans of North and South America to express many concepts. Related to health and wellness, the Medicine Wheel teaches the four aspects of the individual's nature: the physical, the mental, the emotional, and the spiritual. Each of the dimensions must be in balance to be healthy. The Medicine Wheel can

also be used to express the individual's relationship with the environment and the Creator as a dimension of wellness.

Reflect on...

■ patients' expressions of a spiritual or religious cause for their illness. What are your thoughts or feelings regarding these beliefs? What are your own thoughts about spiritual or religious causes of illness?

Dietary Beliefs

Religious beliefs may also dictate dietary practices. Examples of religions that have specific beliefs or laws about diet include Judaism, Islam, and Christianity.

Orthodox Jews observe a kosher diet. **Kosher** means that food is considered clean according to Jewish law. Meat and dairy products must not be eaten at the same meal. If meat is eaten, then bread cannot be buttered and milk or cream cannot be served with tea or coffee. Some meats and fish are prohibited in a kosher diet, for example, lamb, beef, and chicken can be eaten but pork and shellfish are forbidden. Strict observers of Jewish dietary laws require that their meat be slaughtered according to religious tradition. Some Orthodox families will maintain two sets of cooking utensils and china in order to strictly observe the prohibition of mixing meat and dairy. Jews of the Conservative and Reformed belief may vary in their observance of dietary laws. Fasting is required during the high Holy Days of Rosh Hashanah and Yom Kippur. People who are ill are usually excused from fasting requirements. Many hospitals and long-term care facilities will provide kosher meals for patients who observe Jewish dietary laws.

Islamic (Muslim) dietary practices forbid the eating of pork or any meat of the pig. Animals that are being killed for food must be slaughtered according to religious law. The ingestion of alcohol is strictly forbidden. Fasting is required during daylight hours for the entire month of Ramadan.

Christian belief systems vary widely in their dietary requirements. Many people who are Roman Catholics abstain from meat on certain days, such as Ash Wednesday and Good Friday. Some Christian religions encourage fasting on Ash Wednesday and Good Friday or before attending weekly services. Other Christian religions encourage fasting as a way of cleansing the body. Several Christian religions discourage or even prohibit the ingestion of alcohol, others discourage the ingestion of caffeine, and some discourage the ingestion of meat.

It is important for the nurse to determine the dietary requirements of their patients and clients and convey dietary preferences to the dietitian for hospitalized patients or residents of long-term care facilities. When providing health teaching related to diet, religious requirements must be considered and supported.

Pain and Its Spiritual Meaning

Beliefs about and responses to pain vary among people. Spiritual or religious beliefs about pain must be considered in relation to both the actual perception of pain and the meaning or significance of pain to the client and family. Some patients may consider pain a punishment for bad deeds; the individual is, therefore, expected to tolerate pain without complaint in order to atone for sins. People may also use their faith to help manage their pain through prayer and meditation. Spiritual or religious practices that relieve pain should be supported and encouraged, while at the same time the nurse offers medication and other nonpharmacological remedies to alleviate pain.

Childbirth and Perinatal Care

Religious and spiritual beliefs may provide guidance for the management of life events such as the birth of a baby. Christian religions that practice baptism during infancy believe that the infant is born with sin and must be baptized in order to go to heaven. Because of this belief, the infant who is in danger of dying at birth must be baptized shortly after birth. Although it is acceptable for the nurse or other health care provider to baptize an infant with the parents' permission, if the infant is at risk for dying, it is preferable for the family's priest or minister to perform this ritual.

In the Jewish tradition, circumcision is a religious rite performed on the male child eight days after birth. When the boy is circumcised, he receives his Hebrew name. This name will be used at his Bar-Mitzvah, at his wedding, and on his gravestone.

Muslims may wish that the first sounds the newborn baby hears is the call to prayer, which is whispered in each ear. The call to prayer is "Allah is most great. I testify that there is no God but Allah. I testify that Muhammad is the prophet of Allah. Come to prayer. Come to salvation. Allah is most great. There is no God but Allah." Muslim boys must be circumcised between the ages of 7 days and 12 years.

Death and Dying

Religious and spiritual beliefs may also prescribe the care of patients immediately before death, at the time of death, and during the period after death. Beliefs about preparation of the body, autopsy, organ donation, cremation, and prolonging life are closely allied to the person's religion. Autopsy, for example, may be prohibited, opposed, or discouraged by Eastern Orthodox religions, Muslims, Jehovah's Witnesses, and Orthodox Jews. Some religions prohibit the removal of body parts and dictate that all body parts be given appropriate burial. Organ donation is prohibited by Jehovah's Witnesses and Muslims, whereas Buddhists in America consider it an act of mercy and encourage it. Cremation is discouraged, opposed, or prohibited by the Mormon, Eastern Orthodox, Islamic, and Jewish faiths. Hindus, in contrast, prefer cremation and cast the ashes in a holy river. Prolongation of life is generally encouraged; however, some religions, such as Christian Science, are unlikely to use medical means to prolong life, and the Jewish faith generally opposes prolonging life after irreversible brain damage. In hopeless illness, Buddhists may permit euthanasia.

Nurses also need to be knowledgeable about the client's death-related rituals, such as administration of the Sacrament of the Sick (formerly referred to as Last Rites) and Holy Communion, prayer and chanting at the bedside, and other rituals, such as special procedures for washing, dressing, positioning, and shrouding the dead. In some religions, family members of the same sex wash and prepare the body for burial and cremation.

Jews may want to speak the Shema or have it said for them at the time of their death. The Shema is a prayer of praise learned by Jews in childhood, "Hear, O Israel, the Lord our God is one Lord . . ." Autopsy is discouraged. When autopsy is warranted, it must be limited to essential organs or systems, and all body parts must be buried together.

Muslims believe that their deaths are predetermined by Allah, and therefore death should not be feared. The body is ritually washed and wrapped in a linen shroud. Autopsy is permitted only for medical or legal purposes.

Nurses need to ask family members about their preference and verify who will carry out these activities. Burial clothes and other cultural or religious items are often important symbols for the funeral. For example, faithful Mormons are often dressed in their "temple clothes." Some Native Americans may be dressed in elaborate apparel and jewelry and wrapped in new blankets with money. The nurse must ensure that any ritual items present in the health care agency be given to the family or to the funeral home.

Reflect on...

■ spiritual or religious beliefs and practices related to death and dying among people of the different spiritual or religious groups in your community. How can the nurse support the client and family in the performance of death and dying prayers and rituals?

SPIRITUAL DISTRESS

Spiritual distress is defined as "the state in which the individual experiences or is at risk of experiencing a disturbance in his/her belief or value system that is the source of strength and hope" (Carpenito-Moyet, 2003, p. 743). Spiritual distress may be the cause of illness, especially emotional distress, or it may occur as a result of illness as one questions why "God is allowing this (illness) to happen to them." Sometimes people experience a crisis of faith when they question their relationship with God or another Supreme Being. Such questioning can be a part of faith development as the individual progresses from one stage of faith to another. One must remember that faith is belief that is based on something that cannot be observed. When spiritual or religious beliefs that the person has held on faith are being challenged by outside forces, they may become unsure about their beliefs. This may result in a search for new meaning in the spiritual self. The nurse must be aware of patients and families who are experiencing spiritual distress, because this can affect their response to medical treatment.

Spiritual distress can also be a result of physiologic problems, treatment concerns, or situational issues. Physiologic problems include having a medical diagnosis of a terminal illness such as cancer or a debilitating disease such as Parkinson's or Alzheimer's disease. Pain is a physiologic problem that may lead to spiritual distress, especially if the pain is extreme or cannot be relieved effectively. Treatment-related factors include recommendations for treatments that the patient's religious beliefs prohibit, such as blood transfusion, amputation, abortion, organ donation or transplantation, dietary restrictions, or surgery. Religious beliefs may also influence patient and family decisions regarding resuscitative procedures at the end of life. Situational issues that may result in spiritual distress include the death or illness of a significant other, domestic violence, beliefs about sexuality, or the inability to practice one's religious rituals.

PROVIDING SPIRITUALLY COMPETENT CARE

All phases of the nursing process are affected by the client's and the nurse's spiritual beliefs and practices. As the client and the nurse come together in the nurse-client relationship, a unique spiritual environment is created that can improve or impair the client's outcome. Self-awareness of personal biases can enable nurses to modify behaviors or (if they are unable to modify behaviors) to remove themselves from situations where care might be compromised. Nurses can become more aware of their own spiritual values through values-clarification activities.

Spiritual Assessment

To obtain spiritual-assessment data, nurses use broad statements and open-ended questions that encourage clients to express themselves fully. At the assessment stage nurses make no conclusions but obtain information from clients. There are spiritual-assessment tools available. Nurses need to use tools that are appropriate to the situation and adapt them as required. For example, a nurse in the hospital may need a different format than a nurse working in a community setting. It is unnecessary to complete a total spiritual assessment for every client. Instead, nurses need to collect enough basic data to identify spiritual practices that are important to the client especially during illness or crisis. Sometimes, simply asking clients what their spiritual or religious needs are may be sufficient to provide effective spiritual support. Maugans (1996) developed a spiritual assessment method for physicians using the acronym **SPIRIT** (see the box on page 408). This model is useful for all health care providers who want to provide spiritually competent care. The box on page 409 provides guidelines for assessing spiritual needs of clients.

Diagnosing, Planning, and Implementing Spiritually Competent Care

Conclusions based on the spiritual assessment result in identifying nursing diagnoses related to spiritual needs. Three nursing diagnoses have been developed by the North American Nursing Diagnosis Association (NANDA) related to spirituality: Spiritual Distress, Risk for Spiritual Distress, and Readiness for Enhanced Spiritual Well-Being.

Spiritual Distress is defined by NANDA International (2003, p. 177) as "impaired ability to experience

SPIRIT Model for Assessing Spirituality

S = *Spiritual belief system*—What is the client's formal religious affiliation or spiritual belief system?

P = *Personal spirituality*—What are the personal religious or spiritual beliefs of the client and how do they influence daily life?

I = *Integration and involvement in a spiritual community*—Does the client belong to a spiritual or religious group or community? What is the importance of this affiliation for the client? Does the community provide support for the client?

R = *Ritualized practices and restrictions*—Are there specific rituals or practices related to daily life or worship that are important to the client? Are there components of medical care or treatment that are forbidden based on spiritual or religious obligation?

I = *Implications for medical care*—How do the client's spiritual or religious beliefs and practices influence their health care decisions? How can the nurse or physician provide care that is congruent with the client's spiritual or religious beliefs?

T = *Terminal events planning (advance directives)*—Are there specific spiritual or religious beliefs or practices that the client holds in regard to end of life care?

Source: Adapted from "The SPIRITual history," T. A. Maugans, 1996, *Archives of Family Medicine, 5*(1), 11–16.

and integrate meaning and purpose in life through a person's connectedness with self, others, art, music, literature, nature, or a power greater than oneself." Risk for Spiritual Distress is defined as being "at risk for an altered sense of harmonious connectedness with all of life and the universe in which dimensions that transcend and empower the self may be disrupted" (NANDA, 2003, p. 179).

Characteristics associated with Spiritual Distress are as follows:

- Expressions of hopelessness or a lack of meaning and purpose in life
- Expressions of being abandoned by God or the client's identification of a Supreme Being
- Expressions of anger toward a Supreme Being
- Sudden changes in spiritual or religious practices, either decreasing or increasing normal spiritual activities
- Requests to see a spiritual or religious counselor
- Requests for spiritual or religious literature (e.g., Bible, prayer book) or symbols (e.g., rosary, prayer beads, religious medals).

Readiness for Enhanced Spiritual Well-Being is defined as the "ability to experience and integrate meaning and purpose in life through a person's connectedness with self, others, art, music, literature, nature, or a power

greater than oneself (NANDA, 2003, p. 180). Characteristics associated with Enhanced Spiritual Well-Being include having the following:

- The resources to meet spiritual needs
- A sense of inner peace
- A sense of meaning and purpose in life
- A source of love and support, hope, and forgiveness
- A reverence for life
- A sense of relationship with others, including family, friends, community, environment, and a Supreme Being
- A sense of harmony, balance, and connectedness
- The ability to transcend the self

For clients who have a readiness for enhanced spiritual well-being, the nurse's role is to support existing spiritual resources and assist clients in maintaining their spiritual connections and promote further spiritual development. Some people will respond to adversity through an increased spiritual strength that provides hope and comfort.

For clients experiencing spiritual distress, the nurse can plan for and provide an environment and interventions that will help the client to do the following:

- Fulfill religious obligations
- Draw on and use inner resources more effectively

Assessing Spiritual Needs

ENVIRONMENT

- Does the client have religious objects, such as a Bible, prayer book, devotional literature, religious medals, rosary or other type of beads, photographs of historic religious persons or contemporary church leaders (e.g., pope, church president), paintings of religious events or persons, religious sculptures, crucifixes, objects of religious significance at entrances to rooms (e.g., holy water founts, a mezuzah, or small parchment scroll inscribed with an excerpt from the Bible), candles of religious significance (e.g., Pascal candle, menorah), shrine, or other?

- Does the client wear clothing that has religious significance (e.g., head covering, undergarment, uniform)?

- Are get-well greeting cards religious in nature or from a representative of the client's church?

- Does the client receive flowers or bulletins from his or her church?

BEHAVIOR

- Does the client appear to pray at certain times of the day or before meals?

- Does the client make special dietary requests (e.g., kosher diet, vegetarian diet, or diet free from caffeine, pork, shellfish, or other specific food items)?

- Does the client read religious magazines or books?

VERBALIZATION

- Does the client mention God (Allah, Buddha, Yahweh), prayer, faith, church, or religious topics?

- Does the client ask for a visit by a clergy member or other religious representative?

- Does the client express anxiety or fear about pain, suffering, or death?

INTERPERSONAL RELATIONSHIPS

- Who visits? How does the client respond to visitors?

- Does a priest, rabbi, minister, elder, or other religious or spiritual representative visit?

- How does the client relate to the nursing staff? To his or her roommate(s)?

- Does the client prefer to interact with others or to remain alone?

Source: Adapted from *Spiritual Care: The Nurse's Role* (3rd ed.), by Judith Allen Shelly and Sharon Fish. © 1988 by InterVarsity Press, Christian Fellowship of the USA. Used by permission of InterVarsity Press, P.O. Box 1400, Downers Grove, IL 60515.

- Maintain or establish a relationship with a Supreme Being
- Find meaning and purpose in life and in the present situation
- Promote a sense of hope
- Have needed spiritual resources

Nursing actions to help clients meet their spiritual needs include (1) providing presence, (2) supporting religious practices, (3) assisting clients with prayer, and (4) referring clients for spiritual counseling (Blais, 2000, p. 229).

Critical Thinking Exercise

Using the Spiritual Needs Assessment Guidelines above, assess clients of different spiritual or religious belief systems. Based on your spiritual assessment, what needs have you seen in your clients? How will you meet these needs? How do the spiritual needs of one client differ from another?

Providing Presence

The nurse provides presence by communicating a willingness to care, to listen, and to be available to the client. Mauk and Schmidt (2004, pp. 248–249) state that "nurses often provide the greatest amount of spiritual care to patients without employing multiple strategies or interventions but by simply being with the patient. The gift of presence, being with the patient in the time of need, can provide a tremendous spiritual benefit." Combining presence with touch can reassure and provide comfort for clients.

Supporting Religious Practices

The nurse can support the client's religious practices by providing privacy or quiet for the client to observe spiritual or religious observances, including prayer, devotional reading, and rituals. The nurse can call, for example, the client's spiritual counselor, priest, rabbi, or imam, to provide spiritual support. The nurse can ensure that dietary requirements are met by notifying the dietitian or nutritional counselor.

The accompanying box provides strategies for supporting religious practices.

Assisting Clients with Prayer

Prayer involves a sense of love, connection, and a reaching out. It has many health benefits and healing properties (Dossey, 1993). Prayer is defined by Mauk and Schmidt (2004, p. 247) as talking to God. It has also been described as talking with God or a union with God. Prayer offers a means to do the following:

■ Have someone to talk to
■ Promote a sense of being loved unconditionally
■ Provide a sense of serenity and connection with something greater
■ Develop compassionate behavior

Clients may choose to participate in private prayer or want group prayer with family, friends, or a spiritual counselor. The nurse's responsibility is to ensure privacy and a quiet environment. The nurse can also ensure that objects needed for prayer, such as rosaries, prayer beads, or prayer books, are within easy reach.

Supporting Religious Practices

- Create a trusting relationship with the client so that any religious concerns or practices can be openly discussed and addressed.

- If unsure of client religious needs, ask how nurses can assist in having these needs met. Avoid relying on personal assumptions when caring for clients.

- Do not discuss personal spiritual beliefs with a client unless the client requests it. Be sure to assess whether such self-disclosure contributes to a therapeutic nurse-client relationship.

- Inform clients and family caregivers about spiritual support available at your institution (e.g., chapel or meditation room, chaplain services).

- Allow time and privacy for, and provide comfort measures before, private worship, prayer, meditation, reading, or other spiritual activities.

- Respect and ensure safety of client's religious articles (e.g., rosary, prayer beads, medals, amulets, icons, prayer clothing).

- If desired by client, facilitate visitation of minister, priest, rabbi, imam, or other spiritual counselor. Collaborate with chaplain when available.

- Prepare client's environment for spiritual rituals or visitation of spiritual leader or counselor.

- Make arrangements with dietitian so that dietary needs can be met. If institution cannot accommodate client's needs, ask family to bring food if appropriate.

- Acquaint yourself with the religions, spiritual practices, and cultures of the area in which you are working.

- Remember the difference between facilitating/supporting a client's religious practice and participating in it yourself.

- Ask another nurse to assist you if a particular religious practice makes you uncomfortable.

- All spiritual interventions must be done within agency guidelines.

Source: Adapted from Spirituality, by B. Kozier, G. Erb, A. Berman, and S. Snyder, 2004. In *Fundamentals of Nursing: Concepts, Process, and Practice* (7th ed., p. 1004). Upper Saddle River, NJ: Prentice Hall.

Nursing care may need to be adjusted to accommodate for prayer times.

Illness can interfere with some clients' ability to pray. Feelings such as anxiety, fear, guilt, grief, despair, and isolation can produce barriers to relationships in general, and in the relationship the person has with God or their Supreme Being. In these instances clients may ask the nurse to pray with them. Prayers with clients should only be done when there is mutual agreement between the client and those praying with them. If a patient asks the nurse for prayer and the nurse does not feel comfortable, one option may be to suggest a silent prayer. The nurse can stand quietly at the bedside and may even hold the patient's hand. This can provide comfort when no one else is available. When clients are experiencing severe spiritual distress, the nurse should refer them to a chaplain or other spiritual counselor. It is important that nurses not impose their own spiritual beliefs or practices on clients, but rather respond to the spiritual needs expressed or manifested by the client.

Referring Clients for Spiritual Counseling

Referral to a spiritual counselor may be done whenever the client expresses the need for spiritual support. Many clients have their own spiritual or religious support person (e.g., minister, priest, rabbi, imam) in addition to members of their faith community who may provide support and prayer. For clients who do not have a personal spiritual counselor, the agency chaplain may provide spiritual support or obtain an appropriate spiritual support person. If the agency does not employ a chaplain, a list of available spiritual leaders should be kept on the nursing unit. Nurses in home health care or practicing in community settings can check telephone directories, directories of community service agencies, or religious directories to identify an available spiritual support person. Many religious communities will provide support to members of their faith

Critical Thinking Exercise

Identify resources (e.g., churches, synagogues, or mosques) available in your community that will assist health care providers in your health care agency in delivering spiritually competent care. What services are provided? Are services available to clients who are not members of the specific faith community?

who are not members of their specific faith community. For example, a priest may visit a client in the hospital or at home even though the client is not a member of the priest's parish. Often parish nurses, or faith community nurses visit members of their faith community who are ill at home or are hospitalized. In the absence of the spiritual leader, faith community nurses may be permitted to administer religious rituals and other services that the spiritual leader usually provides. In the situation in which there is conflict with prescribed treatment and the client's religious beliefs or practices, the nurse can encourage the client, the client's physician, and the client's spiritual counselor to discuss the conflict and explore alternatives to the recommended treatment. The major roles of the nurse are to provide information and resources so that clients can make an informed decision within the context of their spiritual or religious belief system and to support the client's decision.

EXPLORE MEDIALINK

Questions, critical thinking exercises, essay activities, and other interactive resources for this chapter can be found on the Web site at http://www.prenhall.com/blais. Click on Chapter 22 to select activities for this chapter.

SUMMARY

In viewing people holistically, nurses must consider the spiritual and religious beliefs of clients when providing care. Just as there are diverse cultural groups in the United States and Canada, there is also diversity of spiritual and religious belief systems. Spiritual and religious beliefs can influence clients' beliefs about causes of illness, healing practices, and the choice of health care

provider. Spiritual and religious beliefs can be a source of strength and comfort for clients experiencing illness.

Spirituality, religion, and *faith* are terms often used interchangeably; however, they are different. Spirituality refers to the essence of one's relationship with God or a higher power. Religion is an organized system of beliefs shared by a group of people and the practices,

Bookshelf

Burkhardt, M. A., & Nagai-Jacobson, M. G. (2002). *Spirituality: Living our connectedness.* **Albany, NY: Delmar.**

This text explores foundational concepts in spirituality, including nursing's spiritual heritage, healing and spirituality, healing and spiritual presence, and caring for the nurse's spirit.

Health Ministries Association, Inc. (1998). *Scope and standards of parish nursing practice.* **Washington, DC: American Nurses Publishing.**

For nurses interested in parish nursing, this text integrates the nursing scope and standards of practice (ANA, 2003) with the scope and standards of parish nursing practice to guide nurses in their development as parish nurses.

Henry, L. G., & Enry, J. D. (2004). *The soul of the caring nurse.* **Washington, DC: American Nurses Association.**

This text describes the role of the caring nurse through personal stories. Stories of caring and healing through spirituality and faith are provided by critical care nurses, home care nurses, parish nurses, and nurse educators. The text also explores strategies for nurses to care for themselves.

Mauk, K. L., & Schmidt, N. K. (2004). *Spiritual care in nursing practice.* **Philadelphia: Lippincott.**

This text explores the relationship between health, spirituality, and nursing care from an interdisciplinary perspective. Spiritual development across the life span is discussed and the belief systems of various religious traditions are presented.

---

including worship, related to that belief system. Faith is the belief in something that cannot be directly observed.

Spiritual development is also referred to as faith development and spiritual formation. As with other types of growth and development, spiritual or faith development occurs in a linear fashion and a person can be in more than one stage at a time. The work of Westerhoff and Fowler serve as the foundation of our understanding of spiritual development.

Prayer is a communication or petition to God or a Higher Power in word or thought. Meditation is an internal reflection or contemplation. Spiritual and religious belief systems use prayer and meditation as a means of communication with a Higher Power, either directly or indirectly, and as a means of self-reflection.

Nurses must be knowledgeable about the spiritual and religious belief systems in the communities where they practice. Nurses should be aware of holy days, sacred writings and symbols, beliefs about dress, and spiritual and religious beliefs and practices related to health and nursing care. Spiritual and religious beliefs may influence dietary practices, beliefs and practices about pain and its management, childbirth and perinatal care, and end of life care.

Nurses must be able to recognize spiritual distress and plan nursing care to assist the client. Nurses can assist clients by providing presence, supporting religious practices, assisting clients with prayer, and referring clients for spiritual counseling. Nurses must not attempt to convert clients to another spiritual or religious belief system.

REFERENCES

Andrews, M. M., & Boyle, J. C. (2003). *Transcultural concepts in nursing care* (4th ed.). Philadelphia: Lippincott.

Barnum, B. S. (1996). *Spirituality in nursing: From traditional to new age.* New York: Springer Publishing Company.

Blais, K. (2000). Spirituality. In B. Kozier, G. Erb, A. J. Berman, and K. Burke. *Fundamentals of nursing: Concepts, process, and practice* (6th ed.). Upper Saddle River, NJ: Prentice Hall.

Burkhardt, M. (1993). Characteristics of spirituality in the lives of women in a rural Appalachian community. *Journal of Transcultural Nursing, 4,* 12–18.

Burkhardt, M. A., & Nagai-Jacobson, M. G. (2002). *Spirituality: Living our connectedness.* Albany, NY: Delmar.

Carpenito-Moyet, L. J. (2003). *Nursing diagnosis: Application to clinical practice* (3rd ed.). Philadelphia: Lippincott Williams & Wilkins.

Dossey, B. M., Keegan, L., & Guzzetta, C. E. (2000). *Holistic nursing: A handbook for practice* (3rd ed.). Gaithersburg, MD: Aspen.

Dossey, L. (1993). *Healing words: The power of prayer and the practice of medicine.* New York: Harper San Francisco.

Eerdmans, W. B. (1994). *Eerdman's handbook to the world's religions.* Grand Rapids, MI: William B. Eerdmans Publishing Company.

Fowler, J. W. (1981). *Stages of faith development: The psychology of human development and the quest for meaning.* San Francisco: Harper & Row.

Health Ministries Association, Inc. (1998). *Scope and standards of parish nursing practice.* Washington, DC: American Nurses Publishing.

Henry, L. G., & Enry, J. D. (2004). *The soul of the caring nurse.* Washington, DC: American Nurses Association.

Kozier, B., Erb, G., Berman, A., & Snyder, S. (2004). *Fundamentals of nursing: Concepts, process, and practice* (7th ed.). Upper Saddle River, NJ: Prentice Hall.

Lowe, J., & Struthers, R. (2001). A conceptual framework of nursing in Native American culture. *Journal of Nursing Scholarship, 33*(3), 279–283.

Maugans, T. A. (1996). The SPIRITual history. *Archives of Family Medicine, 5*(1), 11–16.

Mauk, K. L., & Schmidt, N. K. (2004). *Spiritual care in nursing practice.* Philadelphia: Lippincott.

McSherry, W. M. (1998). Nurses' perceptions of spirituality and spiritual care. *Nursing Standard, 13*(4), 36–40.

Meisenhelder, J. B. (2003). Gender differences in religiosity and functional health in the elderly. *Geriatric Nursing, 24*(6), 343–347.

Moschella, V. D., Pressman, K. R., Pressman, P., & Weissman, D. E. (1997, Spring). The problem of theodicy and religious response to cancer. *Journal of Religion and Health, 36*(1), 17–20.

Murray, R. B., & Zentner, J. P. (2001). *Health promotion strategies through the life span.* Upper Saddle River, NJ: Prentice Hall.

NANDA International. (2003). *NANDA nursing diagnoses: Definitions and classification 2003–2004.* Philadelphia: NANDA.

O'Brien, M. E. (1999). *Spirituality in nursing: Standing on holy ground.* Boston: Jones and Bartlett.

Pollock, R. (2002). *The everything world's religions book.* Avon, MA: Adams Media Corporation.

Purnell, L. D., & Paulanka, B. J. (2003). *Transcultural health care: A culturally competent approach* (2nd ed.). Philadelphia: F. A. Davis.

Shelly, J. A., & Fish, S. (1988). *Spiritual care: The nurse's role* (3rd ed.). Downers Grove, IL: InterVarsity Press.

Spector, R. E. (2004). *Cultural diversity in health and illness* (6th ed.). Upper Saddle River, NJ: Prentice Hall Health.

Statistical Abstracts of the United States. (2002). http://www.census.gov/prod/2004pubs/03statab/pop.pdf.

Vardy, L. (1995). *God in all worlds.* Toronto: Vintage Canada.

Westerhoff, J. (1976). *Will our children have faith?* New York: Seabury Press.

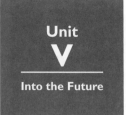

CHAPTER 23

Advanced Nursing Education and Practice

Objectives

■ Discuss education for advanced nursing roles.

■ Differentiate among functional advanced nursing roles, including clinical nurse specialist, nurse practitioner, nurse-educator, and nurse administrator.

■ Describe the historical development of advanced practice nursing.

■ Discuss certification and regulation of advanced practice roles.

■ Compare graduate education programs in advanced practice nursing.

■ Identify international perspectives on advanced nursing practice roles.

M E D I A L I N K

Additional online resources for this chapter can be found on the companion Web site at http://www.prenhall.com/blais.

Graduate education provides specialized knowledge and skill to enable nurses to assume advanced roles in education, administration, research, and practice. It also prepares nurses for advanced practice in a variety of specialized roles in primary, secondary, and tertiary settings. Graduate programs prepare clinical nurse specialists, nurse practitioners, nurse-midwives, and nurse-anesthetists.

Nurses prepared to assume advanced nursing roles bring new ideas, insights, and enlightenment to the total health care system. Their creativity, competence, commitment, and courage will influence the quality of care in a changing health system. Nurses with graduate education can influence the health care system from within by assuming positions of leadership in administration, education, and practice. They can also influence the political system to effect needed change through the research process. The growth of advanced practice nursing occurs through education, professional role advancement, and legislation. Choosing a graduate nursing program involves identifying one's personal career goals and then selecting the best program to enable one to meet those goals.

CHALLENGES AND OPPORTUNITIES

Advanced practice nursing has proliferated in response to managed care. As a result of health care reform, societal changes, an increasing international perspective, and demographic population changes, new advanced practice roles and changes in old ones have evolved. This has challenged the traditional ways of educating nurses and of practicing nursing. The changes in health care delivery continue, and the development of advanced practice roles must also continue to meet new demands.

The opportunities for nursing to redefine its role and practice in response to demands for change are tremendous. The evolution of advanced practice nursing to more autonomous roles needs to be driven by the nursing profession's vision as opposed to being reactive to outside pressures. Nursing education and advanced practice roles will need to develop in tandem if nursing is to be effective in preserving the best of what nursing has been and to take the profession into the future of health care.

ADVANCED NURSING EDUCATION

Historically, basic education in nursing prepared the graduate to be a nurse generalist. Nurses obtained education for specialization after completing the basic program, usually through hospital-based postgraduate courses designed to provide knowledge and skill in a specialized area. This type of specialized preparation in the early part of the twentieth century generally focused on obstetric nursing and private-duty nursing. As nurses acquired a greater body of knowledge in the sciences of anatomy, physiology, microbiology, chemistry, pathophysiology, and pharmacology, they became better able to make assessments about the nature of clients' problems. Nurses' increasing skills enabled them to assume a more active role in the care of their clients. Knowledge and skill that had previously been

the physician's domain gradually crossed over into nursing practice. For example, nurses acquired the skills to conduct in-depth physical assessments, venipuncture, suturing, ordering basic diagnostic studies, and administering life-saving medications under protocols.

As the nurse's role expanded, nurses became more specialized, and standards of practice required greater consistency in what nurses were permitted to do and could be expected to do. As the settings for practice became more specialized, postbasic specialty courses proliferated to include oncology nursing, critical care nursing, recovery room nursing, operating room nursing, rehabilitation nursing, and so on. These developments created a need for more formalized programs of study to ensure consistency of education and skill training.

Preparation for Advanced Clinical Practice

Specialty education provided in universities and colleges at the master's degree level evolved during the 1940s and 1950s. The idea was facilitated by the return of nurses from military service during World War II. These nurses often had GI benefits to return to school for advanced education. Passage of the National Mental Health Act in 1946 provided additional funds for education of nurses in the area of psychiatric/mental health nursing. During a 1952 conference sponsored by the National League for Nursing (NLN), it was agreed that the purpose of baccalaureate education was to prepare nurse generalists, whereas master's education was devoted to the preparation of nurse specialists. Master's level education was envisioned as the appropriate foundation for the preparation of nurses for specialty practice. Early graduate degrees in nursing focused on the functional roles of educator and administrator; for example, the degree offered at Columbia University's Teacher College focused on the preparation of nurse educators. The first clinical master's program was developed in 1954 by Hildegard Peplau at Rutgers University to prepare advanced practice nurses in psychiatric/mental health nursing. At this time, nurses prepared with graduate degrees in clinical specialties were referred to as **nurse clinicians** or **clinical nurse specialists.** The primary purpose of the clinical nurse specialist (CNS) was to improve client care and nursing practice by functioning as an expert nurse in the practice setting. The clinical nurse specialist was considered to be an expert in a specialized area of nursing practice, usually in the acute-care setting, and served as an expert care provider, a resource to novice nurses or general staff nurses for education and development, a consultant to the physician and other health professionals, and an active participant in research related to the specialized area of practice. Some believed that the clinical nurse specialist should not be used as a direct care provider, but rather as a clinical educator, consultant, or researcher. There was also concern that the role of the clinical nurse specialist was not clearly defined because nurses performed different roles and functions (educator, researcher, consultant, direct care provider, administrator) in different settings (Hamric, Spross, & Hanson, 2000).

During the 1960s, the United States experienced a health care personnel shortage as a result of the Vietnam War. Also during this time, a maldistribution of primary care physicians exacerbated the problem. In response to this problem, Dr. Loretta Ford and Dr. Henry Silver (a physician) developed the first nurse practitioner program in 1965 at the University of Colorado focusing on the care of children. Within 9 years, there were 65 nurse practitioner programs in pediatrics; additional programs were developed that focused on women's health or family health.

Because of society's need to meet its health care needs and the lack of graduate-level clinical nursing programs, short-term certificate programs were created to prepare nurse practitioners to meet health care demands. There was no consistency in the educational prerequisites, the length of the program, and the goals and content of the program in these early nurse practitioner programs. Some programs required the nurse to have a baccalaureate degree for admission, whereas others simply required registered nurse licensure and varying numbers of years of nursing experience. Program lengths ranged from a few months to 2 years. Some programs were taught only by physicians; others were taught by both physicians and nurses. Today, most advanced practice education takes place at the graduate level, and American Nurses Credentialing Center (ANCC) certification at the advanced practice levels of clinical specialist and nurse practitioner requires a master's degree.

There remains controversy related to the role of the clinical nurse specialist (CNS) and its differences from and similarities to the role of the advanced nurse practitioner (ANP). The different titles and the various perceptions about these advanced practice roles cause confusion among health care consumers as well as health care professionals. In 1994, the American Asso-

Evidence for Practice

Brown, M. A., & Draye, M. A. (2003). Experiences of pioneer nurse practitioners in establishing advanced practice roles. *Journal of Nursing Scholarship,* *35*(4), 391–392.

A description of pioneers' experience of establishing, building, and maintaining the nurse practitioner (NP) role in a contemporary practice environment was developed through interviews and focus groups with 50 middle-aged women. These women were all currently practicing as advanced practice nurses and began their NP role between 1965 and 1979. Data were gathered about their early experiences and analyzed using interpretive methods of grounded theory.

The central organizing theme that emerged in the data was Advancing Autonomy to Make a Difference. This theme built upon six broad themes: Breaking Free, Molding the Clay, Encountering Obstacles, Surviving the Proving Ground, Staying Committed, and Building the Eldership. The conclusion was that autonomy was requisite for practicing to one's full potential and for maintaining commitment over time. These findings can provide guidance to other beginning NPs in the United States and to NPs in other countries who are just beginning to develop the role.

ciation of Colleges of Nursing (AACN) held a conference on role differentiation of the nurse practitioner and the clinical nurse specialist. At consensus-building work groups, the participants identified the characteristics of the two advanced practice roles, their strengths, and the outcomes that might be expected if the two roles merged or remained separate (see the box on page 418). The reasons cited for merging the CNS and ANP roles included (1) less confusion to the public, (2) clarification of competencies and titles, (3) greater professional and political power, (4) greater marketability of the advanced practice nurse designation, (5) guarantees that preparation of advanced practice nurses would occur at the graduate level, and, perhaps most important, (6) increased benefits to clients resulting from the more comprehensive preparation of their nurses. In a vote taken following the work groups, 68% of the participants voted to merge the ANP and CNS

Comparison of CNS and NP

CLINICAL NURSE SPECIALIST	NURSE PRACTITIONER
Characteristics	**Characteristics**
Expertise in specific populations	Primary care, health-promotion focus
Research projects—team member and evaluator	Client-centered focus
Case management	Diagnosing and prescribing
Staff development and teaching	Case management
Use of systems approach to problem solving	Teacher
Strengths	**Strengths**
Specialized knowledge and skills, in-depth knowledge, expertise	Autonomy of practice
Systems skilled	Cost-effective and reimbursable
Role flexibility—time and practice	Popular with consumers and legislators
	Diagnostician
	Holistic approach (prevention and wellness)

Source: Adapted from *Role Differentiation of the Nurse Practitioner and Clinical Nurse Specialist: Reaching Toward Consensus* (pp. 69–70), by L. R. Cronenwett, December 1994, Proceedings of the Master's Education Conference, American Association of Colleges of Nursing, San Antonio, TX.

roles (AACN, 1994, p. 71). Nursing schools are beginning to merge their existing clinical nurse specialist programs with nurse practitioner programs, providing all graduates with the knowledge and skills to achieve national certification and to be eligible for state licensure at the advanced practice level. (Regulation of advanced practice is discussed later in the chapter.)

The merging of the two roles, often referred to as blended role, is not without controversy. Some argue that the roles are unique and should remain separate. Research comparing the two roles identifies differences in areas of focus and setting of practice even though there are areas of overlap. The Council of Nurses in Advanced Practice of the American Nurses Association (created by the merging of the Council of Clinical Nurse Specialists and The Council of Primary Health Care Nurse Practitioners) surveyed all graduates of CNS and NP programs and found that NP programs placed greater emphasis on history-taking, physical assessment, and pharmacology content, but that other differences were minimal. Practice setting was identified as the defining factor between roles. Concerns about merging the roles involve legislative issues, loss of role identity, increased length of graduate programs to ensure the competencies of both roles, and the ability to safely fulfill

both roles (Lincoln, 2000; Mick & Ackerman, 2000; Williams & Valdivieso, 1994).

Reflect on...

■ how the role of the primary care advanced practice nurse differs from the role of the primary care physician. How does the focus of care differ?

■ the societal benefits of having advanced practice nurses provide primary care.

Master's Degree in Nursing

According to the position statement of the American Association of Colleges of Nursing, advanced practice nursing requires preparation at the master's degree level and may include preparation as a clinical nurse specialist, nurse-anesthetist, nurse-midwife, or nurse practitioner (AACN, 2001a). Most of these advanced practice nurses must have both a graduate degree and certification in the specialty area.

The number of programs offering master's preparation for advanced practice nursing, particularly nurse practitioners, has increased dramatically during the recent past in response to the demand for cost-effective primary care. However, schools of nursing continue to offer specialization in indirect care roles

Evidence for Practice

Lincoln, P. E. (2000). Comparing CNS and NP role activities: A replication. *Clinical Nurse Specialist,* *14*(6), 269–277.

This study replicates a study by Williams and Valdiviesco in 1992 that compared the CNS and NP roles in order to identify trends since the original study. The study included 310 CNSs and 300 NPs practicing in Minnesota randomly drawn from a pool of ANCC certified nurses. Three instruments were used to collect the data: a demographic questionnaire, the Advanced Nursing Practice Survey (ANPS), and the Work Activities Checklist. The ANPS gathered data on clinical activities, values, and working relationships.

Similarities in role function were found between the CNS and NP subjects. Both groups implemented the roles of direct practice, consultation, education, administration, and research. However, the focus of their daily activities differed significantly. CNSs were primarily employed in hospital settings, and most NPs were practicing in ambulatory settings. NPs were located in a wider variety of practice settings, whereas CNSs tended to be in larger cities. The CNS provided less direct care than the NP and more time in such activities as educating staff, consulting with other disciplines, carrying out administrative functions, and participating in research activities.

The author concludes that there are some overlapping roles of the CNS and NP but that each has it own unique contribution to the care of clients. The differences in practice are significant enough that one role cannot be substituted for the other.

In tracking the trends from the original study, it is concluded that the roles have changed to better meet clients' needs, and the evolution has created similarities and overlap. However, the roles continue to have distinct differences in setting, locale, and focus of practice. This study lends support to the continued existence of the two advanced practice roles.

such as management, administration, education, and informatics. These roles will continue to be important as nurses are prepared to be leaders in systems of care (AACN, 2001b).

Regardless of the advanced practice or functional role, the curricula should have a core that is common to all graduate programs. Priorities for the core curriculum include the following (AACN, 2001c):

- Critical thinking and clinical judgment
- Primary health care, patient education, health promotion, rehabilitation, self-care, and alternative methods of healing
- Practice across multiple settings, including nontraditional settings
- Case management, health care policy and economics, research methods, quality indicators, outcome measures, financial management, legislative advocacy, and management of data and technology

Key topics for teaching these requirements include health care policy, organization of the health care delivery system, health care economics and finance, ethical issues in health care, professional role development, theoretical foundations of nursing practice, human diversity and social issues, and health promotion and disease prevention (Robinson & Kish, 2001).

Doctoral Programs in Nursing

The majority of doctoral programs in nursing emphasize clinically relevant research that builds the science for nursing practice and also prepares faculty for academic roles in colleges and universities that offer nursing programs. These doctoral programs must prepare faculty for the future by providing frameworks and tools for moving to new ways of educating for new roles and ways of practice (AACN, 2001c).

Graduates of doctoral programs in nursing are prepared for research, education, and practice and may assume careers as advanced clinicians, administrators, researchers, or public policy makers. The degree granted may be a doctor of philosophy (Ph.D.) in nursing, doctor of nursing science (D.N.S.), or nursing doctorate (N.D.). The differences among these degrees may be minimal in reality but generally reflect a greater emphasis on research (Ph.D.), greater emphasis on the development of nursing science (D.N.S.), or greater emphasis on nursing practice (N.D.). Nurses interested in enrolling in a doctoral program in nursing should review the curriculum plan and philosophy of the selected program to select a match for their professional goals.

ADVANCED NURSING PRACTICE

The number of advanced practice nurses delivering health care in the United States and around the world is increasing. They are delivering cost-effective and high-quality health care to chronically underserved populations in particular. The advanced practice nurse (APN) is an umbrella term for the registered nurse who has met advanced education and clinical practice requirements. This umbrella covers four principal types of APNs: certified nurse-midwives (CNM), clinical nurse specialists (CNS), certified registered nurse-anesthetists (CRNA), and nurse practitioners (NP). Table 23–1 gives examples of the role and scope of each of these four APN roles.

The Strong Model of Advanced Practice identifies five domains of practice, with activities in each practice domain described in accordance with standards of advanced practice. The five domains are: direct comprehensive care, support of systems, education, research, and publication and professional leadership. Within the model, there are unifying strands of collaboration, scholarship, and empowerment describing the attributes of advanced practice, the approach to care, and the professional attitude (Ackerman, Norsen, Weidrich, & Kitzman, 1996).

Much of the primary and preventive care provided traditionally by physicians can be provided by APNs at a lower cost. These nurses work collaboratively with physicians and other health professionals to coordinate health services for the benefit of the client. Each of the 50 states provides regulatory oversight through its board of nursing, which sets competency standards and continuing education requirements. Restrictions on the scope of practice have resulted from the lack of prescriptive authority and lack of eligibility for reimbursement from third-party payers.

Types of Advanced Practice

Advanced practice nursing in the United States has evolved into four main types of advanced practitioners: clinical nurse specialist, nurse practitioner, nurse-midwife, and nurse-anesthetist. As health care delivery systems continue to change and develop, other roles may emerge to meet future needs. Each advanced role

Table 23–1 Examples of the Role and Scope of Advanced Practice Nurses

Advanced Practice Nurses	Application of Advanced Knowledge and Skills	Patient Population Served	Practice Settings
Certified Nurse-Midwives	Well-women health care, management of pregnancy, childbirth, antepartum and postpartum care. Health promotion.	Childbearing women	Homes Hospitals Birthing centers Ambulatory care
Clinical Nurse Specialists	Management of complex patient health care problems in various clinical speciality areas through direct care, consultation, research, education, and administrative roles.	Individuals with physical or psychiatric disability, maternal and child health problems, gerontological problems	Tertiary care Ambulatory care Community care Home health care Rehabilitation
Nurse-Anesthetists	Preoperative assessment, administration of anesthesia, and management of postanesthesia recovery.	Individuals in all age-groups undergoing surgical procedures	Hospital operating rooms Ambulatory care Surgical settings

Nurse Practitioners	Management of a wide range of health problems through physical examination, diagnosis, treatment, and patient/family education and counseling. Primary care and health promotion.	Individuals and families:
		  Women
		  Infants and children
		  Elderly
		  Adults and others
			Primary care
			Long-term care
			Ambulatory and community care
			Tertiary care

Source: From *Certification and Regulation of Advanced Practice Nurses,* by American Association of Colleges of Nursing, 2001, Washington, DC: AACN.

has a distinguishable scope of practice, but knowledge and skills still overlap.

Clinical Nurse Specialist (CNS)

The CNS role evolved as an avenue toward professional advancement for nurses who wanted to remain in clinical practice at the bedside rather than advance to administration or education. Traditionally the role integrates the subroles of expert nurse clinician, consultant, educator, and researcher. These subroles require skill in collaboration, role modeling, patient advocacy, clinical leadership, and being a change agent. The CNS may also assume administrative and management roles, but there is controversy about whether that is appropriate to a role dependent on expertise in clinical practice. The scope of practice is fluid because the subroles are implemented in various ways and as the CNS interacts with other health care professionals. Generally the CNS works with a specific patient population and uses nursing process and theory in practice.

The American Association of Critical-Care Nurses has developed a redefinition of CNS practice presented by the Synergy Model. In this model, the following eight CNS characteristics are applied across three spheres of influence.

1. Clinical judgment
2. Clinical inquiry
3. Facilitator of learning

Interview 23.1 – *Clinical Nurse Specialist*

Sharon S. Cohen, RN, MSN, CEN, CCRN

What was your area of practice before you became a CNS? I was a staff nurse in ICU and in the Emergency Department.

Why did you decide to become a CNS? I'm a creative and self-directed person. I wanted to have greater influence on patient care and staff expertise. So when I got my MSN I felt a CNS role offered me more autonomy than a nurse practitioner role. The inquisitive side of me wanted to incorporate research and that is a part of the CNS role. I basically wanted to elevate the level of expertise at the bedside, and in this role I can see people blossom.

Describe your practice setting and what you do as a CNS. My practice setting is a Level 1 trauma center. I see the patients in the Trauma Resuscitation Unit, Surgical-Trauma ICU, or other floors as needed. I respond to Trauma Alert calls, both pediatric and adult. I am available to staff for questions, particularly clinical questions when the acuity level is high. I am also responsible for program development and CEU offerings and other educational programs. I participate in research and try to get the staff involved in research and in implementing evidence-based practice through policy and protocols.

Describe your best experience as a CNS. The one that really taught me the most involved a 12-year-old girl who was hit by a car while she was crossing the street to get to her school bus. She arrived brain dead and we could do none of our life-saving measures to help her. Her mother was a single mother who was working as a temp; we had no contact information and had to send the police to the agency and then out to find her in the workplace. Before the mother could arrive at the hospital, the PICU nurses had cleaned her up, covered the battered part of her head, and had her looking beautiful when the mother arrived. The little girl had the most angelic expression I have ever seen. After the mother arrived and grieved awhile, she kissed her daughter goodbye. It was at this time I had to approach her about organ donation. I said to her that although I knew this was her worst nightmare, she might be able to help someone else by donating organs. The mother said that there had been an organ-recipient who visited the daughter's school just a few weeks before and told the kids what a wonderful thing it was to receive an organ. The daughter had gone home and told the mother that she wanted to be an organ donor. The mother felt by agreeing to the organ donation she was fulfilling her daughter's wishes. The human contact with that mother taught me so much, and you don't learn those things in textbooks. Those of us who work in trauma become so centered on life saving that we need to remember how to care for the families when we can't save a life.

What encouragement and advice would you give to a nurse considering becoming a CNS? Do your homework on all the advanced practice roles and pick the one that best suits you. I think the CNS role is the hardest because it is more autonomous. You have to want that autonomy to be happy in the role.

4. Collaboration
5. Systems thinking
6. Advocacy or moral agency
7. Caring practices
8. Response to diversity

These characteristics assist the nurse to identify interventions in the three areas of influence: patients and families, nurse to nurse, and individual health care systems (providers and organizations) (Moloney-Harmon, 1999).

The education and expertise should be such that the clinical nurse specialist is eligible for certification in a specialty area. Eligibility requirements vary some-

what from specialty to specialty, and applications are reviewed individually to determine eligibility for certification. The American Nurses Credentialing Center provides national certification of clinical nurse specialists in a number of areas; the certification is valid for a period of 5 years, and renewal requires either a minimum number of continuing education hours or retaking a certification exam.

Nurse Practitioner (NP)

The NP has a wide scope of practice and a more autonomous role using comprehensive assessment, clinical reasoning, and differential diagnosis. NPs have legal authority to implement patient management by ordering

Table 23–2 Certification Available Through American Nurses Credentialing Center

Advanced Practice	Specialty Certification Baccalaureate	Specialty Certification Associate Degree/ Diploma
Nurse Practitioners • Adult Nurse Practitioner • Family Nurse Practitioner • Gerontological Nurse Practitioner • Pediatric Nurse Practitioner • Acute Care Nurse Practitioner • Adult Psychiatric and Mental Health Nurse Practitioner • Family Psychiatric and Mental Health Nurse Practitioner • Advanced Diabetes Management–Nurse Practitioner **Clinical Specialists** • Clinical Specialist in Adult Psychiatric and Mental Health Nursing • Clinical Specialist in Child/Adolescent Psychiatric Mental Health Nursing • Clinical Specialist in Gerontological Nursing • Clinical Specialist in Medical-Surgical Nursing • Clinical Specialist in Home Health Nursing • Clinical Specialist in Pediatric Nursing • Clinical Specialist in Community Health • Advanced Diabetes Management– Clinical Specialist	• Psychiatric and Mental Health Nurses • Medical-Surgical Nurses • Pediatric Nurses • Gerontological Nurses • Perinatal Nurse • Community Health Nurse • College Health Nurse • Cardiac/Vascular Nurse • Informatics Nurse • Home Health Nurse • Nursing Professional Development • Nursing Administration • Nursing Administration, Advanced	• Psychiatric and Mental Health Nurse • Medical-Surgical Nurse • Pediatric Nurse • Gerontological Nurse • Perinatal Nurse • Cardiac/Vascular Nurse

Source: From *ANCC Certification Exams,* by American Nurses Credentialing Center, 2004, http://www.ana.org/ancc/certification/exams.html.

diagnostic tests and treatments and prescribing medications. Health promotion and illness and injury prevention are important focuses. The NP works in a variety of settings, both autonomously and in interdisciplinary groups, providing care for individuals, families, and communities. Table 23–2 shows certification areas available through the American Nurses Credentialing Center.

The **acute-care nurse practitioner** is a registered nurse with a graduate degree in nursing who is prepared for advanced practice using a collaborative model to provide direct services to adult patients who are acutely or critically ill in a variety of settings. They use diagnostic reasoning and advanced therapeutic interventions, and their practice includes independent and interdependent decision making and direct accountability for clinical judgment. The **adult nurse practitioner** is prepared for advanced practice in adult health across the health continuum. The role includes case management, consultation, leadership, education, research, and health policy development. The **family nurse practitioner** is prepared for advanced practice with individuals and families throughout the life span and across the health continuum. The **gerontological nurse practitioner** provides primary care to older adults in a variety of settings and practices, both collaboratively and independently. In this role the NP works to maximize functional abilities; promotes, maintains, and restores health; prevents or minimizes disabilities; and promotes death with dignity. The **pediatric nurse practitioner** provides primary and specialty care for children from birth through 21 years of age. These services are provided within family and developmental contexts to children who are essentially well or who have acute illness, chronic illness, or disabilities. Before December 31, 2000, certification was also offered to school nurse practitioners, but the examination is no longer offered. Previously certified school nurse practitioners can be recertified through continuing education (ANCC, 2000).

Interview 23.2 – *Nurse Practitioner Interview*

Marybeth Thompson, ARNP

What was your area of practice before you became a nurse practitioner? Before I became a nurse practitioner, I was the Nurse Manager of a Diabetes Treatment Center and a hospital educator (concurrently) at two different hospitals, both owned by the same company.

Why did you decide to become a nurse practitioner? Every year I seemed to be moving farther away from interacting with patients. When I was involved with their care, I was frustrated that I couldn't always get the physician's orders I thought were needed. Finally, I realized, "Stop complaining. Just go get the education you need and you can do it yourself!"

Describe your practice setting and what you do as a nurse practitioner. For the last 5 years, I have been associated with two physicians in an internal medicine and gastroenterology practice. I am responsible for the bulk of the internal medicine in the office, but also "work up" the GI cases. On average, I see about 25 patients per day. Most afternoons the physicians are out of the office performing procedures while I continue with office appointments. We receive approximately 100 phone calls daily, most of which I screen. Some can be delegated to my medical assistant; the remainder requires a return call from me. At the end of the day, my two associate physicians and I touch base, usually by phone, to share any pertinent information.

Describe your best experience as a nurse practitioner. My best experience is a relatively simple one. I had just completed the exam portion of a yearly physical on a middle-aged man. I sat down and prepared to go quickly through the requisite preventive health issues for what seemed like the millionth time that day. Instead, I just asked, "What can I say to you to convince you to quit smoking?" He looked at me oddly and said, "I quit smoking 10 months ago. You told me to quit when I saw you last year. No doctor ever told me to before, so I thought it must be pretty important for you to say something." I just looked at him. Sometimes it seems like no one ever listens to my advice. But this guy really did. Wow! I promised myself I would never again underestimate what effect concerned urging can have on a patient's health.

What encouragement and advice would you give to a nurse considering becoming a nurse practitioner? Perseverance is the key. We think we're not smart enough or we're too busy, but these are just the things we tell ourselves, and what other people tell us, that limit our horizons. Do it slowly if you need to, because time will surely pass whether you persevere or not.

Interview 23.3 – *Certified Nurse-Midwife*

Elisa Wolfe, MSN, CNM

What was your area of practice before you became a nurse-midwife? I was a Clinical Nurse Specialist in Obstetrics at a large county medical center, and before that I worked in Labor and Delivery for 12 years.

Why did you decide to become a nurse-midwife? I loved obstetrics and wanted to move ahead in advanced practice nursing. Getting a master's degree in nurse-midwifery just made sense to me.

Describe your practice setting and what you do as a nurse-midwife. I work with a group of physicians and nurse-midwives providing service at a large public institution. We staff the prenatal clinics and do hospital deliveries and make rounds on the patients. I spend sometimes two or three days a week in the clinic and the rest at the hospital. As a nurse-midwife I see low-risk patients, but our population is really not very low risk, so we do a lot of co-management and consultation with the physicians when there is a problem.

Describe your best experience as a nurse-midwife. I'm a relatively new nurse-midwife, and there really isn't just one. I love delivering babies and being with the mother at such a special time in her life. I like seeing them in the clinic. Enjoying the clinic setting as much as I do surprised me; I have always liked being in the hospital and wasn't looking forward to working in an office setting, but at the clinic, there is so much opportunity to talk to the patients and really teach them. However, being able to assist a woman while she is giving birth is very special. It is a moment she will always remember, and it makes me very happy to be a part of it.

What encouragement and advice would you give to a nurse considering becoming a nurse-midwife? If you love obstetrics, just do it! It's hard, but it's fun and well worth the time and effort. You get to be with the mothers in different settings, and there is always something new and changing. I like the fact that I can be in an advanced practice role and remain in the hospital setting. For those who like the fast pace and adrenalin rush of acute care, you can experience that as a nurse-midwife. There is more autonomy for those who want that in their work, but you have to love OB.

Certified Nurse-Midwife (CNM)

The practice of Nurse Midwifery in the United States began in the 1920s and was established by such early leaders as Mary Breckinridge and Hattie Hemschemeyer. Its history is linked to the Frontier Nursing Service. A **certified nurse-midwife** (CNM) is a registered nurse who has advanced educational preparation in midwifery, which includes theory and extensive supervised clinical experiences in prenatal care, management of labor and delivery, postpartum care of the mother and infant, family planning, and gynecological care for well women. The focus of education is on normal obstetrics and newborn care. Most nurses who choose to become nurse-midwives have extensive prior nursing experience in maternity and public health nursing. The majority of nurse-midwifery programs in the United States offer a master's degree, and all are accredited by the American College of Nurse-Midwives (ACNM). The ACNM is also the credentialing organization that sets the standards by which nurse-midwifery is practiced in the United States. Certified nurse-midwives practice in all 50 states in the United States delivering babies in hospitals, in birthing centers, and in the home. Although most nurse-midwives practice independently, providing care for women and children, all maintain an affiliation with a physician specialist in obstetrics and gynecology for consultation and referral of clients with complications.

Nurse-midwives also practice in Great Britain, Canada, Australia, Europe, Africa, and many of the island nations in the Caribbean. The education, regulation, and extent of practice of nurse-midwives vary around the world. The World Health Organization (WHO) has placed increasing emphasis on the role of the midwife in partnership with the International Confederation of Midwives and the International Council of Nurses. The Global Advisory Group on Nursing and Midwifery (GAGNM) was created in response to international concerns about ensuring quality nursing and midwifery services for worldwide populations. The growth, development, and support of these roles are viewed as key in achieving health for all (Thompson, 2002).

Bookshelf

Breckinridge, M. (1981). *Wide neighborhoods: The story of the frontier nursing service.* Lexington, KY: University Press of Kentucky.

The author describes the story of the beginning of the frontier nursing service and of providing nursing and health care to an underserved area of Appalachia. She founded the Frontier Nursing Service by gathering dedicated nurses willing to serve in an isolated area where little health care was available.

Wells, R., & McCarty, P. (1998). *Mary on horseback: Three mountain stories.* New York: Dial Books for Young Readers.

This is a book to recommend to younger readers, grades 2–5. It tells the stories of three families who were helped by Mary Breckinridge, the first nurse to go into the Appalachian Mountains and provide medical care.

Evidence for Practice

Swartz, M. K., Grey, M., Allan, J. D., Ridenour, N., Kovner, C., Walker, P., & Marion, L. (2003). A day in the lives of APNs in the U.S. *The Nurse Practitioner, 28*(10), 32–39.

A national survey of NPs and CNMs collected data on their practice for a typical day. They were asked about hours worked, number of patients seen, practice setting, clinical problems encountered, and other information. A total of 676 Advanced Practice Nurses participated in the study. On a typical day NPs and CNMs spent 7.35 hours seeing an average of 15.35 patients. The average time per visit was 27 minutes. Seventy-eight percent of the nurses practiced in an office or clinic, 12% practiced in a hospital setting, 2% practiced in a nursing home, and 8% identified another type of practice setting. Overall, laboratory studies were requested for 35% of the patients and radiographic studies for 10%. A physician consult was obtained for 15% of the patients, and 8% were referred to a specialist. Forty-two percent of the patients received counseling or patient education and a prescription for one medication. About 16% received prescriptions for two or more drugs. The patients seen by the nurses on that day were racially and culturally diverse, and about two thirds were female. Poor patient adherence to care regimens and patient difficulties with keeping appointments and follow-up visits were among the most challenging clinical problems identified, and these problems were confounded by associated difficulties with patients' financial resources. The results of this survey indicate that NPs and CNMs routinely manage complex caseloads.

Certified Registered Nurse-Anesthetist (CRNA)

The nurse-anesthetist was one of the earliest advanced practice roles in the United States. Nurses started administering anesthesia as early as 1889. A **certified registered nurse-anesthetist** (CRNA) is a registered nurse who has advanced educational preparation, including classroom and laboratory instruction and supervised clinical practice, in the delivery of anesthesia to clients in a variety of practice settings, including hospitals, ambulatory surgical centers, birthing centers, and clinics. The American Association of Nurse Anesthetists, founded in 1931, established a certification program for nurse-anesthetists in 1945 and an accreditation program for educational programs for nurse anesthesia in 1952. In some settings, such as birthing centers and ambulatory surgical centers, nurse-anesthetists may deliver anesthesia independently to clients with uncomplicated vaginal deliveries or minor surgeries.

A CRNA takes care of a patient's anesthesia needs before, during, and after surgery. The tasks they assume in performing the role include the following:

- Performing physical assessment
- Participating in preoperative teaching
- Preparing for anesthetic management
- Administering anesthesia to keep the patient free of pain
- Maintaining anesthesia intraoperatively
- Overseeing recovery from anesthesia
- Following the patient's postoperative course from recovery room to patient care unit

CRNAs practice in traditional operating rooms, ambulatory surgery centers, pain clinics, and physicians' offices. Many practice on a solo basis and have independent contracting arrangements with physicians and hospitals (AANA, 2001). Although CNAs are legally allowed to provide anesthesia in all 50 states, some states require physician supervision.

Interview 23.4 – *Certified Nurse-Anesthetist*

Gerard T. Hogan, Jr., CRNA, MSN, DNSc, ARNP

What was your area of practice before you became a nurse-anesthetist? I was an ICU/CCU nurse. I enjoyed the challenge of taking care of critically ill patients in an acute-care setting. Before I started working in the ICU I spent one year on a surgical floor. That taught me valuable organizational skills that I still use today.

Why did you decide to become a nurse-anesthetist? It seemed like a natural career progression move for me. Nurse-anesthesia builds on the critical care nursing skills developed working in the ICU. It requires vigilance and skill. I had considered becoming an Adult or Acute Care ARNP, but anesthesia fascinated me.

Describe your practice setting and what you do as a nurse-anesthetist. Nurse-anesthetists practice in all 50 states and in the Federal and Military systems. We are responsible for every aspect of anesthesia patient care, from the pre-operative assessment to the Post Anesthesia Care Unit. I currently practice in a 500-bed community/teaching hospital. I conduct preanesthetic interviews, provide general anesthesia, regional anesthesia, and monitored anesthesia care. I follow my patients in the PACU and order medications as needed for them there. Since I am also a faculty member at a local university, I am a clinical instructor to nurse-anesthesia students on a daily basis.

Describe your best experience as a nurse-anesthetist. I think my best experiences as a CRNA happen when I make a connection with patients and put their mind at ease regarding their anesthetic. As nurses we all learn how to communicate, and CRNAs are unique in that they carry these skills with them into the operating room. Taking the time to talk to patients, get to the root of their fears, and then instilling trust, to me is the best experience as a CRNA.

What encouragement and advice would you give to a nurse considering becoming a nurse-anesthetist? Study hard in nursing school and get good grades. Prepare for the GRE and work toward a high score. Admission to a CRNA program is very competitive. Nurse-anesthesia educational programs are very rigorous and demanding, so you need to set your priorities and be totally committed to the goal of becoming a CRNA. Get your finances in order and have a plan on how you will support yourself. All CRNA programs are full-time only and you will have little or no time to work. I think the best advice I can offer is to never forget where you came from. Nursing is an integral part of nurse-anesthesia. Being a CRNA allows me to blend one-on-one patient care with complex monitoring and pharmacology. It was the perfect fit for me.

Reflect on...

■ the specialty practice areas of advanced nurse practitioners and clinical nurse specialists. What are the differences? What are the similarities?

■ client satisfaction with the APN. What client needs does the APN meet that the physician may not meet? What client needs does the physician meet that the APN may not meet?

Regulation of Advanced Practice

The regulation of advanced practice nursing in the United States varies from state to state. Each state has the jurisdiction to determine the requirements for licensure of the APN including the use of a particular title and the definition of the scope of practice. The majority of state boards of nursing use certification examinations for the regulation of APNs and provide coverage under their registered nurse license. Only three states (California, Florida, and New York) provide either dual licenses or separate certification for APNs (Hickey, Ouimette, & Venegoni, 2000).

Various legal titles are conferred by the states to designate the APN, including nurse practitioner, advanced practice registered nurse, advanced practice nurse, and advanced registered nurse practitioner. In addition, certification titles such as certified nurse-midwife, clinical nurse specialist, and certified registered nurse-anesthetist cause confusion in the public's mind about who APNs are and what they do. The state boards of nursing as well as the professional nursing organizations are currently considering this issue of APN titling.

Certification is a voluntary process by which an agency or an association grants recognition to a person who has met specified qualifications. Certification is intended to protect the public by enabling the identification of competent people. It signifies the attainment of specific criteria and knowledge, skills, and abilities in a specific specialty field (ANCC, 2001). Many APNs are certified by national professional organizations that have developed educational and experiential criteria for specialty certification. For example, the Pediatric Nursing Certification Board (PNCB) provides pediatric nurses certification opportunities as certified pediatric nurse practitioners (CPNP) and certified pediatric nurses (CPN). It is the largest certification organization for this specialty and has granted more than 13,000 national pediatric nursing certifications (PNCB, 2003). Most states require certification by a recognized national certification body before a nurse can function at the advanced practice level.

APNs with the assistance of national professional organizations, have fought hard to obtain legal authority to practice, to be directly reimbursed for their service, and to prescribe medications. Whereas most states recognize the nurse-anesthetist, the nurse-midwife, and the nurse practitioner roles, many states do not recognize the clinical nurse specialist as an advanced practice role. Most states require the completion of a master's degree in nursing with an advanced practice specialty for licensure as an APN.

APNs have sought to receive direct reimbursement for their services from private insurers, Medicaid, Medicare, and other governmental funders of health care services. Whereas many states provide for some level of direct reimbursement from governmental sources, usually at a percentage of what a physician will receive for providing the same service, a few states provide full reimbursement for advanced practice nursing services. Some states authorize a percentage of reimbursement (usually around 85%) when the nurse bills directly but will reimburse at 100% if the nurse bills indirectly through a physician/nurse collaboration.

The right to prescribe medications and other therapies is a third area requiring legal authority. The majority of states allow APNs to prescribe, but many require that such prescriptions follow physician protocols and be co-signed by a physician or include the physician's name and drug number on the prescription form. Some states require pharmacist approval. Many states limit the APN's prescriptive authority to certain classifications of drugs, often prohibiting the nurse from prescribing controlled drugs. Some states have developed a formulary of drugs from which nurses can prescribe. Some states grant prescriptive privileges only to nurses who are working in public health clinics, rural health facilities, or other medically underserved settings. In those states where APNs have

some level of prescriptive authority, they may be required to have a course in advanced pharmacology, some specified period of supervised clinical practice, or a master's degree in nursing. Some states mandate continuing education in pharmacology to maintain prescriptive privileges.

The International Prespective

The International Council of Nurses (ICN) established an International Nurse Practitioner/Advanced Practice Nursing Network in 2000 responding to new nursing roles emerging worldwide. To facilitate common understanding and to guide further development, an official ICN position paper was released in 2002 with the following definition:

> A Nurse Practitioner/Advanced Practice Nurse is a registered nurse who has acquired the expert knowledge base, complex decision-making skills and clinical competencies for extended practice, the characteristics of which are shaped by the context and/or country in which s/he is credentialed to practice. A Masters degree is recommended for entry level. (ICN, 2002)

The next step will be the development of scope of practice and standards related to advanced practice roles worldwide.

In Canada, Advanced Nursing Practice (ANP) is an umbrella term describing an advanced level of nursing practice that maximizes the use of in-depth nursing knowledge and skill. ANP extends the boundaries of the scope of practice. The domain of practice is usually direct care but may include education, research, or administration (Canadian Nurses Association [CNA], 2002). Nurse practitioners integrate into their practice diagnosing and treating health problems and prescribing drugs. There is variability as to entry-level requirements for NPs because of the variety of programs developed in the 1980s and 1990s leading to the NP role, although movement is toward graduate education as the minimum level of preparation (CNA, 2003a). The CNS is a registered nurse with a graduate degree and expertise in a specialty area. The role was introduced in the 1960s and comprises five domains: practice, consultation, education, research, and leadership (CNA, 2003b).

The Canadian Nurses Association offers a certification program that provides a clinical credential in a number of clinical specialties. Eligibility for certification is based on experience in the specialty or a combination of experience and postbasic education.

Canadian Nurses Association Specialty Certifications

- Cardiovascular
- Critical Care
- Critical Care—Pediatrics
- Emergency
- Gastroenterology
- Hospice Palliative Care
- Nephrology

- Neuroscience
- Occupational Health
- Oncology
- Perinatal
- Perioperative
- Psychiatric/Mental Health

Source: From *Certification,* Canadian Nurses Association, 2004, http://www.cna-aiic.ca.

Nursing legislation across Canada is built on professional responsibility and accountability, and nurses must not act beyond their individual level of competence and preparation. The accompanying box shows the certification areas provided by the Canadian Nurses Association.

In Australia, there are two levels of nurses: the registered nurse and the enrolled nurse. The registered nurse is a first-level nurse, educated in preregistration degree-level courses in universities. The enrolled nurse is a second-level nurse who provides nursing care within the limits specified by education. They are educated primarily through advanced-certificate or associate diploma–level courses in colleges of technical and further education. In 2001 about 80% of nurses were registered nurses and about 20% were enrolled nurses (Australian Institute of Health and Welfare, 2003).

The Australian Nursing Council, Inc. establishes competency standards for both levels, and these standards assist in establishing the scope of practice. State and territory nurse regulatory authorities establish and maintain standards and processes for the regulation of nursing. The standards cover clinical practice, management of care, counseling, health promotion, client advocacy, facilitation of change, clinical teaching, supervising, mentoring, and research (Australian Nursing Council, Inc., 2000, 2001).

Postgraduate education is available in many areas of specialization such as mental health, community, critical care, emergency care, and many others. Nurse practitioners are authorized to practice by the nurse regulatory authorities and legislation provides NPs the authority to prescribe some medications and initiate some investigations as a member of a multidisciplinary team. Midwifery in Australia is achieved through a postgraduate course, and the midwives are authorized to practice midwifery care from conception to early parenting (Australian Peak Nursing Forum, 2004).

Evidence for Practice

Miles, K., Penny, N., Power, R., & Mercey, D. (2003). Comparing doctor- and nurse-led care in a sexual health clinic: Patient satisfaction questionnaire. *Journal of Advanced Nursing, 42*(1), 64–72.

A questionnaire was distributed to a convenience sample of 132 women attending a nurse-led clinic and 150 women attending a doctor-led clinic in London. The women were seen for sexually transmitted infections and other sexual health problems. Thirty-four items on the questionnaire were rated on a five-point Likert scale. The total satisfaction scores were significantly higher from the women attending the nurse-led clinic. Subscores measuring quality and competence of technical care, provision of information, and overall satisfaction were significantly higher as well. There were no significant differences on subscales measuring service attributes nor on attributes of interpersonal relationships. These patients were more satisfied with the care provided in a nurse-led clinic than that in a doctor-led clinic.

Critical Thinking Exercise

Interview an advanced practice nurse and a nurse working in a traditional role using the criteria on Pavalko's occupation to profession continuum found in Chapter 2 ∞. What differences did you find in the two roles related to the criteria for a profession? Was there a difference in autonomy of practice?

Critical Thinking Exercise

What knowledge and skills are shared by nurses and physicians? Which specific skills fall in the domain of basic nursing practice, which fall into advanced nursing practice, and which are specific to the practice of medicine?

The Future of Advanced Practice Nursing

APNs fill a need for quality primary care services at an affordable cost to clients in both rural and urban settings. Access to affordable care has been one of the driving forces in the increased number of APNs in recent years. That societal need is likely to continue to influence the delivery of health care. Nursing is strategically positioned to be a major player in policy development for the future.

Registered nurses, advanced practice nurses, and professional nursing organizations will need to educate not only the public but also the politicians and legislators about the proper role of the advanced practice nurse. The APN has a major role in preventing illness and promoting health for individuals, families, and communities. As APNs expand their roles and become more autonomous, role conflict with primary care physicians develops. For the advanced practice roles to fulfill their potential, there must be a cooperative and collaborative relationship established with other health care providers, particularly with physicians. The need for further expansion of the scope of practice to include prescriptive privileges and other procedures traditionally performed by physicians will continue into the future.

Professional nursing organizations will need to ensure a high standard for those who aspire to advanced practice certification. Educational institutions will need to collaborate and cooperate with professional nursing organizations and employers of APNs to ensure that the classroom and clinical instructional experiences prepare graduates to assume the APN role effectively. Recently there has been much discussion about merging the role of the advanced nurse practitioner with the clinical specialist to decrease professional and public confusion. Many educational institutions are already changing their curricula to integrate the two roles in graduate education. However, the move has remained somewhat controversial.

Reflect on...

■ the future of advanced practice in your community, state (province, territory), and nation. How do you see APNs solving some of the problems in today's health care system?

■ whether advanced practice is a professional career choice for you. Do you have the assertiveness required to perform in an independent role?

SELECTING A GRADUATE PROGRAM

Choosing a graduate program is an important decision for a nurse who is committed to lifelong work in nursing. Several factors must be considered, including professional career goals, personal and family factors, and characteristics of the proposed program. See the box on page 430.

Professional Career Goals

The nurse must first identify personal career goals. Graduate education is preparation for specialized practice. Not all graduate programs will provide the course work to meet the requirements for all advanced nursing roles and all clinical practice settings. Some graduate schools of nursing focus on nurse practitioner roles; others focus on the roles of nurse educator and administrator. Some schools are highly specialized and may provide only a single program, for example, in nurse-anesthesia. Some schools of nursing have become innovative and offer highly specialized graduate programs of study, such as nursing informatics, aerospace nursing, or forensic nursing. Some graduate schools of nursing integrate advanced clinical practice roles with functional roles of education or administration but still require that the nurse choose an area of

Criteria for Considering a Graduate Program

- Professional career goals
- Personal and family factors
- Program characteristics
    1. Type of graduate programs offered
    2. School's philosophy of nursing and education
    3. Accreditation status
    4. National standing

5. Admission requirements
6. Faculty qualifications
7. Institutional climate
8. Resources
9. Clinical facilities
10. Assistantships and other financial support
11. Program graduation requirements

Source: Adapted from "Graduate Education: Making the Right Choice," by G. W. Poteet, L. C. Hodges, and S. Tate. In *Current Issues in Nursing* (4th ed., pp. 182–187), by J. McCloskey and H. K. Grace (Eds.), 1994, St. Louis: Mosby.

clinical specialization, such as adult health or child health, women's health, gerontology, physiologic health, or psychiatric/mental health. Graduate study may include shared core or common courses that all students take (e.g., nursing theory, nursing research); however, the student must be assured that the program provides the course work and clinical experiences that the student will need to achieve personal goals. For example, the nurse who wants to become a teacher in a school of nursing should take courses in teaching methods, curriculum development, and clinical evaluation of students; the nurse who wants to become a child health nurse practitioner must have clinical experience in pediatrics with appropriate faculty and preceptors.

The nurse must also decide whether to pursue a graduate degree in nursing or a graduate degree in another field. For example, some nurses who want to become administrators in health care organizations may choose a graduate degree in business or health care administration. Nurses in psychiatric/mental health nursing may choose a graduate degree in mental health counseling. Before selecting a non-nursing graduate degree, the nurse should investigate the requirements for nursing licensure and certification in the desired field and consider possible future requirements. Currently, some national certification programs require the graduate degree in nursing (e.g., American Nurses Credentialing Center [ANCC] clinical nurse specialist in medical-surgical nursing or gerontologic nursing), whereas others do not (e.g., Association of Operating Room Nurses [AORN] nurse-anesthesia). Many professional nursing organizations are developing or plan-

ning changes in certification requirements that will mandate the graduate degree in nursing. Many state boards of nursing are also developing rules that will mandate the graduate degree in nursing to practice in an advanced nursing role. Further, the nurse who wants to teach nursing will need to consider employment requirements. Accreditation criteria for schools and colleges of nursing specify that graduate preparation be in the content area being taught. In other words, someone teaching nursing must have an advanced degree in nursing rather than education, psychology, or another discipline.

Clearly defining professional goals enables the nurse to identify those graduate programs that provide the education and experiences to meet those goals. The nurse then considers personal and family factors and program characteristics to determine which program is most appropriate.

Personal and Family Factors

Several personal and family factors may affect a nurse's choice of a graduate nursing program. Is the nurse able to travel or relocate to another city or state to pursue graduate education? If there is a long commute to school, should the nurse relocate to be closer to school and its resources, such as the library or computer laboratories? Must the nurse support self or family while going to school? If so, the availability of employment opportunities is important. If the nurse is working while going to graduate school, the nurse may desire flexible school or work schedules to facilitate balancing study and work time. It may be best for the nurse to select a program that allows part-time study if work and family demands are heavy. When travel opportunity is limited, the nurse may want to investigate available online courses and programs.

The nurse who is married needs the support of spouse and other family members while going to school. Working and going to school may limit the nurse's ability to fulfill spousal and parenting responsibilities. At the same time, children who see their parent continuing professional education have a role model for lifelong learning. The nurse who is returning to school needs to strategize with family members about how to meet family responsibilities.

Program Characteristics

Poteet, Hodges, and Tate (1994, p. 184) identify the following essential elements for assessing a graduate program: accreditation status, national standing, admission requirements, faculty qualifications, institutional climate, resources, clinical facilities, assistantships and other financial support, and program requirements. In addition, they recommend that the nurse should obtain information about what specific programs of study are offered and the school's philosophy of nursing and education. This information may be obtained from the institution's catalog or Web site, a telephone or in-person interview, or through discussion with a current student or graduate.

1. *Programs of study offered.* Does the school offer the specific program of study to enable the nurse to achieve professional goals? Are programs offered on campus only or through distance learning techniques such as video conferencing, community-based learning, Internet courses, or correspondence?

2. *School's philosophy of nursing and education.* Does the school subscribe to the philosophy of one nursing theorist, or do they have an eclectic model, that is, an integration of several theorists? Knowing the school's philosophy helps the prospective student understand the foundational beliefs of the school, its faculty, and the curriculum. Is the school's philosophy of nursing and education consistent with the nurse's philosophy? Inconsistency between the nurse's philosophy and the program's philosophy may interfere with success in the program.

3. *Accreditation status.* Accreditation may be conferred by a state government; by a regional accreditation association, such as the Southern Association of Colleges and Schools (SACS); or by a professional organization, such as the National League for Nursing Accreditation Commission (NLNAC) or American Association of Colleges of Nursing (AACN). Specialty nursing organizations may also accredit specific programs; for example, the American College of Nurse Midwifery accredits graduate programs in midwifery. Graduation from an accredited program may be important for the graduate to meet national certification requirements and to obtain licensure for advanced practice.

4. *National standing.* Programs may have a national reputation for excellence in certain fields of study. This reputation is usually based on the achievements of the faculty, the facilities for learning, and the achievements of its graduates. Attending a program with a national reputation for excellence may enhance the graduate's opportunities for employment.

5. *Admission requirements.* Admission requirements may include a minimum grade-point average (GPA) for undergraduate work, a minimum score on a national entrance examination such as the Graduate Record Examination (GRE) or the Miller Analogy Test (MAT), and successful completion of specific prerequisite courses such as physical assessment, statistics, or computer science. Most graduate nursing programs require completion of a baccalaureate degree in nursing. Some graduate programs allow nurses with a baccalaureate degree in another field to enter the graduate nursing program but require that the student complete any undergraduate nursing courses that were not previously taken (McGriff, 1996, p. 9). Because admission to graduate nursing programs is competitive, students need to be aware of specific admission requirements so that they can take action to meet or exceed the requirements; if they fail to meet the requirements, they may be denied admission. The student who is denied admission should question whether there are any admission waivers under which they might still qualify, such as a minority waiver or conditional admission.

6. *Faculty qualifications.* All faculty who teach at the graduate level should have a doctoral degree and a history of scholarly productivity. Students should expect to be taught by faculty who are experts in their fields. Students should seek a program where there are faculty who have expertise in the area of their interest.

7. *Institutional climate.* Prospective students may want to question students currently in the program

about the climate of the school of nursing and the university/college. Do the university and school of nursing provide an environment of diversity where students can experience the value and strength of human difference? Is there an open climate in the school of nursing and the university community that allows scholarly inquiry without fear of retribution? Are relationships among faculty, students, administration, and other staff open and conducive to learning? Do faculty members have a reputation of being "student friendly"; that is, are they readily available for student consultation, or are they difficult to contact outside scheduled class times? Do faculty members challenge students to achieve their fullest potential in an atmosphere of academic rigor? Do faculty members teach most of the courses, or do teaching assistants or adjunct faculty teach a high percentage of classes?

8. *Resources.* What resources are available to support and enhance student learning? Are library materials adequate, including books and journals to support the student's field of study, computer services, and statistical consultation to facilitate student research? Are study areas, lounges, and dining facilities adequate? Students should also inquire about hours of operation, especially evening, weekend, and holiday hours, to determine whether resources are available when the student needs them. Is there on-campus housing available for the student who must relocate for graduate study?

9. *Clinical facilities.* Are adequate clinical sites and preceptors available to support students, especially those who are in programs preparing the advanced nurse practitioner? Clinical facilities should include primary, secondary, and tertiary settings that provide diverse practice opportunities. Preceptors should be available who are experts in the desired specialty and who like working with students. If this is a nurse practitioner program, is most of the teaching and clinical precepting done by qualified nurse practitioner faculty or is there a heavy reliance on physician preceptors? Clinical practice settings should provide opportunities for graduate students to demonstrate critical thinking in the delivery of care to diverse clients with complex problems. Some graduate programs may provide clinical opportunities that are international in scope, for example, clinical experience study programs to provide primary care in underdeveloped nations.

10. *Assistantships and other financial support.* What is the availability of financial assistance? Many graduate programs provide teaching or research assistantships, in which the student receives tuition assistance in exchange for providing either teaching or research support to faculty. For the student whose professional goals involve teaching or research, assistantships provide an opportunity to gain experience in the role while completing formal graduate education. Many professional nursing organizations provide scholarship assistance for graduate nursing students. Other financial assistance may be available, especially for the student pursuing a graduate degree as an advanced nurse practitioner. Students should inquire about opportunities for financial assistance from their professional organizations, the school of nursing, and the university financial aid office.

11. *Program requirements.* What are the requirements for degree completion? Specifically, how many credit hours, what type of course work, and how many classroom and clinical hours are required? A requirement of nurse practitioner certification, in most clinical areas, is a specified minimal number of hours in clinical practice. Will graduates of the program be eligible to take the national certification exam?

Some graduate programs may be offered in cooperation with another academic discipline; for example, some programs in nursing administration are offered jointly with schools of business. These may result in dual degrees in each discipline; they are typically lengthy because of the need to meet requirements for each discipline. Other programs grant only a nursing degree but cooperate with other schools in offering course content. A joint position statement on nursing administration education by the American Organization of Nurse Executives (AONE) and AACN states that the educational preparation should take place in schools of nursing and include interdisciplinary education in business, economics, and/or health service administration (AACN, 2001d).

EXPLORE MEDIALINK

Questions, critical thinking exercises, essay activities, and other interactive resources for this chapter can be found on the Web site at http://www.prenhall. com/blais. Click on Chapter 23 to select activities for this chapter.

SUMMARY

Advanced practice nursing has evolved from the early 1900s to become a well-defined area of practice that provides services related to disease prevention, health promotion, health restoration, and rehabilitation. Advanced nursing practice includes clinical nurse specialists, nurse practitioners, nurse-midwives, and nurse-anesthetists. APNs work in a variety of practice settings across the health care continuum but are most suited to the delivery of primary care to rural and urban populations, especially underserved populations, such as the poor and the elderly.

In some countries, the CNS role is well established, but the nurse practitioner role is not as widespread. Certification and regulation of advanced practice has been developed by professional nursing organizations and state boards of nursing to ensure safe practice by qualified practitioners. Increasingly, nurses are required to obtain education for advanced practice in graduate programs to be eligible for certification and/or state licensure. The ICN is developing position statements to guide advanced practice in nursing internationally.

The future of advanced practice includes redesign of graduate nursing curricula to incorporate the clinical specialist role with the nurse practitioner role. Continued legislative activity by APNs will be needed to ensure equitable compensation and a broader scope of practice. The advanced practice nurse will be a major contributor to the delivery of quality health care at an affordable cost to clients in a changing health care environment.

Nurses planning to pursue graduate study must determine their professional goals before choosing a program. After identifying specific programs that will enable the nurse to meet desired goals, the nurse needs to evaluate the programs based on personal and family needs and program characteristics. Graduate programs in nursing may focus on nursing education, nursing administration, or advanced practice nursing.

REFERENCES

Ackerman, M. H., Norsen, L., Weidrick, B., & Kitzman, H. J. (1996). Development of a model of advanced practice. *American Journal of Critical Care, 5,* 68–75.

American Association of Colleges of Nursing. (1994). *Role differentiation of the nurse practitioner and clinical nurse specialist: Reaching toward consensus.* Proceedings of the Master's Educational Conference. San Antonio, TX: AACN.

American Association of Colleges of Nursing. (2001a). *Certification and regulation of advanced practice nurses.* Washington, DC: AACN.

American Association of Colleges of Nursing. (2001b). *Nursing education's agenda for the 21st century.* Washington, DC: AANC.

American Association of Colleges of Nursing. (2001c). *A vision of baccalaureate and graduate nursing education: The next decade.* Washington, DC: AACN.

American Association of Colleges of Nursing. (2001d). *Joint position statement on nursing administration education.* Washington, DC: AACN.

American Association of Nurse Anesthetists. (2001). *Questions and answers about a career in nurse anesthesia.* http://www.aana.com/information.

American College of Nurse Midwives. (2003). *The CNM profession.* http://www.acnm.org/educ.

American Nurses Credentialing Center. (2000). *Nurse practitioner certification.* http://www.nursingworld.org/ancc/certify/catalogs/2000/cbt/nursprac.htm.

American Nurses Credentialing Center. (2001). *Frequently asked questions.* http://www.nursingworld.org/ancc/faqs.htm.

Australian Institute of Health and Welfare. (2003). *Nursing Labour Force 2002.* Canberra.

Australian Nursing Council, Inc. (2000). *ANCI national competency standards for the registered nurse and the enrolled nurse.* http://www.anci.org.au/competencystandards.htm.

Australian Nursing Council, Inc. (2001). *Nursing in Australia.* http://www.anci.org.au/nursing.htm.

Australian Peak Nursing Forum. (2004). *Nursing in Australia.* http://www.anc.org.au.

Canadian Nurses Association. (2002). *Position statement: Advanced nursing practice.* http://www.cna-nurses.ca.

Canadian Nurses Association. (2003a). *Position statement: The nurse practitioner.* http://www.cna-aiic.ca.

Canadian Nurses Association. (2003b). *Position statement: The clinical nurse specialist.* http://www.can-aiic.ca.

Cronenwett, L. R. (1994). *Molding the future for advanced practice nurses: Education, regulation, and practice. Role differentiation of the nurse practitioner and clinical nurse specialist: Reaching toward consensus* (pp. 1–20). Proceedings of the Master's Education Conference, American Association of Colleges of Nursing, San Antonio, TX.

Hamric, A., Spross, J., & Hanson, C. (2000). *Advanced nursing practice: An integrative approach* (2nd ed.). Philadelphia: W. B. Saunders.

Hickey, J. V., Ouimette, R. M., & Venegoni, S. L. (2000). *Advanced practice nursing: Changing roles and applications* (2nd ed.). Philadelphia: Lippincott.

International Council of Nursing. (2002). *ICN announces position on advanced practice nursing roles.* Press Release. http://www.icn.ch/pr19_02.htm.

Lincoln, P. E. (2000). Comparing CNS and NP role activities: A replication. *Clinical Nurse Specialist, 14*(6), 269–277.

McGriff, E. P. (1996, January). Graduate education in nursing. *NSNA/Imprint,* pp. 9–11.

Mick, D., & Ackerman, M. (2000). Advanced practice nursing role delineation in acute and critical care: Application of the Strong Model of Advanced Practice. *Heart and Lung, 29*(3), 210–221.

Moloney-Harmon, P. A. (1999). The Synergy Model: Contemporary practice of the CNS. *Critical Care Nursing, 19,* 101–104.

Pediatric Nursing Certification Board. (2003). *PNCB exam information.* http://www.pncb.org/ptistore/control/exams/index.

Poteet, G. W., Hodges, L. C., & Tate, S. (1994). Graduate education: Making the right choice. In J. McCloskey & H. K. Grace (Eds.), *Current issues in nursing* (4th ed.). St. Louis: Mosby.

Robinson, D., & Kish, C. P. (2001). *Core concepts in advanced practice nursing.* St. Louis: Mosby.

Thompson, J. E. (2002). The WHO Global Advisory Group on Nursing and Midwifery. *Journal of Nursing Scholarship, 34*(2), 111–113.

Williams, C. A., & Valdivieso, G. C. (1994). Advanced practice models: A comparison of clinical nurse specialist and nurse practitioner activities. *Clinical Nurse Specialist, 8,* 311–318.

Wilson, D. (1994, December). Nurse practitioners: The early years (1965–1974). *Nurse Practitioner, 19*(12), 26, 28, 31.

Visions for the Future

Objectives

- Identify past events that have shaped and molded nursing.
- Discuss projections of future events that will affect nursing.
- Identify anticipated changes in health care and nursing in the future.

M E D I A L I N K

Additional online resources for this chapter can be found on the companion Web site at http://www.prenhall.com/blais.

There are numerous trends within nursing that are likely to continue and blossom in the years ahead. There will be changes that we are yet to anticipate.

Patricia Benner (2000, p. 35) predicted that in the new millennium nurses will be doing more in the community but also will continue to be even more integral to the provision of intensive care that will increasingly be the focus of hospital care. She advocates that a major task should be to recover the "Nightingale vision of attending to the real world of embodiment, and social, emotional, and physical environments that support well-being and promote health." She expresses the hope that caring practices will be recognized as good in themselves, regardless of more objective and measurable outcomes.

Heller, Oros, and Durney-Crowley (2000) identify 10 trends that will affect the future of nursing education. They are driven by socioeconomic factors, developments in health care delivery, and professional issues unique to nursing:

1. Changing population demographics and increasing ethnic and cultural diversity of nursing students
2. The technological explosion, particularly information technology
3. Globalization of the world's economy and society
4. The era of the educated consumer, alternative therapies and genomics, and palliative care
5. The shift to population-based care and the increasing complexity of patient care
6. The cost of health care and the challenge of managed care
7. The impact of health policy and regulation
8. The growing need for interdisciplinary education for collaborative practice
9. The current nursing shortage and opportunities for lifelong learning and workforce development
10. Significant advances in nursing science and research

Transformations are already taking place in nursing and nursing education based on these trends, and change is expected to continue.

Nursing has a chance to grow and develop its vision for practice and education. Influences on new nursing roles include increasing cultural diversity, reorganization of health care, interdisciplinary functions, managed care, creation and dissemination of nursing research knowledge, and the information superhighway. In the past, patients had to adapt to the culture of health care and, particularly, of hospitals. Now nursing has the opportunity to adapt health care to the culture of the people for whom nurses care.

The rapid changes in health care delivery and changing population demographics have affected supply and demand of nurses. The future will require effective identification and planning for personnel needs. Although enrollments in baccalaureate and master's degree programs have recently begun to increase, the future ability of nursing education to respond to the demand is threatened by a shortage of nursing faculty (American Association of Colleges of Nursing [AACN], 2004). The demand for nurse practitioners will likely continue in the role of primary-care providers, especially in managed-care settings. Nursing administrators will need to ensure adequate staffing of skilled and qualified nurses while maintaining a cost-effective staffing mix (Mailer et al., 2000).

CHALLENGES AND OPPORTUNITIES

In today's health care environment, the nursing profession and nurses as individuals face many challenges. Nursing roles are expanding and developing at a rapidly increasing pace. Old roles and skills are no longer adequate, and education must make adjustments to keep pace and provide leadership. The challenge for nurses is to take control of these changes and become proactive in meeting society's needs for health care now and in the future.

Professional organizations provide an opportunity for nurses to unite in vision and growth for nursing practice and education. There are many opportunities for nurses to grow both professionally and personally. The vast resources of information technology and distance education provide an avenue to continuing development of knowledge, skills, and experiences that can advance nursing in the future.

PAST EVENTS THAT HAVE AFFECTED NURSING

Events That Promoted Nursing's Growth and Development

Many events of the past spurred the growth and development of nursing as a profession; many events and public policy changes that were never intended to help or harm nursing's development nevertheless changed nursing. Social movements and technological advancements also have propelled nursing into both favorable and hazardous positions.

A discussion about nursing's growth must include the impact of World War II on the quantity and quality of nurses in many countries. World War II and the period following were times of major change, both for health care and for women. Major medical and surgical advances were discovered (some by intent, others by accident), and new techniques for care were developed. Women played a major role in the military and performed valiantly in front-line medical units; some served as volunteers in the American and International Red Cross, whereas others entered the workforce in areas they had never before encountered. With most men at war, women were drawn into a work life that was new to them.

Nursing both advanced during this period and suffered. In answering the call to patriotic duty, many women chose nontraditional roles, particularly because the salaries available to "war workers" were higher. The changing work opportunities for women had a negative effect on nursing: The challenge of doing "men's work" attracted many women who might have otherwise pursued nursing. This shift in work choice caused a shortage of nurses in America, even after the war was over. In response to the shortage and in line with the desire of professional nursing organizations in the United States to advance nursing's professional standing, a two-year associate degree nursing program was developed for the junior/community colleges.

Although before World War II nurses were educated primarily in hospitals, the first university baccalaureate degree program in nursing (BSN) in the United States had been in existence since 1909. However, the number of BSN programs has not increased at the same rate as ADN programs. These changes in the education of nurses have significant implications for the future of professional nursing, which is discussed later in this chapter.

Another event that has affected nursing's growth and development is the position paper issued by the American Nurses Association (ANA) in 1965, which suggested that all education for nurses take place in institutions of higher learning. Although both ADN and BSN programs existed throughout the United States at that time, most nurses were prepared in hospital-based diploma programs, and the position paper met with much resistance and even anger. By 1978, the ANA issued another recommendation, one that was even stronger. The ANA recommended there be two levels of nurses prepared in universities or colleges: ADN and BSN nurses. In 1985, the ANA went even further, suggesting different titles for the two levels of nurses. By then, several nursing organizations, including the National League for Nursing (NLN), had joined the movement. However, it was not long before the NLN withdrew its support in an attempt to avoid an intraprofessional fight. In 1995, the ANA reaffirmed its position and encouraged ways to move on the recommendation while preserving the integrity of the profession. As professional nursing moved toward the goal of requiring the baccalaureate degree as the minimum credential for professional practice, RN/BSN transition programs were developed to enable the ADN nurse to move upward. RN/MSN programs have also been developed to enhance career mobility. Although these developments have advanced nursing, the continued inability to reach consensus on the "entry to practice" preparation has resulted in divisiveness among nurses with different educational preparation.

In Canada, two-year programs and four-year degree nursing programs were developed to augment the hospital training schools. In Australia and Great Britain, baccalaureate nursing programs emerged as those nations moved toward the goal of educating nurses in institutions of higher learning. It is interesting to note that individual nurses in the United States, Great Britain, Australia, Canada, and other British Commonwealth nations elected to advance their own professional development by obtaining baccalaureate and master's degrees in other disciplines, most notably education, social work, and health service administration.

Another historical event that has affected nursing, especially in the United States, is the development of the role of the advanced nurse practitioner. This role evolved from two sources: the nurse practitioners and the clinical nurse specialist (CNS). In 1965, Dean Loretta Ford, in collaboration with Dr. Henry Silver (a physician) initiated a new kind of nurse preparation as a solution for the physician shortage in Colorado. Registered nurses were given six weeks of continuing education in which they learned assessment skills and then functioned as physician extenders. Almost immediately that education was increased, and currently most nurse practitioners hold master's degrees and are certified. The CNS role developed within acute-care settings and was found within higher education from the outset. The development of advanced practice is another example of nursing responding to a societal need and is a resulting change in the practice of some nurses. This historical event has been an advancement and a problem: Nursing now struggles for legislation that will enable advanced nurse practitioners to receive third-party reimbursement and prescriptive authority.

In the United States in the mid-1990s, President Clinton's attempts at national health care reform and increases in the number of for-profit health care corporations also affected nursing. In an effort to avoid national regulation and the perceived problems associated with socialized health care in other countries, insurance companies, physicians, and hospitals moved toward a system of managed care. This resulted in redesign of hospital-based client care delivery and consequent downsizing of both professional and support staff. To reduce costs, hospitals have instituted shorter length of stays, integrated systems, case management, and the use of unlicensed assistive personnel (UAPs). Other countries have implemented similar changes to provide their citizens with affordable health care.

A shift from curing illness to promoting health and preventing illness has, however, provided new opportunities for nurses. This shift in health care from the hospital to the community has increased the need for primary practitioners; more opportunities exist for advanced nurse practitioners and other advanced practice nurses, such as nurse-midwives, nurse-anesthetists, and clinical nurse specialists. This trend to involve more nurses in the care of the public outside the hospital setting has major implications for nursing education and for the future utilization of nurses (Bower, 1997).

Events That Have Indirectly Affected Nursing

Medical advances (e.g., new surgical procedures, the proliferation of diagnostic and monitoring instrumentation, and new pharmacological preparations) have changed not only the physician's practice but also nursing practice. In the past, the nurse's hands, eyes, and ears were the principal tools for assessing clients; today, the nurse augments these tools with data from monitoring equipment that can provide more subtle and accurate information. Some of these advances have made the nurse's job easier; others, such as the development of new and more powerful drugs, have broadened the nurse's responsibilities. Knowing the drug's expected action, adverse effects, and compatibility with other drugs is a complicated responsibility. Nurses have significantly more responsibility and accountability today than they had in the past and this increase is likely to continue.

Cost-containment measures instituted by hospitals in many countries have also changed nursing practice. Changes that began as downsizing, or a reduction in staff to save money, quickly became a redesign of the entire hospital delivery system. Cross-training, focusing on the client, streamlining processes using continuous quality improvement (CQI), and the increased use of unlicensed assistive personnel (UAPs) or minimally trained support staff are only a few of the outcomes of the redesign. In some cases, the result was a redesign of the nurse's role; in other instances, an elimination of RN positions. RN and LPN/LVN ratios were shifted, and more management and delegation skills were required of the RN. Some RN activities were delegated to other, "cross-trained" health care workers (paramedics, respiratory therapists, phlebotomists, ECG technicians), and the RN was educated to assume additional responsibilities. Some RNs, for example, have returned to school to become respiratory therapists so that they might be able to provide total care to clients who have respiratory disorders or are ventilator dependent.

Managed care in the United States has been another cost-containment method that has affected the nurse's role. Managed care refers to a system in which hospitals (with subsidiary clinics, home care, skilled nursing facilities, and so on) and physician groups provide comprehensive care for groups of people who purchase their insurance and agree to use the program for health services. It is expected that free-market competition will provide the system with the lowest cost for care. And because the price for that care is based on the total number of members, the cost of caring for those who need care will be balanced by those members who are well and do not require services. Keeping members well so that they do not need the system is how costs are contained. Thus there is a new focus on wellness.

Case managers are needed as "gatekeepers" of the system so that only care that is deemed essential is provided. Cost for the care is determined proactively, so the system must be careful not to spend more than it is paid by capitation (numbers of those insured). Thus, in the new managed care environment nurses must have case management, coordination, assessment, health promotion, illness prevention, and cost-containment skills. The goal of keeping people focused on staying well and out of the hospital constitutes an entirely new paradigm of care. The way the goal is met and funded affects the role expectations and responsibilities of the nurse.

Public policy has changed everyone's lives. Informed consent laws have increased the public's knowledge about and participation in decisions about their health care. The Self-Determination Act of 1991 has allowed people to make decisions in advance about their future health care, before they are unable to make such decisions. People have more choice about how and when health care will be delivered. These laws have also affected the role of the nurse. Monitoring the procedures for gaining consent and implementing procedures to ensure that the client's living will or durable power of attorney for health care is understood and documented are now a part of the nurse's responsibility. Issues such as the "right to die," assisted suicide, and other ethical dilemmas are of daily concern to the nurse in all practice settings. These and other added duties change the nurse's role, both in scope and accountability (Bower, 1997).

Social Movements and Technological Initiatives That Have Affected Nursing

The women's movement that began in the 1960s has had a major impact on nursing. Predominantly a woman's profession (about 10% of nurses are men), nursing has benefited from the recognition of women as a force for social change. As a result of the gains made by the feminist movement, nurses have gained better salaries, better working conditions, access to higher education, and access to opportunities as middle managers and executives in many occupations as well as nursing. Nurses have recently seized the opportunity to become entrepreneurs. Many nurses would have been unlikely to rise to such challenges if the women's movement had not opened the door to opportunity.

No discussion of the changes in nursing would be complete without indicating the impact of the information age and the way that computers have changed daily life. Computer technology is influencing health care by improving storage of and access to health care information. Nurses will be able to access and input client information at bedside computers or in the client's home through portable laptop computers. Computers will improve the accuracy and efficiency of documentation. By touching the computer screen, nurses record client information and make it available to the physician, the pharmacy, and any other service that is online.

Clients can carry a card that contains information about their insurance coverage, status, medical history, medications, and demographic information. Insertion of this card into a computer sends that information to all who need to know; as a result, traditional health and medical records and files may soon become unnecessary. Instead of spending hours on manual recording, the nurse can spend that time with the client. Because the computer is often in the hospital room, at the clinic, or even in the home, the client can also share and participate in the development of the record.

The personal digital assistant (PDA) is among the newest tools being used. It is a hand-held computer that has an operating system designed to work with a personal computer. Some accept data from a keyboard, and others have a graffiti board and stylus used to write on the screen. It can provide an access point to the Internet and personal and office e-mail. Health care professionals use it as a resource by downloading books and protocols and to organize patient data, track patient care visits, and transmit prescriptions. Downloaded pharmacy programs enable providers to check drug doseages, side effects, contraindications, and insurance plan coverages. Charting can be done on a PDA and later downloaded to the patient's medical record. Home health nurses have been able to store information in a portable manner. A major concern about the use of PDAs in health care is security of data and the device itself. In

the near future, voice recognition may be available so that the voice of the user is registered and will be recognized before records are accessed. There are also patient uses for the PDA in the self-management of chronic illness. For example, someone with diabetes could log in blood glucose measurements, insulin doses, amount of exercise, and dietary information, and then use the PDA to inform them of necessary steps to take in managing the disease. Applications for PDAs will likely increase in the future to the point where nurses will view them as a necessity for everyday practice.

Computers have also affected nursing education. Computer technology has facilitated supervision of students at a distance. PDAs provide information to students visiting clients in the home and act as vehicles for distributing client data to the college or clinic. Computerized instruction allows faculty to focus on the student's ability to think critically rather than on the ability to accumulate facts. A major advantage of computer technology is that it enables students to interact with information, classmates, faculty, and other nurses online at home, in the computer laboratory or library, in the classroom, or in the clinical setting. Thus, computerized instruction expands the instructional environment so that learning is portable, accessible, and always available. There are no constraints of time, person, or place. These advances in computer technology and their application to nursing and health care require that nurses broaden their knowledge still further, so that they become computer literate.

Through technology and travel, the world has become a smaller place. Immigrants and refugees readily cross national borders to seek opportunity in new lands. Nurses are more able to move rapidly to assist with the delivery of care to victims of natural and man-made health disasters. The shrinking of the worldwide community requires that nurses become more knowledgeable about and accepting of cultural difference. Nurses need to be aware of different beliefs about health and illness and different cultural healing practices. The nurses of tomorrow need to be more than culturally aware—they need to strive for cultural competence in providing nursing care.

This overview of changes that have affected nursing and nursing practice is not meant to be comprehensive; there are many more good examples of events that have directly or indirectly changed nursing. Rather, this overview was intended to show that any changes in nursing in the past were usually linked to professional or societal change. As one considers the future, it is important to keep this point in mind (Bower, 1997).

Reflect on...

- how the changes in health care financing have affected your own health care. What has been gained from these changes? What might have been lost from health care?
- how the information technology advances have affected nursing practice. Do some nurses have a more difficult time adapting to these changes? What might be some helpful strategies for nurses to adapt to the changes?
- the societal changes in population demographics as they relate to health care. How has nursing adapted to these changes? What related needs might have gone unmet or been undermet?

FUTURE EVENTS THAT WILL AFFECT NURSING

During the past century, there have been tremendous advances in health care, such as immunizations and antibiotics, and these have contributed to a greatly increased life expectancy. The 2000 census, for the first time, had a three-digit space for age. In the 1900s, when pneumonia and tuberculosis were the leading causes of death, no one could have forecast the advances that would be developed to manage these diseases as well as other health problems. The threat of bioterrorism after September 11, 2001, has influenced health care planning. The future will no doubt present anticipated challenges based on what society is experiencing at the present, as well as unanticipated ones.

The drivers of change in the future of health care are likely to include consumerism, the disarray of managed care, biotechnological innovation, information technology, and community focus (Morrison, 2000). Consumerism is likely to become a force as the public becomes more discontent with the current state of health care. Some key factors in consumer discontent are a better-educated public, intensive media coverage of health care issues, activities of advocacy groups, and the emergence of complementary alternative medicine. Managed care has lost favor with health care consumers due in part to the lack of choice in providers and services. The pharmaceutical industry and the medical technology industries have made great investments that will continue to create innovations. The Internet and health-related portals bring information technology to the public as never before, and tele-

Evidence for Practice

Artinian, N. T. (2001). Effects of home telemonitoring and community-based monitoring on blood pressure control in urban African Americans: A pilot study. *Heart and Lung, 30*(3), 191–199.

This study tested the hypothesis that persons who participate in nurse-managed home telemonitoring (HT) plus usual care or who participate in nurse-managed community-based monitoring (CBM) plus usual care will have greater improvement in blood pressure from baseline to three months than will persons who receive usual care only. An experimental design was used with random assigment of subjects to one of three groups: HT, CBM, and usual care. The groups were stratified (matched proportions) by use or nonuse of antihypertensive medication. One-way analysis of covariance, controlling for age and body weight, analyzed changes in blood pressure from baseline to 3 months.

Both the HT and the CBM groups had clinically and statistically significant drops in both systolic and diastolic blood pressure readings, with the HT group having the greatest drop. There was little change for the usual care group.

These results support the effectiveness of both home telemonitoring and community-based monitoring in developing new health care delivery strategies in the future.

health and remote telemetry are changing the way health care is delivered. Focus on communities as a point of entry into health care, and delivery of services is increasing along with the recognition of the important role the community can play in health.

Computer Technology and Its Effect on Health and Nursing Care

The computer systems of tomorrow will require that all health care providers be knowledgeable and practiced in the use of computers. It will take more than being computer literate to function in the computer world of tomorrow. Knowledge of word processing using several software packages, the ability to use spreadsheets, and the ability to adapt to ever-changing computer systems will be necessary. For a while, health care facilities will need to train their personnel, but eventually all workers will be expected to have computer skills when hired. This means that schools of nursing and other departments of colleges and universities will need to ensure that all graduates of their programs are able to access computers and obtain the information needed.

Some of the projections can be provocative, particularly those that relate to innovative technology. The use of virtual computerization in the learning environment is one of those. Much of that technology has been applied to games, but not to education.

> Imagine wearing a headset with two small screens, located in front of your eyes, used to project computer graphic images, and earphones to receive computer-generated sound. On your hands you wear data gloves, which contain position sensors. These sensors tell the computer exact positions, especially of your body and arms. The computer responds to the movement of your head, eyes, hands, and arms. It might even have voice recognition and respond to your commands. (Justice, 1999, p. 14)

Any number of clinical scenarios could be displayed in this virtual world, allowing students and nurses to learn skills and refresh previously learned ones. A trainer may be involved for guidance and may even control the progression of the scenario to assess the ability to respond to changes and crises and fit the experience to the learner's level of expected performance. The computer can be programmed to score the performance, providing new avenues for testing skills and perhaps even testing for licensure.

The three-dimensional images can be made even more lifelike by the use of head-mounted displays, allowing total visual immersion, and of auditory feedback in response to the viewer's movements and contact with virtual objects. Pilot training has used flight simulators for some time, but the use of this technology has been fairly limited in other contexts. This advancement is likely to affect education and perhaps even the practice of nursing in the future, particularly if the technology were to be applied to client education.

More applications for online services will be implemented in the future. Patient information sources will be used to an even greater degree, creating a more educated health care consumer. Nurses can be developers of these information services, as well as referral agents. Online continuing education and formal education will probably continue as a trend in the near future, creating new opportunities for nurses to update their own knowledge base and advance their careers. Programs using digital interactive television that offers two-way communication are being piloted and have tremendous opportunity for creative applications in health care.

Telehealth is a recent advance that will continue to grow and expand in the future. Synonymous with telemedicine, online health, and e-health, it is an umbrella term encompassing health activity that involves distance. It can be applied to home nursing, health monitoring, consultation, and many other aspects of health care. It holds promise of improving access to health care in areas where there are geographical barriers, and it can reduce costs associated with travel. An exemplar of telehealth is Alberta Wellnet in Canada. This project has multimedia videoconferencing units in health centers throughout the province that are linked. There are five priorities for this program: expansion of telemental health, teleultrasound, teleradiology, telegeriatrics, and telerehabilitation. The network provides access to education, clinical consultation, and conduct of business. It links nurses with other nurses and with other health care providers. It improves access to peers and to specialists for both health care providers and for patients (Anderson, 2002).

Physician and nonphysician offices should soon be able to access the hospital system so that they do not need a paper trail or their own electronic system. With managed care, the system should expand to connect the hospital, the insurance company (or payer), and the physician and nonphysician care providers. Soon, with a tap of the finger, a client's record can be accessed from any of those entities.

It will not be long before nurses will carry pocket computers on their uniform belts to record data and make assessments at the site of the client (whether in hospital, home, school, or job). These data will simultaneously be entered in the client's personal record and be available to any department in the hospital as long as the client is there. This capacity for simultaneous entry and distribution is already possible in restaurants, where the server enters the order in the computer at tableside, records it, and notifies the kitchen without ever going near the kitchen until the order is ready. That same entry creates a bill that is ready for customers when they leave.

Similar activities will soon be part of every health care facility to ensure smooth, quick care and accurate accounting. The capacity is there; all that is necessary is to find ways to fund the systems and to put them in place so they "talk" to one another.

Robotics is another area of advanced technology that could affect the practice of nursing. There have

Evidence for Practice

Baker, L., Wagner, T. H., Singer, S., & Bundorf, M. K. (2003). Use of the Internet and e-mail for health care information: Results from a national survey. *Journal of the American Medical Association, 289*(18), 2400–2406.

A survey sample drawn from a panel of more than 60,000 U.S. households consisted of 4764 respondents who were 21 years of age or greater and were self-reported users of the Internet. Approximately 40% of these respondents reported using the Internet for advice or information related to health or health care during the previous year. Six percent had used e-mail to contact a health care professional. Only one third of those using the Internet for health reported that the Internet use made a difference in a decision about health care, and very few reported that Internet use had any impact on health care utilization. High percentages (93 and 94%, respectively) said that Internet use had no effect on number of physician visits they had or on the number of telephone contacts. About 5% reported use of the Internet to obtain prescriptions or purchase pharmaceutical products.

Although many people use the Internet for health information, its use may be somewhat less than anticipated. The use is not yet universal, and there is room for development of approaches to Internet utilization for health care.

been applications of early robotic technology to the use of programmable machines for the delivery of supplies and even trays within hospitals, but thus far uses have been fairly limited. Speculation about future applications can conjure up images of robotic nurses in the image of R2D2 and C3P0 from the *Star Wars* movies, but other possibilities may be closer to implementation. Some medical and surgical procedures could be robotically assisted. Robotic devices are likely to become more integrated into rehabilitation and prosthetics.

Technologies have changed the practice of nursing in the recent past, and that trend is expected to continue. More and more sophisticated devices for monitoring and administering care have made the delivery of care very different in recent decades. With the shortage of highly skilled nurses that are needed for the high-tech environments, aggressive recruitment and retention strategies are being implemented. The unique body of knowledge needed for these roles is not acquired in undergraduate nursing programs as they are now taught. This has led to a new model of offering speciality education in some Canadian schools. A partnership among Queen Elizabeth Hospital II, the Health Science Center, and Dalhousie University School of Nursing will provide a strategy for specialty education at three educational levels in acute-care nursing. The areas offered are emergency, critical care, and perioperative nursing (Robertson, 2000). Nursing education will need to adapt to prepare nurses for practice in the future, and new templates will emerge.

Responses to demographic and societal changes within the changing paradigms of health care delivery create challenges to the public's health, both now and in the future. Leaders at the Centers for Disease Control and Prevention have identified at least ten future health challenges. These challenges encompass not only the changes in health care delivery and the aging of society, but also such things as risks imposed by lifestyles, the environment, and new scientific frontiers, such as the brain and human behavior and genome mapping (Koplan & Fleming, 2000). These challenges for the future include the following:

1. Instituting a rational health care system that balances equity, cost, and quality
2. Eliminating health disparities by improving access to health care using innovative community-based strategies tailored to a diverse population
3. Focusing on children's emotional and intellectual development, as well as physical health, to permit them to achieve full potential
4. Achieving a longer "health span" so that people are not merely living longer
5. Integrating physical activity and healthy eating into daily lives to counteract the trend toward obesity and its consequences for health
6. Cleaning up and protecting the environment, which is likely to be increasingly challenged
7. Preparing to respond to emerging infectious diseases resulting from microbial adaptation and antibiotic resistance
8. Recognizing and addressing the contributions of mental health to overall health and well-being
9. Reducing the toll of violence in society
10. Using new scientific knowledge and technological advances wisely by applying them equitably, ethically, and responsibly

Some of these challenges have strategies that can easily be identified and evolved from earlier attempts to improve health and health care. Others need an approach that is less clear and may create controversy or even divisiveness in the planning. Nevertheless, there are valuable opportunities to make a difference in future health.

Many factors will affect nursing in the future. What nurses do, how they are educated, and where they practice will undoubtedly change. Nurses need to embrace the changes and be a part of shaping the future.

Reflect on...

■ the rapid changes in technology that have come about since you have been a nurse. Were these changes embraced by everyone when they were new? Has practice improved because of them?

■ the changes in the nurse-client relationship that has been associated with new nursing roles and the use of technological advances. How does the nurse maintain a therapeutic relationship with the client when machines take over some of the nursing functions?

■ the skills you believe will be important in the future. What are they and how should they be taught?

Health Care System Changes

As the health care system struggles to provide care for all people at a reasonable cost, it will undergo many changes. Although managed health care is only the latest attempt to reverse the escalating costs of care, time and the outcomes will determine its impact. However, while managed care is available, there will be fewer professional nurses in hospitals and more multiskilled workers supervised by professional nurses. The term *multiskilled worker* refers to a person who is prepared to provide basic care under supervision but who is not licensed. Basic care will also change as technology takes over the measuring of vital signs and other parameters of assessment. The client's history, which is already on the client's personal computer card, will need revising only as new events occur and information is added to the computer record.

Because the length of stay for a hospitalized person will become shorter, the care provided will address the very acute phase of the illness episode and will be directed toward pain management, respiratory facilitation, cardiac support, and neurological monitoring. Preparing the client for recovery at home will be a major aspect of the nurse's role. To plan and implement effective care, nurses will need to maintain and increase their knowledge of physiologic and psychologic functioning, technological monitoring systems, client care, and computer systems.

Seriously ill clients confined to a hospital bed will require intensive care administered by professionals who will administer medications using equipment that is computer driven. There will be less worry about turning clients because the hospital beds of tomorrow will be designed to rotate the occupant periodically so that skin integrity is preserved. The professional nurse will assign dressing changes and other treatments to the multiskilled workers, so the cost of care will be contained by the number and level of the workers assigned to the units. Self-directed work teams made up of cross-trained professionals and multiskilled workers will direct, provide, and evaluate the care.

One of the most exciting possibilities for what might occur in the United States is described by Jeffrey Bauer (1994), who proposes that the health care system be changed by breaking the monopoly held by physicians over the delivery of health care to American citizens. Bauer proposes that health care costs will not decrease until citizens are allowed to select the provider they want. He proposes that health care be placed on the free market so that maximum choice and quality competition are available. He believes we must "take the shackles off America's many competent non-physician providers and allow the American consumer free access to their services" (Bauer, 1994, p. 19).

If Bauer's plan were to come into being—and there are good reasons to believe that it will—then advanced nurse practitioners, certified nurse-midwives, dentists, pharmacists, certified nurse-anesthetists, physical therapists, occupational therapists, and respiratory therapists, to name only a few, would be able to respond directly to the public's needs. The consumer would be free to choose from an expanded menu of qualified providers, a development that would bring the cost of care down while providing quality care for all. Nurses will be needed in increasing numbers in ambulatory surgical centers, diagnostic centers, home care, nursing homes, and skilled nursing facilities as hospitals become smaller and health care moves to the community. Those nurses with baccalaureate and master's degrees will have first choice as nonphysician providers because they are the best prepared for the role required of the nurse in the community. The nurse's role will include direct and indirect care; nurses will care for and manage others who provide care. In rural areas, advanced nurse practitioners will act as primary care providers as they assess, treat, and follow up on common, ordinary health care problems. Problems that require surgery or specialty consultation will be referred to physicians and other nonphysician providers. Physicians, nurses, and other health care providers will work together as interdisciplinary teams providing the consumer with the expertise of many care providers. Collaborative efforts will be necessary as the world of health care becomes more complex and technology continues to improve and change. The anticipated changes in the health care delivery system of the future require that everyone, health professional and consumer alike, must change his or her expectations and behaviors. The changing health care system requires more personal health responsibility on the part of the consumer and greater responsiveness on the part of health care providers.

The association of nursing with complementary alternative medicine is a trend that is likely to continue into the future. As nurses move into greater roles in case management, they will need to understand which therapies are appropriate for each client, and when nontraditional therapies are appropriate, nurses will assist clients in making decisions regarding alternative treatments.

Regulatory Changes

In the future there probably will be some major changes in the regulation of physicians and nonphysician health care providers. The National Council of State Boards of Nursing (which is composed of representatives from each state's board) has proposed that there be national standards for licensing entry-level nurses and measuring the competency of nurses over time. The PEW Health Professions Commission (1995) went even further, proposing that the regulation of all physician and nonphysician health care providers be carried out at the national level and that the approach be an interdisciplinary one.

What would this mean? It could mean that regulations would be competency based, broad enough to allow for change, and yet definitive enough to assure the public that the provider, regardless of title, is qualified to offer the service. It could mean that quality control would be the key ingredient in determining universal standards for all health care providers, no matter where they practice or what title they hold. The state could provide the entry examination, and the professions could be held legally and financially responsible for the conduct of their members under state and federal guidelines based on general norms set across all health care disciplines. Would this work? Several professional organizations believe so, and there is enough

pressure from legislators to indicate that this kind of modification could occur.

The value of this approach to regulation is that competency standards, not titles, would drive decisions; as a result, nonphysician providers would be considered equal partners in health care delivery. Having the state control entry to practice based on national standards and the profession control certification based on their own specific practice expectations for general and advanced practice results in more meaningful recertification of providers with the least amount of government intrusion. These radical changes are becoming necessary to the removal of traditional practice barriers among physicians, nurses, and other health care providers. Advanced nurse practitioners have demonstrated that they are excellent primary caregivers, but most state regulations, which generally are influenced by physician lobbyists, have kept legislators from making the changes needed for the legitimate use of advanced nurse practitioners. The argument of cost could be used to make the case for national, standardized regulation, but the argument that advanced nurse practitioners are adequately prepared and have demonstrated their value as primary care providers is a better one.

Continued Medical, Surgical, and Pharmacological Advances

The list of advancements in medicine is a long one. For example, it is possible to clone people (although whether to do so is an ethical controversy); treat highly infectious diseases with potent chemicals; keep people alive with machines that breathe for them and keep the heart pumping; and remove, sterilize, and replace a person's bone marrow to cure disease. It is possible to perform surgery while the client's blood is cycled through an artificial heart and lungs, transplant organs from human and animal donors, and replace old, worn-out joints with new artificial ones. It is possible to save the life of a 26-week premature infant through mechanical breathing, intravenous feedings, and highly potent drugs. It is possible to replace amputated limbs with artificial ones and to provide computer and mechanical support that can enable a paralyzed person to pursue a career and be self-supporting.

The development of medications that produce desired physiologic effects and change psychologic moods has prolonged life, made it more comfortable, and enhanced people's ability to enjoy it. Drugs can be a vital part of healthy living for those with chronic physiologic or psychologic illnesses. Some drugs, however, have also caused dependence, making people less able to cope or function without them.

Medical treatment of chronic conditions and acute phases of infection and much posttrauma care often centers around pharmacological therapy. Furthermore, the number of nonprescription medications has increased as the Food and Drug Administration (FDA) releases many prescription drugs for over-the-counter purchase. The consumer now has even more choices than before. A trip to the drugstore or local supermarket or discount store allows the consumer access to a vast variety of remedies for a stuffy nose, sore throat, respiratory congestion, bowel problems, joint aches, heartburn, urinary discomfort, worry, or whatever else is causing distress. It is very easy to acquire drugs, and the public uses many drugs; in fact, polypharmacy has become a major problem in America because many people combine prescription drugs and nonprescription drugs in a haphazard manner.

Pharmacological advancements have also had a significant impact on nursing. Nurses have had to expand their knowledge base of pharmacology and their skills in caring for clients who have had surgery or who are undergoing medical treatment. Keeping informed about the newest drugs means the nurse must consult the National Drug Formulary or other drug references more often. Moreover, it is becoming even more urgent for nurses to face the inevitable ethical dilemmas. The need for more information and more discussion about ethical issues will continue and escalate as health care in hospitals becomes more acute, as arguments rage over the distribution of financial resources for expensive "experimental treatment" (e.g., complex organ transplants) versus less expensive preventive care (childhood immunizations), and as more nonphysician providers deliver care in homes, malls, offices or places of work, schools, churches, clinics, ambulatory centers, and nursing homes.

In the past, nurses have responded to the events that confront them; no doubt they will again. In the 21st century, however, nurses' responses will need to be quicker and more flexible. This means nurses will need more education and a greater understanding of the community and aggregate care. Nurses will also have to see themselves as "knowledge workers" and facilitators of care rather than individual caregivers. This is a major paradigm shift.

Teaching, preparing educational materials, and teaching others how to teach will consume more of a nurse's time. Interactive video, distance learning, and using computers and other audio-visual equipment for learning will expand the market for instructional materials and good teachers. Because people will learn in their homes and at work, instructional materials will need to be portable and self-contained. Group learning will become as common as individual learning, and the use of the "information highway" will be a key mode of delivery. With satellites available and cables throughout the United States, North America, and the world, disseminating information will not be difficult.

Surgical procedures, medical treatment, and pharmacological therapies will continue to advance. In fact, there is every reason to believe the advancements will develop even more rapidly, so that only those who are continuous learners will be able to keep pace. Nurses will have to be continuous learners if they expect to have a place in the new health care paradigm.

Historically, nurses have cared for the sick. In the new paradigm, nurses will focus on wellness and prevention. The nurse will be the primary person who works to help individuals stay well and do things that promote health. Nurses will have to increase their knowledge base about nutrition, exercise, vitamin replacement, and the effects of cigarette smoking and the use of alcohol. As "models of good health," some nurses will have to adopt healthier behaviors and lifestyles. They will also have to keep abreast of the most recent research in the prevention and treatment of cancer, AIDS, and other infections.

Nurses will also need to take an active role in preparing healthy citizens for the future by teaching children about exercise, nutrition, safety, and other habits for healthy living, at a time when lifelong habits are learned. Teaching children about sex, sexually transmitted diseases, alcohol, and drug abuse will also be a challenge. Pressures from parents and organized religion have made it difficult to offer sex education in public and private schools. Nurses must be advocates for children and actively work to see that sex education becomes part of the school curriculum.

For much of the history of Western-trained nursing, nurses have focused on the physical body of patients. Nurses are now being faced with encountering patients in virtual environments where they are not physically present. The challenge for nurses will be to address the difference between live sight and touch of the patient to visibility through a medium. It challenges traditional ideas of presence, physical proximity, and physical ministrations. Nurses should be interested in how the new technologies enhance nursing practice but also how they might undermine the

Critical Thinking Exercise

After reading the quotation by Margaret Sandalowski below, identify your concerns about how this would affect quality of health care delivered by nurses. Using two columns, write in column one the ways you feel health care might be compromised. In column two, list at least one action a nurse or nurses could take to address that concern in a positive way.

presence of a nurse. Both will need to be considered in determining the best use of teletechnologies.

> The patient is no longer necessarily the corporeal person in the bed or on the examinining table, but rather the hypertexted, hyperreal representation on screen in the form of a rhythm strip; black-and-white or colorized image; or numeric, graphic, digital, schematic, or other visual display. The clinician, in turn, is no longer necessarily the flesh and blood person next to the bed or examining table, but rather a voice on the telephone, an e-mail correspondent, an on-line presence, or the tele-image of a face or hand holding a medical instrument. (Sandelowski, 2002, p. 66)

PAST LESSONS THAT CAN HELP NURSES IN THE FUTURE

From what has happened in health care, nurses can learn many lessons that may help them deal with the future.

1. The health care delivery system in the United States is remarkably flexible. Since the 1800s, the U.S. health care system has responded quickly to changes in technology, scientific discoveries, and new health threats. Medical science has undergone several revolutionary redefinitions; many infectious diseases have been conquered, and new ones have taken their place; more of the population has been able to survive to old age; the hospital has been redefined from a place for the poor to die to a place for anyone to be restored to health. For those who do die, the causes of death have changed. One hundred years ago, the leading killers were polio and infectious diseases. Today's leading killers are heart disease, tobacco, AIDS, and violence. Health insurance, which was instituted in the early part of the century to support personal payment, now has become the main source of payment for health care.

2. Changes in the health care system have always occurred rapidly and sometimes without warning. Most of the changes outlined in this chapter took place quickly, and many of the advancements in medicine were unexpected or the result of war. Government and society did not set out to initiate Medicare or to institute diagnosis-related groups (DRGs) or, for that matter, to turn to managed care. These developments happened quickly as a way to solve an immediate problem. Clearly, the system is not driven by tradition or "cast in stone."

3. No one entity is in control of the health care system. Only a brief scan of any newspaper will reveal that no one body—not physicians, federal or state governments, insurers or payers—controls the system, as President Clinton discovered when he tried to reform the system in the mid-1990s. Consumers are becoming more interested in how the system works and how to change it because it is their tax dollars that support it.

4. Health care providers, especially nurses, have made major strides each time the system changed. These most recent changes have clearly presented great opportunities for nurses and other nonphysician caregivers. New roles, roles most appropriately played by providers with an interest and preparation in prevention, are waiting to be filled by nurses.

As soon as one understands these lessons, the possibilities for the future become apparent. For example, it is possible for anyone to influence the development of tomorrow's health care system. Modifications will undoubtedly occur quickly and repeatedly as nations seek ways to provide quality health care for all. Control of the system will shift from one source to another. Because control has thus far resided with government, professionals, and insurance companies, it seems likely that consumers may be the next group to want and assume control (Bower, 1997).

VISIONS OF TOMORROW

Throughout this chapter several themes have emerged that provide the framework for a vision of tomorrow.

Health care will be provided mostly in the community. Whereas acute and critical phases of illness will be attended to in hospitals, most health care will be delivered within the community. During the 1960s, the number of hospitals grew rapidly because funding was available and because it was believed that the best care could be provided there. It has since been learned that hospital care is very costly, disrupts the family, and focuses on cure, not prevention. In the 2000s, care will be delivered primarily outside the hospital. Schools, churches, the workplace, home clinics, skilled nursing facilities, and nursing homes will be the sites for care.

Care is already provided in clinics, in nursing homes, in the home, and at skilled nursing facilities. More health care will also be provided in schools and in the workplace. The rise of alcohol and drug abuse in the young, the increasing incidence of HIV in adolescents and young adults, and the increasing number of teenage pregnancies will require more preventive care in the school setting. The same is true of the workplace: Occupational health care is growing because prevention is less costly than illness care. Reducing absenteeism and tardiness increases productivity. Also, employees will avail themselves of services that are easy to access; accessing care on the job is often preferable to taking time from work to visit a clinic.

Churches and other faith communities are natural places for health care, especially if there is a holistic approach. Much of what ails people is tied into their sense of self and how they cope. For many people, religious and spiritual resources can be integral to their ability to cope with illness or the threat of a health condition. Parish nursing is a new but growing field of nursing and has been particularly helpful in rural regions.

Healthmobiles will bring primary health care and dental services and screening to special locations, such as farmworkers' camps, retirement communities, and inner-city neighborhoods. Education to prevent problems will be a major focus for the homebound and the poor.

As the population grows older, Americans will receive more long-term care at home. Electronic monitoring equipment will be attached to telephones to allow those who are homebound to relay medical information to clinics or home health agencies. An increasing amount of follow-up will be done by telephone as reimbursement systems switch from fee-for-service to managed care and capitation.

Independent nonphysician providers, particularly nurses, will deliver a significant proportion of the nation's primary care. Because advanced nurse practitioners have responded so well to the country's need for more primary care providers, they will deliver a significant portion of the nation's primary care. Advanced nurse practitioners educated as family, pediatric, and geriatric care practitioners will complement physician family practitioners as the backbone of the nation's health care system. This linking will occur both in nurse-only practices and in collaborative practice arrangements with physicians. Nurse-midwives will take over many of the primary care functions of obstetricians/gynecologists, including the management of low-risk pregnancies. Physicians will continue to do what they have been doing, but there will be much more collaborative practice with nurses and other nonphysician providers. The clinical nurse specialist role and the nurse practitioner role will continue to blur as advanced practice nurses provide care in communities as specialists in health promotion.

Nurses will work collaboratively with physicians and other nonphysician providers. These groups of providers will offer their services in retail locations as small businesses (a major reason why all nurses will need a business education). Health "stores" will vary in size from small basic care operations located in shopping malls to free-standing buildings with huge clinics offering everything from dentistry and family medical care to physical therapy and life-saving emergency services.

The new providers (nurses, physicians, and other nonphysicians) will be much more attuned to what the consumer wants. The hours of service will change so the consumer can access the services in the evenings and on weekends. The larger locations will offer comprehensive wellness programs promoting healthy lifestyles, provide facilities for weight control and exercise, and offer programs about nutrition and exercise. Illness care will be available, but the major emphasis will be on health promotion.

Nurses will take the lead in the development of these "health centers" because the framework for nursing throughout its history has been holistic and comprehensive. Nurses have always promoted health and focused on the prevention of illness. Moreover, nurses can lead the way to better health and cut costs by helping the public assume responsibility for their lives as healthy individuals.

Physicians will assume roles as coproviders, specialty-care providers, and consultants. Although many physicians may express serious concern about what is happening and will happen in the future, nurses and consumers can expect that many physicians will quietly lead the way into the new system. Many physicians will remain as specialty-care providers because there will still be a need for physicians who are prepared to care for specific health care problems, such as oncologists, orthopedists, neurologists, psychiatrists, cardiologists, and so on. Other physicians will join collaborative practices with advanced nurse practitioners to provide comprehensive basic care. Some physicians will seize the opportunity to enter entrepreneurial businesses. There will be plenty to do in the new system, but everyone will need to change their expectations and responsibilities.

Physician activity will affect nursing as nurses seize opportunities for collaborative practice. Advanced practice nurses will need physician consultation in their independent practices, especially for their clients with more complex problems. Over time, physicians and nurses will work together in more ways and in better ways as it becomes more clear how the new system will unfold.

Informed consumers will become more self-directed and assume more responsibility for their health. One of the most exciting advances in the future will be one-stop diagnostic centers. Like a full-service gas station, these diagnostic centers will provide informed consumers access to urinalysis, blood tests, throat cultures, and even some radiographic tests. These diagnostic centers will be electronically linked to large, fully equipped laboratories for confirmation of diagnoses and to health databases that store consumer records. Educational services will also be available through interactive computer programs and video libraries.

Computer terminals in pharmacies will help consumers find answers to questions regarding health and illness. Pharmacists will be able to diagnose such common ailments as throat infections and skin rashes with the help of computer protocols and over-the-counter diagnostic tools. Women already can diagnose pregnancy at home using a simple diagnostic package purchased at a supermarket, pharmacy, or discount store.

For easy access, diagnostic centers will be located in health care clinics, supermarkets, shopping malls, and department stores. Consumers will also be able to authorize a pharmacist to access their personal medical records to check for allergies to prescriptive drugs or other medications. It is easy to see that consumers will have much more control, involvement, and accountability in their health care. This is perhaps the most exciting aspect of the new system.

Access to health care/consultation will resemble the market for other services and products. Because health care/consultation will be easy to access, it will resemble other kinds of services the consumer uses. The clinics, pharmacies, and diagnostic centers will remain open nights and weekends; some may even remain open 24 hours a day. Clearly, tomorrow's health care agencies will be much more attuned to the needs of the customer. Larger agencies will offer comprehensive wellness programs that promote healthy lifestyles, including good nutrition and proper exercise.

Education and prevention will be the major product lines of the retail health and medical stores of the future. The focus of the new clinics will be on keeping people healthy and diagnosing and treating people who are ill. The dream of comprehensive care will finally become a reality.

Education for nurses will reflect the changes in the health care delivery system and the application of new educational technologies. Nurses' education, consistent with these many changes, will also change and will use virtual reality, simulators, and Web-based/enhanced classes. The focus of the programs (regardless of the level) will be on the community and on prevention. Nurses will continue to teach how to care for the sick, but the major emphasis will be how to keep people well. Teaching, consulting, and learning referral skills will be essential for the nurses of the future, therefore, much more time will be spent on helping students learn these skills.

Group work and a focus on working with aggregates will supersede the time spent on individual care. Because nurses will be in the community and focusing on prevention, it will be imperative that they can work with groups. Being able to work with parents, abused women, persons with AIDS, people with cardiovascular problems, and any number of other groups will be necessary if the nurse is to use time efficiently and spend it with the individuals who need the care. This means that the educational program must devote more time to developing nurses' group process skills.

Nursing students and nurses will also need computer skills. They will need not only word processing and spreadsheet skills but also the ability to use virtual reality equipment. Computer competence will probably become a prerequisite for admission to a nursing program in the future.

An important new focus for nursing education at all levels will be on the community. Although students live in a community and read about communities, until they understand that a community is more than a geographic boundary, they will not be prepared for the health care of tomorrow. Much more time will be spent on the study of community and its impact on the health of the citizens. Nurses will also need to become more aware of the global community and become more geographically knowledgeable and culturally competent.

Nursing practice will have a global focus. As geographic barriers become more passable, immigrants and refugees will move from areas with limited resources to areas with more opportunity. These immigrants will bring beliefs and practices about health care that are culturally driven; they also will bring illnesses that may be unique to their race or geographic homeland. Nurses will need to become more aware of global health problems and their impact on nursing practice. Through advances in technology, nurses have a greater ability to communicate or travel to other countries and continents and are better able to network with the global nursing community.

Through technology, students will probably learn more at home than at the college or university. Student access to technology at home and the use of virtual reality will also change faculty behavior. Faculty will need to know how to manage distance education and keep abreast of ever-changing computer and video technology and the broadening concepts of community, prevention, health promotion, and the globalization of America.

An important and imperative looming change is a decision on the basic preparation of nurses. The ANA, NLN, and other specialty-nursing organizations will take the lead and determine the basic preparation of professional nurses. This action will not only help correct the confusion for potential students, but also lay the foundation for advanced practice. Legislators, other professional groups, and the public will finally know the scope of basic professional nursing practice. Statutes will be more clear, and regulations governing practice will be consistent. Nothing the profession can do will be as important or as necessary as this action.

The world of tomorrow is exciting. Health promotion, rather than medical care, will finally be the focus. With these changes will come a challenge for nursing. Nursing will need to grasp the opportunity and be-

Critical Thinking Exercise

Compare and contrast your own vision for the future of health care with the author's vision. Include your thoughts about nursing in your community, your nation, and the world. Are the views consistent? Do you see different or additional changes that have not been discussed here? If yes, what are they? What trends cause you to forecast these changes?

come the leader in the movement toward providing care that creates a better life for each citizen. Clearly there will be a need for more nurses prepared at the baccalaureate and master's levels to meet the demands of a community-based consumer population. New technologies will be available for nurses' use. The system is now ready and able to respond to the need, and the public is ready for the new ways. Nursing education and practice must seize the opportunity to make the necessary changes (Bower, 1997).

EXPLORE MEDIALINK

Questions, critical thinking exercises, essay activities, and other interactive resources for this chapter can be found on the Web site at http://www.prenhall.com/blais. Click on Chapter 24 to select activities for this chapter.

Bookshelf

Reich, R. B. (2001). *The future of success.* **New York: Alfred A. Knopf.**
The former secretary of labor under President Clinton presents the notion that technological advances and innovations are why Americans are working longer hours than ever before. He examines what success has come to mean and offers options to reestablish balance.
Schwartz, P. (1996). *The art of the long view: Planning for the future in an uncertain world.* **New York: Doubleday and Company, Inc.**
This book discuss the ability to visualize different kinds of futures incorporating what the author refers to as

"the intangibles": our hopes and fears, our beliefs and dreams. Stories and scenarios are used to present the ideas.
Fukuyama, F. (2003). *Our posthuman future: Consequences of the biotechnology revolution.* **Picador USA.**
The author, a social philosopher, raises concerns about how biotechnology threatens human nature and human dignity. He looks at the possible dangers of continued and uncontrolled technology in the future as it affects humanity.

SUMMARY

Nursing has faced many changes in recent years, and change will continue in the future. There are many opportunities for nurses to take charge of the coming changes and help design the future of health care. The growth and development of nursing as a profession have been driven by social movements and technological advances. This includes the movement of nursing education into higher education, expanded practice within nursing roles, and the development of the nurse practitioner role. Medical advances and cost-containment strategies have contributed to changes in nursing practice. The women's movement changed the way nursing is perceived, and information technology and computers have also had an impact on the evolution of health care practitioners.

In the future, we will see an older population needing health care, and we will encounter a new level of consumerism. Complementary alternative medicine will continue to be aligned with nursing and a more holistic approach to care. Computer technology will make information more accessible but will also alter the way in which care is delivered. The health care provider may be receiving information via telecommunications and in return delivering care using that medium rather than in a face-to-face setting. Physician and nurse working relationships will become more collegial, and care will be multidisciplinary. Technology will continue to increase and will demand changes in practice in ways we have yet to see.

Several themes emerge in a vision of the future. Health care will be more community focused. Nonphysician providers will increase in numbers and level of responsibility for primary care. Practice will be shaped by consumer demands and become more consumer-oriented. Informed consumers will become more responsible for the provision of their own health care. Education for nurses will change to meet these new demands for practice and performance of roles. Health care and the nursing profession will assume a more global orientation. The nature of the future will demand a decision on the basic level of preparation for nurses.

REFERENCES

American Association of Colleges of Nursing. (2004). *Thousands of students turned away from the nation's nursing schools despite sharp increase in enrollment.* Washington, DC: AACN.

Anderson, C. (2002). Benefits of telehealth. *Alberta RN, 58*(8), 7.

Bauer, J. (1994). *Not what the doctor ordered.* Chicago: Probus.

Benner, P. (2000). Shaping the future of nursing. *Nursing Management, 7*(1), 31–35.

Bower, F. (1997). Looking into the future. In B. Kozier, G. Erb, & K. Blais, *Professional nursing practice: Concepts and perspectives* (3rd ed.). Menlo Park, CA: Addison Wesley Longman, Inc.

Heller, B., Oros, M. T., & Durney-Crowley, J. (2000). The future of nursing education: 10 trends to watch. *Nursing and Health Care Perspectives, 21*(1), 9–13.

Jenkins, R. (1997). Superhighway for the future of nursing: Signposts. *Nurse Educator, 22*(3), 44.

Jones, C. H. (1998). The future of nursing and complementary alternative health-care. *New Mexico Nurse, 43*(3), 17.

Justice, D. (1999). Virtual nursing. *Nursing Standard, 14*(8), 14–15.

Koplan, J. P., & Fleming, D. W. (2000). Current and future public health challenges. *Journal of the American Medical Association, 284*(13), 1696–1698.

Mailer, S. S., Charles, J., Piper, S., Hunt-McCool, J., Wilborne-Davis, P., & Baigis, J. (2000). Analysis of the nursing work force compared with national trends. *Journal of Nursing Administration, 30*(10), 482–489.

Morrison, I. (2000). *Health care in the new millennium: Vision, values, and leadership.* San Francisco: Jossey-Bass.

PEW Health Professions Commission. (1995). *Licensure and regulation of health care providers.* San Francisco: UCSF Center for the Health Professions.

Robertson, K. A. (2000). Clinical major option: A model for implementing critical care nursing into baccalaureate preparation. *Canadian Critical Care Nurse, 11*(3), 22–24.

Sandelowski, M. (2002). Visible humans, vanishing bodies, and virtual nursing: Complications of live, presence, place, and identity. *Advances in Nursing Science, 24*(3), 58–70.

Index